Women's health in general practice
2e

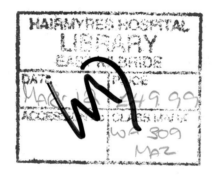

Women's health in general practice
2e

Danielle Mazza

MBBS MD FRACGP DRANZCOG Grad Dip Women's Health

Associate Professor, Department of General Practice,
School of Primary Health Care, Faculty of Medicine, Nursing and Health Sciences,
Monash University, Melbourne
Senior Medical Staff, Royal Women's Hospital, Melbourne
General Practitioner, Melbourne

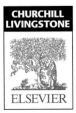

CHURCHILL
LIVINGSTONE

ELSEVIER

Sydney   Edinburgh   London   New York   Philadelphia   St Louis   Toronto

Churchill Livingstone
is an imprint of Elsevier

Elsevier Australia. ACN 001 002 357
(a division of Reed International Books Australia Pty Ltd)
Tower 1, 475 Victoria Avenue, Chatswood, NSW 2067

National Library of Australia Cataloguing-in-Publication Data

---

Mazza, Danielle.
Women's health in general practice / Danielle Mazza

2nd ed.
9780729538718

Women – Diseases.
Gynecology.
Women's Health Services.
Family medicine.

616.0082

Publisher: Sophie Kaliniecki
Developmental Editor: Neli Bryant
Publishing Services Manager: Helena Klijn
Project Coordinator: Karen Griffiths
Edited by Carol Natsis
Proofread by Sarah Newton-John
Illustrations by Alan Laver and TNQ
Cover and internal design by Darben Design
Index by Cynthia Swanson
Typeset by TNQ
Printed by CTPS

Contents

Foreword

As general practitioners we need to have detailed knowledge of the breadth of clinical conditions if we are to provide effective healthcare and advice to all our patients. The diversity of new findings in areas of women's health can be overwhelming for the busy general practitioner as we each try to develop a balanced, informed and practical approach to providing up-to-date quality care in our daily clinical settings.

This second edition of *Women's Health in General Practice* provides an ideal resource for meeting our needs. This is an invaluable 'one-stop shop' covering the breadth of women's health issues that are seen in general practice. Danielle Mazza's approach to this key area of general practice combines her extensive practical clinical knowledge with the approach of a dedicated and respected teacher.

Each of the milestones in women's lives that can impact upon their health and wellbeing are covered in a very practical manner. Danielle's experience as a leading general practitioner working in women's health has ensured that all key areas of women's health are covered, while maintaining the focus on the daily realities of general practice.

Danielle's experience as a teacher has ensured that the key learning objectives are at all times in the foreground, and readers will value the use of effective education tools such as case studies, frequently asked questions, high-quality images, clear tables and graphic highlighting of key clinical points within the body of the text.

But what good is practical experience without a sound knowledge base? Fortunately for busy clinicians, Danielle's experience as a leading researcher in this field has ensured that this text is evidence-based, assuring the reader that the information and learning acquired from *Women's Health in General Practice* is relevant, and will assist us to continue to improve the quality of women's healthcare that we provide to our patients.

In this new edition, Danielle has reviewed and revised each chapter and incorporated recent developments in each clinical topic area, up-to-date references and, where available, the details from new relevant evidence-based guidelines.

Women's Health in General Practice is an immensely useful contribution to the body of knowledge for general practice. Not only does it deserve to become an essential part of our reference libraries, but I suspect that there will be many copies sitting permanently on desks in front of general practitioners around the world and being referred to on a daily basis as we strive to provide the best quality service to the people who trust us for their medical care and advice.

Professor Michael Kidd AM
MBBS MD FRACGP Dip RACOG
President-elect, World Organization of Family Doctors
Sydney 2010

Preface

In revising *Women's Health in General Practice,* I have been amazed at developments in the field over the last few years and how far the evidence base has moved forward. Areas where dramatic change has occurred include the role of hormone replacement therapy, human papilloma virus vaccination and the availability of new contraceptive delivery methods. We also have a much better understanding of complex issues such as premenstrual symptoms, polycystic ovary syndrome, perinatal depression, violence against women and female sexuality.

Randomised controlled trials and longitudinal studies have revolutionised our day-to-day approach to many women's health issues, and there are increasingly more relevant systematic reviews and evidence-based guidelines available for use. Despite this, general practitioners will agree that many of the dilemmas we face in practice remain unanswered by current research and, even when information exists, it is often hard to access. My hope is that the second edition of this book will provide the user with a useful amalgamation of the evidence in order to better manage sexual and reproductive health issues in women in primary care.

Almost every chapter of this second edition has involved a major rewrite of contents, with the addition of new references, tables and figures. I have however, kept the original accessible style, endeavouring wherever possible to answer the difficult clinical questions that I myself encounter in daily practice.

It has been an honour to have *Women's Health in General Practice* nominated as a recommended text for the vocational training of general practitioners and used in examination settings in Australia.

I hope that the learnings the book provides prove beneficial not only to the readers, but ultimately to the patients they serve.

Danielle Mazza
Melbourne 2010

Acknowledgments

The first edition of this book was the result of a suggestion by Professor John Murtagh that I collate my writings into a textbook on women's health for general practitioners. Some of the work has therefore been published in other formats in *Australian Family Physician and Australian Doctor*.

I would like to thank John for his encouragement and for introducing me to his publishers. I would also like to thank my family for their support and the space they gave me to write this book.

Danielle Mazza, 2010

Reviewers

Jill Benson, MBBS, DCH, FACPsychMed, MPH
Director, Health in Human Diversity Unit, Discipline of General Practice, University of Adelaide, South Australia, Australia

Jenny Westgate, MBChB, MRCOG, FRANZCOG, DM
Associate Professor in Obstetrics and Gynaecology, University of Auckland, New Zealand
Clinical Director of Gynaecology, Waitemata District Health Board, New Zealand

Ian Symonds, BMedSci(Hons), MBBS, MMedSci(Ed), DM, FRCOG, FRANZCOG
Professor of Obstetrics and Gynaecology, University of Newcastle, New South Wales, Australia
Senior Staff Specialist, John Hunter Hospital, Newcastle, New South Wales, Australia
Adjunct Professor, University of New England, New South Wales, Australia

William Liley, BPhty, DipEdSt, MBBS(UQ)
Intern, Cairns Base Hospital, Cairns, Queensland, Australia

1

Adolescent gynaecology

OBJECTIVES

- To understand normal pubertal development in girls
- To know when and how to investigate girls presenting with primary amenorrhoea
- To understand the mechanisms responsible for the development of primary dysmenorrhoea
- To understand the mechanisms responsible for the development of dysfunctional uterine bleeding in an adolescent
- To appropriately manage primary dysmenorrhoea and dysfunctional uterine bleeding in adolescent girls

PUBERTAL DEVELOPMENT AND PRIMARY AMENORRHOEA

What is puberty and when does it occur?

Puberty is the physical, emotional and sexual transition from childhood to adulthood. It involves five changes: breast, pubic hair, axillary hair development, the growth spurt and the onset of menstruation. In girls pubertal development commences at around 8–9 years of age and lasts for 4–5 years. Precocious puberty is said to have occurred if pubertal development commences before then.[1]

What determines the onset of puberty?

The actual endocrine events that initiate puberty are unknown. It appears that puberty is held in check by higher central nervous system controls, but the restraint can be eliminated by injury or tumour growth, both of which can result in premature puberty. Gonadal steroids are produced as a result of increased gonadotrophin stimulation, and secondary sexual development follows a well-described pattern of changes.[2]

Puberty involves five changes: breast development, pubic hair development, axillary hair development, the growth spurt and the onset of menstruation.

What is the sequence of events that occurs during puberty?

Usually there is a distinct chronological sequence to pubertal development. The first event to occur

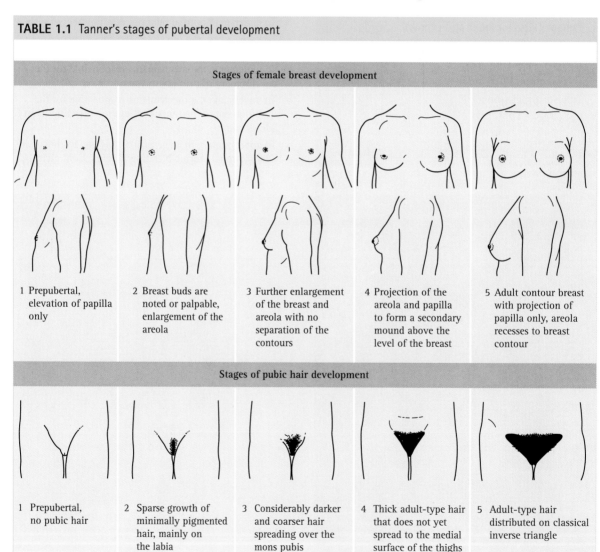

TABLE 1.1 Tanner's stages of pubertal development

Stages of female breast development

1 Prepubertal, elevation of papilla only

2 Breast buds are noted or palpable, enlargement of the areola

3 Further enlargement of the breast and areola with no separation of the contours

4 Projection of the areola and papilla to form a secondary mound above the level of the breast

5 Adult contour breast with projection of papilla only, areola recesses to breast contour

Stages of pubic hair development

1 Prepubertal, no pubic hair

2 Sparse growth of minimally pigmented hair, mainly on the labia

3 Considerably darker and coarser hair spreading over the mons pubis

4 Thick adult-type hair that does not yet spread to the medial surface of the thighs

5 Adult-type hair distributed on classical inverse triangle

CASE STUDY: 'She still hasn't got her periods.'

When you look at children aged 11 or 12, what strikes you very quickly is the great disparity in development between children of a similar age. It is therefore not surprising that GPs often see an anxious parent worried about why their daughter is not as developed as her peers. Helen was one such parent. She presented one morning with her daughter Annie in tow. Annie, she said, had recently turned 15 and still hadn't had a period. Apparently all the other girls in her class were menstruating and Helen wondered if there was anything wrong.

While Helen was talking, the GP glanced down at Annie's file. There wasn't much of note. There were no major childhood illnesses, no relevant family history and only a couple of episodes of mild asthma. Looking over at Annie, the GP immediately took note of several things. First, she appeared to be a normal-looking girl. At 15 she was as tall as her mother and seemed to have normal breast development from what could be seen through her clothes. The GP said to her, 'I'm going to ask you some funny-sounding questions. Do you mind?' She shook her head so the GP went on, 'Annie have you got hair under your arms yet?' She nodded. 'And do you have pubic hair yet?' Again she nodded. 'When did you get as tall as your mum?' Helen intervened and said

that Annie seemed to go through a growth spurt about a year ago, but that she thought that she was still growing as her brothers and father were all over 180 cm and she had just got to 165 cm. 'And how old were you when you started getting your periods Helen?' 'I think it was when I turned 16', the girl's mother replied.

In order to know whether or not Helen had a cause for concern, it was necessary to accurately stage where Annie was in the pubertal cycle.

On examination, Annie had normal sexual development. There was no evidence of any underlying issues and, since her mother had not menstruated until the age of 16, Helen could therefore be reassured that menarche was probably quite imminent. Annie could be reviewed again in 6 months, during which time her first period would most likely occur. It would also be important to tell her that it was possible that Annie's periods would be irregular for the first few months as her hormonal system settled into a regular pattern.

Several months later Helen came in with Annie to get some advice about the young woman's acne. Helen said, 'We were very relieved. Annie got her first period a couple of months after we last saw you. Now she's like all the rest of her friends'.

is breast budding followed by sexual hair growth, the growth spurt and finally menarche. Tanner has described this sequence and in girls takes into account both breast and pubic hair development (Table 1.1).[3] Axillary hair becomes evident approximately at Tanner's stage 3, while the growth spurt occurs between Tanner's stages 2 and 5, peaking at the onset of Tanner's stage 4. Girls undergo this growth spurt on average two years earlier than boys and reach a peak growth velocity of 8 cm/year before the production of oestrogen eventually closes the epiphyses.[4] Figure 1.1 shows the timing of pubertal events in graph form.

What is the average age of menarche?

Over the last century the average age of menarche has dropped by 3 years[5] and now stands at 12.7 years.[6] Factors contributing to this change include public health successes such as improved childhood nutrition and health status through reduction in childhood infections.[7] While decreases in age at menarche until the mid-1960s resulted from 'positive' changes, such as better nutrition, it has been suggested that decreases since that time are related to 'negative' changes, such as overeating and decreased physical activity, and that these negative changes have brought about a disparity

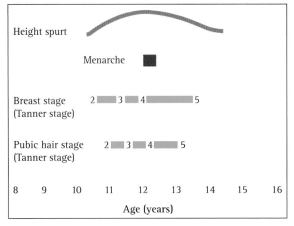

FIGURE 1.1 Timing of pubertal events in girls (Adapted from Kidson[10])

between physical and psychosocial maturity as well as a potential for increased rates of breast cancer later in life.[8]

What is a 'normal' adolescent menstrual pattern?

Most adolescent cycles range from approximately 20 to 45 days and last 2–7 days, even in the first gynaecological year. Cycles become more regular with increasing age and gynaecological age. By the third gynaecological year, 60–80% of cycles are 21–34 days long and a young woman's 'normal' cycle length is established by approximately the fifth or sixth gynaecological year, or by age 19–20.[9] It is important to note, however, that she may well have started some form of hormonal contraception by then and may never have had the opportunity to experience her 'normal' cycle.

The five-stage system established by Tanner should be used to describe normal pubertal development.

When is a girl considered to have primary amenorrhoea?

Absence of periods is called primary amenorrhoea and should be investigated if there is a failure to establish menstruation by the age of 14 years in girls without signs of secondary sexual development, or by the age of 16 in the presence of normal secondary sexual characteristics.[4] These age limits, while arbitrary, allow for variability in the normal rates of sexual maturation and the increasingly lower mean age of menarche.

Primary amenorrhoea can be classified according to the presence or absence of secondary sexual characteristics. The onset of menstruation should usually occur within 2 years of the onset of breast development, pubic and axillary hair development and the growth spurt.[10] Box 1.1 lists the possible causes of primary amenorrhoea when secondary sexual characteristics are present and Table 1.2 shows the causes of primary amenorrhoea when secondary sexual characteristics are absent. In this latter situation, classification is assisted by consideration of height.

BOX 1.1 Causes of primary amenorrhoea when secondary sexual characteristics are present (Adapted from Edmonds[54])

- Constitutional delay
- Pregnancy
- Genitourinary malformation
  Imperforate hymen
  Transverse vaginal septum
  Absence of a vagina and/or of a functioning uterus
- Androgen insensitivity
  XY female
  Testicular feminisation
- Resistant ovary syndrome

TABLE 1.2 Causes of primary amenorrhoea when secondary sexual characteristics are absent (Adapted from Edmonds[54])

Normal stature	Short stature

• Hypothalamic dysfunction
    Chronic illness
    Anorexia, weight loss, exercise
    'Stress'
• Isolated gonadotrophin-releasing
• Hormone deficiency
    Kallman's syndrome
    The olfactogenital syndrome
• Hyperprolactinaemia
• Ovarian dysgenesis/agenesis
• Premature ovarian failure
• Galactosaemia
• Gonadal dysgenesis
	• Hydrocephalus
	• Trauma
	• Empty sella
	    syndrome
	• Tumours
	• Turner's syndrome

What is the GP's role when a patient presents with primary amenorrhoea?

A GP's main task is to determine whether puberty is pathologically as opposed to physiologically delayed.

What history needs to be taken?

At the initial presentation, a history detailing the following issues needs to be taken:

- family history of:
  - delayed puberty
  - genetic anomalies
- symptoms associated with possible causes of the amenorrhoea, for example:
  - cyclical lower abdominal pain, possibly suggesting haematocolpos (accumulation of menstrual blood in the vagina)
  - symptoms of hypothyroidism
  - absence of a sense of smell, which may be associated with gonadotrophin deficiency
  - presence of chronic illness such as diabetes, coeliac disease or chronic renal or heart disease
  - history of chemotherapy
  - recent emotional upsets or change in body weight
  - level of exercise.

Absence of periods (primary amenorrhoea) should be investigated if there is a failure to establish menstruation by the age of 14 years in girls without signs of secondary sexual development, or by the age of 16 in the presence of normal secondary sexual characteristics.

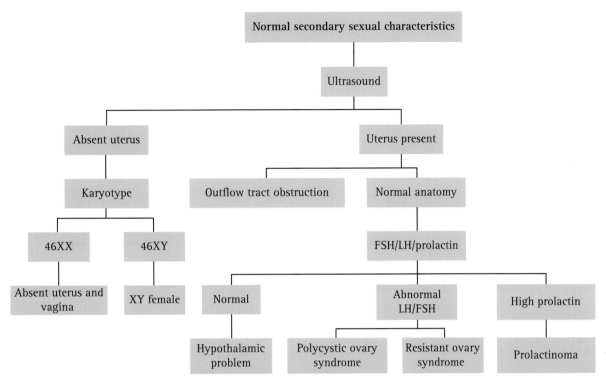

FIGURE 1.2 Investigative pathway for primary amenorrhoea when the patient has normal secondary sexual characteristics (Adapted from Edmonds[54])

What are the essential features of the examination during this consultation?

During examination, height and weight should be assessed in order to calculate the girls' body mass index. The presence of secondary sex characteristics (such as breast tissue, and pubic and axillary hair) should be noted, as should features of Turner's syndrome, signs of androgen excess, thyroid disease and galactorrhoea. It is important, however, not to examine the breasts if it is likely that prolactin estimation will be needed, as the level may then be falsely elevated. The external genitalia should be examined to look for clitoromegaly (indicating virilisation) and imperforate hymen (particularly if there is a history of cyclical pain). A pelvic examination to assess whether or not a uterus is palpable is inappropriate in young women who are not sexually active and can be assessed later using ultrasound if necessary. Pregnancy, however, must be excluded.

What kind of investigative pathway should be followed?

If, when examining a young girl with primary amenorrhoea, normal secondary sexual characteristics are present but there is no family history of delayed menarche, the investigative pathway shown in Figure 1.2 should be followed. If, on the other hand, no secondary sexual characteristics are seen, GPs should assess height and follow the investigative pathway given in Figure 1.3 (p 6).

What common causes of primary amenorrhoea will a GP encounter?

From a general-practice or primary-care perspective, the most common cause of primary amenorrhoea is constitutional delay. This delay is caused by an immature pulsatile release of gonadotrophin-releasing hormone (GnRH), which eventually matures spontaneously. There is often a family history of delayed menarche or puberty in these girls.[11] After constitutional delay, Turner's syndrome and, more rarely, an absent vagina with a non-functioning uterus are the next most common causes of primary amenorrhoea seen in general practice.

The most common causes of primary amenorrhoea seen in general practice are:

- constitutional delay
- Turner's syndrome
- absent vagina or uterus.

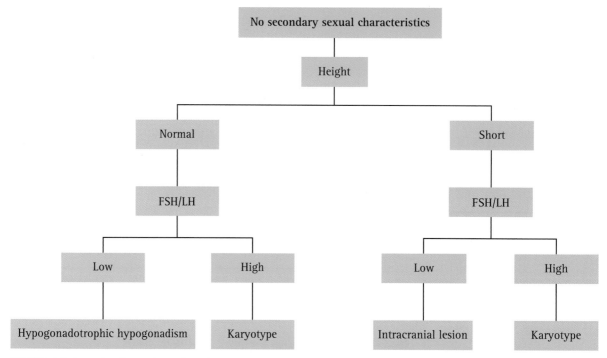

FIGURE 1.3 Investigative pathway for primary amenorrhoea when the patient has no secondary sexual characteristics (Adapted from Edmonds[54])

Turner's syndrome is caused by a chromosomal abnormality, whereby there is either complete absence or a partial abnormality of one of the two X chromosomes. The incidence of this syndrome is 1 in 2000 female births.[12] The features of Turner's syndrome are variable; they may include short stature, webbed neck, lymphoedema, a shield chest with widely spaced nipples, scoliosis, a wide carrying angle, coarctation of the aorta and streak ovaries.

Rokitansky-Kuster-Hauser syndrome is the name given to a condition where there is either partial or complete absence of the vagina, and a rudimentary uterus. It accounts for up to 15% of primary amenorrhoea cases.[13] While ovarian development is normal, up to 40% of girls with this syndrome have associated renal tract abnormalities and 12% have skeletal abnormalities.[14]

Summary of key points
- Puberty in girls usually begins at approximately 8–9 years of age and lasts 4–5 years.
- Pubertal development follows an orderly pattern, as set out by Tanner's stages of pubertal development.
- Menarche should occur within 2 years of the onset of breast development, pubic and axillary hair development and the growth spurt.

- When a patient presents with what appears to be delayed puberty, height measurement and noting the presence or absence of secondary sexual characteristics are essential parts of the examination.
- From a general-practice or primary-care perspective, the most common cause of primary amenorrhoea is constitutional delay.

PRIMARY DYSMENORRHOEA

Why is it important to differentiate between primary and secondary dysmenorrhoea?

Dysmenorrhoea literally means painful menstrual flow and refers to cramping lower abdominal pain occurring with the onset of menstrual flow. In cases of primary dysmenorrhoea, the initial onset of pain commences usually 6–12 months after menarche, with the onset of ovulatory cycles,[15] and occurs in the absence of any pelvic disease. In contrast, secondary dysmenorrhoea usually commences later in life and results from some kind of underlying problem, such as endometriosis.

In primary dysmenorrhoea the initial onset of pain usually commences 6–12 months after menarche.

CASE STUDY: 'She gets terrible period pain.'

Tania accompanied her 13-year-old daughter into the consultation. Sally looked pale and a little distressed. Tania explained that Sally had started menstruating some 8–9 months ago. Initially things hadn't been too bad, but the last three periods had been woeful. Sally had had dreadful period pain. Paracetamol had not helped at all and Tania had found her daughter clutching her lower abdomen, rolling around on the bed and whimpering on several occasions. Sally had also missed 3 days of school with each of her last few periods. Tania was convinced that there was something terribly wrong with her daughter, as she had never experienced that degree of pain with her own periods.

How common is primary dysmenorrhoea?

The prevalence of period pain has been shown to be up to 90% in women aged 18–45 attending primary care practices.[16] In a prospective study of teenage women at a US college,[17] menstrual pain occurred in 71.6% of menstrual bleeds, most commonly beginning on the first day of the menses. A total of 60% of women reported at least one episode of severe pain, while 13% reported severe pain more than half the time. Just over 40% of the women studied reported absenteeism or the inability to participate in an activity on at least one occasion owing to the pain.

In an Australian study of year 11–12 high-school girls, the prevalence of dysmenorrhoea was 80%, with 53% of girls with dysmenorrhoea reporting that it limited their activities. In particular, 37% said that dysmenorrhoea affected their school activities.[18] In school-aged girls menstrual pain was significantly associated with school absenteeism and decreased academic performance, sports participation, and socialisation with peers.[19] School administrators, therefore, have a vested interest in providing health education on this topic to their students.[18]

What does the pain feel like?

Period pain usually starts with menstrual flow and lasts for 1–3 days, peaking at the time of the heaviest flow. There is a background dull ache in the suprapubic area, with sharp, intermittent spasms of pain. The pain can also radiate to the lower back and the upper thighs and be associated with nausea, vomiting, diarrhoea, fatigue, headache and hyperventilation.

What actually causes it?

Women who suffer from period pain have increased levels of uterine tone and uterine muscular activity. Myometrial contractions are stimulated by prostaglandins, in particular $PGF_{2\alpha}$. This prostaglandin and PGE2 have been found in elevated levels in women suffering from dysmenorrhoea, compared with controls.[20] This would explain why prostaglandin synthetase inhibitors are effective in treating dysmenorrhoea. More controversial is the role of vasopressin in the aetiology of dysmenorrhoea.[21] Vasopressin causes myometrial hyperactivity and vasoconstriction, with resultant uterine ischaemia and pain. Elevated plasma levels of vasopressin have been found in women with primary dysmenorrhoea.[22] Thankfully, primary dysmenorrhoea is significantly reduced after pregnancy. An increase in uterine vascularity or a decrease in uterine innervation may be responsible for this decrease.[23]

Primary dysmenorrhoea is significantly reduced after pregnancy.

Are there any particular risk factors for period pain?

Research shows that the following factors are significantly associated with period pain:[24,25]

- duration of menstrual flow
- younger average menarche
- smoking
- obesity
- alcohol consumption
- high levels of stress
- depression
- anxiety
- disruption of social networks.

How do I tell if it is primary or secondary dysmenorrhoea?

The diagnosis of primary dysmenorrhoea is one of exclusion. The young woman gives a history of the onset of period pain soon after menarche in which pain occurs with each period and is restricted to the first 1–3 days of the period. This focused history and a normal examination differentiate between primary and secondary dysmenorrhoea (Table 1.3, p 8).

In contrast, because secondary dysmenorrhoea can be caused by many different conditions (Table 1.4, p 8), sufferers complain of other, varying symptoms. For example, complaints of heavy bleeding may be associated with uterine pathology. Dyspareunia (if the young woman is sexually active) or pain occurring at other times in the menstrual cycle is suggestive of endometriosis, and fever and malaise with an inflammatory process such as pelvic infection. Co-existing infertility is also a pointer to these latter disease processes. Another pointer to secondary dysmenorrhoea is non-responsiveness to first-line therapies such as non-steroidal anti-inflammatories (NSAIDs) and the combined oral contraceptive pill (COCP).

If period pain fails to respond to therapy with non-steroidal anti-inflammatory drugs (NSAIDs), the diagnosis of primary dysmenorrhoea should be reconsidered.

What first-line treatments should be used?

NSAIDs and the oral contraceptive pill are very effective first-line agents for the treatment of primary dysmenorrhoea. NSAIDs work by inhibiting the production of the prostaglandins that are the cause of the pain and should be used in sufferers when contraception is not required.

The different formulations of NSAIDs all have similar efficacy for dysmenorrhoea, and pain relief is achieved in approximately 70% of women.[26] Compared with placebo treatment, the number needed to treat is 2.1 for at least moderate pain relief over 3–5 days.[26]

Interestingly, young women are unaware of which medication is most effective for treating period pain. The most common medication used by those reporting dysmenorrhoea is simple analgesics (53%) followed by NSAIDs (42%). More than a quarter of young women (27%) are unaware that NSAIDs are a possible treatment option for dysmenorrhoea.[18] Even when they do use NSAIDs, adolescents do not use effective treatment regimens, with about a quarter using less than the recommended dose of these medications and 43% failing to reach the maximum daily frequency.[27]

It is therefore important to explain to adolescents that NSAIDs act to prevent pain, rather than as an analgesic. For this reason, the following advice needs to be given to young women who require NSAIDs:

- Start taking the NSAIDs as soon as you know that your period is imminent or as soon as the bleeding starts.
- Because these tablets prevent pain, you need to take them at the correct dose on a regular basis for the first 1–3 days of your period.

While dosing may be a factor in the choice of which NSAID to recommend (as it varies between

TABLE 1.3 Distinguishing between primary and secondary dysmenorrhoea on history

	Primary dysmenorrhoea	Secondary dysmenorrhoea
Age at symptom onset	Adolescence	Mid to late 20s
Duration	First 2–3 days of period	Persists beyond first 2–3 days of period
Pain at other times of menstrual cycle?	No	Yes
Other types of pain?	No	Dyspareunia (pain with intercourse)

TABLE 1.4 Causes of secondary dysmenorrhoea

Uterine	Extra-uterine
• Adenomyosis	• Endometriosis
• IUD	• Pelvic inflammatory disease
• Fibroids	• Functional ovarian cysts
• Cervical stenosis	• Benign or malignant tumours
• Cervical polyps	• Inflammatory bowel disease

NSAIDs), the choice of which NSAID to take is less important than using them in the correct way. This involves commencing just before the onset of menstruation (when this can be predicted) and using the right dose and frequency usually for the first 2–3 days of a period. Fortunately the incidence of side effects is low, probably because of the intermittent and short-term nature of use.

In the treatment of dysmenorrhoea, the choice of which NSAID to take is less important than using them in the correct way.

It is difficult to state the efficacy of oral contraceptives in reducing dysmenorrhoea because research in this area is of poor quality.[28] While oral contraceptives probably work through reducing the menstrual fluid volume and by suppressing ovulation,[29,30] about 30% of users report no relief from dysmenorrhoea.[31] There is some controversy as to whether monophasic oral contraceptives are more effective than triphasics.[29,30] Progestogen-only pills (the mini-pill) should theoretically also be more effective, as they reduce menstrual flow; however, the intermittent and unpredictable bleeding that occurs with this form of contraception limits its use in management of dysmenorrhoea. NSAIDs can also be used by women taking oral contraceptives to help prevent any residual pain (an important point to highlight when counselling patients and their mothers about pain management).

Are there any non-pharmaceutical options for management?

Alternative therapies such as thiamine, pyridoxine, magnesium, fish oil and vitamin E may have some efficacy.[32] Other non-pharmaceutical approaches that have some support include a low-fat vegetarian diet,[33] exercise,[34] acupuncture[35] and heat therapy.[36] Transcutaneous electrical nerve stimulation (TENS) has been found to be effective in reducing pain associated with primary dysmenorrhoea, with one study showing that it worked faster than Naproxen.[37]

What can be offered to women with refractory pain?

If primary dysmenorrhoea is not controlled by either NSAIDs or the combined oral contraceptive pill (COCP), or both, then the diagnosis should be questioned. Endometriosis can occur in adolescence, and one study has shown that the mean delay in diagnosis for this condition from the time of the onset of pain is 12 years.[38] However, it is fair to say that about 10–20% of young women will be refractory to first-line treatment. Other treatments described in the research literature include the following:

- The administration of exogenous nitric oxide. This has successfully resulted in uterine relaxation in a variety of obstetrical/gynaecological disorders. Transdermal glyceryl trinitrate (a source of exogenous nitric oxide) has been found to be useful as a modulator of uterine contractility and therefore is a new and mechanistically different therapeutic alternative for the management of primary dysmenorrhoea.[39]
- Uterine nerve ablation (UNA) and presacral neurectomy (PSN) are two surgical treatments that have been increasingly used in recent years. However, a recent Cochrane review has found that there is insufficient evidence to recommend the use of nerve interruption in the management of dysmenorrhoea, regardless of cause.[40]
- Significant amounts of leukotrienes have been identified in the endometrium of women with primary dysmenorrhoea who do not respond to treatment with antiprostaglandins. Leukotriene receptor antagonists (which have recently been promoted for the treatment of asthma) may have potential use in the management of primary dysmenorrhoea (especially in patients who are not responding to the traditional treatment using PG synthetase inhibitors).[41]
- Other agents that have been trialled in the treatment of dysmenorrhoea include calcium channel blockers such as nifedipine and diltiazem. These agents block uterine contractions, but patients experience side effects such as headache, flushing and palpitations.[42,43]
- Menstrual cycle suppressants, such as progestogens, danazol and gonadotrophin-releasing hormone analogues, may be considered for resistant dysmenorrhoea, but should normally be used only on specialist advice.[15]

Summary of key points
- Dysmenorrhoea is caused by the production of prostaglandins.
- Dysmenorrhoea in adolescence is usually primary—that is, it is not due to pelvic pathology.
- Many adolescent girls and their mothers treat dysmenorrhoea inadequately with over-the-counter preparations.
- NSAIDs and the COCP are highly effective first-line agents in the treatment of dysmenorrhoea.
- About 30% of women have inadequate relief from the COCP when used to treat dysmenorrhoea and 10% are refractory to both NSAIDs and the COCP.

DYSFUNCTIONAL UTERINE BLEEDING IN ADOLESCENCE

Why does dysfunctional uterine bleeding occur in adolescence?

Dysfunctional uterine bleeding (DUB) is irregular bleeding arising from anovulation (Box 1.2, p 10). After menarche, the hypothalamic–pituitary–ovarian axis can take several years to mature, resulting in anovulatory, and therefore irregular, cycles.[44] Anovulation occurs in 55% to 82% of cycles in adolescents between the time of menarche and for 2 years after menarche, in 30% to 45% of cycles from 2–4 years after menarche and in no more than 20% of cycles from 4–5 years after menarche.[45] During an anovulatory cycle, the corpus luteum fails to form, causing failure of normal cyclical progesterone secretion. This results in continuous unopposed production of oestradiol, stimulating overgrowth

CASE STUDY: 'The blood just gushes away.'

Jane's mother rings as soon as your clinic opens requesting an urgent appointment for her 14-year-old daughter. When they arrive you are told that Jane began to menstruate about a year ago, but when her period started yesterday the bleeding seemed excessively heavy and she was forced to change her pads every 1–2 hours. Overnight, when she woke to go the toilet she found blood all over the sheets and felt a flood of blood gush away from her as she stood. This morning, the bleeding has continued to be very heavy with clots and quite severe cramping pain.

Further questions reveal that Jane's periods have been quite irregular since she started menstruating. While initially they came every 30–35 days, she has not bled for the last 3 months. Jane has previously been well, has no history or family history of bleeding disorders and is not sexually active. Examination is unremarkable and her pulse and blood pressure are normal, with no postural drop.

After explaining that the most likely diagnosis is dysfunctional uterine bleeding secondary to anovulation, you order a full blood examination (FBE). You then start Jane on a monophasic 30 μg COCP and some mefenamic acid, and ask her mother to call the next day to let you know how things are going. When she does she sounds relieved and tells you that the bleeding has slowed down a lot. You inform her of the normal blood test results and ask her to return with Jane after she has taken the 21 active pills in the pack so that you can discuss whether or not Jane will continue on the COCP.

BOX 1.2 Definition of terms

Term	Definition
Dysfunctional uterine bleeding (DUB)	Irregular bleeding from anovulation
Oligomenorrhoea	Bleeding intervals greater than 35 days
Polymenorrhoea	Bleeding intervals fewer than 21 days
Menorrhagia	Regular, normal bleeding intervals but excessive flow and duration
Metrorrhagia	Irregular intervals, excessive flow and duration
Amenorrhoea	Bleeding intervals greater than 6 months

of the endometrium. Without progesterone, the endometrium grows thicker and thicker, eventually outgrowing its blood supply and leading to necrosis. The result is very heavy bleeding. A similar situation can arise in women with polycystic ovary syndrome and during the perimenopause.

Most adolescent girls will develop ovulatory cycles within 2 years of menarche.

Is there anything else I need to check for?

While the great majority of non-pregnant adolescents suffering from DUB have anovulatory cycles, studies have shown coagulopathies in up to 20% of those admitted to hospital.[46,47] The most common of these are thrombocytopenia and von Willebrand's disease (which occurs in 1% of the population[48]). Coagulation problems are typically associated with heavy but regular monthly bleeding. Most adolescents have bleeding that lasts 3–7 days; bleeding for longer than 7 days is uncommon and merits evaluation.[49] Severity of menstrual loss is not predictive of a bleeding disorder; however, a careful personal and family history of bruising and bleeding should be taken in all teenagers who present de novo with menorrhagia, with routine screening in all patients with a positive family history.[46]

In general practice, an FBE to check for anaemia is warranted when a patient presents with DUB that has occurred on several occasions. If medical management is not effective, coagulation studies and thyroid hormone studies and a prolactin level test should be undertaken. Pelvic examinations are not necessary in those adolescents who are not sexually active or who are still within 2 years of menarche.[50] In sexually active teenagers, however, a pelvic examination, pregnancy test, Pap smear and investigations for sexually transmitted infections (STIs) should be undertaken.

Dysfunctional uterine bleeding is the most common cause of abnormal uterine bleeding in adolescence.

How do I know if emergency treatment is required?

Emergency treatment is required when the patient presents hypovolaemic, or with uncontrollable bleeding or a very low haematocrit.

What management should be instituted in emergency settings?

For some young women, admission, intravenous fluids, blood transfusion and fresh frozen plasma may be required. Beyond this, however, there is no consensus or evidence-based approach to their management.[51] Because some patients with heavy bleeding may have scant endometrial tissue, high-dose oestrogen has been recommended for those requiring hospitalisation. Conjugated equine oestrogen (Premarin) is given either orally 2.5 mg q.i.d. or intravenously 25 mg every 2–4 hours for 24 hours. Bleeding will usually cease after the first intravenous dose, after which the patient can be changed over to oral oestrogen for 21 days, with the addition of 10mg daily of medroxyprogesterone acetate for the last 7 days. However, this approach is not commonly used.[51]

What treatment can be commenced in the general practice setting?

Patients who are not hypovolaemic and who have a stable haematocrit level can be treated in the general practice setting. The choice of agents to manage the menorrhagia is similar to those used in older women. NSAIDs can reduce menstrual loss by on average 30%, and may be of assistance, but are less effective than the antifibrinolytic medication tranexamic acid (1g four times daily, on days of heavy bleeding), which has been demonstrated to reduce menstrual loss by 50%.[52]

The COCP will also reduce menstrual loss and can be used in a continuous fashion, running packets back to back.[53] Any of the low-dose, monophasic combined oral contraceptive pills can be used. Bleeding usually ceases in 12–24 hours. However, because a large amount of endometrium may be in place, the initial withdrawal bleed that occurs after taking the 21 active pills may still be heavy. If the oral contraceptive is continued over the next 2–3 months, the endometrium will be better controlled, resulting in much lighter withdrawal bleeds.

Dysfunctional uterine bleeding can usually be managed confidently by administering the combined oral contraceptive pill.

Summary of key points
- Dysfunctional bleeding in adolescence is due to anovulatory cycles.
- If medical management is not effective, a pathological cause, such as a bleeding disorder, should be sought.
- Most adolescents will respond promptly to a 30 µg COCP.
- In emergency situations, admission and fluid replacement may be required.

TABLE 1.5 Periods in adolescence: what to expect

	Normal	Abnormal	
Normal onset of pubertal development	8–9 years	Precocious puberty	≤7 years
Average age of menarche	12–13 years	Absence of menstruation in girls *without* signs of secondary sexual characteristics	≥14 years
Onset of menarche	Within 2 years of onset of breast development, pubic and axillary hair development and the growth spurt	Absence of menstruation in girls *with* signs of secondary sexual characteristics	≥16 years
Adolescent cycle range	20–45 days		
Normal duration of menstruation	2–7 days		
Menstrual flow	Average tampon or pad lasting 3–4 hours	Heavy menstrual flow	Changing pad or tampon more than once or twice in a 2–4 hour period
Presence of dysmenorrhoea	Up to approximately 80% of young women	Amenorrhoea	No periods for >90 days

- Most young women will achieve regular ovulatory cycling within 2 years of menarche, although in some it may take up to 5 years.

TIPS FOR PRACTITIONERS

- In cases of primary amenorrhoea pregnancy must be excluded.
- If a young woman with primary amenorrhoea presents accompanied by her mother, ask the mother about her own menstrual history.
- A pelvic examination to assess whether or not a uterus is palpable is inappropriate in young girls who are not sexually active and can be assessed later using ultrasound if necessary.
- Menarche should occur within 2 years of the onset of breast development, pubic and axillary hair development and the growth spurt.
- It is important to advise adolescents and their mothers about the nature of adolescent periods (Table 1.5), especially that periods can be irregular for the first few months after menarche as the hormonal system settles into a regular pattern and finally produces regular cycles.
- When treating dysmenorrhoea, encourage correct use of NSAIDs to obtain maximal effect. This consists of commencing the NSAID when menstruation is imminent (not when it has already begun) and using correct dosages.
- Packets of combined oral contraceptive pills can be used back to back (skipping the sugar pills and therefore skipping menstruation) to manage dysmenorrhoea (see contraceptive chapter for further advice) and dysfunctional uterine bleeding in adolescence.
- In cases of dysfunctional uterine bleeding in adolescence, make sure that the family history is explored for bleeding disorders.

REFERENCES

1. Carel J-C, Leger J. Precocious puberty. N Engl J Med 2008; 358(22):2366–2377.
2. Styne DM. Physiology of puberty. Horm Res 1994; 41(Suppl 2):3–6.
3. Tanner JM. Growth at adolescence. Oxford: Blackwell Science; 1962.
4. Edmonds DK. Gynaecological disorders of childhood and adolescence. In: Edmonds DK, ed. Dewhurst's textbook of obstetrics & gynaecology for postgraduates. 6th edn. Oxford: Blackwell Science; 1999:12–16.
5. Bellis MA, Downing J, Ashton JR. Adults at 12? Trends in puberty and their public health consequences. J Epidemiol Community Health 2006; 60(11):910–911.
6. DiVall SA, Radovick S. Pubertal development and menarche. Ann N Y Acad Sci 2008; 1135:19–28.
7. Gluckman PD, Hanson MA, Gluckman PD, et al. Evolution, development and timing of puberty. Trends Endocrinol Metab 2006; 17(1):7–12.
8. Herman-Giddens ME. The decline in the age of menarche in the United States: should we be concerned? J Adolesc Health 2007; 40(3):201–203.
9. Adams Hillard P. Menstruation in adolescents: what's normal? Medscape J Med 2008; 10(12):295.
10. Kidson W. How to investigate the patient presenting with delayed puberty. Modern Medicine of Australia February 1997; 120–126.
11. Rosenfeld RG. Constitutional delay in growth and development. Semin Adolesc Med 1987; 3:267–273.
12. Saenger P. Turner's syndrome. New Engl J Med 1996; 335:1749–1754.
13. Pletcher JR, Slap GB. Menstrual disorders: amenorrhea. Pediatr Clin North Am 1999; 46:505–518.
14. Griffin JE, Edwards C, Madden JD, et al. Congenital absence of the vagina. The Mayer-Rokitansky-Kuster-Hauser syndrome. Ann Intern Med 1976; 85:224–236.
15. Proctor M, Farquhar C, Proctor M, et al. Diagnosis and management of dysmenorrhoea. BMJ 2006; 332(7550):1134–1138.
16. Jamieson DJ, Steege JF. The prevalence of dysmenorrhea, dyspareunia, pelvic pain, and irritable bowel syndrome in primary care practices. Obstet Gynecol 1996; 87:55–58.
17. Harlow SD, Park M. A longitudinal study of risk factors for the occurrence, duration and severity of menstrual cramps in a cohort of college women. BJOG 1996; 103:1134–1142. [Published erratum in BJOG 1997; 104:386.]
18. Hillen TI, Grbavac SL, Johnston PJ, et al. Primary dysmenorrhea in young Western Australian women: prevalence, impact, and knowledge of treatment. J Adolesc Health 1999; 25:40–45.
19. Banikarim C, Chacko MR, Kelder SH. Prevalence and impact of dysmenorrhea on Hispanic female adolescents. Arch Pediatr Adolesc Med 2000; 154:1226–1229.
20. Lumsden MA, Kelly RW, Baird DT. Primary dysmenorrhoea: the importance of both prostaglandins E2 and F2 alpha. BJOG 1983; 90:1135–1140.
21. Valentin L, Sladkevicius P, Kindahl H, et al. Effects of a vasopressin antagonist in women with dysmenorrhea. Gynaecol Obstet Invest 2000; 50:170–177.
22. Akerlund M. Vascularization of human endometrium. Uterine blood flow in healthy condition and in primary dysmenorrhoea. Ann N Y Acad Sci 1994; 734:47–56.
23. Sjoberg NO. Dysmenorrhoea and uterine transmitters. Acta Obstetricia et Gynaecologica Scandinavica 1979; Supplement 87:57–59.
24. Sundell G, Milsom I, Andersch B. Factors influencing the prevalence and severity of dysmenorrhoea in young women. BJOG 1990; 97:588–594.
25. Wang L, Wang X, Wang W, et al. Stress and dysmenorrhoea: a population based prospective study. Occup Environ Med 2004; 61(12):1021–1026.
26. Marjoribanks J, Proctor ML, Farquhar C. Nonsteroidal anti-inflammatory drugs for primary dysmenorrhoea. Cochrane Database Syst Rev 2003; 4:CD001751.
27. Campbell MA, McGrath PJ. Use of medication by adolescents for the management of menstrual discomfort. Arch Pediatr Adolesc Med 1997; 151:905–913.
28. Proctor ML, Roberts H, Farquhar CM. Combined oral contraceptive pill (OCP) as treatment for primary dysmenorrhoea. Cochrane Database Syst Rev 2001; 4:CD002120.
29. Milsom I, Sundell G, Andersch B. The influence of different combined oral contraceptives on the prevalence and severity of dysmenorrhoea. Contraception 1990; 42:497–506.

30. Nabrink M, Birgersson L, Colling-Saltin AS, et al. Modern oral contraceptives and dysmenorrhoea. Contraception 1990; 42:275–283.
31. Robinson JC, Plichta S, Weisman CS, et al. Dysmenorrhea and use of oral contraceptives in adolescent women attending a family planning clinic. Am J Obstet Gynecol 1992; 166:578–583.
32. Proctor ML, Murphy PA. Herbal and dietary therapies for primary and secondary dysmenorrhoea. Cochrane Database Syst Rev 2001; (3):CD002124.
33. Barnard ND, Scialli AR, Hurlock D, et al. Diet and sex-hormone binding globulin, dysmenorrhea, and premenstrual symptoms. Obstet Gynecol 2000; 95(2):245–250.
34. Daley AJ, Daley AJ. Exercise and primary dysmenorrhoea: a comprehensive and critical review of the literature. Sports Med 2008; 38(8):659–670.
35. Proctor ML, Smith CA, Farquhar CM, et al. Transcutaneous electrical nerve stimulation and acupuncture for primary dysmenorrhoea. Cochrane Database Syst Rev 2002; 1:CD002123.
36. Akin MD, Weingand KW, Hengehold DA, et al. Continuous low-level topical heat in the treatment of dysmenorrhea. Obstet Gynecol 2001; 97(3):343–349.
37. Milsom I, Hedner N, Mannheimer C. A comparative study of the effect of high-intensity transcutaneous nerve stimulation and oral naproxen on intrauterine pressure and menstrual pain in patients with primary dysmenorrhoea. Am J Obstet Gynecol 1994; 170(1 Pt 1):123–129.
38. Hadfield R, Mardon H, Barlow D, et al. Delay in the diagnosis of endometriosis: a survey of women from the USA and the UK. Hum Reprod 1996; 11:878–880.
39. Moya RA, Moisa CF, Morales F, et al. Transdermal glyceryl trinitrate in the management of primary dysmenorrhoea. Int J Gynaecol Obstet 2000; 69:113–118.
40. Wilson ML, Farquhar CM, Sinclair OJ, et al. Surgical interruption of pelvic nerve pathways for primary and secondary dysmenorrhoea. Cochrane Database Syst Rev 2000; CD001896.
41. Abu JI, Konje JC. Leukotrienes in gynaecology: the hypothetical value of anti-leukotriene therapy in dysmenorrhoea and endometriosis. Hum Reprod Update 2000; 6:200–205.
42. Andersson KE. Calcium antagonists and dysmenorrhea. Ann N Y Acad Sci 1988; 522:747–756.
43. Sandahl B, Ulmsten U, Andersson KE. Trial of the calcium antagonist nifedipine in the treatment of primary dysmenorrhoea. Arch Gynecol 1979; 227:147–151.
44. Lavin C. Dysfunctional uterine bleeding in adolescents. Curr Opin Pediatr 1996; 8:328–332.
45. Adams Hillard PJ. Menstruation in young girls: a clinical perspective. Obstet Gynecol 2002; 99(4):655–662.
46. Jayasinghe Y, Moore P, Donath S, et al. Bleeding disorders in teenagers presenting with menorrhagia. Austr N Z J Obstet Gynaecol 2005; 45(5):439–443.
47. Bevan JA, Maloney KW, Hillery CA, et al. Bleeding disorders: a common cause of menorrhagia in adolescents. J Pediatr 2001; 138(6):856–861.
48. Werner EJ, Broxson EH, Tucker EL, et al. Prevalence of von Willebrand disease in children: a multiethnic study. J Pediatr 1993; 123(6):893–898.
49. ACOG Committee on Adolescent Health Care. ACOG Committee Opinion No. 349, November 2006: Menstruation in girls and adolescents: using the menstrual cycle as a vital sign. Obstet Gynecol 2006; 108(5):1323–1328.
50. Hillard PJ, Rebar RW. Abnormal uterine bleeding needs a special approach. Contemp Obstet Gynecol 1990; 51–68.
51. Grover S. Bleeding disorders and heavy menses in adolescents. Curr Opin Obstet Gynaecol 2007; 19(5):425–419.
52. Lethaby A, Augood C, Duckitt K, et al. Nonsteroidal anti-inflammatory drugs for heavy menstrual bleeding. Cochrane Database Syst Rev 2007; 4:CD000400.
53. Archer DF. Menstrual-cycle-related symptoms: a review of the rationale for continuous use of oral contraceptives. Contraception 2006; 74(5):359–366.
54. Edmonds DK. Primary amenorrhea. In: Edmonds DK, ed. Dewhurst's textbook of obstetrics & gynaecology for postgraduates. 6th edn. Oxford: Blackwell Science; 1999: 34–42.
55. Adams Hillard PJ. Menstruation in adolescents. Ann N Y Acad Sci 2008;1135:29–35.

2

Menstrual problems

OBJECTIVES

- To know the prevalence and current understanding of the aetiology of premenstrual syndrome (PMS)
- To understand the impact of psychosocial issues on the presentation and management of PMS
- To be aware of the evidence regarding the therapeutic efficacy of the various agents used to treat PMS
- To develop a diagnostic approach to the presentation of secondary amenorrhoea
- To be aware of the implications of secondary amenorrhoea with regard to fertility and long-term oestrogen deficiency
- To be aware of the risk factors for endometrial hyperplasia and know when to refer for endometrial assessment
- To initiate and undertake the medical management of menorrhagia

PREMENSTRUAL SYNDROME

What is the difference between premenstrual tension, premenstrual syndrome and premenstrual dysphoric disorder?

While premenstrual tension (PMT) is the term commonly used by women to describe the constellation of symptoms some experience prior to periods, premenstrual syndrome and premenstrual dysphoric disorder (PMDD) are medically defined terms. Premenstrual syndrome is a diagnosis in the *Tenth Revision of the International Classification of Diseases* (ICD-10). The only criterion for this diagnosis is that there should be a history of a single physical or mood symptom occurring in a cyclical basis.[1] Premenstrual dysphoric disorder is a much more specific condition listed by the American Psychiatric Association in the *Diagnostic and Statistical Manual of Mental Disorders* (DSM-IV) and supersedes the condition 'late luteal phase dysphoric disorder' listed in the DSM-III.[2] The diagnostic criteria for PMDD are listed in Box 2.1.

What symptoms do women complain of when they have PMS?

Women complain of many different kinds of symptoms when they have PMS. Premenstrual symptoms are commonly experienced as disturbances of affect, cognition and performance, and as somatic discomforts. Table 2.1 outlines the various symptoms and symptom clusters experienced. A woman tends to have the same set of symptoms from one cycle to the next.[3]

CASE STUDY: 'I get terrible PMT.'

Joan, aged 36, presents to you for a routine smear. As you are taking her menstrual cycle history she mentions that actually she wants some advice about 'premenstrual tension'. Over the past year or so she says that she has found it very hard to cope in the week before her period. She finds herself very irritable with her husband and two children and bursts into tears for no reason. She also complains of feeling headachy and having very sore breasts. Her girlfriend has recommended evening primrose oil to her and she has started using it.

After taking the smear, you talk to Joan about her premenstrual symptoms. She acknowledges that, while she has had some symptoms premenstrually since menarche, they have been more severe in the past year since she returned to full-time work because of her husband's unemployment. She is finding it difficult juggling work and the demands of her family. You satisfy yourself that Joan has no symptoms of depression and explain to her a little about PMS and why her symptoms might be severe at this point in time. You also tell her that evening primrose oil has not been found to be particularly effective but advise her to continue with it if she finds it useful. You ask her to return in 3 months with a symptoms chart.

She returns 3 months later with a chart that is typical of PMS. At that time you counsel her regarding the introduction of lifestyle measures that may assist her and provide her with some written information about the aetiology and treatment of PMS. She returns with one of her children 2 months later for another matter, at which time Joan reports that the symptoms have subsided somewhat.

TABLE 2.1 Premenstrual syndrome symptom clusters

Affective	Cognitive or performance	Fluid retention	General somatic
• Depression or sadness • Mood instability or mood swings • Irritability • Tension • Anxiety • Tearfulness • Restlessness • Anger • Loneliness • Appetite change • Food cravings • Changes in sexual interest • Pain • Headache or migraine • Back pain • Breast pain • Abdominal cramps • General or muscular pain	• Difficulty in concentrating • Decreased efficiency • Confusion • Forgetfulness • Accident-prone • Social avoidance • Temper outbursts • Energetic	• Breast tenderness or swelling • Weight gain • Abdominal bloating or swelling • Swelling of extremities	• Fatigue or tiredness • Dizziness or vertigo swings • Nausea • Insomnia

BOX 2.1 DSM–IV TR criteria for premenstrual dysphoric disorder (PMDD) (From American Psychiatric Association[2])

A
At least five of the following symptoms (one of which must be 1, 2, 3 or 4, below) must be present in the majority of menstrual cycles in the last year. Symptoms should be isolated to the late luteal phase of the menstrual cycle and remit within days of onset of the menses.

1. Markedly depressed mood, feelings of hopelessness, self-deprecating thoughts
2. Marked anxiety, tension, feelings of being 'keyed up' or 'on edge'
3. Marked affective lability
4. Persistent and marked anger or irritability or increased interpersonal conflicts
5. Decreased interest in usual activities
6. Subjective sense of difficulty concentrating
7. Lethargy, easy fatigability, marked lack of energy
8. Marked change in appetite

9. Marked change in sleep pattern
10. Subjective sense of being overwhelmed or out of control
11. Physical symptoms (e.g. breast tenderness or swelling, headaches, joint or muscle pain, sensation of bloating, weight gain)

B
Symptoms cause marked interference with work, school, usual social activities or relationships with others.

C
The problem is not an exacerbation of the symptoms of a chronic condition (e.g. major depressive disorder).

D
The above criteria must be confirmed by prospective daily ratings during at least three consecutive symptomatic cycles to confirm a provisional diagnosis.

How common is it?

While many women complain of PMS or PMT, studies suggest that only 5–8% of women with hormonal cycles have moderate to severe symptoms.[4] Premenstrual symptoms such as breast fullness and tenderness, bloating and irritability can in fact be considered as physiological, with up to 90% of women experiencing some cyclical variation in mood and physical symptoms, and 50% of women claiming to have PMS.[5] Some 35% of women with the condition will seek medical treatment[6] and up to 20% of all women of fertile age have premenstrual complaints that could be regarded as clinically relevant.[7] A diagrammatic model that is useful in explaining this concept to patients is given in Figure 2.1.

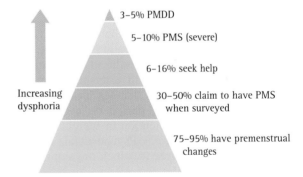

Most women suffer from premenstrual symptoms, but only 3–5% suffer from the extreme form of premenstrual syndrome—namely premenstrual dysphoric disorder.

What causes PMS?

In the past various hypotheses regarding the aetiology of PMS were upheld. These are listed in Box 2.2 (p 18). Because the symptoms of PMS are

FIGURE 2.1 A diagrammatic representation of the prevalence of premenstrual symptoms in women (From Vanselow[10])

Increasing dysphoria

- 3–5% PMDD
- 5–10% PMS (severe)
- 6–16% seek help
- 30–50% claim to have PMS when surveyed
- 75–95% have premenstrual changes

linked to the menstrual cycle, researchers believed for a long time that there must be some kind of hormonal imbalance at the root of PMS. However, multiple studies failed to demonstrate a link between PMS and circulating oestradiol or progesterone.[8]

The most recent theories[9] suggest the following:

- The disorder is related to enhanced sensitivity to progesterone in women with underlying serotonin deficiency. The importance of serotonin for the regulation of mood and aggression, the probable role of serotonin in modulating sex-steroid-driven behaviour as well as the effectiveness of selective

---

BOX 2.2 Previously held beliefs regarding the aetiology of PMS

- Psychological
- Progesterone deficiency
- Hormonal 'imbalance'
- Sex-hormone-binding globulin (SHBG) deficiency
- Sodium and water retention
- Prolactin excess
- Pyridoxine deficiency
- Endorphins
- Diet

Research has found that a large number of women who present with symptoms of PMS do not have the condition at all. One study found that 20.5% did not have a symptom-free period in the follicular phase, 20.1% had another psychiatric condition, 16.6% had menstrual irregularities, 10.2% were menopausal or perimenopausal and 8.4% had other medical disorders.[12]

Women presenting with premenstrual complaints often have psychiatric, medical and/or gynaecological comorbidity.

serotonin reuptake inhibitors (SSRIs) in the management of PMS suggest that serotonin could be involved in the pathophysiology of PMS.

- Dysregulation of allopregnanolone (a progesterone metabolite) and GABA systems may play a role in premenstrual syndrome.
- Endogenous opioids may be involved, as women with PMDD appear to have lower pain thresholds and lower pain-tolerance times than controls.
- Genetic factors may also play a role.

It is controversial whether the somatic symptoms of breast tenderness, bloating and joint and muscle pains result from a reduced tolerance to physical discomfort while in a dysphoric mood state, or are caused by changes in hormone-responsive tissues in the periphery, there being no evidence of water retention or weight gain in the premenstrual phase.[4] Psychosocial factors may influence the degree to which the symptoms interfere with daily life.

Do any conditions masquerade as PMS?

PMS is probably best dealt with in the general practice context because intercurrent illness, be it psychiatric, medical or gynaecological, can contribute to premenstrual symptoms and may present as 'PMS'. Difficulties in the social context, such as with a partner or children or at home, are probably the most common precipitating causes of presentation.[10]

Links have been found between PMS and sexual abuse, as well as with posttraumatic stress disorder.[11] It is therefore important to identify these issues, together with any current or previous intimate partner violence. Concurrent alcohol and drug use to alleviate symptoms of depression and anxiety may also be an issue.

To produce a successful outcome, therefore, the astute practitioner needs to ensure that any comorbid conditions are detected and managed. This is particularly so because PMS may be the label a woman has given to symptoms she does not understand. One study, for example, found that the majority of women who referred themselves to a PMS clinic met the diagnostic criteria for affective disorders—most commonly major depression or anxiety disorders.[13]

Are there any investigations to carry out?

While no discrete investigations will assist GPs in diagnosing PMS, careful consideration of the symptoms via a thorough history and examination is necessary. This entails finding out:

- what the major presenting symptoms are
- how the timing of symptoms relates to the patient's menstrual cycle
- what symptoms are troubling to the patient
- what, if any, symptoms are unrelated to the menstrual cycle.[14]

There are no investigations that will help with forming a diagnosis of premenstrual syndrome.

Symptom charting will help to clarify what the major symptoms are and whether they are indeed cyclical in nature. It needs to be carried out prospectively before a diagnosis of PMS or PMDD can be made. An example of a symptom chart is given in Figure 2.2.

It is important to detect and treat any underlying psychopathology. A history of mood disorder, trauma, unresolved losses or ongoing threats of

Daily Symptom Calendar
In the chart below write down what you feel each day over three months
A = no symptoms
B = some symptoms
C = severe symptoms
Also be sure to shade the days you menstruate.

Day of the month	1	2	3	4		2 7	2 8	2 9	3 0	3 1
Depressed or sad										
Tense and irritable										
Insomnia										
Poor concentration										
Anxious or feeling 'on edge'										
Angry or short–tempered										
Tearful										
Tender, full breasts										
Bloated abdomen										
Swelling of hands or feet										
Generalised aches and pains										
Headaches										
Tiredness										
Increased or decreased appetite										
Food cravings										
Other (specify)										

FIGURE 2.2 A symptom chart for prospective recording of symptoms thought to be related to PMS.

harm (e.g. violence, abandonment, incarceration, homelessness, hunger or job loss) raises the likelihood of an affective diagnosis.[15] Simple depression questionnaires administered premenstrually and in the follicular phase can also assist in diagnosing underlying depression.

What general approach can GPs use when managing women with PMS?

Once other pathologies have been ruled out, management can focus on the following principles:

- providing reassurance and empathy
- increasing the patient's threshold for symptoms by increasing the woman's understanding of the condition and making sure she has adequate levels of support
- addressing lifestyle issues in order to decrease stressors
- implementing specific therapies directed at providing symptomatic relief
- if necessary, altering the patient's hormonal status in order to eradicate cycles.

A recurrent complaint of women with PMS is that they feel they are not believed.[16] Often a sympathetic ear and a good explanation are all that is required,

together with some reassurance that many women suffer from PMS to a certain degree.

GPs should approach premenstrual complaints through reassurance, empathy, addressing lifestyle issues and targeted therapy.

The next step is to explain the causation of PMS to the patient. When doing so, a helpful concept to discuss is that of the 'symptom threshold'. This can be explained as follows:

- Most women suffer from some symptoms premenstrually.
- Stressors may make women more vulnerable to PMS when otherwise they would not suffer to the same degree.
- Personality factors, coping style, learnt behaviour and negative attitudes towards menstruation may mean that 'ill health' is more likely to manifest itself premenstrually.
- Treatment should focus on enhancing the woman's ability to deal with the stress she is experiencing in her life and enhancing her ability to take control.

A healthy lifestyle will help to overcome the condition and gain wellbeing and self-confidence. The positive effects of moderate exercise on mood and general health are well documented,[17] and women engaging in moderate aerobic exercise at least three times a week have significantly fewer premenstrual symptoms than sedentary women.[18,19] Learning and implementing relaxation techniques such as yoga or meditation can also be helpful because they give the patient time to herself to unwind and 'de-stress'.[20] Eating a healthy, low-fat, high-fibre diet, with adequate vitamins and minerals and reduced salt, alcohol, sugar and caffeine intake, is good general advice to give too.

Which specific treatments are effective in treating PMS?

Because SSRIs reduce both mood symptoms and somatic complaints, as well as improving quality of life and social functioning, many believe that SSRIs should be regarded as first-line treatment for PMS patients with severe mood symptoms.[21] The most recent Cochrane systematic review confirms that SSRIs are highly effective in treating physical, functional and behavioural symptoms.[22] All SSRIs (fluoxetine, paroxetine, sertraline, fluvoxamine, citalopram) are effective in reducing premenstrual symptoms and can be prescribed as either luteal phase only (intermittent) or by continuous administration.[22]

The fast onset of action of SSRIs in the management of PMS renders intermittent treatment, from midcycle to menses, a feasible alternative to continuous therapy.

When counselling women regarding the use of SSRIs in the management of PMDD, it is important to cover the points listed in Box 2.3.

BOX 2.3 Prescribing advice regarding use of SSRIs to treat moderate–severe premenstrual symptoms (From Yonkers et al[4])

- The beneficial effect of SSRIs for PMS begins rapidly (compared with the antidepressant effect, which is slow in onset)
- The fast onset of action in PMS renders intermittent treatment, from midcycle to menses, a feasible alternative to continuous therapy.
- Even brief periods of active treatment are more effective than a placebo.
- While most women with PMS prefer intermittent to continuous treatment, SSRIs administered intermittently seem less effective for somatic symptoms than for mood symptoms, and less effective than continuous treatment for somatic symptoms.[23]
- Side effects of SSRIs are usually mild.
- Nausea is very common during the first days of treatment, but vanishes after a few days. It usually does not reappear, even when the treatment is intermittent.
- Reduced libido and anorgasmia are common, and often persist for the duration of treatment, but are not present during the drug-free intervals of intermittent treatment.
- SSRIs are not addictive; discontinuation symptoms may occur when continuous use is stopped suddenly. With intermittent use of SSRIs, discontinuation symptoms are seldom a problem, suggesting that 2 weeks (the luteal phase of the cycle) is too short an exposure period to elicit withdrawal symptoms.

Because, until recently, the aetiology of PMS has been so unclear, all kinds of other therapies have been promoted as cures for PMS. Despite the publication of systematic reviews of the evidence behind these 'cures', [24–26] women continue to use unproven treatments, often on prescription or the recommendation of their GP.

A systematic review of randomised, controlled trials (RCTs) of complementary and alternative therapies for PMS[24] reviewed the evidence for the therapies shown in Box 2.4. Disappointingly, the authors concluded that on the basis of current evidence, none of the complementary/alternative therapies listed could be recommended as a treatment for premenstrual syndrome.

In a review of the efficacy of progesterone and progestogens in the management of PMS,[26] its authors found no evidence to support the claimed efficacy of progesterone in the management of premenstrual syndrome and insufficient evidence to make a definitive statement about progestogens (current evidence suggesting that they are not likely to be effective).

Vitamin B_6 (pyridoxine) is a cofactor in neurotransmitter synthesis and is therefore thought to be helpful in treating mood-related disorders. A systematic review by Wyatt et al[25] concluded that randomised, placebo-controlled studies of vitamin B_6 treatment for premenstrual symptoms were of insufficient quality to draw definitive conclusions. There was limited evidence to suggest that a dose of 100 mg of vitamin B_6 daily (and possibly 50 mg) is likely to be beneficial in the management of

---

BOX 2.4 Therapies of no proven benefit for the treatment of PMS

Herbal medicines
- Chaste tree (*Vitex agnus castus*)
- Gingko biloba
- Evening primrose oil

Homeopathy

Dietary supplements
- Calcium supplementation
- Magnesium supplementation
- Vitamin E
- Multinutrient supplement
- Carbohydrate drink

Relaxation

Massage

Reflexology

Chiropractic

Biofeedback

premenstrual syndrome. In particular, vitamin B$_6$ was significantly better than a placebo in relieving overall premenstrual symptoms and depression associated with premenstrual syndrome, but the response was not dose-dependent. Importantly, no conclusive evidence was found of neurological side effects with these doses.

Evening primrose oil, another very popular therapy among women, contains the essential fatty acids linoleic and gammalinolenic acid. These are precursors of prostaglandins. Most women use evening primrose oil in an attempt to alleviate premenstrual breast symptoms. Large quantities are recommended in the order of eight 500 mg capsules a day. A review of RCTs that compared evening primrose oil with a placebo failed to show any significant benefit.[27]

Evening primrose oil does not have any significant benefit over a placebo for management of premenstrual symptoms

Another option is to totally suppress ovulation in an effort to alleviate premenstrual emotional and physical symptoms. However, the use of medications such as the gonadotrophin-releasing hormone agonists leads to prolonged low oestrogen levels and cardiac and osteoporotic health risks. When using this medication, women will experience hot flushes and sweats, but these may be preferable to the cyclical depression, irritability and headaches of PMS. Add-back hormone replacement therapy (HRT), in which women take oestrogen in order to overcome the oestrogen-lowering side effect of gonadotrophin-releasing hormone, may be required. Danazol can also be used to treat PMS, acting by inhibiting pituitary gonadotrophins, but its side effects include androgenic and virilising effects. When used only during the luteal phase, side effects are minimised. However, while mastalgia may be relieved, the general symptoms of PMS are not.[28]

Another hormonal option is the use of oestradiol implants to suppress ovulation. This reduces symptoms of PMS, but the uterus must be protected from unopposed oestrogen. While using oral progestogens for this purpose may result in a return of troublesome symptoms, another option is to insert Mirena, the levonorgestrel-releasing intrauterine device (IUD).

The humble oral contraceptive pill (COCP) can also suppress ovulation and so should theoretically improve PMS. However placebo-controlled studies have been few and mostly negative.[4] A recent Cochrane review found that the new 24-day drospirenone plus EE 20 mcg COCP may help to treat premenstrual symptoms, but studies showed a large placebo effect. Further studies are necessary to clarify whether the COCP works beyond three cycles for women with less severe symptoms, and whether the drospirenone COCP is better than other COCPs in treating premenstrual symptoms.[29]

For specific symptom control, bromocriptine is effective in alleviating cyclical mastalgia.[30]

An option for patients who have expectations of negative symptoms or of impaired performance around the menses is cognitive behavioural therapy.[31]

Summary of key points
- Up to 90% of women experience some cyclical symptoms, but only 3–5% of women have the severe form of PMS called premenstrual dysphoric disorder.
- The aetiology of PMS is complex and multifactorial and not simply related to sex-steroid-hormone levels.
- Medical, gynaecological and psychiatric conditions often masquerade as PMS.
- Treatment focuses on reassurance and empathy, decreasing stressors and if necessary specific therapies targeting specific symptoms.
- Randomised, controlled trials have found complementary therapies, progesterone, vitamin B$_6$ and evening primrose oil to be no better than placebos in the management of PMS.
- SSRIs are very effective in treating severe mood symptoms of PMS when used either intermittently or continuously.

SECONDARY AMENORRHOEA

What is secondary amenorrhoea?

Secondary amenorrhoea is defined as the absence of menstruation for 6 consecutive months in a woman who previously had regular periods.[32] It does not include the physiological causes of amenorrhoea—namely pregnancy, lactation and menopause.

Pregnancy needs to be excluded in women presenting with secondary amenorrhoea.

CASE STUDY: 'The pill has made me infertile.'

Marie was a 25-year-old woman who had been on the pill since she was 18. After breaking up with her boyfriend, she had decided to stop the pill and was surprised to find that after the initial withdrawal bleed she did not get her periods. She did a home pregnancy test, which was negative, and 6 months later went to see her GP. After explaining the situation, she told the GP, 'Mum says it's because I've taken the pill for so long it's made me infertile!'

Marie's case is one of 'post-pill amenorrhoea', a term that family planners abhor. 'Post-pill amenorrhoea' is the period of time it takes for the hypothalamic–pituitary–ovarian axis to return to its normal functioning after being suppressed by the synthetic hormones in the combined pill. In most women, 'post-pill amenorrhoea' is either non-existent or of 1–2 months duration. If women experience amenorrhoea for longer, it is usually because some organic cause is halting normal menstruation, usually polycystic ovarian syndrome (PCOS). It is likely that taking the pill was actually disguising the problem, which then emerged on discontinuation.

In contrast, the majority of women using the progestogen-only contraceptive agent Depo-Provera® or the levonorgestrel intrauterine device will become amenorrhoeic after 6–9 months use of these agents. This is a direct result of the progestogen that thins the endometrial lining and, in the case of Depo-Provera® (and in some women the progestogen-only pill), suppresses ovulation. In these women normal menstruation and fertility returns after discontinuation of these agents (in the case of Depo-Provera® in an average of 9 months after the last injection), unless there is an underlying organic problem.

Marie by definition had secondary amenorrhoea.

How is secondary amenorrhoea different from primary amenorrhoea?

Primary amenorrhoea occurs when there is failure to establish menstruation and is generally regarded as abnormal by the age of 14 years in girls without signs of secondary sexual development or by the age of 16 in the presence of normal secondary sexual characteristics.[33] (For further information on primary amenorrhoea, see Chapter 1.)

How common is secondary amenorrhoea?

In general, secondary amenorrhoea (prevalence of 1–3%)[34] is much more common than primary amenorrhoea (prevalence of about 0.3%).[35] However, when considering certain population groups, such as the infertile (10–20%),[36] competitive runners training 130 kilometres per week (up to 50%)[32]

and ballet dancers (up to 44%),[32] the prevalence of amenorrhoea is much higher.

What are the common causes of secondary amenorrhoea seen in general practice?

From a clinical perspective, GPs should firstly rule out the possibility of pregnancy and ensure that it is secondary amenorrhoea and not primary amenorrhoea that they are dealing with. The majority of cases are then accounted for by one of four conditions: polycystic ovary syndrome (PCOS), hypothalamic amenorrhoea, hyperprolactinaemia or ovarian failure.[37]

The most common cause of secondary amenorrhoea in women attending general practice is PCOS.

PCOS is present in approximately 30% of women with amenorrhoea[38] but is of itself more likely to cause oligomenorrhoea (76%) than amenorrhoea (24%).[39]

Up to one-third of cases of secondary amenorrhoea are caused by a prolactin-secreting adenoma.[40] In women with amenorrhoea associated with hyperprolactinaemia, the main symptoms are usually those of oestrogen deficiency.[41] Galactorrhoea is found only in up to one-third of hyperprolactinaemic patients, although its appearance is not correlated either with prolactin levels or with the presence of a tumour.[42]

Ovarian failure or menopause is considered premature if it occurs before the age of 40. In 20–40% of cases it is caused by autoantibodies;[43,44] however, other causes include mumps, surgery, radiotherapy or chemotherapy.

In order to sustain a normal menstrual cycle, a woman's body mass index needs to be >19 (normal = 20–25 kg/m^2).[32] Amenorrhoea is induced when a woman loses 10–15% of her normal weight for height.[32] This weight loss can be due to a number of causes, from illness to anorexia to exercise. Exercise-induced amenorrhoea is found in women undertaking endurance events, such as long-distance running, and in those who participate in activities where appearance is important, such as ballet and gymnastics.

What history should be covered when dealing with a case of secondary amenorrhoea?

- Previous menstrual, obstetric and gynaecological (endometrial curettage, oophorectomy) history
- Recent contraceptive use, i.e. progestogens or COCP

TABLE 2.2 Causes of secondary amenorrhoea when there are no features of androgen excess present (From Balen[32])

Physiological
- Pregnancy
- Lactation
- Menopause

Uterine
- Cervical stenosis
- Asherman syndrome (intrauterine adhesions secondary to instrumentation)

Ovarian
- Premature ovarian failure
- Resistant ovary syndrome

Hypothalamic
- Weight loss
- Exercise
- Psychological distress
- Chronic illness
- Idiopathic

Pituitary
- Hyperprolactinaemia
- Hypopituitarism
- Sheehan's syndrome

Causes of hypothalamic/pituitary damage
- Tumours
- Cranial irradiation
- Head injuries
- Sarcoidosis
- Tuberculosis

Systemic disease
- Chronic illness
- Hypo/hyperthyroidism

Iatrogenic
- Post-pill and Depo-Provera® injection (temporary)
- Radiotherapy
- Chemotherapy

↓or normal FSH (62%)	↑Prolactin (14%)	↑FSH (12%)
Chronic anovulation (PCOS)	Radiographic evaluation necessary for prolactinoma	Ovarian failure
Functional hypothalmic anovulation		

FIGURE 2.3 Use of FSH and prolactin to determine possible cause of amenorrhoea (relative frequency in clinical practice) (From Reindollar et al[38])

- Risk of pregnancy
- Associated symptoms, e.g. galactorrhoea, hirsutism, hot flushes and/or dry vagina, symptoms of thyroid disease
- History of an eating disorder, recent change in body weight or emotional upsets
- Level of exercise
- Previous abdominal, pelvic or cranial radiotherapy or history of chemotherapy
- Family history of early menopause

What are the important aspects of the examination in cases of secondary amenorrhoea?

- Height and weight
- Hirsutism, acne or signs of virilisation, such as deep voice or clitoromegaly
- Signs of thyroid disease or galactorrhoea
- Acanthosis nigricans (hyperpigmented thickening of the skin folds of the axilla and neck), which is a sign of profound insulin resistance and is associated with polycystic ovarian syndrome
- Fundoscopy and assessment of visual fields if a pituitary tumour is suspected
- Pelvic examination for enlarged polycystic ovaries

What investigations should be undertaken?

Since the commonest cause of amenorrhoea is pregnancy, *always* do a pregnancy test before proceeding with other investigations. If this is negative, then the estimation of follicle-stimulating hormone (FSH), thyroid-stimulating hormone (TSH) and prolactin will identify the most common causes of amenorrhoea (Fig 2.3).[37]

The thyroid function tests will rule out both hyper- and hypothyroidism. Prolactin levels may be moderately and transiently elevated in response to stress, a breast examination and venepuncture, returning to normal levels (<400 mU/L) within 48 hours. Dopamine antagonists such as many antipsychotic drugs are also associated with raised prolactin levels. More permanent elevation at levels >700 mU/L can result from PCOS or pronounced hypothyroidism (thyrotrophin-releasing hormone stimulates the secretion of prolactin). A prolactin level above 1000 mU/L on two occasions warrants further investigation (e.g. CT or MRI scan of pituitary fossa) and is suggestive of a microadenoma; a level greater than 5000 mU/L is usually associated with a macroadenoma.[32]

The third step is to assess the woman's oestrogen status. Serum oestradiol levels can be misleading and are not generally recommended.[45] A progestogen challenge test is a more reliable way of assessing oestrogen status and is carried out by giving the woman oral medroxyprogesterone acetate in a dose of 5–10 mg for 5–7 days. Women with adequate circulating oestrogen and a normal genital outflow tract will have a withdrawal bleed (positive test) usually two days after discontinuing the progestogen. If no withdrawal bleed occurs (negative test), oestrogen levels are likely to be low. A negative test can also result from destruction of the endometrium (Asherman syndrome) or an outflow obstruction. These possibilities may be indicated by the history and can be confirmed by the use of a cyclic oestrogen and progestogen challenge (i.e. giving the woman a COCP to take for 1–2 months) or by hysteroscopy.

Serum gonadotrophin levels (FSH and LH) are used to distinguish between hypothalamic or pituitary failure and gonadal (ovarian) failure. Four common pictures emerge. These are summarised in Table 2.3. An elevated FSH of >50 IU/L is an indication of ovarian failure or premature menopause. Low FSH and low LH levels in the presence of a negative progestogen challenge is an indication of amenorrhoea secondary to exercise, low weight and/or stress. Normal or mildly raised gonadotrophin levels, particularly with a raised LH:FSH ratio, in the presence of a positive progestogen challenge test and mildly elevated androgens is indicative of PCOS.

What issues need to be covered when managing secondary amenorrhoea in general practice?

When a woman presents with amenorrhoea, GPs should:

- treat any underlying causes where possible
- take preventive action against complications arising from long-term oestrogen deficiency
- consider, detect and manage unopposed oestrogen production (e.g. endometrial hyperplasia and neoplasia)
- give advice about future fertility and address any psychological distress.

What is the management of hyperprolactinaemia?

Hyperprolactinaemia is probably best dealt with in consultation with a specialist endocrinologist. MRI is recommended to diagnose a prolactinoma.[37] Bromocriptine is very effective and reduction in tumour volume is seen within 6 weeks of commencing therapy.[32] Cabergoline is more expensive than bromocriptine but is easier to administer, usually better tolerated and effective in patients who do not have a response to bromocriptine. Surgery is reserved for cases of drug resistance.

What is the management of polycystic ovary syndrome?

Most management of PCOS is symptom-oriented.[46] For further information on PCOS, see Chapter 6.

BOX 2.5 Causes of secondary amenorrhoea when androgen excess is present

- Polycystic ovary syndrome
- Late-onset congenital adrenal hyperplasia
- Adrenal or ovarian androgen-producing tumour

TABLE 2.3 Laboratory findings in common causes of secondary amenorrhoea

	FSH	LH	Prolactin	Testosterone	Oestrogen status
Hyperprolactinaemia	Normal or low	Normal or low	High	Normal	Low
Polycystic ovarian syndrome	Normal	Raised in 40%	Normal or moderate rise in 5–30%	Slightly raised	Normal
Premature menopause	Very high	High	Normal	Normal	Low
'Hypothalamic', i.e. associated with weight loss, exercise or stress	Low or normal	Low or normal	Normal	Normal	Low or normal

What is the management of weight-related amenorrhoea?

Weight-related amenorrhoea is very challenging to treat, given the fact that in many women an underlying eating disorder may be present. Referral to a psychiatrist may be helpful in these cases, as would the assistance of a dietician.

What advice can a GP give about premature ovarian failure?

Premature ovarian failure is said to have occurred when amenorrhoea, persistent oestrogen deficiency and elevated FSH levels occur before the age of 40. Possible causes include fragile X syndrome carriers and other genetic abnormalities and autoimmune disorders, as well as iatrogenic causes such as chemotherapy and radiation therapy for malignancy (both of which have some potential for recovery). It is important to be aware that ovarian function may fluctuate, with increasingly irregular menstrual cycles occurring before the final depletion of oocytes and permanent ovarian failure result. Because of this fluctuation, undertaking a single FSH to diagnose premature ovarian failure is unreliable.

Are there any times that a GP should refer the patient to a specialist?

In secondary amenorrhoea, GPs should refer:

- patients with hyperprolactinaemia for CT or MRI imaging
- patients with mildly raised testosterone levels who do not have PCOS and patients with testosterone levels in the normal male range
- patients with POF for screening for autoimmune disease (e.g. Addison's disease when this is clinically indicated); chromosomal analysis may also be considered for those under 30 years of age
- patients with low gonadotrophin levels that cannot be explained by stress, exercise and weight loss.

What risks are there to the woman as a result of secondary amenorrhoea?

In situations where the woman has a normal oestrogen status but is anovulatory, she is at risk of endometrial hyperplasia (because of the unopposed oestrogen). Using progestogens for 10–14 days of every month or a COCP will decrease this risk.

When the woman is hypo-oestrogenic (where amenorrhoea is due to hyperprolactinaemia, premature ovarian failure, weight loss or exercise) a different set of problems arise, the most important being the risk of osteoporosis and the next being cardiovascular disease.

Women suffering from secondary amenorrhoea may suffer from the consequences of long-term oestrogen deficiency and will have problems with fertility.

Compared with women who have normal menstrual cycles, a 10–20% decrease in lumbar bone density has been found in women with hypo-oestrogenic amenorrhoea, irrespective of the cause.[47,48] Oestrogen replacement should therefore be given to all women who have been amenorrhoeic for longer than 6 months. It is most appropriately and conveniently given in the form of the COCP.[49] Calcium supplementation (1500 mg/day) is also recommended[50] as is maintaining normal vitamin D levels.

Another concern for hypo-oestrogenic women is the risk of cardiovascular disease. There have been few studies to date evaluating this risk, however. One small study looking at lipids in women with hypothalamic amenorrhoea (HA) found that in contrast to menopausal oestrogen deficiency, young women with HA and oestrogen deficiency have increased levels of HDL and no increases in TC, LDL and triglycerides.[51] This study suggests that the negative effects of oestrogen deficiency on cardiovascular risk factors may be modified in women with hypothalamic amenorrhoea.

Women with PCOS also have an increased risk of developing cardiovascular disease, hypertension and diabetes. It is believed that the main underlying disorder is insulin resistance and this results in an associated dyslipidaemia (with raised triglycerides, raised LDL levels and reduced HDL levels) and elevated plasminogen activator inhibitor-1 levels.[52]

What advice can be given about future fertility?

Amenorrhoea is a sign for a woman that 'something' is not working properly. It can therefore be associated with considerable anxiety, altered self-image and loss of self-esteem. It is important to advise women with secondary amenorrhoea that pregnancy is still a possibility if there is any sporadic ovulation occurring. Contraception should therefore be used if they do not wish to conceive. For most however, the concern is that of future fertility. Reassuringly, treatment of the underlying cause of the amenorrhoea is usually all that is required to restore fertility.

Summary of key points
- When a woman presents with secondary amenorrhoea, pregnancy must be excluded.
- The most common cause of secondary amenorrhoea in women presenting to GPs is PCOS.

- The three key issues in managing women with secondary amenorrhoea are to treat underlying causes, prevent complications arising from oestrogen deficiency and to counsel the woman regarding future fertility.

MENORRHAGIA

What is menorrhagia?

Menorrhagia is the medical term used for heavy periods. Research involving the collection of pads and tampons to measure blood loss has shown that on average women lose 35 mL of blood with each period. Menorrhagia has been defined as a loss of ≥80 mL of blood in a period, this level being above the 90th percentile.

How common is it?

Population studies have demonstrated that 10% of menstruating women lose >80 mL of blood.[53] Recent studies show that subjective estimation of loss by women correlates with the measured loss better than previously believed.[54]

How commonly do women present with menorrhagia to their GP?

Given that approximately 5% of women aged 30–49 consult their GP about heavy bleeding each year,[55] menorrhagia is a condition that GPs need to be able to manage effectively and well. This is especially so since until recently the risk of hysterectomy (primarily for menstrual disorders) by the end of reproductive life was 20%.[56]

What do women understand about menorrhagia and what do they want from their GP?

An interesting study recently looked at women's perceptions of menorrhagia, their understanding of the mechanisms behind it and their expectations of medical professionals regarding this problem.[57] The study involved interviews with women who had presented to their GP with 'heavy periods'. The researcher found that women had a precise understanding of their complaint. A change in cycle was indicative of a problem to many women, without reference to outside criteria. Women attached particular importance to how they felt and to their ability to function, and they rejected the medical emphasis on blood-loss evaluation. Many women were dissatisfied with the GP consultation and felt that doctors were dismissive of their problem. They were seeking an explanation for the change in their periods and had concerns that related to their

CASE STUDY: 'I'm completely exhausted.'

Beth, 42, gave a fairly classical history of menorrhagia. Over the last year her periods had been getting heavier and heavier and lasting for up to 10 days at a time. More recently she had been experiencing very heavy periods, passing clots, staining the sheets at night and generally feeling exhausted at 'that time of the month'.

Initially she went to see her GP, who ordered an Hb and iron studies. These came back borderline low and so Beth was started on iron tablets. The GP then referred her to a gynaecologist, hoping that the specialist would institute the appropriate management. The trouble was that in the time between Beth's first visit to her GP and her appointment with the recommended specialist she had had another two horrible, heavy periods. At the gynaecologist's, a full history was taken and Beth had a thorough examination, and was then referred for a vaginal ultrasound. Before she returned to see the gynaecologist she had had another awful period. So when, at the second and subsequent appointment, after learning that Beth didn't want any children, the gynaecologist suggested that a hysterectomy was the way to go, Beth didn't hesitate.

The problem was that because of medical insurance qualifying periods her operation was not for another 3 months. This meant that, despite having consulted two doctors and having been investigated, she was still not getting any immediate management and was suffering unnecessarily as a result. Given that medical management could only have helped Beth's symptoms, not worsen them, there was no reason for not introducing them at the first consultation (as long as there were no contraindications). Had Beth felt more 'in control' of her symptoms, she might well have opted to manage slightly heavier periods that she could nevertheless cope with rather than undergo a hysterectomy.

understanding of menstrual bleeding. Interviewees were unsure whether period problems could be described as illness, and what range of disturbance was normal.

GPs should therefore consider menstrual blood loss to be excessive when it interferes with the woman's physical, emotional, social and material quality of life, whether it occurs alone or in combination with other symptoms. Any interventions should therefore be measures aimed at improving quality of life.[58]

What approach should a GP use for a woman complaining of heavy menstrual blood loss?

Recent evidence-based guidelines[58] suggest a new approach to heavy menstrual loss in the general practice setting. This approach is summarised in the algorithm in Figure 2.4

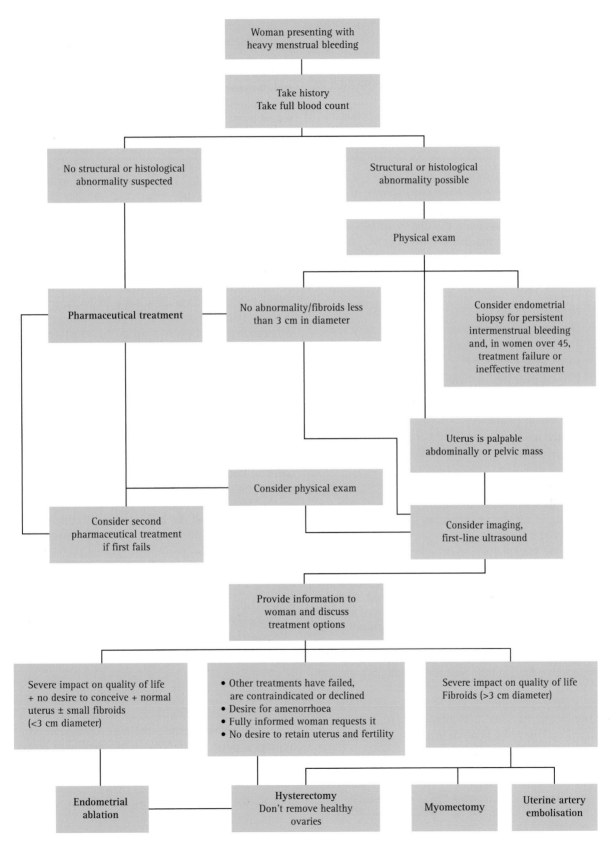

FIGURE 2.4 A care pathway for heavy menstrual bleeding (From NICE[58])

This pathway suggests that as a first step GPs should consider:[58]

- the nature of the bleeding
- related symptoms that might suggest structural or histological abnormality
- impact on quality of life and other factors that may determine treatment options (such as presence of co-morbidity).

What key questions should be asked when taking a history from a patient complaining of heavy periods?

The first issue is to assess the degree of blood loss. Women may find this difficult to quantify. Instead of measuring blood loss by collecting sanitary pads, GPs use 'proxies' of measurement by asking questions such as:

- How many pads or tampons would you use a day?
- Do you pass any clots?
- Do you ever use a tampon *and* a pad and still worry about leaking?
- Do you ever feel like you are flooding?

Clots, flooding and the need for simultaneous use of pads and tampons are good indicators of menorrhagia.

It is then important to clarify whether or not the bleeding is regular or irregular. This will point to whether the bleeding is associated with ovulatory cycles or anovulatory cycles, both of which can be associated with dysfunctional uterine bleeding. In women in their late 30s and 40s, excessive menstrual loss is usually ovulatory and brought about by fibroids. Between 80% and 90% of women with heavy menstrual bleeding have regular cycles (lasting 21–35 days).[59] Women with prolonged irregular bleeding or intermenstrual bleeding are reported to have submucous fibroids or endometrial polyps in 25–50% of cases, albeit in highly selected populations.[60] The incidence of polyps or submucous fibroids in women with regular heavy menstrual bleeding is unknown.

Irregular or intermenstrual bleeding as compared with regular heavy bleeding may be an indicator of underlying pathology.

It is very rare to find haemostatic causes of menorrhagia. Laboratory-based research has found, however, that in women with menorrhagia the endometrium has increased fibrinolytic activity[61] and increased production of prostaglandins.[62] These observations point the way to some of the more recent management options that are being offered to women.

The third issue that needs to be addressed is to what degree the symptoms are interfering with the woman's daily life? Is she able to cope with work, family and daily life when she has her periods? Does she need to make sure she is always near a bathroom and a toilet to attend to the bleeding? This will give the GP a guide to the urgency of the situation.

Finally the GP needs to address the possibility of anaemia. One consequence of excessive menstrual loss is iron deficiency anaemia, resulting in complaints of exhaustion and lethargy. In the Western world, menorrhagia is the most common cause of iron deficiency anaemia, and low haemoglobin concentrations may objectively predict heavy menstrual loss.[63]

What features in the history should make a GP suspicious of underlying pathology?

Structural abnormalities of the uterus such as endometrial polyps, adenomyosis and leiomyomata are well known to be causative factors of excessive uterine bleeding. GPs need to be alert to features in the history that are suggestive of underlying pathology as well as malignancy, as the risk of endometrial cancer starts to rise when women are in their 40s.

Risk factors for endometrial hyperplasia in premenopausal women include:

- infertility and nulliparity
- exposure to unopposed endogenous or exogenous oestrogen/tamoxifen
- polycystic ovarian syndrome
- obesity
- family history of endometrial and colonic cancer.[64]

In percentage terms, the risk of endometrial hyperplasia or carcinoma in women with heavy menstrual bleeding is:

- 4.9% for all women
- 2.3% for women <45 years and <90 kg
- 13% for women >90 kg
- 8% for women >45 years.[65]

Increasing age and obesity are important risk factors for endometrial hyperplasia and cancer.

If the history suggests heavy menstrual bleeding without structural or histological abnormality, pharmaceutical treatment can be started without carrying out a physical examination or other investigations at the initial consultation in primary care, unless the treatment chosen is the levonorgestrel-releasing intrauterine system (LNG-IUS) or a pap smear is due. However, if the history suggests heavy menstrual blood loss with symptoms such as intermenstrual or postcoital bleeding, pelvic pain, dyspareunia and/or pressure symptoms, a physical examination and/or other investigations (such as ultrasound) should be performed[58] to exclude pathology and the presence of malignancy.[66]

When should a GP undertake an examination?

Many would argue the old adage, 'if you don't look you won't find', and recommend examination for all women with menorrhagia.

The NICE guidelines[58] specify, however, that examination is necessary if:

- a GP considers there are features in the history suggestive of underlying pathology (such as risk factors for endometrial hyperplasia)
- the woman has decided to go ahead with a LNG-IUS (to assess the uterus for suitability for the device)
- the woman is to be referred for further investigations, such as ultrasound or biopsy.

Those who have fibroids that are palpable abdominally or who have intracavitary fibroids and/or a uterine length >12 cm when measured at ultrasound or hysteroscopy should be offered immediate referral to a specialist.[58]

Are there any laboratory tests a GP should order in women complaining of menorrhagia?

While numerous investigations are available, GPs should consider the fact that in 40–60% of women with menorrhagia no underlying cause is found (these women are said to have dysfunctional uterine bleeding (unexplained menorrhagia)) and think about the rationale for each investigation before it is undertaken (Box 2.6).

As symptoms and signs of anaemia do not correlate well with the haemoglobin level until the patient is moderately-to-severely anaemic, a full

> **BOX 2.6 Recommendations regarding commonly performed investigations for menorrhagia (From NICE[58])**
>
> - A full-blood-count test should be carried out in all women with HMB. This should be done in parallel with any HMB treatment offered. [C]
> - Testing for coagulation disorders (for example, von Willebrand's disease) should be considered in women who have had HMB since menarche and have a personal or family history suggesting a coagulation disorder. [C]
> - A serum ferritin test should not routinely be carried out in women with HMB. [B]
> - Female hormone testing should not be carried out in women with HMB. [C]
> - Thyroid testing should only be carried out when other signs and symptoms of thyroid disease are present. [C]

blood count should be performed in all women complaining of heavy menstrual bleeding to aid recognition of the severity of menstrual blood loss. It is not recommended that iron studies are performed routinely, as the haematological indices usually give some indication of the iron stores.[58] Women who are severely anaemic (<80 g/L) should be referred to a specialist immediately because of the increased likelihood of pathology.[67] Tests for coagulopathies should be undertaken only in those who have experienced heavy bleeding since menarche or who have a personal or family history suggesting a coagulation disorder. It is not useful to carry out female hormone testing. Thyroid testing should be carried out only when other signs and symptoms of thyroid disease are present.[58]

In cases of menorrhagia, a serum ferritin does not really give any additional information beyond that obtained with a full blood count.

What is the role of ultrasound in the investigation of women with heavy bleeding?

Highest-level evidence supports the use of ultrasound as the first-line diagnostic tool for identifying structural abnormalities. It is a non-invasive, non-painful method of selecting those women who need further diagnostic evaluation. It can identify endometrial thickness (the limit of normal is 10–12 mm in premenopausal women), polyps and fibroids, and in menopausal women has a sensitivity of more than 96% for detecting endometrial cancer by measurement of the endometrium in menopausal women.[68,69]

High-level evidence supports the use of transvaginal ultrasound as the first line diagnostic tool in the investigation of women with menorrhagia

It should therefore be undertaken when:

- the uterus is palpable abdominally
- vaginal examination reveals a pelvic mass of uncertain origin
- pharmaceutical treatment fails.[58]

What is the role of hysteroscopy and biopsy?

Hysteroscopy should be used as a diagnostic tool only when ultrasound results are inconclusive—for example, to determine the exact location of a fibroid or the exact nature of the abnormality.[58]

Biopsy is necessary to exclude endometrial cancer or atypical hyperplasia. Indications for a biopsy include:

- persistent intermenstrual bleeding
- treatment failure or ineffective treatment in women aged 45 and over.[58]

Dilatation and curettage alone should not be used as a diagnostic tool.[58]

Which women should be referred for endometrial assessment?

Exactly which women should undergo endometrial assessment and what the nature of that assessment should be remains controversial. New Zealand guidelines[65] recommend a transvaginal ultrasound (TVS) of the endometrium in women:

- whose weight is >90 kg
- whose age is >45 years (UK guidelines[70] recommend further assessment in women >40 years)
- who have other risk factors for endometrial hyperplasia or carcinoma, such as known POS, infertility, nulliparity or exposure to unopposed oestrogens, or a family history of endometrial or colon cancer.

If the endometrial thickness on TVS is >12 mm, an endometrial sample should be taken to exclude endometrial hyperplasia. If TVS is not available, then an endometrial sample should be taken. Hysteroscopy and biopsy is indicated for women with erratic menstrual bleeding, failed medical therapy or a TVS suggestive of intrauterine pathology such as polyps or submucous fibroids. Hysteroscopy with biopsy detects more pathology when compared directly with dilatation and curettage (D&C) as a diagnostic procedure.[71] An alternative to hysteroscopy is the use of the 'pipelle' as a method of endometrial sampling (biopsy). The procedure is done 'blind' and, while it is a more acceptable procedure for women, the question of whether it can be substituted for a formal hysteroscopy and still achieve high degrees of sensitivity and specificity remains unresolved.

Endometrial thickness of >12 mm may indicate endometrial hyperplasia.

Should all women with menorrhagia be started on iron tablets?

During normal menstruation, bleeding typically lasts for 4 ± 2 days, during which an average of 35–40 mL blood is lost, an amount equivalent to 16 mg of iron. The recommended dietary intake of iron is adequate to compensate for a monthly loss of 80 mL, but the diet of the average woman is iron deficient, allowing anaemia to manifest with menstrual volumes of more than 60 mL per month.[53] In many instances, the principal symptom experienced by women with abnormal uterine bleeding is fatigue, secondary to anaemia. As a result, a daily dose of 60–180 mg of elemental iron should be used to treat the anaemia.

What other management can GPs institute for patients with menorrhagia?

Pharmaceutical treatment should be considered where no structural or histological abnormality is present, or for fibroids less than 3 cm in diameter that are causing no distortion of the uterine cavity.[58]

As the case study demonstrates, GPs should institute some kind of management for women to lessen their blood loss before they are seen by a gynaecologist, if this is ultimately necessary. Many medical management options are available to GPs, including non-steroidal anti-inflammatory drugs (NSAIDs), hormonal therapies such as the COCP or cyclical progestogens, tranexamic acid and even the levonorgestrel-releasing intrauterine system

TABLE 2.4 A comparison of medical therapies for the treatment of heavy menstrual bleeding (From National Advisory Committee on Health and Disability[65])

Drug	Mean reduction in mean blood loss, 80 mL/cycle) %	Women benefiting (proportion with blood loss) %
Levonorgestrel IUS	94	100
Oral progesterone (days 5–25)	87	86
Tranexamic acid	47	56
NSAIDs	29	51
Combined oral contraceptive pill	43	50
Danazol	50	76
Oral progesterone (luteal phase, days 12–26)	24	18

(LNG-IUS) Mirena. The comparative efficacy of available medical therapies for menorrhagia is given in Table 2.4. If pharmaceutical treatment is required while investigations and definitive treatment are being organised, either tranexamic acid or NSAIDs should be used.

Medical management of menorrhagia is very effective and should be introduced by GPs.

Several factors will influence treatment choice:

- the presence of ovulatory or anovulatory cycles
- the need for contraception or a wish to conceive
- the patient's preference (particularly whether she is happy using hormonal therapy)
- contraindications to treatment.

If history and investigations indicate that pharmaceutical treatment is appropriate and either hormonal or non-hormonal treatments are acceptable, treatments should be considered in the following order:[58]

1. levonorgestrel-releasing intrauterine system (LNG-IUS), provided long-term use(at least 12 months) is anticipated
2. tranexamic acid, non-steroidal anti-inflammatory drugs (NSAIDs) or combined oral contraceptives (COCPs)

BOX 2.7 Prescribing tips in relation to pharmaceutical options for the treatment of HMB (From NICE[58])

- Women offered an LNG-IUS should be advised of anticipated changes in the bleeding pattern, particularly in the first few cycles and perhaps lasting longer than 6 months. They should therefore be advised to persevere for at least six cycles to see the benefits of the treatment.
- When HMB coexists with dysmenorrhoea, NSAIDs should be preferred to tranexamic acid.
- Ongoing use of NSAIDs and/or tranexamic acid is recommended for as long as the woman finds them to be beneficial.
- Use of NSAIDs and/or tranexamic acid should be stopped if there is no improvement of symptoms within three menstrual cycles.
- When a first pharmaceutical treatment has proved ineffective, a second pharmaceutical treatment can be considered rather than immediate referral to surgery.
- Oral progestogens given during the luteal phase only should not be used for the treatment of HMB.

3. norethisterone (15 mg) daily from days 5 to 26 of the menstrual cycle, or injected long-acting progestogens.

Danazol should not be used routinely for the treatment of heavy menstrual bleeding. Further prescribing tips in relation to pharmaceutical options for the treatment of heavy menstrual bleeding can be found in Box 2.7

Two main first-line treatments for menorrhagia are non-hormonal—the antifibrinolytic tranexamic acid (Cyklokapron) and NSAIDs. The effectiveness of these treatments has been shown in randomised trials[72–74] and reported in systematic reviews of treatment.[75,76]

The levonorgestrel-IUS should be recommended as a first-line treatment for women with menorrhagia who do not want to conceive and for whom medical management is appropriate.

As a rule of thumb, GPs can say to their patients that tranexamic acid reduces menstrual loss by about a half and NSAIDs by about a third. For many of the women that GPs see, these figures approximate to the fact that a woman may return to what her 'normal' periods were like, doing away with the need for surgery. Both kinds of drugs have the advantage of being taken only during menstruation itself (an aid to compliance) and are particularly useful for those women who either do not require contraception or do not wish to use a hormonal therapy. They are also of value in treating excessive menstrual blood loss associated with the use of non-hormonal intrauterine contraceptive devices.

How does tranexamic acid work and what are the contraindications and side effects?

Tranexamic acid works by depressing the fibrinolytic activity of peripheral blood through the inhibition of plasminogen activation. Reviews estimate that correct use of tranexamic acid (commenced with the onset of bleeding: two to three tablets are taken four times a day for the first 4 days of the period) reduces menstrual blood loss by 34–59% over two to three cycles, and that 12% of women report adverse events, such as nausea, vomiting, diarrhoea and dyspepsia.[77,78] Unlike NSAIDs, tranexamic acid has no effect on dysmenorrhoea. The risks associated with this drug are related to thrombosis. Contraindications include a past history of venous thromboembolism (VTE) or stroke, and a problem with colour vision that developed after birth.

It is important also to note that tranexamic acid:

- does not reduce dysmenorrhoea/pain associated with bleeding, so advice on suitable pain relief may be required
- is not a contraceptive, so advice on suitable contraception may be required
- does not regulate cycles, so advice and suitable additional treatment should be given, if required.

How should NSAIDs be prescribed for the treatment of menorrhagia?

Any NSAID can be used, but the most common ones prescribed are probably:

- mefenamic acid (Ponstan) 500 mg t.d.s.
- diclofenac (Voltaren) 50 mg t.d.s.
- naproxen (Naprosyn) 250–500 mg t.d.s.

The woman should take the tablets only during the menses but, as with the management of dysmenorrhoea, she should try to commence the medication when she knows that menstruation is imminent to maximise the effectiveness of the medication. GPs should be wary of the contraindications to NSAIDs. They are:

- current GI bleeding or ulceration
- inflammatory bowel disease
- history of hypersensitivity (asthma, angio-oedema) precipitated by aspirin or NSAID
- renal or hepatic impairment.

How useful are hormonal therapies?

Traditionally hormonal therapy for menorrhagia has consisted of progestogens given during the luteal phase of the cycle.[79] Despite the fact that such treatments have been found to be ineffective, they remain the first choice of many general practitioners and gynaecologists.[80] Progestogens are effective in reducing blood loss only when given for 21 days in each cycle, but the side effects may be such that patients would not choose to continue with treatment.[81]

The COCP is probably the treatment with which GPs will feel the most familiar and, provided that there are no contraindications, it is useful in the management of menorrhagia. Not only will it provide contraception; it will significantly reduce the amount of blood loss that a woman is experiencing. The GP can then also change the pill to suit the woman; for example, if a levonorgestrel pill is not reducing the bleeding enough, then one that contains norethisterone or a third-generation progestogen pill can be tried. The GP can also suggest that the woman tricycles the pill—that is, that she leaves out the sugar pills in the three-pill packets and takes the hormone pills continuously so that she can have a real break from her periods. The pill is also useful in anovulatory bleeding because it imposes a 'cycle'.

The final and preferred[58] 'medical' option, due to its cost-effectiveness when long-term use is concerned, is the levonorgestrel-releasing intrauterine system (Mirena) consisting of a T-shaped intrauterine device sheathed with a reservoir of levonorgestrel that is released at the rate of 20 mg daily. This low level of hormone minimises the systemic progestogenic side effects, and patients are more likely to continue with this therapy than cyclical progestogen therapy. It exerts its clinical effect by preventing endometrial proliferation and consequently reduces both the duration of bleeding and the amount of menstrual loss.[82] For up to 6 months, patients may experience irregular bleeding or spotting, especially in the first 3 months, but by 12 months most women have only light bleeding and a major proportion are amenorrhoeic.[70] Many of the potential problems of bleeding and spotting can be overcome by thorough pretreatment counselling.

What about surgery?

Medical management of menorrhagia in no way precludes the option of surgery further down the track, but it does give the woman some time to recover from the 'heavy periods' she has been experiencing and to consider all her options, including surgery. If medical management is not instituted, women may well feel that surgery is the only way to get themselves out of the difficult situation they find themselves in. Indeed, for many women a hysterectomy may be the best option, ending the need for continuing management of the menorrhagia.

Summary of key points
- One-third of women complain of heavy periods but only 10% have menorrhagia.
- Until recently, 20% of women had had a hysterectomy by the end of their reproductive years.
- The most common causes of heavy bleeding are ovulatory cycles and fibroids.
- Risk factors for endometrial hyperplasia and cancer in premenopausal women include infertility and nulliparity, exposure to unopposed endogenous or exogenous oestrogen/tamoxifen, polycystic ovarian syndrome, obesity and a family history of endometrial and colonic cancer.
- A full blood count should be carried out in all women with menorrhagia.
- Endometrial assessment is necessary in obese women, those over 45 and those with a risk factor for endometrial hyperplasia and/or cancer.
- Medical management of menorrhagia is very effective.
- Tranexamic acid reduces menstrual loss by about a half and NSAIDs by about a third.
- Progestogens are effective in treating menorrhagia only if used for a minimum of 21 days.
- The COCP or the Mirena levonorgestrel-releasing IUS is also effective in the management of menorrhagia.
- If history and investigations indicate that pharmaceutical treatment is appropriate and either hormonal or non-hormonal treatments are acceptable, the levonorgestrel-releasing intrauterine system (LNG-IUS) is the preferred option, provided long-term use is anticipated.

TIPS FOR PRACTITIONERS

- When considering a patient with PMS, an important question to ask is 'what caused you to come about this today?' This question will help uncover recent stressors that may have altered the woman's ability to cope with premenstrual symptoms. Addressing these stressors will be an important step in the therapeutic process.
- GPs should emphasise the positive effects of moderate exercise on mood and general health, as well as recommending relaxation techniques

such as yoga or meditation to assist women in dealing with their stressful lives.
- When women present with secondary amenorrhoea, always be sure to exclude pregnancy prior to further investigation.
- Asking the patient if they ever 'flood', pass clots or need to wear a tampon as well as a pad because of worries of leakage gives a useful indication of the heaviness of blood flow during menstruation.
- While only 12–14 days/month of progestogen are required to prevent endometrial hyperplasia where there is unopposed oestrogen, a minimum of 21 days of progestogen/month is necessary to treat menorrhagia effectively.

REFERENCES

1. World Health Organization. Mental, behavioural and developmental disorders. In: Tenth revision of the International Classification of Diseases (ICD-10). Geneva: World Health Organization; 1996.
2. American Psychiatric Association. Diagnostic and statistical manual of mental disorders. 4th edn. Washington DC: American Psychiatric Association; 2000.
3. Bloch M, Schmidt PJ, Rubinow DR. Premenstrual syndrome: evidence for symptom stability across cycles. Am J Psychiatry 1997; 154(12):1741–1746.
4. Yonkers KA, O'Brien PM, Eriksson E. Premenstrual syndrome. Lancet 2008; 371(9619):1200–1210.
5. Sveindottir H, Backstrom T. Prevalence of menstrual cycle symptom cyclicity and premenstrual dysphoric disorder in a random sample of women using and not using oral contraceptives. Acta Obstet Gynecol Scand 2000; 79: 405–413.
6. Hylan TR, Sundell K, Judge R. The impact of premenstrual symptomatology on functioning and treatment-seeking behavior: experience from the United States, United Kingdom, and France. J Womens Health Gend Based Med 1999; 8: 1043–1052.
7. Borenstein JE, Dean BB, Endicott J, et al. Health and economic impact of the premenstrual syndrome. J Reprod Med 2003; 48(7):515–524.
8. Roca CA, Schmidt PJ, Bloch M, et al. Implications of endocrine studies in premenstrual syndrome. Psychiatr Ann 1996; 26:576
9. Henshaw C. PMS: diagnosis, aetiology, assessment and management: revisiting premenstrual syndrome. Adv Psychiatr Treat 2007; 13:139–146.
10. Vanselow W. A comprehensive approach to premenstrual complaints. Aust Fam Physician 1998; 27:354–361.
11. Perkonigg A, Yonkers KA, Pfister H, et al. Risk factors for premenstrual dysphoric disorder in a community sample of young women: the role of traumatic events and posttraumatic stress disorder. J Clin Psychiatry 2004; 65(10):1314–1322.
12. Mortola JF. Applications of gonadotropin-releasing hormone analogues in the treatment of premenstrual syndrome. Clin Obstet Gynecol 1993; 36:753–763.
13. Keenan PA, Stern RA, Janowsky DS, et al. Psychological aspects of premenstrual syndrome. I. Cognition and memory. Psychoneuroendocrinology 1992; 17:179–187.
14. Daugherty JE. Treatment strategies for premenstrual syndrome. Am Fam Physician 1998; 58:183–192, 197–198.

15. Bancroft J, Rennie D, Warner P. Vulnerability to perimenstrual mood change: the relevance of a past history of depressive disorder. Psychosom Med 1994; 56:225–231.
16. Leather AT, Holland EFN, Studd JW, et al. A study of the referral patterns and therapeutic experiences of 100 women attending a specialist premenstrual syndrome clinic. J R Soc Med 1993; 86:191–201.
17. Byrne A, Byrne DG. The effect of exercise on depression, anxiety, and other mood states: a review. J Psychosom Res 1993; 37:565–574.
18. Johnson WG, Carr-Nangle RE, Bergeron KC. Macronutrient intake, eating habits, and exercise as moderators of menstrual distress in healthy women. Psychosom Med 1995; 57:324–330.
19. Prior JC, Vigna Y, Alojada N. Conditioning exercise decreases premenstrual symptoms: a prospective controlled three-month trial. Eur J Appl Physiol 1986; 55:349–355.
20. Goodale IL, Domar AD, Benson H. Alleviation of premenstrual-syndrome symptoms with the relaxation response. Obstet Gynecol 1990; 75:649–655.
21. Steiner M, Pearlstein T, Cohen LS, et al. Expert guidelines for the treatment of severe PMS, PMDD, and comorbidities: the role of SSRIs. J Women's Health (Larchmt) 2006; 15(1):57–69.
22. Brown J, O'Brien PM, Marjoribanks J, et al. Selective serotonin reuptake inhibitors for premenstrual syndrome. Cochrane Database Syst Rev 2009; 2:CD001396.
23. Landen M, Nissbrandt H, Allgulander C, et al. Placebo-controlled trial comparing intermittent and continuous paroxetine in premenstrual dysphoric disorder. Neuropsychopharmacology 2007; 32(1):153–161.
24. Stevinson C, Ernst E. Complementary/alternative therapies for premenstrual syndrome: a systematic review of randomized controlled trials. Am J Obstet Gynecol 2001; 185:227–235.
25. Wyatt KM, Dimmock PW, Jones PW, et al. Efficacy of vitamin B6 in the treatment of premenstrual syndrome: systematic review. Br Med J 1999; 318:1375–1381.
26. Wyatt K, Dimmock P, Jones P, et al. Efficacy of progesterone and progestogens in management of premenstrual syndrome: systematic review. Br Med J 2001; 323:776–780.
27. Budeiri D, Li Wan Po A, Dornan JC. Is evening primrose oil of value in the treatment of premenstrual syndrome? Control Clin Trials 1996; 17:60–68.
28. O'Brien PM, Abukhalil IE. Randomized controlled trial of the management of premenstrual syndrome and premenstrual mastalgia using luteal phase-only danazol. Am J Obstet Gynecol 1999; 180:18–23.
29. Lopez LM, Kaptein AA, Helmerhorst FM. Oral contraceptives containing drospirenone for premenstrual syndrome. Cochrane Database Syst Rev 2009; (2):CD006586.
30. Mansel RE, Dogliotti L. European multicentre trial of bromocriptine in cyclical mastalgia. Lancet 1990; 335:190–193.
31. Christensen AP, Oei TP. The efficacy of cognitive behaviour therapy in treating premenstrual dysphoric changes. J Affect Disord 1995; 33:57–63.
32. Balen AH. Secondary amenorrhea. In: Edmonds DK, ed. Dewhurst's textbook of obstetrics & gynaecology for postgraduates. 6th edn. Oxford: Blackwell Science; 1999: 42–61.
33. Edmonds DK. Primary amenorrhea. In: Edmonds DK, ed. Dewhurst's textbook of obstetrics & gynaecology for postgraduates. 6th edn. Oxford: Blackwell Science; 1999:34–42.
34. Pettersson F, Fries H, Nillius SJ. Epidemiology of secondary amenorrhea. I. Incidence and prevalence rates. Am J Obstet Gynecol 1973; 117:80–86.
35. Singh KB. Menstrual disorders in college students. Am J Obstet Gynecol 1981; 140:299–302.
36. Franks S. Primary and secondary amenorrhoea. Br Med J (Clin Res Ed) 1987; 294:815–819.
37. Practice Committee of American Society for Reproductive Medicine. Current evaluation of amenorrhea. Fertil Steril 2008; 90(5 Suppl):S219–S225.
38. Reindollar RH, Novak M, Tho SPT, et al. Adult-onset amenorrhea: a study of 262 patients. Am J Obstet Gynecol 1986; 155(3):531–543.
39. Bili H, Laven J, Imani B, et al. Age-related differences in features associated with polycystic ovary syndrome in normogonadotrophic oligo-amenorrhoeic infertile women of reproductive years. Eur J Endocrinol 2001; 145(6):749–755.
40. Schlechte J, Sherman B, Halmi N, et al. Prolactin-secreting pituitary tumors in amenorrheic women: a comprehensive study. Endocrinol Rev 1980; 1:295–308.
41. Jacobs HS. Management of prolactin-secreting pituitary tumours. In: Studd J, ed. Progress in obstetrics and gynaecology. Edinburgh: Churchill Livingstone; 1981; 1:263–276.
42. Jacobs HS, Franks S, Murray MA, et al. Clinical and endocrine features of hyperprolactinaemic amenorrhoea. Clin Endocrinol 1976; 5:439–454.
43. Alper MM, Garner PR. Premature ovarian failure: its relationship to autoimmune disease. Obstet Gynecol 1985; 66:27–30.
44. Damewood MD, Zacur HA, Hoffman GJ, et al. Circulating antiovarian antibodies in premature ovarian failure. Obstet Gynecol 1986; 68:850–854.
45. Kiningham RB, Apgar BS, Schwenk TL. Evaluation of amenorrhea. Am Fam Physician 1996; 53:1185–1194.
46. Balen AH. Pathogenesis of polycystic ovary syndrome—the enigma unravels? Lancet 1999; 354:966–967.
47. Biller BM, Baum HB, Rosenthal DI, et al. Progressive trabecular osteopenia in women with hyperprolactinemic amenorrhea. J Clin Endocrinol Metab 1992; 75:692–697.
48. Drinkwater BL, Nilson K, Chesnut CH 3rd, et al. Bone mineral content of amenorrheic and eumenorrheic athletes. N Engl J Med 1984; 311:277–281.
49. Seeman E, Szmukler GI, Formica C, et al. Osteoporosis in anorexia nervosa: the influence of peak bone density, bone loss, oral contraceptive use, and exercise. J Bone Miner Res 1992; 7:1467–1474.
50. Skolnick AA. 'Female athlete triad' risk for women. JAMA 1993; 270:921–923.
51. Miller KK, Grinspoon S, Klibanski A. Cardiovascular risk markers in hypothalamic amenorrhoea. Clin Endocrinol (Oxf) 2000; 53:359–366.
52. Hopkinson ZE, Sattar N, Fleming R, et al. Polycystic ovarian syndrome: the metabolic syndrome comes to gynaecology. Br Med J 1998; 317:329–332.
53. Hallberg L, Hogdahl A, Nilsson L, et al. Menstrual blood loss, a population study: variation at different ages and attempts to define normality. Acta Obstet Gynecol Scand 1966; 45:320–351.
54. Warner PE, Critchley HO, Lumsden MA, et al. Menorrhagia I: measured blood loss, clinical features, and outcome in women with heavy periods: a survey with follow-up data. Am J Obstet Gynecol 2004; 190(5):1216–1223.
55. Vessey MP, Villard-Mackintosh L, McPherson K, et al. The epidemiology of hysterectomy: findings in a large cohort study. BJOG 1992; 99:402–407.
56. Coulter A, McPherson K, Vessey M. Do British women undergo too many or too few hysterectomies? Soc Sci Med 1988; 27:987–994.
57. O'Flynn N, Britten N. Menorrhagia in general practice—disease or illness. Soc Sci Med 2000; 50:651–661.
58. NICE (National Institute of Health and Clinical Excellence). NICE clinical guideline 44. Heavy menstrual bleeding. London: NICE; 2007. Online. Available: http://www.nice.org.uk/nicemedia/pdf/CG44NICEGuideline.pdf [accessed 23.06.09].

59. Coulter A, Bradlow J, Agass M, et al. Outcomes of referrals to gynaecology outpatient clinics for menstrual problems: an audit of general practice records. BJOG 1991; 98:789–796.

60. Nagele F, O'Connor H, Davies A, et al. 2500 outpatient diagnostic hysteroscopies. Obstet Gynecol 1996; 88:87–92.

61. Dockery CJ, Sheppard B, Daly L, et al. The fibrinolytic enzyme system in normal menstruation and excessive uterine bleeding and the effect of tranexamic acid. Eur J Obstet Gynaecol Reprod Biol 1987; 24:309–318.

62. Smith SK, Abel MH, Kelly RW, et al. Prostaglandin synthesis in the endometrium of women with ovular dysfunctional uterine bleeding. BJOG 1981; 88:434–442.

63. Janssen CA, Scholten PC, Heintz AP. A simple visual assessment technique to distinguish between menorrhagia and normal menstrual blood loss. Obstet Gynaecol 1995; 85:977–982.

64. Farquhar CM, Lethaby A, Sowter M, et al. An evaluation of risk factors for endometrial hyperplasia in premenopausal women with abnormal menstrual bleeding. Am J Obstet Gynecol 1999; 181:525–529.

65. National Advisory Committee on Health and Disability. Guidelines for the management of heavy menstrual bleeding. New Zealand: NACHD; 1998.

66. Osei J, Critchley H. Menorrhagia, mechanisms and targeted therapies. Curr Opin Obstet Gynecol 2005; 17(4):411–418.

67. Fraser IS, McCarron G, Markham R, et al. Measured menstrual blood loss in women with menorrhagia associated with pelvic disease or coagulation disorder. Obstet Gynecol 1986; 68: 630–633.

68. Vercellini P, Cortesi I, Oldani S, et al. The role of transvaginal ultrasonography and outpatient diagnostic hysteroscopy in the evaluation of patients with menorrhagia. Hum Reprod 1997; 12(8):1768–1771.

69. Smith-Bindman R, Kerlikowske K, Feldstein VA, et al. Endovaginal ultrasound to exclude endometrial cancer and other endometrial abnormalities. JAMA 1998; 280(17): 1510–1517.

70. Royal College of Obstetricians and Gynaecologists. The initial management of menorrhagia. Evidence-based clinical guidelines, No 1. London: RCOG; 1998.

71. Goldrath MH, Sherman AI. Office hysteroscopy and suction curettage: can we eliminate the hospital diagnostic dilatation and curettage. Am J Obstet Gynecol 1985; 152:220–229.

72. Preston JT, Cameron IT, Adams EJ, et al. Comparative study of tranexamic acid and norethisterone in the treatment of ovulatory menorrhagia. BJOG 1995; 102:401–406.

73. Andersch B, Milsom I, Rybo G. An objective evaluation of flurbiprofen and tranexamic acid in the treatment of idiopathic menorrhagia. Acta Obstet Gynecol Scand 1988; 67:645–648.

74. Bonnar J, Sheppard BL. Treatment of menorrhagia during menstruation: randomised controlled trial of ethamsylate, mefenamic acid, and tranexamic acid. Br Med J 1996; 313:579–582.

75. Cooke I, Lethaby A, Farquhar C. Antifibrinolytics for heavy menstrual bleeding. In: Cochrane Collaboration, eds. Cochrane Library, Issue 1. Oxford: Update Software; 1999.

76. Lethaby A, Augood C, Duckitt K. Nonsteroidal anti-inflammatory drugs for heavy menstrual bleeding. In: Cochrane Collaboration, ed. Cochrane Library, Issue 1. Oxford: Update Software; 1999.

77. Lethaby A, Augood C, Duckitt K, et al. Nonsteroidal anti-inflammatory drugs for heavy menstrual bleeding. Cochrane Database Syst Rev 2007; 4:CD000400.

78. Wellington K, Wagstaff AJ. Tranexamic acid: a review of its use in the management of menorrhagia. Drugs 2003; 63(13):1417–1433.

79. Lethaby A, Irvine G, Cameron I. Cyclical progestagens for heavy menstrual bleeding. In: Cochrane Collaboration, ed. Cochrane Library, Issue 1. Oxford: Update Software; 1999.

80. Farquhar CM, Kimble R. How do NZ gynaecologists treat menorrhagia? Aust N Z J Obstet Gynaecol 1996; 36:1–4.

81. Irvine GA, Campbell-Brown MB, Lumsden MA, et al. Randomised comparative trial of the levonorgestrel intrauterine system and norethisterone for the treatment of idiopathic menorrhagia. BJOG 1998; 105:592–598.

82. Silverberg SG, Haukkamaa M, Arko H, et al. Endometrial morphology during long-term use of levonorgestrel releasing intra-uterine devices. Int J Gynecol Pathol 1986; 5:235–241.

3

Contraception

CHAPTER CONTENTS

OBJECTIVES

- To be aware of the legal issues concerning the provision of contraception to adolescents
- To be able to explain the relative benefits and disadvantages of the various contraceptive methods
- To be able to counsel women effectively regarding their contraceptive options, especially in relation to their life stage
- To be able to start women on hormonal contraception
- To understand how to manage the common problems that arise when women use contraception
- To be able to explain to women how to use the combined oral contraceptive pill (COCP) to avoid menstruation and the risks and benefits of avoiding menstruation using the COCP
- To be able to instruct patients about effective condom use
- To be able to counsel patients about diaphragms and caps
- To understand the principles of natural family planning
- To be aware of contraceptive factors that aid or detract from compliance
- To be able to counsel women regarding use of emergency contraception
- To understand the advantages and disadvantages of the different methods of sterilisation

GOOD PRACTICE IN CONTRACEPTIVE COUNSELLING

If sexual and reproductive health are considered to be a right for both women and men, then good practice in contraceptive counselling must involve providing women with informed choice. This means that GPs must be abreast of the range of contraceptive options open to women and men and be able to outline confidently the benefits and risks of each of these for the patient's particular situation. Practising clinicians can be surprised by the choices women make with regard to contraception, as these choices do not always fit with the stereotypes we may have. What suits one woman may not suit another in similar circumstances.

An approach that is useful is the 'life-stage approach', which incorporates the issue of 'how important is it for you not to get pregnant at this point in time?'. This question recognises the fact that, for younger women who are not in committed relationships, pregnancy may be the last thing they desire, and so very effective forms of contraception that are not user-dependent may be favoured. For women who are in their late 20s or early 30s, however, the issue might be appropriate pregnancy spacing rather than whether or not they get pregnant, and less effective forms of contraception may be more readily accepted.

Whatever type of contraception is chosen, it is important that women feel informed, supported and able to use it effectively. Time needs to be taken to allay fears, dispel myths and provide the necessary knowledge and skills. Back up written information should be provided and opportunities for questions and follow up and review given. Contraceptive counselling is a very challenging part of sexual and reproductive healthcare, especially because you are assessing the risk of unplanned pregnancy and sexually transmitted diseases and dealing with the topic of the patient's sexuality and sexual practice all at the same time. Nevertheless, providing a woman with the capacity to control her reproductive functions and therefore the direction of her life can be one of the most rewarding aspects of clinical practice.

COMBINED HORMONAL CONTRACEPTION

Contraception for adolescents

Are there any legal issues to consider when prescribing the pill to adolescents?

While exceedingly common, this kind of consultation poses a dilemma for many GPs. Sarah is under age and yet she has acted responsibly in seeking out

---

CASE STUDY: 'I know we're going to have sex soon, so I want to start the pill.'

Sarah, 15 years, attended her family's GP requesting contraception. She had no significant past history or family history and was yet to become sexually active. She had come with a girlfriend from school and asked the GP not to tell her mother about the appointment.

On further questioning, Sarah said she had been with her current boyfriend for 2 months and knew they were going to have sex soon, so she wanted to do the right thing and make sure she was 'protected'. While she was aware from school sex education classes of the need to use condoms, she also wanted to get 'the pill' just to be sure she didn't fall pregnant. She begged the GP not to tell her parents as they were very religious and she was scared about what they would do if they knew she was going to have sex. After further discussion, the GP felt that Sarah was a responsible girl who was well aware of the potential repercussions of unprotected sex.

The GP spent the rest of the consultation showing Sarah how to use a condom and allowing her to practice the technique on a plastic model. After taking Sarah's blood pressure, she prescribed her a low-dose combined oral contraceptive and explained how to use it correctly and when she would be safe from a contraceptive point of view. Sarah was given a follow-up appointment for 2 weeks to review the information given at this initial consultation and to follow up with further information. She was also given written information to take away on safe sex, emergency contraception and contraception in young people.

---

contraception before becoming sexually active. She is also seeking the GP's confidentiality and is fearful of the consequences of her parents finding out that she has come to see the GP, let alone the fact that she is planning to become sexually active.

Unfortunately, many young women fall pregnant before starting contraception, as they tend to wait several months after commencing sexual activity before presenting to a doctor. Indeed, adolescents have little knowledge of the medical system and are generally apprehensive about seeing GPs whom they have seen with their parents for childhood illnesses for fear of disclosure.

In Sarah's situation, the 'mature minor rule' applies and is based on an English legal precedent called the Gillick case. This case ran in the English courts in 1985. Mrs Gillick was a Roman Catholic mother of 10 children, who was affronted by the prospect of one of her under-age daughters being prescribed the oral contraceptive pill without her mother's consent.

When dealing with adolescents requiring contraception, a GP should assess whether the young woman is a 'mature minor'—that is, whether she understands the consequences of her actions.

The final judgment in this case went 3–2 against Mrs Gillick. The conclusion was that there was no provision to hold that a girl under 16 lacked the legal capacity to consent to contraceptive advice, examination and treatment, provided that she had sufficient understanding and intelligence to know what they involved. It was agreed, however, that it would still be most unusual for a doctor to give such advice and treatment without the consent of the parents. In the situation where the girl refused either to tell her parents herself or allow the doctor to do so, the doctor would be justified in proceeding without the parents consent, or even their knowledge, provided that he was satisfied that:

- the girl would understand his advice
- he could not persuade her to inform her parents or allow him to do so
- she was very likely to have sexual intercourse with or without contraceptive treatment
- unless she received contraceptive advice or treatment, her physical or mental health, or both, were likely to suffer
- her best interests required him to give her contraceptive advice, treatment or both without parental consent.

The Gillick case also held that a doctor would not be criminally liable for aiding in the offence of carnal knowledge by prescribing contraceptives or giving contraceptive advice.

What form of contraceptive would you choose?

While this may be the start of sexual activity for Sarah, one should not assume that her partner has yet to become sexually active. Her GP should therefore recommend to her the 'belt and braces' approach to contraception, otherwise known as 'double Dutch'. Sarah requires an effective contraceptive to prevent pregnancy, as well as condoms to prevent her catching a sexually transmitted disease (STD).

GPs should encourage all sexually active young people to pursue a 'double-Dutch' approach to contraception by using condoms and hormonal methods simultaneously.

Many would argue that Sarah should just use a condom with emergency contraception as a back up (see p 46). However, even in experienced users, condoms can break and/or spillage occur. In the inexperienced hands of teenagers, where lubrication is not always prevalent, condom failure is likely to occur more often. Sarah may also have problems in getting her partner to accept condom use. Sex may also occur after alcohol or drug use. For all of these reasons, Sarah is best off using hormonal contraception as well as condoms. However, GPs should make adolescents aware of the existence of emergency contraception and how to access it, should they need it in the future.

Sarah would therefore benefit from hormonal contraception either in the form of a combined oral contraceptive pill (COCP) or a long-acting reversible contraceptive (LARC) such as Implanon® or Depo Provera®. While the COCP has both contraceptive and non-contraceptive benefits (Table 3.1), LARCs offer higher efficacy because they are not as user-dependent. It is important, however, to offer Sarah a choice of contraceptive methods so that she is informed and able to choose the method that suits her best. For example, if she has a chaotic lifestyle or a poor memory and is fearful of forgetting to take the pill every day (especially if the packet has to be kept out of sight of her parents), then Depo-Provera® or Implanon® is probably the more suitable alternative.

TABLE 3.1 Benefits of the combined oral contraceptive pill

Contraceptive benefits	Other benefits

• Highly effective
• Convenient
• Reversible
	• Beneficial for menstruation
	  – less heavy bleeding
	  – less anaemia
	  – less dysmenorrhoea
	  – regular bleeding with ability to manipulate timing of menstruation
	  – less PMS symptomatology
	  – no ovulation pain
	• Less pelvic inflammatory disease
	• Less extrauterine pregnancies
	• Less benign breast disease
	• Less functional ovarian cysts
	• Decrease in ovarian and endometrial cancers
	• Less sebaceous disorders
	• Protection from osteoporosis and control of menopausal symptoms in older women
	• Reduction in the rate of endometriosis

If she wanted to use the COCP, which pill would she start with?

When prescribing hormonal contraception, a general rule of thumb is to use the lowest possible dose of hormones to attain both contraception and cycle control. Possible pills to use in Sarah's case are a monophasic (either a 20 mg or 30 mg ethinyloestradiol pill) or a triphasic low-dose pill. These pills are low-dose, cheap and easy to use. Monophasic pills have a greater margin for error than their triphasic counterparts. They are also easier to manipulate, should the young woman want to delay her period because she is going swimming, camping or on holiday, and are therefore probably a better option. A monophasic COCP containing levonorgestrel is a good first choice, although pills with different types of progestogen can be used initially, or introduced later if there are side effects.

Summary of key points

- The 'mature minor' rule (based on legal precedent) states that as long as a minor is mature enough to understand the consequences of her actions a doctor may treat her in the same way as an adult patient (i.e. prescribe contraception to her without informing her parents).
- Contraception for adolescents should take the 'double-Dutch' approach of concomitant use of condoms and hormonal contraception to protect against STDs and pregnancy.
- All adolescents who are sexually active or about to become so should be made aware of the availability of emergency contraception.
- Long-acting reversible contraceptives are a good option for adolescents who are at risk of contraceptive failure due to poor compliance.
- First-choice combined oral contraception for a young woman is a low-dose (20 mg or 30 mg) monophasic pill.

Dispelling myths about the pill

How commonly are myths about the pill believed?

Wide-ranging misconceptions about the pill exist among women. Many believe that oral contraceptive use is more dangerous than childbirth, that the pill has substantial health risks and that the pill causes cancer.

Women are often surprised to hear that the pill actually has benefits in addition to being a contraceptive. One hopes that this information, once given, will spread through the schoolyard and back to mothers, so that siblings will not grow up learning

---

CASE STUDY: 'I've heard the pill causes cancer.'

Jodie is 17 years old and is completing her final year of high school. She has been sexually active for 2 years and so far she has been using condoms as contraception. In the last 6 months she has needed to use emergency contraception twice. On one occasion the condom broke and more recently she didn't use a condom at all. Thankfully, both times the emergency contraception has been successful.

This visit was the follow-up consultation 4 weeks after she had taken the emergency contraception. It's not often that a GP actually gets to see young women at this stage. They are usually reassured by having got their period and don't bother to turn up for the follow-up visit. Jodie, however, was one of the more conscientious ones, returning for her pregnancy test and STD check.

Now was the perfect time to talk to her about contraception. Her chosen method (condoms) had let her down twice and she may now be more amenable to some information about adding more foolproof forms of contraception. A consultation involving a negative pregnancy test is therefore an ideal time for contraceptive counselling. Before arriving, Jodie was probably nervous and thinking about the possible consequences of an unplanned pregnancy. She would have run through the various scenarios facing her and perhaps made a mental decision to use a different form of contraception. The challenge for the practitioner is to grab this opportunity and use it.

A useful opening line to someone like Jodie, with the pregnancy test sitting squarely on the desk facing both GP and patient, is: 'What are you thinking about contraception for the future?' It is usually at this stage that GPs hear a barrage of misinformation about the pill. As it turns out, a lot of it comes from schoolyard talk with girlfriends, but a lot also originates from the mouths of mothers. Perhaps mothers say these things in order to dissuade their daughters from becoming sexually active and thereby unwittingly encourage unprotected sex.

'I've heard the pill causes cancer.'

'I don't want to put on any weight.'

'I've heard that if your periods aren't regular when you go on the pill, then they'll never be regular when you want to stop.'

'My skin is pimply enough as it is and I don't want it to get worse.'

Another common objection is from young women who have been experimenting with speed, ecstasy and cocaine who say that they don't want to go on the pill because they don't want to put chemicals in their body.

the same falsehoods. GPs should make it a practice to discuss the non-contraceptive benefits of the pill routinely with women presenting for a discussion about their contraceptive options.

The first issue to highlight is that whenever they think of the side effects of contraception they should be comparing these to the side effects of pregnancy. In 90% of cases women who are sexually active without contraception will fall pregnant within a year. Yet doctors rarely speak about the mortality and morbidity associated with pregnancy and the fact that these are much higher than the morbidity and mortality associated with the use of oral contraception.

When explaining the risks and benefits of the combined oral contraceptive pill to a patient, it is useful to compare the risks to those incurred by pregnancy.

It is important also to explain to young women why it is that all these myths have arisen about the pill. The pills that women take today are not the same as the ones taken by their mothers. The dosage has come down from 100 mg of oestrogen, which used to make women vomit and was related to strokes and heart disease, to 30 mg or less. The COCP is one of the most researched pharmaceutical products in the world. Provided women are healthy, have normal blood pressure and do not smoke, these events are no more likely to occur than if they were not on the pill.[1]

How safe is the pill?

An British study of 46,000 women (which began in 1968) tracked users of oral contraceptive pills containing 50 mg of oestrogen for 25 years.[2] This study showed that over the entire follow-up period the risk of death from all causes was similar in never-users of the pill to ever-users. For women who had stopped using the pill more than 10 years previously, there were no significant increases or decreases either overall or for any specific cause of death.

Does the pill cause cancer?

The pill acts in a preventive fashion against ovarian and endometrial cancer. Use of combined oral contraception decreases the risk of a woman developing ovarian cancer by 40%. The longer a woman uses the pill, the greater the effects. Ovarian cancer is associated with many factors, such as family history, decreased parity, late age of menopause and early menarche. It is thought that women who do not bear children have a 2–2.5-fold increased risk of developing ovarian cancer, and this is perhaps because of the increased opportunities for monthly follicular development. The pill suppresses follicular activity and is therefore associated with a relative risk of 0.6 in ever-users and 0.4 in women who use the pill for >5 years.[3] The increasing protection with increased duration of use has been confirmed in other studies.[4]

Endometrial cancer occurs in 0.1 per 100,000 women aged 20–24 and in 12 or more women per 100,000 in those aged 40–44. The risk factors for this cancer are similar to those of ovarian cancer and include obesity, nulliparity, early menarche and late menopause, and the administration of unopposed oestrogen. The effect on endometrial cancer of taking the pill is similar to that of ovarian cancer, with use of the pill decreasing risk of endometrial cancer by 50%. This effect is maintained for at least 20 years after discontinuation of the pill.[4]

While the explanation is unclear, several studies have found that ever-users of the COCP have a 60% reduction in bowel cancer.[5]

Unfortunately, use of the pill may increase the risk of a woman developing breast cancer. The relationship between breast cancer and the pill has now been the subject of numerous studies. Collectively they suggest the following:[6]

- Past users (>10 years since use) are at no increased risk for breast cancer.
- Current and recent users (<10 years since stopping) have a small increase in the risk of breast cancer, which is not related to duration of use.
- The small excess risk seems largely confined to tumours localised in the breast. Such tumours have a better prognosis than those that have spread beyond the breast.
- A family history of breast cancer, duration of use, age at first use and the dose and type of hormone had no additional effect in the risk of developing breast cancer once the length of time since the last use was taken into account.[7]

It is important to assist women to gain some perspective about this increased risk, given the degree of awareness of breast cancer in the community. This can be done using the information given in Table 3.2 (p 42). Given that the incidence of breast cancer increases with age naturally (1 in 500 women have breast cancer by age 35 compared with 1 in 100 by age 45 and 1 in 12 by age 75), the risk attributable to COCP use by women increases in older women.[7]

The COCP appears also to increase the risk of cervical cancer (five extra cases per 100,000 women per year), but it is unclear whether this is a causal relationship.[8] Long-duration follow-up studies certainly show a clear effect of duration of pill use, with the odds ratio of developing cervical cancer being 2.9 after 4 years of COCP use and 6.1 after 8 years.[4] Despite this, it is important to remember that HPV is the primary carcinogen and that smoking is probably a more important co-factor than the COCP.[9]

Regarding other cancers, liver cancer might be increased by the pill (but it is a rare cancer anyway), and the role of the COCP in the development of malignant melanoma remains controversial.[7]

Use of the COCP results in decreased risk of ovarian, endometrial and bowel cancers, but increased risk of breast, cervical and liver cancers.

Are women who take the pill at increased risk of adverse cardiovascular events?

In general women are at low risk of adverse cardiovascular (CVS) events before the menopause. This is even truer for *young* women, who are the usual COCP users. The risks of myocardial infarction, ischaemic stroke, haemorrhagic stroke and venous thromboembolism in COCP users are related to:

- personal or family history
- smoking
- elevated blood pressure
- increased age
- diabetes.

The COCP magnifies all of these underlying risks and usage of the pill should be carefully considered in women who have any of these risk factors.[6]

What long-term health benefits result from using the pill?

Some long-term health benefits of the pill proved by research include a decrease in menstruation-related disorders, pelvic inflammatory disease and benign breast disease. Possible effects attributed to pill use include protection against the development of benign ovarian cysts, fibroids and osteoporosis.

The COCP results in improvements in acne, menstrual disorders and benign breast disease and decreased rates of pelvic inflammatory disease (PID).

TABLE 3.2 Excess number of breast cancer cases/10,000 women who had used the COCP for 5 years and were followed up for 10 years after stopping, compared with never-users (From Collaborative Group on Hormonal Factors in Breast Cancer[98])

COCP use for 5 years up to age:	Excess cases of breast cancer in 10,000 women
20	0.5
25	1.5
30	5
35	10
40	20
45	30

However, GPs should note that most of the findings described above were associated with use of the 50 mg oestrogen pills, while most women these days are on lower dose pills.

Is the pill associated with weight gain?

Another major misconception held by young women concerns weight. Every patient can recount stories of friends who put on 'massive' amounts of weight when on the pill. A recent systematic review, however, has found no evidence supporting a causal association between combination oral contraceptives, or a combination contraceptive skin patch, and weight gain.[10]

What about acne?

Doctors should explain to teenagers that most COCPs will actually improve acne. If, in rare cases, acne is worsened on a levonorgestrel-containing pill, it is worth trying the norethisterone-containing pills or a third-generation pill containing one of the newer progestogens. COCPs containing cyproterone acetate actually target acne more specifically because of their anti-androgenic action, as do COCPs containing drospirenone (Yasmin and Yaz). The benefits may take up to 6 months to take effect, however, and the woman should be warned that on stopping the pill her acne might recur.

In conclusion

Explaining the beneficial effects of COCP use is only one aspect of contraceptive counselling. It is important to take the time to explain the mechanism of action of the pill and to ensure that the woman knows how to take it correctly and understands the importance of not missing pills. What to do when a pill is missed should be explained, together with the fact that the most dangerous ones to miss are the hormone pills taken immediately before and after the sugar pills. This information should be accompanied by written instructions that the woman can refer to in a time of need.

Given that many women discontinue the pill during the first year of use (stopping and starting as they go in and out of relationships), advice about the non-contraceptive benefits of the pill and the lack of long-term morbidity should reassure women that they can continue to take the pill even when they are not sexually active. This will then bring to an end another commonly held myth about the pill 'that you need to take a break from it every now and then' and perhaps succeed in preventing what is often a consequence of pill cessation – an unplanned pregnancy.

A common myth is that women need to take a break from the pill every now and then.

Summary of key points

- Women have many misconceptions about the risks of using the COCP.
- Benefits of the COCP include its efficacy, convenience and reversibility.
- Health benefits of the COCP include reduction in menstrual disorders, pelvic inflammatory disease, benign breast disease and ovarian cysts.
- With regard to cancer, the COCP protects against endometrial, ovarian and colorectal cancers, but appears to be related to increased risk of breast, cervical and liver cancers.
- The COCP is not contraindicated in women with past treatment of CIN lesions, with the benefits outweighing the risks (WHO classification 2); however, women should be encouraged to undergo regular cervical cancer screening and to have the human papillomavirus (HPV) vaccine.
- Women should be advised to compare the risks of morbidity and mortality associated with COCP use with those associated with pregnancy.
- Personal and family history, smoking, blood pressure and increasing age are major determinants in elevating the risk of adverse CVS events occurring in COCP users.

Starting a woman on the pill

CASE STUDY: 'I want to go on the pill.'

Tina is 18 years old and is asking to start on the pill. Having checked her past and family history, ascertained that she is a non-smoker and checked her blood pressure, you now commence counselling her about how to take the pill. How do you go about this and what points need to be stressed?

What are the contraindications to the pill?

Before starting a woman on the pill, a GP must rule out any contraindications to its use. These contra-indications have been classified by the World Health Organization[11] into four categories (Box 3.1, p 44).

What examination needs to be carried out before a woman starts the pill?

The only examination routinely required prior to first prescription of the COCP is blood pressure. In asymptomatic women, breast and pelvic examinations are unnecessary. Blood tests are also unnecessary unless there is a specific clinical indication.[12]

What messages need to be conveyed to women starting the COCP for the first time?

Many young women are familiar with the pill before they even get to the consulting room. Information has already been obtained from girlfriends who may be using it, from sex education at school or from reading magazines.

It is important to do a couple of things in addition to counselling the patient. The first is to tell them not to be scared about what they read in the product information, which is based on medicolegal necessities and is not altogether representative of what they will experience. The second important thing is to give the patient an objective source of information that has in writing what you are about to tell them.

The following points are a summary of important issues to cover (and assume you are starting the woman on a 28-pill packet).

The quick-start method

Traditionally women have been told to wait until their next period to begin the COCP in order to ensure that they are not pregnant when they start. Waiting makes women vulnerable to pregnancy, however, and may discourage women from starting contraception because of the need to wait.

To overcome this problem the 'quick-start' method has been devised.[13] It involves starting the

---

BOX 3.1 Contraindications to use of the COCP (From WHO[11])

CATEGORY FOUR: conditions in which the health risk increases unacceptably if the contraceptive method is used
- Breastfeeding and less than 6 weeks postpartum
- Cerebrovascular or coronary artery disease
- Hypertension with blood pressure >160/100 mmHg
- Hypertension with vascular disease
- Migraine with focal neurological symptoms
- Diabetes with vascular complications (including hypertension, nephropathy, retinopathy, neuropathy) or of >20 years' duration
- Past or present evidence of deep venous thrombosis or pulmonary embolism
- Complicated valvular heart disease
- Acute liver disease
- Malignant liver tumour
- Breast cancer in the past 5 years
- Smoking 15 or more cigarettes per day in women aged 35 or more
- Severe decompensated cirrhosis
- Benign liver tumour

CATEGORY THREE: conditions where the theoretical or proven risks usually outweigh the advantages of using the method
- Breastfeeding from 6 weeks to 5 months postpartum
- Hypertension with BP 140–159/90–99 mmHg
- History of hypertension where blood pressure cannot be evaluated

- Known hyperlipidaemia
- Migraine without focal neurological symptoms in women aged 35 or more (if it develops during use of COCPs, it becomes category 4)
- History of breast cancer with no evidence of disease for past 5 years
- Smoking less than 15 cigarettes per day in women aged 35 or more
- Chronic liver disease other than severe cirrhosis, including mild cirrhosis
- Symptomatic gallbladder disease

CATEGORY TWO: conditions where the advantages of using the method generally outweigh the theoretical or proven risks
- Smoking in women under 35 years old
- Migraine without focal neurological symptoms in women under 35 years old (if it develops during COCP use, it becomes category 3)
- Diabetes without vascular complications
- Family history of venous thromboembolism (first-degree relative)
- Superficial thrombophlebitis
- Uncomplicated valvular heart disease
- Cervical intraepithelial neoplasia
- Undiagnosed breast mass
- Asymptomatic gallbladder disease
- Sickle-cell disease

CATEGORY ONE: conditions for which there are no restrictions on the use of the contraceptive method

---

COCP on the day of the consultation, regardless of the patient's menstrual cycle day, and means that no counselling about when to begin is necessary. The woman swallows her first pill in the clinic immediately after prescription, and continues to take a pill each day. All patients who receive the first pill during the clinic visit first undergo a urine pregnancy test and emergency contraception if needed and receive at least one pack of the COCP so that they do not have to go to a pharmacy to fill a prescription before beginning. The quick-start method is outlined in Box 3.2.

Understanding how the pill works

Most young women do not understand how the pill works. They believe that since they are getting a 'period' every month they must be having a normal cycle and so they talk about having premenstrual symptoms even when they are taking the pill, despite the fact that they are not cycling. Ask them to show

you the most dangerous time to miss a pill. They will often point to midway through the packet, showing their lack of understanding of the mode of action of the pill. It is therefore important to explain to a young woman that the COCP in essence puts the ovaries to sleep and that if taken correctly, no eggs are released and that is why she will not fall pregnant. Explain that when first starting the pill it takes 7 days to put the ovaries to sleep and that therefore she is not safe from a contraceptive point of view until she has taken seven active pills. Subsequent pills taken keep the ovaries asleep (quiescent).

Missed pills

After asking the young woman to show you the most dangerous times to miss a pill, explain that this is in fact immediately before and after the sugar pills. This fits in nicely with the analogy of putting the ovaries to sleep. If the pills before or after the sugar pills are missed, the 'pill-free interval' is lengthened, thereby

1. Ascertain low pregnancy risk (one or more of the following): the woman should:
   - have had no intercourse since the last period
   - have used another method
   - be within 7 days of the onset of menstruation, miscarriage or termination of pregnancy
   - have used emergency contraception
   - be fully breastfeeding less than 6 months post-partum
   - have a negative urine pregnancy test.
2. Begin with an active tablet during the consultation.
3. Advise the woman to use condoms for the first 7 days of pill use.
4. Follow up with a urine pregnancy test in 4–6 weeks.
5. Provide written information to take home.

BOX 3.3 Benefit of a 4-day pill-free interval

Yaz is the first COCP to be manufactured with a 4-day pill-free interval rather than seven. Shortening the pill-free interval gives the user a greater margin of error should she forget to recommence her next pill packet on time (i.e. if she misses the first pill of her next pack).

BOX 3.4 Missed pills

One pill missed (late by up to 24 hours)
1. Take the pill as soon as you remember.
2. Take the next pill at the usual time.
3. Keep taking active pills as usual.

More than one pill missed (>24 hours)
As well as 1–3 (above), avoid sex or use condoms for 7 days.

If pills are missed in week 1 (days 1–7) (because the pill-free interval has been extended), emergency contraception should be considered if unprotected sex occurred in the pill-free interval (sugar pills) or in week 1, restarting the COCP with the next active pill within 24 hours of taking emergency contraception.

If pills are missed in week 3 (days 15–21) (to avoid extending the pill-free interval) finish the pills in current pack and start a new pack the next day, thus omitting the pillfree interval (sugar pills).

allowing the ovaries to wake up and release an egg. (The pill-free interval has been set arbitrarily at 7 days by manufacturers in order to replicate a normal 28-day cycle, except for Yaz, which has a 4-day pill-free interval—see Box 3.3.) If more than 7 days go by (i.e. if more than seven pills are missed), there is a chance that ovulation, and therefore pregnancy, could occur.

There has recently been some controversy over whether advice to women regarding missed pills should differ according to the oestrogen dose in the pill.[9,14] The simplest advice (erring on the side of caution) for pills that have the traditional 21 active pills and 7 sugar pills is outlined in Box 3.4 and Figure 3.1 (p 46). Where a pill like Yaz (24 active pills and 4 sugar pills) is used, the advice for missed pills is dependent on whether more than 7 pills have been missed.

It is also important to stress that a 'period' on the pill is only in fact a withdrawal bleed (and not related to having a normal cycle). Draw diagrams of the endometrium being nurtured and sustained by hormones, only to shed away when the hormones are not present.

When starting a woman on the pill, a GP should explain that the pill 'puts the ovaries to sleep' and that when starting the pill it takes 7 days for this to happen.

In a case of vomiting or diarrhoea
Should a woman vomit within 2 hours of taking a pill, the absorption of the hormones is questionable and another active pill should be taken (from the end of the pack). If the replacement pill and a second one taken 25–26 hours later fails to stay down then the missed pill rules should be followed. Diarrhoea without vomiting is not a problem unless it is 'cholera-like'.[9]

When antibiotics are prescribed
No study has reliably investigated if the efficacy of the COCP is reduced with concurrent antibiotic use. Short-term antibiotic use alters gut flora and reduces the enterohepatic circulation of oestrogen. Gut flora recovers after 3 weeks of antibiotic use.[15]

If a woman starting the COCP has been using a non-liver-enzyme-inducing antibiotic for ≥3 weeks,

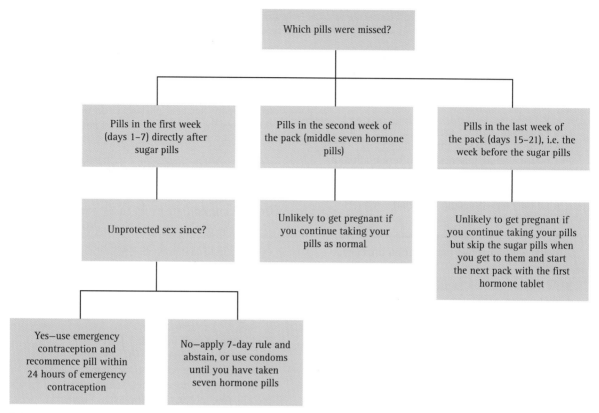

FIGURE 3.1 Flow chart for management of missed pills (when using a 28-day pack)

no additional contraceptive behaviour is required unless the antibiotic is changed, when it should be managed as for short courses (<3 weeks) of antibiotic use. Women using the COCP who are given a short course (<3 weeks) of non-liver-enzyme-inducing antibiotics should be advised to use additional contraceptive protection while taking the antibiotic and for 7 days after stopping the antibiotic.[16]

Side effects

One of the most common reasons women avoid using the pill is fear of weight gain. This is especially true of adolescents, who can sometimes be obsessed with their weight and dieting. While progestogens such as levonorgestrel may stimulate the appetite, young women starting contraception are often at the end of their pubertal growth spurt and may be putting on weight anyway. In a study of women who used the COCP for 12 cycles, approximately equal numbers of women gained or lost more than 2 kg in weight, with the majority (74%) being unchanged or within ± 2 kg of their baseline weight before starting the COCP.[17] Other side effects, such as nausea and break-through bleeding, usually lessen with time, and young women starting the pill should be advised to continue for at least 3 months in order

to see whether commonly experienced side effects dissipate. Many young women chop and change their pills too quickly. Such moves result in added problems that make them declare that they are unable to use the pill. This is a shame, as they have 30 or so potentially reproductive years ahead of them and may well need to use the pill in the future.

Another common side effect is the change in appearance of menstrual flow that younger women, especially, are not prepared for and may think is abnormal. Menstrual flow is usually reduced and may become quite dark in appearance. If women are not prepared for this, they may take it as a sign of illness or infection.

Young women starting out on the pill should be advised to continue for at least 3 months in order to see whether commonly experienced side effects dissipate.

Emergency contraception

Counselling regarding use of any form of contraception is incomplete without giving details to the woman of emergency contraception. As mentioned earlier, missed pills either before or after the sugar pills may result in the need for emergency contraception.

Summary of key points
- GPs need to rule out contraindications to COCP use prior to prescribing.
- Apart from taking the woman's blood-pressure, no other routine examinations or investigations are necessary before starting a woman on the pill.
- Patients need to be advised about the following issues before starting the pill:
  - the fact that the pill puts the ovaries to sleep so that ovulation does not occur
  - what to do if they miss pills
  - what to do if they have vomited or are prescribed broad-spectrum antibiotics
  - side effects of the pill
  - the availability of emergency contraception.

Drug interactions with the pill

Consumer medicine information found in a COCP packet is quite specific. Under the heading 'Taking other medicines' instructions similar to the following are found:

> Tell your doctor if you are taking any other medicines including medicines you buy without prescription from a pharmacy, supermarket or health food shop. There may be interference between —— and some other medicines including:
>
> - antibiotics such as rifampicin, ampicillin and tetracyclines
> - medicine for epilepsy (such as phenytoin)
> - phenylbutazone
> - griseofulvin
> - barbiturates (phenobarbitone)
> - primodone
> - carbamazepine.
>
> These medicines may affect how well —— works. You may need to use an additional form of contraception (such as condoms or a diaphragm) while you are taking the other medicine and for 7 days following. Your doctor may also advise you to skip the 7 pill-free days (the pill-free days are when you would normally be taking the green pills). If you take —— you may need to use additional contraception for 4 weeks after finishing the course of ——.

BOX 3.5 Antibiotics that interact with the pill

- Rifampicin
- Griseofulvin
- Ampicillin and derivatives
- Tetracyclines
- Cephalosporins

CASE STUDY: 'That must be how I got pregnant!'

When counselling a young woman and her relatively young mother about the pill, the GP mentioned to them that antibiotics might decrease pill absorption and lead to pill failure. At that point the mother said, 'Is that so? No one ever told me that. That must have been how I got pregnant with her!'

The issue of what advice to give women about the interaction between broad-spectrum antibiotics and the COCP is important for two reasons: firstly because the COCP is one of the most popular forms of contraception and is used by millions of women around the world, and secondly because of the very serious consequences of having an unwanted pregnancy.

What is the background efficacy of the pill?

When considering drug interaction, it is important to know what the efficacy of the pill really is. The failure rates in clinical trials have been shown to be as low as 0.1/100 woman years. Typically, however, these very low rates of pregnancy are not achieved because of 'user failure'. Time and again studies have shown the difficulty in remembering to take a pill every day and so, with typical usage, up to 5% of women will have an unintended pregnancy during their first year of COCP use. The possibility of interactions with broad-spectrum antibiotics should therefore be looked at with this figure in mind.

What is the mechanism of drug interaction with the pill?

There are several ways that drugs can potentially interact with the COCP, including inducing liver enzymes and reducing the enterohepatic recirculation of oestrogen.

Some anticonvulsants are well known to induce liver enzymes that cause the breakdown of oestrogens

CASE STUDY: 'I'm not taking any medication but I'm on the pill.'

Melanie was 27 years old and had a history of sinusitis. This particular day she came in requesting a script for some antibiotics. She had a fever and was complaining of maxillary and frontal pain. Not having met her before, the GP asked her if she was allergic to anything, to which she answered 'No'. The GP then asked if she was taking any medication, to which she again answered 'No'. The GP turned to the computer and started using the script-writing software. As the GP double-clicked on 'cefaclor', a warning sign flashed up on the screen: 'Warning: potential drug interaction between antibiotics and the combined oral contraceptive pill! Do you wish to proceed?' The GP turned back to Melanie and said, 'The computer is telling me you are taking the pill'. 'Oh yeh, sorry', she answered. 'I've been on it for ages. I don't really think of it as medication …'

The GP continued with the prescription and, on handing it to Melanie, thought about the options—should she be allowed to walk out without further advice, or should the possibility of decreased efficacy of the pill when using antibiotics be mentioned? The decision is made even more difficult knowing that the latter option entails giving a mini-lecture that goes something like

this: 'Now, you know that the pill may not be as effective when you are taking antibiotics. If you want to be 100% safe, you need to use condoms or abstain from having sex while you're taking the antibiotics and for 7 days afterwards. You should still continue taking your pills as normal, but if you get to the sugar pills during that time just skip them and go straight onto the next lot of hormone tablets. That'll mean that you won't have a period this month, but that doesn't matter. Any questions?'

Not only is this a mouthful, but it is quite complicated. It takes a good deal of time to demonstrate with a sample pack of pills and all the while the woman is looking at the GP astounded because she has probably not been given this advice on the numerous occasions when she has taken antibiotics in the past. This will either be because the GP wasn't aware that she was on the pill or was hedging his/her bets and didn't give the warning.

Would that have been such a bad thing to do? Especially when the rather complicated set of instructions that have to be given may well lead to patient confusion, poor compliance and a higher 'user failure rate' of the pill?

---

and progestins. Anticonvulsants most likely to have this effect are:

- phenobarbital
- phenytoin
- carbamezipine
- primidone
- ethosuxamide.

Drug interactions occur with the pill through two mechanisms: liver enzyme induction and interactions with gut flora.

Sodium valproate, clonazepam, clobazam and the newer anti-epileptics (including vigabatrin and lamotrigine) do not have this effect. In cases where women are taking anticonvulsants that interact with the pill, the contraceptive efficacy of the pill is reduced, especially with 'low-dose' pills. The solution is therefore to use a pill that contains 50 mg of oestrogen.

Rifampicin and griseofulvin have similar enzyme-inducing effects, particularly rifampicin, which is very potent in this regard. Even if it is given only as a short-term dose (as is the case for prophylaxis

against meningitis), increased elimination of the pill components must be assumed for 4 weeks afterwards. This necessitates the use of alternative forms of contraception for all of this time.

When the pill is taken, the progestogen component is 80–100% bioavailable from the upper part of the small bowel. Ethinyloestradiol, however, is subject to the 'first-pass' phenomenon. This means that the oestrogen is conjugated with sulfate in the gut wall and carried in the hepatic portal vein to the liver. The liver metabolises the steroid-forming glucoronides. The metabolites are then excreted via the bile back into the gut, where bowel flora remove the sulfate and glucoronide groups and the oestrogen is reabsorbed.

Theoretically, broad-spectrum antibiotics can eradicate the gut flora responsible for the deconjugation of the ethinyloestradiol metabolites and therefore reduce the amount of reabsorption that occurs during short-term antibiotic use or during the initial days of long-term antibiotic use before resistant gut flora emerge. In practice, however, the evidence backing this theory remains unclear, with one study showing increased faecal excretion of conjugated metabolites but no demonstrable reduction in plasma unconjugated oestrogen concentrations.

The argument becomes interesting because the bioavailability of orally administered ethinyloestradiol is usually 40%, but varies markedly from 20% to 65% in different individuals. This variation in initial bioavailability may account for the sporadic cases of pregnancy that occur with concurrent antibiotic use. For example, if the woman had a low background availability of ethinyloestradiol, coupled with a large enterohepatic circulation and gut flora sensitive to the antibiotic being prescribed, she might be more likely to fall pregnant. The problem is that the very small subgroup of women who may have all these factors concurrently cannot be identified by any routine diagnostic tests.

What other factors may be implicated in the interaction between broad-spectrum antibiotic use and the COCP?

Other factors that may be implicated in the interaction between broad-spectrum antibiotic use and the COCP include:

- when there is antibiotic-induced vomiting or diarrhoea, causing a decrease in the amount of hormones initially absorbed
- when the symptoms of the illness requiring antibiotics, or the side effects of the antibiotics themselves, make women less consistent in pill taking
- what stage the woman has reached in the COCP packet when she starts and finishes taking the antibiotics, especially if this is directly before or after the sugar pills.

The research on these issues is not very directive. Large retrospective studies of women sampled from dermatology clinics have lacked control groups and mainly report on women using long-term antibiotics for acne control.

A small number of prospective studies have looked at the issue pharmacologically, taking blood tests of hormone levels and doing studies of cervical mucus while women on the COCP took short courses of antibiotics. These studies, while reporting the enormous inter- and intra-individual variation in plasma levels of oestrogen and progestogen, found that none of the women ovulated.

So what can GPs conclude from this muddled picture?

Well, there are several lessons to be learned:

- Always ask female patients if they are using hormonal contraception. Simply asking if they are taking any medications will not necessarily tell you that they are on the pill.

- Given the serious consequences of unwanted pregnancy, being cautious and recommending additional or alternative forms of contraception during short courses of broad-spectrum antibiotics and the initial weeks of long-term antibiotics may be justified to protect the few unidentifiable women who may be at risk. If you are going to give this advice, then it is worth doing it properly. Written advice such as that given in Figure 3.2 is useful.

- If you are not going to recommend use of alternate contraception during a short course of antibiotics in COCP users, then prescribe a specific antibiotic rather than a broad-spectrum antibiotic like ampicillin or amoxicillin.

- Hormonal contraception is more effective if women understand how it works.

Summary of key points

- When asking women if they are taking any medication, ask specifically about hormonal contraception, as many women don't consider contraception to be medication.
- Drug interactions with the pill are important to consider because of the high prevalence of COCP use by women and because of the serious nature of unintended pregnancy.
- The exact mechanism of antibiotic interactions with the pill remains unclear.
- Women using the COCP should be given clear, written advice about the use of extra precautions when taking broad-spectrum antibiotics.

The pill is one of the most effective forms of contraception available to women. However, there is a small failure rate of 1–3% in healthy women, usually because some pills have not been taken (usually the ones either before or after the sugar pills).

Millions of women using the pill take antibiotics each year. In a small number of cases, broad-spectrum antibiotics may reduce the efficacy of the pill. If you want to be absolutely safe you need to use condoms or abstain from having sex while you're taking the antibiotics and for seven days afterwards.

You should still continue to take your pills as normal but if you get to the sugar pills during that time just skip them and instead go on to the next lot of hormone tablets. That may mean that you don't get a period that month, but that's okay.

FIGURE 3.2 Instruction sheet for women on the COCP who need antibiotics

Third-generation oral contraception

What is the difference between second- and third-generation pills?

All pills contain the same synthetic oestrogen: ethinyloestradiol. The difference between second- and third-generation pills lies in the type of progestogen they contain. Second generation pills contain either levonorgestrel or norethisterone. Third-generation pills contain the newer progestogens desogestrel and gestodene. Levonorgestrel and norethisterone 'oppose osetrogenicity'[9] and therefore can be considered to be more progestogenic in nature, whereas desogestrel and gestodene are more 'oestrogenic' progestogens.

What in real terms are the risks associated with third-generation pills?

Since 1995, a cloud has hung over the first-line use of third-generation contraceptives because of a slight increase in the risk of thromboembolism associated with the newer (third-generation) progestogens such as gestodene and desogestrel.

The increased risk is relatively small, however. Third-generation contraceptives probably double the risk of non-fatal thromboembolism (20–30 instances per 100,000 woman-years), when compared with low-dose second-generation (levonorgestrel and norethisterone) pills (15 instances per 100,000 woman-years). This risk is still less than that incurred when using high-dose oestrogen pills (50 mg) and far less than the risk of a deep vein thrombosis (DVT) occurring during pregnancy (60 instances per 100,000 woman-years).[6]

As with the prescription of any medication, the key to oral contraceptive prescribing, is to rule out absolute contraindications (see Box 3.1) and, in the case of third-generation pills especially, to minimise concomitant risks such as:

- smoking
- hypertension
- strong family history of thromboembolism (even if a thrombophilia screen is negative)
- overweight with a body mass index >30 kg/m²
- severe varicose veins
- genetic thrombophilias: protein C, protein S and antithrombin III deficiencies and factor V Leiden mutation (which affects 5% of the white population).

What are the indications for preferential use of a third-generation pill?

At present the major barrier to first-line use of third-generation COCPs in some countries (such as Australia) is cost. Women who are currently using second-generation pills should continue to do so. Third-generation pills should be kept in reserve for occasions where the woman suffers from progestogenic side effects, such as breakthrough bleeding, acne or weight gain.

Summary of key points

- Pills containing gestodene and desogestrel are considered to be 'third-generation' progestogen pills.
- These pills are associated with a slightly higher risk of venous thromboembolism and so should probably not be prescribed first line.
- Third-generation pills can be used preferentially when a woman suffers from progestogenic side effects such as breakthrough bleeding, acne or weight gain.

CASE STUDY: Cost considerations

Suzy comes from New Zealand and has been on Marvelon for the last 5 years. She is surprised when you advise her of the added cost in Australia of using these pills and asks you if there is any benefit in her continuing on Marvelon if there are other cheaper pills available. She is a student and hasn't much money to spare.

Sorting out problems with the pill

Breakthrough bleeding

Breakthrough bleeding (BTB) is one of the more common side effects experienced by women starting on the COCP and one of the major reasons why women discontinue the COCP.[18] When counselling women about BTB, it is important to emphasise that BTB is at its greatest in the first three months after starting the COCP and that it usually decreases and stabilises by the end of the fourth cycle. Secondly, the occurrence of BTB does not in itself necessarily mean reduced efficacy, for the following reasons:

- Current low-dose pills are remarkably effective, if taken correctly. As a backup to cessation of ovulation, the progestogen content of the pill thickens cervical mucus, preventing sperm penetration.
- The bleeding itself may temporarily enhance the anti-implantation effects of the pill.
- When BTB occurs, sex probably occurs with less frequency.

If BTB occurs after having well-controlled menstrual cycles on the COCP, then causes not related to the pill need to be considered, such as pregnancy, cervicitis, smoking (it is unclear if this is causally related or due to other factors, such as increased rates of poor compliance) or interactions with medications. Lack of adherence to the pill is the most common cause of BTB and emphasises the fact that as GPs we should ensure that patients understand and can follow pill-taking instructions before we decide change the type of pills or method of contraception.

A useful list of questions to use during a consultation for 'unscheduled bleeding' is given in Box 3.6.

A good way to conceptualise things is by remembering that oestrogens build up the endometrium and progestogens stabilise it and that the oestrogen–progestin balance is more important than the absolute level of oestrogen.[20]

If BTB occurs for the first time when the woman has just started on the pill and lasts longer than 3 months, the following options can be tried (in this order):

1. If she is taking a monophasic pill, try changing to a triphasic pill.
2. Consider switching to a pill with a higher ethinyl-oestradiol: progestin ratio, either by increasing the ethinyloestradiol dose (from 20 µg to 30 µg) or decreasing the relative progestin dose.
3. Change the progestin in the pill — gestodene, in particular, provides good cycle control.
4. Try an alternative delivery mode, such as a NuvaRing®.

Acne

Acne that appears for the first time or is exacerbated while using the pill occurs because the progestogen content of the pill brings about androgenic side effects. There are several options: a more oestrogen-dominant COCP such as Marvelon, or a COCP such as Diane (Brenda) can be tried. The latter is a monophasic COCP containing 35 mg of ethinyloestradiol and 2 mg of cyproterone acetate, an anti-androgen. More recently pills containing drospirenone have been introduced (Yasmin and Yaz). This progestogen also has anti-androgenic effects and can be useful for management of acne.

A previous conception on the pill

Unfortunately for some women, despite correct use of the COCP they have still ovulated and conceived. This has occurred because the pill-free interval of 7 days is too long for these women and their ovaries 'wake up' and ovulate during this time. An alternative contraceptive option for them is the highly efficacious Depo-Provera® or Implanon. However, should they wish to continue on the pill they must either:

- shorten their pill-free interval (i.e. either by decreasing the number of sugar pills they take each month from 7 to 3–4 in a standard 28-day pack, or by using Yaz, a drospirenone-containing COCP with only 4 sugar pills in a 28-day pack)
- or tricycle the pill (so that they skip three out of four withdrawal bleeds) and take only 3 sugar pills instead of 7.

BOX 3.6 Points to cover in the clinical history taken from a woman using hormonal contraception who presents with unscheduled bleeding (From Faculty of Sexual and Reproductive Healthcare Clinical Effectiveness Unit[19])

The clinical history should include an assessment of:
- the woman's own concerns
- current method of contraception and the duration of use[a]
- use of the current contraceptive method[b]
- use of medications (including over-the-counter preparations) that may interact with the contraceptive method, or any illness that may affect the absorption of orally administered hormones

- cervical screening history[c]
- risk of sexually transmitted infections (i.e. for those aged <25 years, or women at any age with a new partner, or with more than one partner in the last year)
- bleeding patterns before starting hormonal contraception, since starting and currently
- any other symptoms suggestive of an underlying cause (e.g. abdominal or pelvic pain, postcoital bleeding, dyspareunia, heavy bleeding)
- the possibility of pregnancy.

[a]Progestogen-only methods are more likely to present with unscheduled bleeding than combined hormonal methods, and bleeding with progestogen-only pills is less likely to settle than bleeding with the progestogen-only injectable.

[b]For example, missed pills.

[c]A woman presenting with abnormal bleeding who is participating in a national cervical screening program does not require a cervical screen unless one is due.

Nausea

Nausea occurs in some women as a direct result of the oestrogen in the pill. Should the nausea continue beyond the third packet, the woman can either lower the dose of oestrogen by switching to a 20 mg pill, change to a more progestogenic pill such as Microgynon 30 (Nordette 30), or change to a progestogen-only method.

Decreased libido

Again, this side effect is predominantly due to progestogen, although libido is a construct of many psychosocial issues that must be explored before simply positing a biomedical cause. The more oestrogenic pills, however, will sometimes improve these symptoms. These pills include those containing norethisterone or gestodene.

Amenorrhoea

Many women are concerned when their bleeds consist of a dark-brown smudge and are very anxious if they have no bleeding at all, as they think they may be pregnant. The cyclic build-up of the endometrium when a woman is on the pill is almost always less than that occurring during normal cycles. This is particularly so with norethisterone-containing pills.

If women prefer to have a withdrawal bleed that appears more 'normal' they should use triphasic pills or third-generation pills.

Conversely, it is important to be aware that women who present with amenorrhoea may be pregnant.

Headaches in the pill-free interval

Some women suffer from 'withdrawal headaches'. These can be diagnosed when the woman complains of headaches that occur on a monthly basis when she starts the sugar pills in the packet. The way to avoid this problem is to tricycle the packets, thereby avoiding the withdrawal headaches for 3 out of every 4 months. Another option is to use a 0.625 mg conjugated oestrogen tablet (oestrogen-replacement therapy) daily during the sugar pills of the pack.

CASE STUDY: Always consider pregnancy.

A patient attended for a repeat prescription of the pill and said that she had had a period some 2 weeks previously. On closer questioning, she revealed that her last three periods had been lighter than usual, that she had developed new stretch marks and nocturia. On examination she was found to be 16 weeks pregnant. Despite having been very careful about taking her COCP she had suffered a vomiting illness some months earlier, resulting in ovulation and conception.

Concurrent use of anti-epileptics

Except for sodium valproate, clonazepam, clobazam, vigabatrin and lamotrigine, anti-epileptics are liver-enzyme inducers, and reduce levels of circulating hormones and therefore the efficacy of the COCP. Women on these medications should therefore be prescribed COCPs with 50 mg of ethinyloestradiol, tricycle their packets and reduce the pill-free interval to 3–4 days. This will ensure more stable levels of hormones and reduce the frequency of epileptic attacks that may occur in the pill-free interval. Alternative forms of contraception may be more appropriate, however, such as the IUD or Depo-Provera®. The efficacy of progestogen-only injectables is unaffected by liver-enzyme inducers and women taking these medications can continue with the usual injection interval of 12 weeks for DMPA (contrary to what was previously advocated).[14]

Summary of key points

- Most side effects of the pill settle after three months of consecutive use of a COCP, so women should be encouraged to persist with their current pill for at least that period of time before changing formulation.
- Oestrogenic side effects of the pill such as nausea can be reduced by decreasing the oestrogen dose from 30 mg to 20 mg or by using a more 'progestogenic' pill (one containing levonorgestrel).
- Progestogenic side effects such as breast tenderness, bloating and acne can be reduced by using more oestrogenic progestogens (norethisterone) or third-generation progestogens.
- Breakthrough bleeding can be controlled by changing to a triphasic pill, changing to a third-generation progestogen pill, increasing the dose of oestrogen in the pill or changing the delivery method to the NuvaRing®.

Delaying or preventing menstruation

Menstruation has traditionally been seen as an unquestionably natural, normal and beneficial state. Monthly menstruation for decades on end has not been the historical norm, however. Because of later menarche, earlier and more numerous pregnancies and higher rates of breastfeeding, the historical average was 160 ovulations per lifetime. For modern women the current average is 450.

From the time of menarche, women learn to expect their period once a month. Those whose periods are less frequent often worry that something is wrong. Bleeding also often relieves women of their premenstrual discomforts, leading them to think that bleeding is beneficial. Many perceive menstruation to be a process that 'cleanses' the womb and 'proof' that they are not pregnant.

In what circumstances should menstruation be avoided?

Most GPs will have had consultations in which women request a method of delaying their periods or altering the timing of when they occur. This is chiefly because the woman does not want to bleed when she is on holiday or during her honeymoon or when she has to compete in athletics or swimming. There are many other reasons, however, that women would want to decrease the frequency of their periods or temporarily stop menstruating altogether. Periods are often a nuisance, requiring women to plan ahead to have the necessary pads and/or tampons available. These products are expensive and often inadequate, resulting in leakage and staining. Women may also suffer from the discomfort of dysmenorrhoea or premenstrual symptoms that are debilitating and may require time off work or school. Menstrual disorders are also the leading cause of gynaecological morbidity, outnumbering the nearest competitor (adnexal masses) by a factor of three.[21] Eradicating menstruation or even decreasing the frequency of bleeds would therefore assist in decreasing the morbidity experienced by women. Several conditions, such as epilepsy and headaches, are often worsened premenstrually or menstrually. In women with these conditions, the eradication of menstruation on an ongoing, albeit temporary, basis would assist clinically.

How can menstruation be avoided?

The easiest way to decrease the frequency of menstruation, or to avoid it completely, is to 'tricycle' pill packets by taking the hormone tablets in a pill packet continuously and without a break for 3 months. This entails leaving out the sugar pills of three packets and taking a hormone tablet every day. The length of time women can continue in this fashion (not taking the sugar pills in the packet) and not get BTB is variable and depends on the individual woman and the type of pill she is taking.

Which is the best pill to use for this technique?

The best type of pill to use to avoid menstruation is a monophasic pill, as this will deliver a constant dose of oestrogen and progestogen to the patient. Most women will not have BTB if they tricycle on a 30 mg (ethinyloestradiol) pill and may even be able to go on for longer, such as for 6–12 months. However, BTB may occur in those taking the 20 mg pill. If

> **CASE STUDY: 'Don't I have to have a period every month?'**
>
> Jane was 19 and presented requesting the pill. I started her on a 20 mg combined pill and went through my routine 'starting out on the pill' consultation. As I usually do, I ended by explaining that she could delay her bleeds and need not bleed every month if she didn't want to. She looked at me surprised and asked, 'But don't I have to have a period every month?' 'No,' I answered. 'When you take the pill, the lining of the uterus builds up less than when you are not using the pill, because you are not ovulating. You bleed only when you start taking the sugar pills because you are withdrawing the hormones. It is therefore an artificial period.' Jane smiled slowly, happy to have this kind of information, and asked me to explain exactly how she could suppress her periods.

BTB occurs on one brand of pill, changing the type of pill to one that contains another progestogen may stop the bleeding. Those progestogens least likely to bring about BTB are the third-generation progestogens such as gestodene and desogestrel.

Women who suffer from menstrual complaints or who do not wish to menstruate can suppress menstruation by taking a monophasic combined oral contraceptive pill continuously.

Is avoiding menstruation in this way safe?

Delaying or eradicating menstruation in this way, without any 'clinical' reason for doing so, is a fairly new concept, and one that has created considerable controversy.[22–25] Some sociologists might argue that making menstruation optional would pathologise menstruation by making it unnecessary. It could also result in discrimination against those women who choose not to suppress their menstrual cycles and therefore take time off work or school because of premenstrual or menstrual symptoms. Others point to the fact that the oral contraceptive pill is not licensed for this purpose, making the prescriber vulnerable to legal action.

Of greater concern, however, is the fact that women who choose to utilise these methods are being exposed to an increase in the total dose of exogenous hormones. When they are tricycling, women use 17 packets of the pill a year, as opposed to the 13 packets they use when taking the COCP in the normal fashion. This is an increase of 30% in the annual hormone load. The oral contraceptive pill is known to have deleterious effects on lipid metabolism and vascular disease. Studies to date have shown that by the end of the 7-day pill-free interval there is a reversal of the HDL suppression caused by use of combined oral contraception,[26] but it is unclear whether this is of clinical significance. Also unknown is what effect tricycling may have on breast cancer risk. Recent publications have advised that current users of the pill are at a slightly increased risk of breast cancer; when they are told about this risk, most women accept it for the sake of contraception.

The fact that women can suppress their periods on an ongoing basis remains one of medicine's best-kept secrets. If women were told that this option exists, many would choose to take it up. This information should become a routine part of contraceptive counselling.

Summary of key points

- Most women are unaware that they can use the combined oral contraceptive pill to avoid menstruating.
- Women suffering from premenstrual or menstrual exacerbations of epilepsy and/or headaches may benefit from avoiding menstruation.
- Avoiding menstruation is best achieved by 'tricycling' a monophasic COCP.
- BTB may occur in some women who tricycle their COCP.
- A theoretical risk is posed by increasing the amount of exogenous hormones ingested annually, although this is probably less significant if woman are using a 20 mg pill.

The NuvaRing®

What is the NuvaRing®?

The NuvaRing® is a vaginal ring made out of the same polymer as the Implanon rod. It contains both oestrogen and progestogen and is therefore best thought of as being the pill in a new delivery mode (Fig 3.3). As such, it has the same contraindications and implications as the COCP. The ring is placed in the vagina for 3 weeks (just as hormone pills are taken for 3 weeks) and then removed for a week (just as sugar pills are taken for a week). Start-up instructions are similar to those for the COCP.

How should it be put in and removed?

Holding the NuvaRing® between thumb and index finger, press the sides together while lying down, squatting, or standing with one leg up—whichever

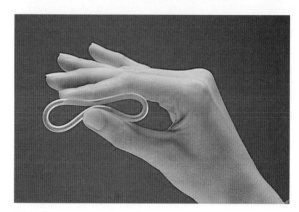

FIGURE 3.3 A NuvaRing®

is most comfortable. Gently push the folded ring into the vagina. The exact position of NuvaRing® is not important for it to be effective, but if it is correctly placed it should not be felt. Once inserted, the NuvaRing® should stay in place for 3 weeks in a row and then be removed 3 weeks after insertion on the same day of the week. This can be done by hooking the index finger under the forward rim or holding the rim between index and middle finger and gently pulling out the NuvaRing®. To continue to have pregnancy protection, a new ring must be inserted 1 week after the last one was removed, even if menstruation has not stopped.

Are there any ways the woman can remember when the 3-week deadline is up?

The manufacturers have devised several options to help women remember when to remove and reinsert their NuvaRing®. The packet comes with diary stickers and an icon can be downloaded onto the woman's computer that can provide a reminder. In addition women can log on to the manufacturer's website and provide their mobile phone number and day of first insertion and then they will be sent an SMS reminder.

How effective is it?

NuvaRing® is just as efficacious as the COCP, and probably even more so, as it is not as user-dependent as oral contraception (the user does not have to remember to take it every day). Like the COCP it suppresses ovulation.

What are the benefits of vaginal administration?

The oestrogen and progestogen in the NuvaRing® are steadily and effectively absorbed directly into the bloodstream through the vaginal wall. This allows for the NuvaRing® to be the lowest dose of combined hormonal contraception currently available on the market.

TABLE 3.3 Questions commonly asked by patients about the NuvaRing®

Question	Response
How do I know if it's in the right place?	Like a tampon if it is positioned properly you shouldn't be able to feel it. If it feels uncomfortable, try gently pushing it in a bit further.
Do you leave it in when you have sex?	Yes
Will he feel it?	During intercourse, some sexual partners may feel the ring in the vagina, but the majority (90%) don't find it a problem. The ring usually lies flat in the vagina and the penis will slide over the top or underneath it.
What happens if it comes out?	Expulsion can occur. Give it a rinse in warm water and place it back inside the vagina straight away (not more than three hours) to maintain contraceptive efficacy
What happens if I am late in taking it out?	There is a week's leeway, so if the NuvaRing® has been left in for more than 3 weeks (but less than 4 weeks), remove it immediately and insert a new ring after a 1-week ring-free break. If it has been left in place for more than 4 weeks, however, it should be considered like a late start on the COCP. If unprotected sex has occurred, the woman should have emergency contraception and then immediately insert a new NuvaRing®, with a follow-up pregnancy test 4–6 weeks later. If unprotected intercourse has not occurred, additional contraception, such as a condom, should be used until the NuvaRing® has been in place for 7 days in a row.
What happens if I am late putting it back in?	After 3 weeks of use, the NuvaRing® should be removed for a 1-week break and then a new one should be inserted no more than 7 days later. If the ring-free interval has been extended beyond 1 week, the possibility of pregnancy should be considered, and, as with missed pills, an additional method of contraception should be used until NuvaRing® has been in place for 7 days in a row.
Is there a way I can avoid getting a period when I use the NuvaRing®?	Like tricycling the pill, the NuvaRing® can be run back to back, with a new ring replacing the old one straight away, instead of waiting 7 days.
What if I get thrush while I am using the ring?	The side effect profile of NuvaRing® is similar to that of the COCP. Thrush creams have no impact on the efficacy of the NuvaRing® and can be used at the same time.
Will it make me put on weight?	The ring does not appear to be associated with weight gain.

It also means that issues such as interactions with broad-spectrum antibiotics and gastrointestinal upsets are avoided, as is first-pass hepatic metabolism, allowing for the lower dose of hormones. There is also no need for daily interaction with the device, potentially increasing user compliance.

One of the major benefits of NuvaRing® is that, despite its low dose of estrogen, it provides excellent cycle control compared with standard COCPs[27–29] and is a serious option to offer women on the COCP who complain of BTB.

Who is it best suited to?

NuvaRing® should really be offered to all women in whom the COCP is a suitable option. Whether or not women are interested in a vaginal ring will depend very much on their own comfort level with their genitalia and the concept of using a vaginal ring, but also on the manner in which it is presented to them and the comfort level of the GP with the idea. One way of framing it is by suggesting that if a woman feels comfortable using a tampon she will probably be able to use the vaginal ring.

Common questions that patients ask and the answers to those questions are given in Table 3.3.

With which COCP is the NuvaRing® comparable?

The NuvaRing® cannot be compared to any specific COCP currently available on the market. The lower dose of hormones in the product and their vaginal absorption directly into the bloodstream makes this method unique.

PROGESTOGEN–ONLY CONTRACEPTION

The mini-pill

Common progestogen-only pills or mini-pills (POP) contain levonorgestrel (e.g. Microlut) or norethisterone (e.g. Noriday) but there are others. The main mode of action of the mini-pill is in the alteration of cervical mucus, making it impenetrable to sperm, but there is also a variable effect on ovulation—hence the possibility of varying patterns of bleeding in users of the mini-pill. The efficacy in situations of ideal use varies, with a risk of pregnancy of 0.3–4 per 100 woman-years, and correlates with a woman's age and therefore her background rate of fertility.

> The mini-pill is a good option for breastfeeding women and those with contraindications to oestrogen.

CASE STUDY: Contraception during lactation

Prue is 32 and currently pregnant with her second child. She asks you what she can use for contraception once the baby is born, as this pregnancy occurred 8 months after the birth of her first child despite the fact that she was still breastfeeding. She intends to breastfeed this baby as well.

During lactation what contraceptive options are there?

There are several options: lactational amenorrhoea, the mini-pill, Depo-Provera®, Implanon, an IUD, barrier methods, tubal ligation, or vasectomy for her partner.

Why is the combined oral contraceptive not a good idea when breastfeeding?

The oestrogen in the COCP reduces the amount and constitution of milk produced during lactation. This is especially important during the first 6 weeks postpartum, when lactation is being established, as it may increase the chances of failure to establish lactation.

What are the guidelines for use of lactational amenorrhoea in the postpartum period?

'Breastfeeding provides more than 98% protection from pregnancy in the first 6 months' following a birth.[30] This statement holds true provided the following conditions are met:

- The woman is not menstruating.
- The woman is fully breastfeeding (i.e. the infant's diet is not supplemented).

How is the POP packaging different from the COCP?

It is important to point out to the user (especially if she has used the COCP in the past) that the mini-pill pack is designed differently from COCP packs. It contains no sugar pills and therefore every pill is an active hormone tablet. She should therefore commence use with a tablet corresponding to the day of the week and take a pill every day, swapping over to her next packet as soon as she finishes the first one.

Are there any contraindications to the use of progestogen-only contraception?

The major contraindications to the use of progestogen-only contraception are pregnancy and coexistent unexplained bleeding (Box 3.7).

When should a postpartum woman commence use of the mini-pill?

The mini-pill does not affect lactation or increase the risk of thrombosis in the postpartum period, so it can be started as soon as the woman feels she would like to become sexually active. However, there is some evidence to show that, if started prior to 4 weeks postpartum, there is an increased likelihood of bleeding problems.

How long does it take to become effective?

The hostile mucus effect is maximal and sustained within 48 hours of commencement. If it is commenced on:

- the first or second day of menstruation
- on about day 21 postpartum if the woman is not lactating, and about 4 weeks after delivery if breastfeeding
- on the same or next day after an abortion or a miscarriage
- after switching over from a COCP

then no extra precautions are necessary and the contraceptive benefits can be said to be immediate.

BOX 3.7 Contraindications to progestogen-only contraception

- Past severe arterial disease or current exceptionally high risk of the same—the reason for this being the decrease in HDL associated with levonorgestrel and norethisterone
- Any serious side effect occurring when on the COCP and not clearly due to oestrogen
- Recent trophoblastic disease
- Undiagnosed abnormal genital tract bleeding
- Actual or possible pregnancy
- Active liver disease
- Sex-steroid-dependent cancer
- Past severe endogenous depression

If the woman is going on the mini-pill after not using any hormonal contraception, she should use condoms or abstain for 48 hours. Patients should be warned that this advice differs from that printed on the patient information sheet in the pill packet.

Within how many hours do you have to remember to take it?

Mini-pill use requires obsessional pill taking. The user has only 3 hours in which to remember to take the mini-pill. This is because the major contraceptive effect is through production of hostile mucus that is very dependent on progestogen levels.

What do you do if you miss a pill?

The pill should be taken when remembered and condoms should be used, or the couple should abstain until 48 hours have passed and the contraceptive effect returns.

What medication may interfere with the effectiveness of the mini-pill?

Enzyme inducers such as rifampicin, barbiturates, phenytoin, carbamazepine, griseofulvin and spironolactone will all interfere with the progestogen levels and therefore the contraceptive efficacy of the mini-pill. Unlike the COCP, drugs that alter bowel flora have no effect on the efficacy of the progestogen-only pill; therefore the woman need not worry about interactions with antibiotics unless the drug is an enzyme inducer.

What time of day should a woman take the POP?

The worst time of day to take the mini pill is just before the most common time for intercourse. This is because at approximately 22 hours after taking the mini-pill, the hostility of the mucus to sperm is starting to wear off. It is therefore advisable for the woman to take the mini pill with breakfast if she mainly has intercourse in the evening, as by that time the mucus will be at its most hostile.

What side effects are there?

As with all progestogen-only contraception, the major problem with the mini-pill is irregular bleeding. The reason for this is the variable effect that the mini-pill has on the individual woman in terms of inhibiting ovulation. About 40% of women on the mini-pill will have normal cycles, with normal ovulation and menstruation. It is these women who are most at risk of pregnancy when taking the mini-pill. About 44% of women on the mini-pill will have irregular cycles, with resultant irregularity in their menstrual cycle. The remaining 16% have ovaries that are suppressed by the exogenous progestogen and so fail to ovulate

or menstruate on the mini-pill. It is these women who are at least risk of pregnancy on the mini-pill.[31]

The other major side effect is the functional ovarian cysts experienced by a small number of women. These are most likely to occur in those women who have irregular cycles when on the mini-pill and may be associated with some pain.

Pregnancies in mini-pill users are more likely to be ectopic although the mini-pill does not actually increase the risk of ectopics occurring compared with the incidence in the general population.

Minor side effects reported include 'bloatedness', breast-tenderness and acne. Some women complain of decreased libido and depression when using the mini-pill.

Are there any new developments in POPs?

A new POP containing desogestrel is available in some countries. This POP is slightly different from its predecessors in that anovulation occurs in 97% of cycles, making it more reliable and efficacious. This also means that rather than having only a 3-hour leeway for a missed pill, this particular POP has a 12-hour leeway. Cerazette, as it is called, still gives some problems with irregular bleeding, but this has been seen to improve with extended use, with 50% of users having either amenorrhoea or only one or two bleeds over a 90-day period.[32]

Are there any concerns about the efficacy of the POP in women who are overweight?

In the last few years, some opinion leaders have been advocating the use of two POPs in women who are >70 kg. However, the UK Faculty of Family Planning Guidelines state that 'There is no evidence that the efficacy of progestogen-only pills (*traditional* or desogestrel-only) is reduced in women weighing >70 kg and therefore the licensed use of one pill per day is recommended'.[33]

Summary of key points

- The POP works primarily through thickening the cervical mucus to make it impenetrable to sperm.
- The POP is ideal for breastfeeding women.
- The POP is taken every day and must be taken within the same 3-hour time period in order to maintain its efficacy.
- Progestogen-only pills may result in irregular bleeding in some women.

Depo–Provera®

Some GPs feel uncomfortable recommending Depo-Provera® to their patients, probably because of their unfamiliarity with it. Many women coming from countries such as New Zealand and Sweden are surprised at the discomfort seen on the faces of their doctor when they ask for a repeat injection, as in these countries Depo-Provera® is considered to be a 'first-line' contraceptive.

Initially, the medical community was wary of this injectable form of progestogen-only contraception, mainly because of an alleged association with breast cancer in research done on beagles. The research was later discounted because beagles are predisposed to breast cancer, with or without the use of Depo-Provera®.

The next assault on the use of Depo-Provera® has come from feminists, who worry about the potential for its abuse by the medical profession. They point to doctors' ability to force contraception onto vulnerable women in our community, such as intellectually disabled and women of non-English-speaking background. There is no denying, however, that Depo-Provera® can be of great assistance to these particular groups of women, as well as to others as a tool in managing menstrual difficulties and problems such as recurrent candidiasis.

What basic information needs to be provided when counselling a new patient about Depo-Provera®?

Efficacy

Depo-Provera® is one of the most efficacious contraceptives available, with a failure rate of 0–1/100 woman-years. This rate, better than the efficacy of the COCP, is due to the fact that there is no risk of user error, because, once injected, the drug is effective for up to 14 weeks (it is a long-acting reversible contraceptive (LARC))

Depo-Provera® is one of the most efficacious forms of contraception currently available.

Mode of action

The major contraceptive effect of Depo-Provera® is the suppression of ovulation. Other contraceptive actions include its progestogenic effect on cervical mucus and on the endometrium

Dosage and timing

Depo-Provera® consists of 150 mg of depot medroxyprogesterone acetate (DMPA) given by injection into the buttock every 12 weeks. The patient can receive the injection either 2 weeks earlier or up to 2 weeks late and still ensure contraceptive efficacy.

> **CASE STUDY: Depo-Provera®**
>
> Jenny is 15 years old. She has been sexually active for 3 months. She wants contraception but is frightened that her mother will find her pill packet, as she knows that her parents regularly search her room because they believe she is using marijuana. Her friend gets 'the needle' and she wants to know if she can get it too.

Benefits

Depo-Provera® is highly effective, convenient (as it is not related to intercourse) and reversible. It also results in reduced menstrual bleeding and less dysmenorrhoea. Like all progestogen-only contraceptives, it reduces the risk of PID because of the changes it causes in cervical mucus and is protective against endometrial cancer. There is also a reduction in the rate of endometriosis.

Disadvantages

The major disadvantage of Depo-Provera®, especially to weight-conscious young women, is weight gain. This is due to a stimulation of appetite rather than fluid retention, and users can expect to gain approximately 1 kg annually.[34]

The other major disadvantage (as with other forms of progestogen-only contraception) is bleeding pattern disturbance. If women are warned about this and expect it to happen, then fewer will discontinue use. For the majority of new users, Depo-Provera® causes an increased number of days where light bleeding or spotting occurs. They should be warned that the bleeding will probably require them to wear a panty liner every day but rarely a pad. For the first two or three injections most women will also get their normal periods. By the third injection however the majority will become amenorrhoeic. This frightens many women who like to use their period as a reassuring sign that they are not pregnant. For others, on the other hand, the convenience of not having to deal with monthly periods is a welcome change and a reason why they choose to continue with Depo-Provera®. In short, at the end of 1 year, 30% of users will have regular cycles, 25% will be amenorrhoeic and the rest will have irregular bleeding. However, after 5 years, only 17% of users have regular cycles, the majority (80%) will be amenorrhoeic and the remaining 3% will have irregular bleeding.

Eventually women will become amenorrhoeic if they continue on Depo-Provera® long enough.

Another possible disadvantage for some women is the delayed return to fertility after using Depo-Provera®. Women can expect to be cycling normally on average some 9 months after their next injection would have been due. Depo-Provera® does not cause permanent impairment to the woman's fertility.

The minor side effects (but sometimes not so minor for patients) include lassitude, depression, loss of libido, vaginal dryness, bloating, dizziness, breast tenderness, leg cramps and headaches.

A summary checklist of the minimum information to be conveyed at counselling is given in Box 3.8

When during the menstrual cycle can Depo-Provera® be commenced?

In menstruating women, the first injection should be given before day 5 of the cycle. The onset of action is immediate.

Depo-Provera® can be used for postpartum women, but commencement is best postponed until 5–6 weeks after the birth in order to decrease the likelihood of heavy and prolonged bleeding.

After a miscarriage or termination of pregnancy, the injection can be used with immediate effect within 7 days of the procedure.

Can you give a test dose or try a woman on a mini-pill first if women do not like the idea of 3 months of irreversible hormone administration?

A test dose is not advisable, as the contraceptive efficacy may not be equivalent: that is, giving 50 mg by injection may not suppress ovulation nor last for a month. Neither oral provera nor the mini-pill is equivalent to intramuscular Depo-Provera® and so cannot be used to test the patient's reaction.

Does Depo-Provera® cause osteoporosis?

Studies to date suggest that long-term use of Depo-Provera® can be associated with a reduction in bone density. This occurs because of the suppression of the ovaries by Depo-Provera® and the resultant low levels of endogenous oestrogen. One small study has found that bone density may rise again after discontinuation of Depo-Provera®. However, concerns over osteoporosis are particularly pertinent for adolescent users, who would normally be laying down bone at this time. It is therefore recommended that there be 'a careful re-evaluation of the risks and benefits in all those who wish to continue use for more than two years'.[35]

Which injection site should be used?

Injectable contraception should be given by deep intramuscular injection into the gluteal or deltoid muscle or the lateral thigh.[35]

A small proportion of women experience heavy bleeding soon after commencing Depo-Provera®. How can this problem be managed?

The reason for the heavy bleeding is because the endometrium has thinned too much as a result of the Depo-Provera®. Contrary to instances of heavy menstrual bleeding in which oestrogen has caused a large build-up in the endometrium and progestogens are needed to stabilise it, the administration of progestogens would make the bleeding worse. Hence, administration of the next dose of Depo-Provera® early is not the answer. Oestrogen is what the patient needs and this can be given in any convenient form, for example, as a 30 mg combined oral contraceptive. This will supply enough oestrogen to build up the endometrium. After 2–3 weeks of therapy, the oestrogen can be discontinued and the patient observed. If her bleeding has settled, she may be able to continue using the Depo-Provera®.

Some patients present late for their repeat injections (i.e. longer than 2 weeks after the injection was due). Will the Depo-Provera® still be effective?

Late presentation is very common in younger Depo users who may be living a chaotic lifestyle (IV drug users, for example), and in patients with a psychotic illness, who often use injectable contraception. In these situations, the advice given in Table 3.4 (p 60) should be followed.

If pregnancy does occur, the best advice available is that there is no evidence of an increase in ectopics or miscarriage. No serious malformations have been associated with Depo-Provera® use, although masculinisation of the female fetus (particularly transient enlargement of the clitoris) and an increased incidence of hypospadias has been reported.

BOX 3.8 Summary checklist for DMPA counselling (Adapted from Guillebaud[9])

- Effects of a single dose last at least 12 weeks.
- Amenorrhoea can occur and women should be reassured that a 'monthly clean out' is not necessary for a woman's good health.
- Frequent irregular bleeding is possible.
- Weight gain is likely.
- Fertility return is delayed.
- There is a theoretical long-term risk of osteoporosis.

TABLE 3.4 Summary of indications for emergency contraception following late progestogen-only injectable injections[a] (From FSRH[99]. Reproduced with permission of the Faculty of Sexual and Reproductive Healthcare.)

Timing of injection	Has unprotected sex occurred?	Can the injection be given?	Is emergency contraception indicated?	Is additional contraception or abstinence advised?	Should a pregnancy test be performed?
Up to 14 weeks after last IM DMPA injection	Not applicable, as long as next injection is given 14 weeks after the last IM DMPA injection or before	YES	NO	NO	NO
When an injection is overdue, e.g.: >14 weeks +1 day or more since last IM DMPA injection	NO (abstained or used barrier methods)	YES	NO	YES, for the next 7 days	NO, if abstained- YES, if used barrier methods, but at least 21 days later
	YES, but only in the last 3 days	YES	YES, should offer progestogen-only EC or a copper IUD	YES, for the next 7 days	YES, at least 21 days later
	YES, but only in the last 4–5 days	YES	YES, should offer a copper IUD	NO, if opts for copper IUD	YES, at least 21 days later
	YES, more than 5 days ago	NO	NO	YES, for 21 days until a pregnancy test is confirmed negative, and for a further 7 days after giving progestogen-only injection	YES, at the initial presentation and at least 21 days later

[a]If EC is refused, decisions about ongoing use of DMPA should be tailored to the individual woman. Alternative methods, if required, should then be considered.
DMPA = depot medroxyprogesterone acetate; EC = emergency contraception; IM = intramuscular; IUD = intrauterine device

Summary of key points
- Depo-Provera® is a useful contraceptive for those who find compliance with pills difficult.
- Depo-Provera® is one of the most efficacious contraceptives currently available.
- Users may initially experience irregular bleeding.
- A side effect of Depo-Provera® is weight gain, secondary to appetite stimulation.

Implanon

What is Implanon?
Implanon is a subdermal implant containing a metabolite of desogestrel, the third-generation progestogen contained in some COCPs. The rod is inserted in the medial aspect of the upper arm (Fig 3.4) and slowly and steadily releases the hormone over the 3 years of its use.

How efficacious is it?
The risk of pregnancy with Implanon is lower than the risk after sterilisation procedures. Part of the reason for its efficacy is that because it is an implant it is not dependent on user compliance or motivation. Implanon works by inhibiting ovulation. However, some follicular activity is still seen, resulting in physiological levels of oestradiol. This means that, unlike Depo-Provera®, there are no concerns about osteoporosis with long-term use. Serum levels are reduced, however, in women taking enzyme-inducing drugs such as rifampicin, griseofulvin, phenytoin and carbamazepine, and the pregnancies that do occur with Implanon are either due to interaction with enzyme inducers or failure to insert the Implanon correctly.

The rod must be replaced every 3 years to retain contraception.

Is it reversible?
The rod can be removed at any time. Serum levels drop quickly after removal of the rod, with 94% of women ovulating within 1 month of removal.[36]

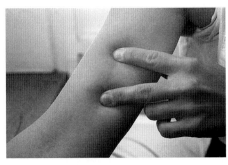

FIGURE 3.4 A contraceptive implant in situ: its position is illustrated by the patient's fingers (From Greer et al[93])

CASE STUDY: Implanon

Belinda, 33 years old, presents wanting to change her form of contraception. Having completed her family some 3 years ago, she has been on the COCP since then. While she has no side effects from taking the COCP, she has found that since returning to work she has had trouble remembering to take the pill and wonders if there is anything else she can try. She and her husband are not prepared to undergo sterilisation procedures, as they still feel too young, and she does not want to have an IUD because she had one between her first and second children and didn't like it. Her friend has recently had Implanon inserted in her arm and she wonders if this form of contraception would be suitable for her.

All types of progestogen-only contraception are plagued with irregular bleeding or spotting, at least in the first few months of use.

For whom is it suitable?

Implanon is an ideal contraceptive for young women who have difficulty remembering the COCP. Many women who have an unplanned pregnancy resulting in an abortion choose to have an Implanon inserted at the time of the procedure. It is also a good option for a woman who has completed her family and does not want to consider sterilisation or an IUD.

Are there any concerns regarding the efficacy of Implanon in women who are overweight?

While blood levels of progestogen may be lower in women who are overweight, Implanon has a very high margin of efficacy, so much so that even in women with a BMI >30 Implanon is classified as a category I contraceptive (no restriction – always usable).[9]

What are the possible side effects?

Like other progestogenic contraceptives, Implanon will affect bleeding patterns. It is difficult to predict in an individual woman what her bleeding pattern will be like but:

- 21% of cycles will be amenorrhoeic
- 26% of cycles will involve infrequent bleeding
- 35% of cycles will be normal
- 18% will involve frequent or prolonged bleeding.[37]

Women should be advised that 20% of users will have no bleeding, while almost 50% will have infrequent, frequent or prolonged bleeding and that bleeding patterns are likely to remain irregular.

If women are counselled and given adequate information about the likelihood of bleeding changes with Implanon, they may be more accepting of these changes. For some women, though, (especially those with religious restrictions during menstruation) irregular unpredictable bleeding is not acceptable.

A key issue to ask women considering Implanon is the importance to them of good cycle control.

In general, other side effects are limited, with some benefits in dysmenorrhoea and acne.

Importantly, there appears to be no change to the balance between coagulation and fibrinolysis, in common with other progestogen-only contraceptives.[38]

While some women experience weight gain while using progestogen only implants there is no evidence to support a causal association between progestogen-only implants and weight change, mood change, loss of libido or headache.[39]

If a woman complains about the bleeding she has with Implanon, can she take anything to improve it?

If a woman has prolonged or untenable bleeding with Implanon, it is unlikely that this situation will change. Some clinicians try 3 months of a desogestrel-containing COCP, and a recent trial has shown that doxycycline 100 mg b.d. for 5 days is more effective than a placebo[40]; however, the problem bleeding tends to recur.

Kylie is 17 years old and presents requesting an abortion because of an unplanned pregnancy. When you ask about her experiences with contraception, she tells you that she was prescribed the COCP but kept on forgetting to take it and had breakthrough bleeding, so she stopped using it. She had been seeing her current boyfriend for two months. She described trying to get him to use a condom, but he had told her that he would withdraw in time. She knew, however, that on a couple of occasions his 'timing' hadn't been good. She was not aware that she had any other contraceptive options apart from the COCP and condoms. When you describe to her the availability and attributes of Implanon, she looks interested but says that that having found herself in this difficult situation she doubts whether she will be sexually active for a while and anyway she doesn't like the sound of having a big needle inserted in her arm. You explain that the Implanon insertion could be done at the same time as the abortion and that if she didn't like it she could always have it removed. Kylie considers your opinion and agrees to go ahead with Implanon at the time of the procedure.

Where does a woman go to have Implanon inserted and removed?

Implanon needs to be inserted and removed by a trained doctor. Training courses are run by the manufacturer, usually through local family planning associations. The main focus of training is to ensure that the device actually ends up in the woman's arm (and not on the floor) and that placement is superficial, as this makes it easy to locate for removal. If there are problems locating the device, removal can occur under ultrasound guidance. All GPs should consider doing Implanon training, as the increased familiarity with the device and the ability to insert and remove mean that Implanon is a more readily accessible contraceptive option to women in general.

Summary of key points
- Implanon is a single rod, subdermal, contraceptive implant containing etonogestrel (a metabolite of desogestrel).
- It is inserted into the upper medial aspect of the arm.
- It provides highly efficacious contraception for 3 years.
- Implanon inhibits ovulation.
- As with other progestogen-only contraceptives, Implanon is associated with irregular bleeding.

INTRAUTERINE DEVICES (IUDS)

Prevalence
Why are IUDs not used more often in Western countries?

Intrauterine devices are extremely effective, useful and well tolerated. Despite this, they are not often used in Western countries. In the most recent study of contraceptive prevalence in Australia, for example, more than 44% of all women aged 18–49 years reportedly used a method of contraception. The most commonly reported methods were the pill (60%) and condom (27%); IUD and natural methods accounted for less than 5% each.[41]

There are several reasons why IUDs remain unpopular. First, many myths exist about IUDs, the two most important being that they bring about abortion and that they cause pelvic inflammatory disease (PID) and subsequent infertility. The second set of reasons for the unpopularity of IUDs concerns doctors and includes lack of familiarity with IUDs, lack of opportunities for training and high insurance costs.

Myth 1: IUDs abort pregnancies

Many patients, and indeed clinicians, remain confused about exactly how IUDs act. A common myth is that an IUD allows fertilisation to occur but not implantation, and that it is therefore an abortifacient. The evidence clearly contradicts this view. The main effects of an IUD are (a) to interfere with sperm migration and sperm function, and (b) to block fertilisation.

The copper in copper-containing IUDs is found in high concentrations in cervical mucus and impairs sperm migration.[42,43] This is demonstrated by the fact that fewer sperm are present in the tubes of IUD users than non-users.[44] Furthermore, the sperm that are recovered from the fallopian tubes of IUD users have been found to be damaged and incapable of fertilisation.[45] When the tubes and uterine cavities of women using IUDs have been flushed in studies, fertilised ova have never been found.[46] One particular study monitored 30 women using IUDs by measuring serial beta-human chorionic gonadotrophin levels for 30 months and did not observe any changes in levels,[47] particularly the rise followed by an abrupt drop in levels characteristic of pregnancy interruption.

In contrast the levonorgestrel IUS, like other progestogen-containing forms of contraception, is believed to have a contraceptive action through thickening cervical mucus, making it impenetrable to sperm.

Myth 2: IUDs cause PID

The legacy of the Dalkon shield, used in the 1970s, has been that IUDs have been associated in the minds of clinicians and women in general with pelvic infection and infertility. However, the early studies looking at this issue had serious methodological flaws. Choices of inappropriate comparison groups, overdiagnosis of salpingitis in IUD users and an inability to control for the confounding effects of sexual behaviour exaggerated the apparent risk.[48] Studies have since shown that the risk of upper genital tract infection is confined to the first 20 days after insertion[49] and that after that the risk of contracting PID is the same as in controls.

IUDs do not abort pregnancies or cause PID.

System issues

The other barriers hindering GPs from recommending or inserting IUDs are more 'system-related' than anything else. Few GPs actually insert IUDs in their practice. This may be related to medical insurance coverage, as some companies charge much higher premiums when GPs undertake IUD insertions.

GPs are not familiar with IUDs. As most IUDs are inserted in family-planning clinics or the private rooms of gynaecologists, few GPs are taught how to undertake the procedure. Neither are they familiar with removal techniques and, because the rates of IUD use are so low, GPs are not accustomed to managing any side effects or complications that may occur. This lack of familiarity leads to decreased confidence when advising patients, with the result that GPs do not recommend the IUD to their patients. These same issues are also faced by gynaecologists[50] and have been reported among British GPs.[51]

Recommending an IUD

When should an IUD be recommended to a patient?

GPs should always mention the IUD as an option when a patient requires contraception. This strategy will inform women of the availability of IUDs and allow them to come back to this method when they are ready.

While an IUD is ideally suited to women who have already had a child, nulliparity is not a contraindication. However, the most common demographic profile of women using IUDs in the Western world are either women who have just had a child, are breastfeeding or want to space their family, or those who have completed their families and neither they nor their partners want sterilisation.

CASE STUDY: IUDs for nulliparous women?

Susan is a 25-year-old G_1P_0 who had an abortion for an unplanned pregnancy last year. She has been in her current relationship for the past 6 months. Her older sister had an IUD inserted soon after the birth of her first child and has recommended it to Susan.

Would you recommend an IUD to a nulliparous woman?

Until recently, nulliparous women were not encouraged to use IUDs because with a nulliparous cervix and generally smaller uterus the IUD is more difficult to insert and rates of expulsion may be higher. Younger unmarried women were also thought to be unsuitable for IUDs because they were not in stable monogamous relationships and therefore more at risk of STDs. It was thought that this put them at increased risk of developing PID and subsequent infertility, which if they have not yet had a child might be a more difficult burden to bear. However, a systematic review[48] (Table 3.5) has found that IUDs do not facilitate PID or make STDs easier to catch.

The UK medical eligibility criteria classify both parous and nulliparous women >20 years as category 1 (they should have unrestricted access to this form of contraception), and young women aged between menarche and 20 years as category 2 (the benefits outweigh the risks).[52]

What benefits would Susan obtain from using an IUD?

IUDs are now the most cost-effective reversible form of contraception available.[53] The many benefits of an IUD are listed in Box 3.9 (p 64).

The introduction of the levonorgestrel-releasing intrauterine system (LNG-IUS) called Mirena (a system rather than a device) has widened the spectrum of women who would benefit from this type of contraception. At present, the IUS has two major indications, contraception and the management of menorrhagia or dysfunctional uterine bleeding.[54] Recent studies have begun to explore the efficacy of this product in the management of other menstrual complaints such as dysmenorrhoea[55] and endometriosis and in the provision of endometrial protection for women using oestrogen replacement therapy.[56]

TABLE 3.5 A summary of the evidence on IUDs, STDs and pelvic infection (From Grimes[48])

Issue	Highest level of evidence	Strength of conclusion	Conclusion
IUD as cause of PID	II-2	A	Risk related to insertion process
Tailstring as cause of PID	I	A	Monofilament tailstring not a vector for infection
IUD insertion in presence of gonorrhoea or *Chlamydia*	II-2	C	Limited data, but no evidence of increased risk compared with gonorrhoea or *Chlamydia* without an IUD insertion
Acquisition of *Chlamydia* by IUD user	II-2	B	No increase in risk
Acquisition of gonorrhoea by IUD user	II-2	C	Limited data
Levonorgestrel-releasing IUS and upper genital tract infection	II-2	C	Conflicting data on protection against PID
Treatment of PID with IUD in situ	I	B	No impaired response to antibiotic therapy
Infertility after discontinuation	II-2	B	No substantial increase in risk

BOX 3.9 The benefits of using IUDs

- Effective
  - Comparable with efficacy of female sterilisation
  - Can be used as emergency contraception up to 5 days after unprotected intercourse
- Safe
  - Mortality 1:500,000
  - No known unwanted systemic effects
- Independent of intercourse
- Motivation is only required at time of insertion
- Cheap and easy to distribute
- Does not influence milk volume or composition
- Continuation rates are very high
- Reversible form of contraception

Choice of IUD

Which one is preferred: the Mirena, Multiload or the Copper T?

With the availability of the Mirena IUS, GPs recommending or inserting IUDs need to decide which device to use, either the non-hormonal IUDs or Mirena. If there are no therapeutic reasons to use Mirena (e.g. menorrhagia), then on the basis of cost and longevity a Copper T380A would be preferred. Indeed, the Copper T380A is now considered to be the 'gold standard' among copper devices.[31] However, if the patient is concerned about the possible side effects of heavier bleeding and dysmenorrhoea with a non-hormonal IUD, she may prefer to use Mirena. Table 3.6 compares and contrasts the Copper T380A

with Mirena. Figures 3.5 and 3.6 show what the various IUDs look like and their relative sizes.

Patients should be advised of potential side effects. The most important of these is the impact of Mirena on bleeding patterns. While initially they may experience some irregular bleeding, after 6 months the majority of women will experience amenorrhoea.

The Mirena levonorgestrel-releasing intrauterine system is an ideal form of contraception for women in their 40s, as it will also assist in the management of menorrhagia.

Should Mirena be preferred over other progestogenic forms of contraception?

All forms of progestogenic contraception affect bleeding patterns and some, like Depo-Provera®, stop ovulation. If Depo-Provera® is used long-term, there are concerns about inducing a prolonged hypo-oestrogenic state and the effect this will have on a woman's bones. In contrast, the levonorgestrel released by Mirena acts only locally, with little systemic effect. Ovulation continues, despite the fact that the woman may become amenorrhoeic owing to the thinning of the endometrium by the local release of levonorgestrel.

A patient decides she wants to go ahead and use an IUD for contraception. What should you do at the initial consultation?

It is important to take a thorough medical and sexual history to exclude contraindications to the

TABLE 3.6 A comparison between the Copper T380A and Mirena

	Copper T380A IUD	Mirena IUS
Active ingredient	Copper	Levonorgestrel
Size	Slimmer (4 mm in diameter)	Thicker (5 mm in diameter)
Cumulative failure rate at 10 years	1.4/100 woman-years	0.2/100 woman-years
Side effects	Increased dysmenorrhoea Heavier periods	Initial irregular bleeding and spotting Amenorrhoea after 6–12 months of use
Indications	Contraception	Contraception First-line management of menorrhagia Endometrial protection for concurrent use of oestrogen postmenopausally

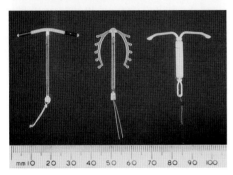
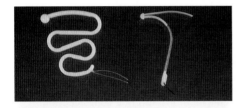

FIGURE 3.5 Intrauterine contraceptive devices: (upper row) Lippes loop and Copper 7 IUDs, which are no longer available; (bottom row, left to right) Copper T and Multiload IUDs and the Mirena IUS (From Greer et al[93])

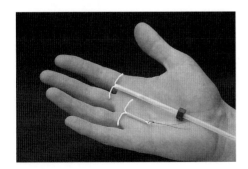

FIGURE 3.6 The Mirena IUS shown with its introducer; note the size of the device relative to an adult hand (From Greer et al[93])

BOX 3.10 Permanent absolute contraindications to IUDs

- Markedly distorted uterine cavity
- Known true allergy to a constituent
- Wilson's disease (for copper devices only)
- Past attack of bacterial endocarditis or of severe pelvic infection in a woman with an anatomical lesion of the heart or after any prosthetic valve replacement

use of an IUD. There are few permanent absolute contraindications to its use (Box 3.10).

Temporary absolute contraindications are those that require sorting out and treatment before an IUD can be inserted. They include undiagnosed genital tract bleeding, suspicion of pregnancy, postseptic abortion, current or suspected pelvic infection, significant immunosuppression or malignant trophoblastic disease with uterine wall involvement.

The examination should include a careful speculum and bimanual examination to check for abnormalities of the cervix and in the size, shape and position of the uterus (it is difficult to insert an IUD into a markedly retroverted uterus).

A Pap smear should be taken, because if colposcopy or laser treatment is necessary it should be performed before the IUD is inserted (otherwise the laser can burn off the strings).

The most recent guidelines[57] advise that only women at higher risk of STIs (i.e. aged <25 years, or >25 years with a new sexual partner or more than one partner in the last year, or if their regular partner has other partners) should be tested for

Chlamydia trachomatis (as a minimum) in advance of insertion. If results are unavailable before insertion, prophylactic antibiotics (at least to cover *C. trachomatis*) may be considered. The same guidelines advise that there is no indication to test or treat other lower genital tract organisms or delay insertion in asymptomatic women attending for insertion of intrauterine contraception

Naproxen given before the procedure may assist with any discomfort that may be experienced.

Issues that a GP should discuss when counselling a patient about use of an IUD are listed in Box 3.11.

Insertion and removal

How are IUDs inserted?

IUDs should be inserted by trained doctors. Generally it is advisable to insert an IUD during a period, as then you are certain the woman is not pregnant and the cervix may be a little more open and the device easier to insert. If it is not inserted during a period, the doctor must be sure that the woman is not pregnant and that she has been using contraception. A speculum is used to visualise the cervix and the anterior lip of the cervix is held with a tenaculum. The uterus is then sounded prior to the device being inserted. Once the IUD is in place, its strings are cut to an appropriate length (usually 2–3 cm) and the instruments are removed. Instrumentation of the cervix causes discomfort and pain and once the IUD is placed in the uterus there is also some cramping. The woman may feel faint and should rest in the waiting room for half an hour after the procedure. The procedure can be done under local anaesthetic, but some argue that this is more painful than just doing the procedure.

What advice should be given after insertion?

The patient should be told to expect some light bleeding for the next few days, with some cramping as the uterus adjusts to having the IUD in situ. She should return about 4–6 weeks after the insertion for a check-up. At this time she will have experienced her first menstruation with the IUD in situ and should have checked that she could feel the strings after that period and every subsequent period. She should be told to return sooner if she develops continuing or increasing pain, malodorous discharge, heavy bleeding or fever, as these may be symptoms of increasingly severe endometritis.

Annual follow-up is not routinely recommended; women should attend at any time if problems arise.[57]

> **BOX 3.11 Issues to be discussed when counselling a patient about use of an IUD (From Faculty of Sexual and Reproductive Healthcare Clinical Effectiveness Unit[57])**
>
> - Mode of action of a Cu-IUD is primarily to prevent fertilisation and the LNG-IUS is to prevent implantation.
> - Failure rates at 5 years' use are low: less than 2% for Cu-IUDs (380 mm^2) and less than1% for the LNG-IUS.
> - Duration of use is 8 years for a CuT380A and 5 years for a LNG-IUS, after which time they should be changed.
> - Uterine perforation is uncommon (up to 2 per 1000 insertions).
> - Expulsion occurs in around 1 in 20 women, is most common in the first year of use and particularly within 3 months of insertion.
> - The risk of ectopic pregnancy is reduced with intrauterine contraception when compared to using no contraception.
> - There is no delay in return to fertility after removal of intrauterine contraception.
> - There is a sixfold increase in the risk of pelvic infection in the 20 days following insertion of intrauterine contraception, but thereafter the risk is the same as in the non-IUD-using population.
> - Bleeding and pain are common causes of discontinuation. Spotting, light bleeding or heavy or prolonged bleeding is common in the first 3–6 months of Cu-IUD use. Irregular bleeding and spotting is common in the first 6 months after insertion of the LNG-IUS. By 1 year after LNG-IUS insertion, amenorrhoea or oligomenorrhoea is usual.
> - Hormonal side effects can be due to systemic absorption of progestogen, but few women discontinue use of the LNG-IUS for this reason and discontinuation rates are not significantly different from those of Cu-IUD users.
> - The insertion procedure and likely discomfort during and after intrauterine contraceptive insertion should be discussed with women and oral analgesia can be advised before insertion.

A patient returns to see you 3 months after insertion of her IUD at a family planning clinic. She was unable to feel her strings after her last period and is worried the IUD may have 'fallen out'. What should you do?

If a woman is unable to feel the strings, then one's first thought must be whether or not the IUD has unknowingly been expelled and whether or not the patient is pregnant or at increased risk of becoming pregnant.

The following steps should be followed:

- Visualise the cervix and see for yourself whether the strings are visible.
- Do a bimanual examination for tenderness and to help exclude pregnancy.
- If no strings are readily seen, explore the cervical canal with narrow artery forceps. An alternative is to use a cytobrush (used normally for taking Pap smears) and rotate it in the endocervical canal to see if you can bring down the strings.
- If no strings are found, do a urinary pregnancy test.
- An ultrasound scan should be performed. If the IUD is visualised in the uterus, no further action is needed.
- If no IUD is seen in the cavity, an X-ray should be carried out to localise the IUD in the pelvis or the abdominal cavity or to confirm that it has truly been expelled.

The presence of Actinomyces is sometimes reported on smears of IUD users. What significance does this have?

Actinomyces israeli is a bacterial commensal of the gut that is found in the lower genital tract only in the presence of a foreign body. The prevalence of *Actinomyces* in IUD users is directly related to the duration of use of the IUD. After 1 year's use, about 1% of smears show *Actinomyces* and this rises to 8–10% after 3 years and 20% at 5 years.

The concern for the patient is that, rarely, *Actinomyces* has been associated with pelvic infection. Despite this the consequences can be severe. If the woman is symptomatic of pelvic infection the IUD is best removed, sent for culture (culture for *Actinomyces* must be specifically requested and generally takes up to 2 weeks) and the woman treated with penicillin.

If, however, the patient is asymptomatic, the IUD can remain in situ after endocervical swabs are taken, provided the woman is counselled about the risk and is told to come back quickly if symptoms appear. Previously, the advice was to remove the IUD, treat and replace, or just replace, but the rate of re-infection with these courses of action was high.

How are IUDs removed?

The simple answer to this is to pull. An IUD should be removed either during or directly after a period. Once the strings are visualised on

speculum examination, sponge forceps can be used to grip the IUD. Gentle traction should be applied after warning the woman that she may feel some discomfort and cramping as the IUD comes out and for some minutes after. Removal of the IUD is much like pulling on the umbilical cord to deliver a placenta; firm downward pressure should be applied. The woman can expect to have some bleeding for a few days, but she is immediately able to conceive.

What other IUDs are currently available or in the pipeline?

A frameless IUD (FlexiGard, Cu-Fix or Gyne-fix) is a single monofilament polypropylene string, knotted at both ends. Six copper bands surround the thread. The knot at the top of the string is embedded 9–10 mm into the myometrium at insertion and the string dangles freely in the uterine cavity. This IUD will therefore be more suited to nulliparous women and those with smaller endometrial cavities. The FibroPlant levonorgestrel IUS has been clinically developed since 1997 and is a further development of the 'frameless' anchoring IUD concept.

Summary of key points
- The IUD is the cheapest, most effective form of reversible contraception available.
- The risk of PID with an IUD is limited to the first 20 days after insertion.
- The availability of the levonorgestrel intrauterine releasing system (Mirena) has widened the indications for use of the IUD.
- Mirena can also be considered in women requiring management of menorrhagia and dysmenorrhoea, for those requiring endometrial protection when using oestrogen replacement therapy and possibly in women suffering from endometriosis.
- While Depo-Provera® causes anovulation, Mirena has few systemic effects.
- Women should not be discouraged from using an IUD because of nulliparity.

BARRIER METHODS

Condoms

The advent of safe hormonal forms of contraception meant that barrier methods such as condoms and diaphragms became a bit passé in the 1960s and 1970s. However, the fear of HIV has brought back into prominence one of the oldest forms of contraception, the condom.

How can GPs encourage condom use in their patients?

In this day and age, contraceptive counselling needs to be provided hand-in-hand with advice regarding the transmission of sexually transmitted diseases. Unfortunately, the most effective forms of contraception in existence today—the combined oral contraceptive pill, injectable contraception such as Depo-Provera®, the IUD and sterilisation—offer no protection from STDs.

GPs should now be recommending the 'double-Dutch' approach to patients who are not in long-term monogamous relationships. This involves using a condom to protect against STDs as well as some other form of contraception as a back-up against the risk of pregnancy.

What advantages are there to condom use?

Condoms have a lot of advantages over other forms of contraception.

- They are harmless to either partner.
- They are easily obtained—no contact with a doctor is required, neither is a prescription.
- They are immediately effective.
- They are the only method of contraception providing STD protection.
- They are the only form of contraception for which a man is responsible.
- They do not interfere with medications.
- They are safe duirng breastfeeding.

What barriers exist to the use of condoms by young people?

For young people, condom use poses many difficulties. Girls, especially, are reticent to carry them, as they feel that this may be interpreted as being readily available for sex. They are also embarrassed at having to buy them from the supermarket, petrol station or chemist, especially in rural areas where they know the shop owners and are frightened that gossip will be spread about their sexual activity.

The most difficult issues to overcome are actually learning how to use condoms and dealing some of the myths associated with them. It is not unusual to find that this sort of counselling needs to be undertaken with people of all ages. While young people sometimes receive this information as part of sex education (depending on the school they go to), it is not uncommon to come across recently divorced older men and women who are contemplating condom use for the first time with a new sexual partner.

Having the various forms of condoms available to show patients is helpful. It can also be useful to go through instructions on how to use them successfully and prevent breakage (Fig 3.7).

1. A new condom should be used for each episode of sex.
2. Check the packet for relevant safety markings and the 'use by' date.
3. Remove the condom from the packet, taking care not to damage it with fingernails, teeth or jewellery.
4. Find the closed end (teat) of the condom; squeeze the teat using your forefinger and thumb to expel any air. Trapped air can cause condoms to burst.
5. Condoms should be placed on the penis when it first becomes erect and before there is any contact with the genital area or vagina.
6. Roll the condom down the erect penis to its base.
7. The use of lubricant is advised when using condoms for anal sex.

   - As soon as the man has ejaculated, and before the penis goes soft, hold the condom firmly in place while pulling out. Do this slowly and carefully so that no semen is spilled.

   - Take the condom off away from the vagina, anus and genital area.

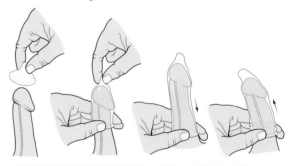

The steps are as follows:

1. Check the use by date of the condom and make sure that it has been stored in a cool, dry and dark place away from sunlight.
2. Open the packet carefully so as not to tear the condom itself – in other words don't use your teeth.
3. Wait until the penis is erect and put it on before there is any contact between the penis and the woman's genitalia.
4. Take the condom out of the packet and hold the teat between two fingers to expel any air.
5. Still holding the teat, roll the condom down the penis to the base.
6. Make sure you have rolled it down as far as it will go.
7. Use some water-based lubricant either on the penis or apply it to the woman's genitalia, to help prevent breakage.
8. After orgasm, hold the condom rim firmly onto the penis as the penis is withdrawn from the vagina. This is where problems occur as often men wait until the penis becomes flaccid before withdrawing. This can result in the condom slipping off and being 'left behind' in the vagina with resultant leakage of semen.
9. Roll the condom off away from your partner.
10. Throw the condom away in the garbage.

FIGURE 3.7 Instructions for condom use (From Faculty of Family Planning and Reproductive Health Care Clinical Effectiveness Unit [63])

- Make sure that the man's penis does not touch the genital area again. If having sex again, use a new condom.
- Do not flush condoms down the toilet. Wrap up the used condom (e.g. in tissue) and put the condom in the bin.

Problems

- If, when putting the condom on, it does not reach the base of the penis, then it is likely that the condom is inside out. The condom should be removed and replaced with a fresh one.
- If the condom rolls up during sex, roll the condom back down.
- If the condom slips off during sex, it should be replaced with a new one immediately.
- If there is any suspicion of possible condom failure (e.g. if the condom bursts, slips or leaks), there may be a risk of pregnancy and/or sexually transmitted infection.

Emergency contraception can be used to reduce the risk of pregnancy and should be taken as soon as possible after a condom accident or episode of unprotected sex. Emergency contraceptive pills are available over the counter at pharmacies in Australia (there is no need for a prescription).

Tests for sexually transmitted infections can be performed if there is any concern about infection.

Where should condoms be stored?

Condoms should be stored in a cool, dry and dark place away from sunlight. Heat may cause the rubber to weaken, so condoms should not be stored in hot places. Keeping a condom in a wallet in a back pocket has been discouraged in the past because of the presumed increased risk of breakage due to mechanical stress and heat, but studies have shown that it is safe to use a condom that has been carried in a wallet for up to a month. [58]

A lot of patients say their condoms break. Is this true?

Despite best intentions and manufacturer's testing, condoms do occasionally break. However, only about one-third of condom breaks occur at the tip of the condom.[59] The majority of breaks occur as a tear along the rim or along the side of the condom, reducing the risk of semen leakage.

One study of young men between 17 and 22 years of age, showed that 23% had experienced at least one broken condom in the past 12 months and 2.5% of all condoms used had broken.[60] Interestingly, increased experience, sex education and higher levels of income were associated with less breakage. In

another French study, the rate of breakage during last intercourse was 3.4% and slippage rate was 1.1%.[61]

What instructions should be given to patients, should breakage or slippage occur?

The first step should be to immediately insert some spermicidal foam or gel into the vagina (if available and if you have not already done so). Second, patients should be instructed to obtain and use emergency contraception within 72 hours of the incident. The sooner that the emergency contraception is taken after the incident, the more effective it will be. Ideally, condom manufacturers should put a packet of emergency contraception in each box of condoms sold, but this development has yet to occur.

Women should be aware of or be given emergency contraception if they are reliant on the use of condoms or diaphragms.

Many people are unaware of the fact that lubrication is one of the key factors to successful condom use. Without lubricant, a fifth of condoms break during anal sex.[62] It is also important to point out that applying lubricant to the tip of the penis under the condom increases the risk of condom slippage.[62] While many condoms are prelubricated, several are not. Also, by the time sexual activity is interrupted to put the condom on, natural lubrication may be lost. Therefore it is important to advise about the type of lubrication that should be used. The lubricant must be water-based, not oil-based as this may erode the condom and increase the risk of breakage. KY jelly is the old standard, but many new water-based lubricants are on the market. Table 3.7 lists safe and unsafe lubricants.

TABLE 3.7 Safe and unsafe products to use as lubricants with condoms

Safe	Unsafe
• KY jelly	• Baby oils
• Contraceptive foams (e.g. Delfen, Orthogynol)	• Burn ointments
• Saliva	• Coconut oil/butter
• Water	• Edible oils (e.g. olive, peanut, sunflower)
• Egg white	• Fish oils
	• Haemorrhoidal ointments
	• Margarine
	• Petroleum jelly (Vaseline)
	• Suntan oil
	• Vaginal creams (e.g. Monistat, Premarin, Vagisil)

Do people use condoms as much as they say they do?

Condoms are very effective if used consistently and correctly. Often, when asking about condom use, GPs will hear patients say, 'Yes, I use condoms'. It is a good idea to then ask, 'Is that every time or most times?' You might be surprised at how often the response is 'Most times'. An estimate of how condom use compares in efficacy to other forms of contraception is given in the Table 3.8. It is important to realise that the 3% failure rate translates to the fact that of 100 couples who use condoms perfectly for 1 year, only three couples will experience an accidental pregnancy. If each of the couples had intercourse on average twice a week for the year, then the 100 couples would have had sexual intercourse 10,400 times over the year. Three pregnancies occurring from 10,400 acts of condom use during sexual intercourse is a remarkably low pregnancy rate (0.03%) when calculated on a per condom basis.

Are condoms that contain a spermicide more effective?

While some condoms contain a spermicide (nonoxyl-9) in their tip, there is no evidence to suggest that the spermicide provides any additional protection against pregnancy or STIs compared with condoms lubricated with a non-spermicidal lubricant.[63]

My female patients complain that their partners refuse to use condoms because they feel too tight

Most complaints about condoms are with regard to size and decreased sensitivity during intercourse. Condoms can be straight-sided or tapered towards the closed end. Unfortunately, there is no getting away from the fact that the ring needs to be firm to hold the condom in place. Most condoms are about 170 mm long, 50 mm and 0.03–0.1 mm thick, although there is some variation.

What about female condoms?

The female condom (Fig 3.8) is made of polyurethane and is shaped like a sock with an inner ring at the closed end that helps with insertion and keeps the female condom in place. The larger, thinner outer ring remains outside the vagina once the condom is inserted. Insertion can take place several hours before sexual activity or immediately before intercourse. It does not have to be removed immediately after intercourse.

Its efficacy in terms of pregnancy prevention is similar to that of other barrier methods.

TABLE 3.8 A comparison of the failure rates and continuing use of various forms of contraception (From Trussell et al[96])

Method	Women experiencing an accidental pregnancy within the first year of use (%)		Women continuing use after one year (%)
	Typical use	Perfect use	
Withdrawal	19	4	
Diaphragm with spermicide	18	6	58
Condom: male	12	3	63
Condom: female	21	5	56
The pill	3		72
• Progestogen-only pill		0.5	
• Combined oral contraceptive pill		0.1	
Implanon[a]	<0.1	<0.1	
NuvaRing®[b]	1		
IUD			
• Copper T380A	0.8	0.6	78
• Levonorgestrel-releasing IUS	0.1	0.1	81
Depo-Provera®	0.3	0.3	70
Female sterilisation	0.4	0.4	100
Male sterilisation	0.15	0.10	100

[a]Information from manufacturer (not available from Trussell)
[b]Information from manufacturer[91] (not available from Trussell)

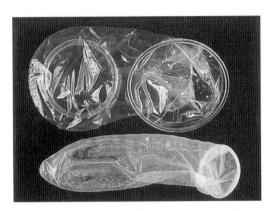

FIGURE 3.8 Female (top) and male (bottom) condoms (From Rymer et al[95])

Female condoms allow women to take control of STD prevention and contraception simultaneously.

Do condoms protect against all STDs?

With increasing knowledge about STDs, particularly viral ones such as herpes and warts, we have to accept that condoms will not protect against all STDs. Protection occurs only in terms of (a) what is covered and (b) the prevention of the exchange of bodily fluids. Recent research that shows that the HPV and HSV viruses are shed from all parts of the genital skin (not just where obvious lesions occur) means that there are no absolute guarantees regarding prevention of disease transmission. The fact that HSV can be shed from the skin at times other than when lesions are present is also a concern. However, at present, condoms provide the best form of protection from STDs that there is, unless abstinence is preferred.

Summary of key points
- Condoms protect against STDs and pregnancy.
- Condoms are very effective if used consistently.
- It is important to teach patients how to use condoms correctly.

Diaphragms and caps

What are the advantages of using a diaphragm or a cap?

Many women like the 'idea' of using a diaphragm or a cap, as these devices do not interfere with the menstrual cycle, have few side effects and are immediately reversible. Once purchased, they can be used for 2 years and are therefore relatively inexpensive. They are also totally under the woman's control and can be used in combination with natural family planning and or condom use.

What are the disadvantages?

What few women consider until they become familiar with diaphragms and caps is that their success at preventing pregnancy is almost totally dependent on user motivation. They should ideally be inserted before intercourse and this requires some forethought as to when sex may occur. For best effect, they should also be used in conjunction with spermicides. Many women feel that spermicides are messy and smelly, however, and this may decrease motivation to use diaphragms properly. Initially, a doctor or nurse must fit the correct size of diaphragm and the woman needs to be refitted after childbirth or if she gains or loses more than 4–5 kg in weight.

Every GP should have the resources necessary to provide adequate contraceptive counselling. This can be achieved by:
- purchasing a contraceptive counselling kit from the Family Planning Organisation in the area. This kit is a box containing an IUD, different kinds of diaphragms, caps and condoms, tubes of spermicidal cream, plastic models for demonstrating condom application, a plastic female pelvis and other relevant material.
- telephoning your local pharmaceutical representative and trying to convince them to provide you with a sample or out-of-date IUD, NuvaRing® and Implanon. If suppliers want women to use their products, they need to provide GPs with samples to use for patient education.
- learning how to fit diaphragms. It is not very difficult and once learned, never forgotten. GPs should obtain a set of fitting rings to keep in their rooms to assist them in choosing the right diaphragm for their patient.

Often as GPs we assume that patients are aware of the full range of contraception available to them. You may be surprised, however, at how many women have ruled out certain contraceptives because of the myths and false information they have heard from their girlfriends or mothers. GPs need to take the opportunity to explore with all women the contraceptive choices available and make sure that the woman has enough information to choose the right contraceptive for her at that point in her life.

The GP can play an important role in advising a woman of her potential risk of failure when using a barrier method. Characteristics associated with a higher than average risk are:[64]

- frequent intercourse (>3 times a week)
- age <30 years

CASE STUDY: 'I didn't realise I had any other option.'

Margie was 27 with three children; the youngest child was just 6 months old. She had presented the week previously to her usual GP asking for her diaphragm to be 'refitted'.

It was interesting to find out that Margie had had her first child at 22 and her next at 24. The most recent pregnancy had been unplanned (her diaphragm had stayed in the bedside table drawer—as often happens) and, although she was happy enough to have a third child, she definitely didn't want any more—at least in the short term. So her plan was to get her diaphragm refitted and to use it for contraceptive purposes more frequently.

She took her diaphragm out of her handbag; she had had it for 5 years and was shocked to hear that the current recommendation was to use it for only 2 years before replacing it.

As in most consultations to do with contraception, the most important question to ask Margie was 'How important is it for you not to get pregnant again soon?' Margie responded, 'Very'. She explained that she had considered a more permanent form of contraception, such as a tubal ligation, but felt she was still too young. The GP therefore engaged her in the reasons why she wanted to continue using a diaphragm at this point in time, particularly because it had not been effective when she last used it. It seemed that Margie really wasn't aware of her alternatives. She wasn't keen on hormones, and wasn't very good at remembering to take pills anyway,

particularly with a new baby occupying her time. Her husband didn't like condoms, so she wasn't sure that she had any choice but to use a diaphragm.

At that point the GP asked her if she had considered an IUD. 'Oh', she replied, 'not really. I don't really like the whole idea of them'. Luckily the GP had one in the drawer and brought it out to show to her. Margie's first reaction was to comment on how small it was, much less scary than she had imagined. The GP suggested that she was an ideal candidate for an IUD: she had already had children, needed long-term but reversible contraception and was in a monogamous relationship. The GP pointed out that current IUDs were able to provide up to 8–10 years of contraception, that she wouldn't have to worry about contraception once it was in and that she could get it removed at any time by a GP. She also had a choice of either the progestogen-releasing IUS (Mirena), which would ultimately make her 'period-free', or the Copper T or Multiload IUD. The GP explained to her that a diaphragm was OK to use if she didn't really mind getting pregnant again, as even when well used it would result in a pregnancy in 12% of women using it. The IUD, on the other hand, had a failure rate of only 2%.

With information in her hand and having seen the IUD, Margie was very interested and went home to speak to her husband about it. Soon after she came back and had a PV, smear and swabs taken, and returned later for an IUD insertion.

- personal style or sexual patterns that make consistent use difficult
- previous contraceptive failure
- ambivalent feelings (patient or partner) about the current desirability of a pregnancy
- intention to delay rather than prevent pregnancy.

What types of diaphragms are there?

There are three types of diaphragms. The flat spring variety is the one most commonly fitted. Coil spring diaphragms are more suitable for women with strong vaginal muscles and arcing diaphragms for those women with poor vaginal tone.

Do they need to be used with spermicide?

There is a significant difference in efficacy of pregnancy prevention between using and not using spermicide with a diaphragm. One study found that the typical user failure rate for diaphragms alone was 28.6%, whereas when diaphragms were used with spermicide the failure rate dropped to 21.2%.[65]

For this reason, spermicide should always be used concurrently with a diaphragm. The woman should be instructed to place about half a teaspoon on the concave surface that will sit against the cervix and to place a little around the rim (this will assist in lubrication as she inserts the diaphragm into the vagina).

Does using a diaphragm and spermicide increase risk of UTIs?

Some women are plagued by recurrent urinary tract infections (UTIs). These women should be advised to use another form of contraception, as the risk of developing a UTI with diaphragm and spermicide use is 2–3.5 times greater than for sexually active women who do not use a diaphragm and spermicide.[66] This may be either because ill-fitting diaphragms impinge on the urethra or because of a possible effect of spermicide on vaginal flora.[67]

Use of diaphragms may be associated with increased risk of UTIs.

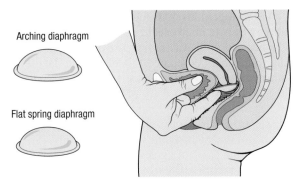

FIGURE 3.9 Use of a diaphragm (From Sundquist[97])

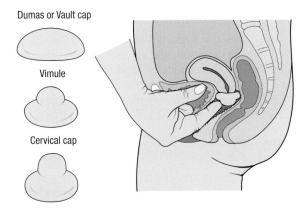

FIGURE 3.10 Use of a cap (From Sundquist[97])

What tips for diaphragm use can a GP give a patient?

Instructions for use of a diaphragms are given in Figure 3.9. However, the following tips are worth emphasising to patients.

- Always make sure you can feel the cervix behind the rubber.
- If it is uncomfortable, it probably is not in the right place.
- Use spermicide and renew with each act of intercourse.
- Leave the diaphragm in situ for a minimum of 6 hours from last act of intercourse.
- Use it every time you have sex.

When should a cap and not a diaphragm be recommended?

Caps are used less frequently than diaphragms. They are preferred when:

- a diaphragm causes dragging and discomfort
- a partner can feel the diaphragm rim
- a closely fitting diaphragm cannot be fitted
- a woman develops recurrent UTIs.

What kinds of caps are there?

Three types of caps are available (Fig 3.10). The cervical cap is thimble-shaped and suitable for those with poor muscle tone. Fitting is unaffected by the size or shape of vagina but it is not suitable for women with a short or badly torn cervix. The Dumas or Vault cap is a hemispherical bowl and is best for those who are not suitable for a cervical cap. The Vimule is a combination of cervical and vault cap and is suitable for patients with a very long cervix.

Summary of key points

- Ideally diaphragms and caps should be used in conjunction with spermicides to achieve maximum efficacy.
- Women who are prone to recurrent UTIs should not use a diaphragm.
- A diaphragm should be replaced every 2 years and refitted after the birth of a child or if the woman gains or loses >5 kg in weight.
- The efficacy of diaphragms and caps depends on user motivation to insert the device before every act of intercourse.

ADDRESSING NON-COMPLIANCE WITH CONTRACEPTION

In the USA, half (48%) of all pregnancies are unintended and it is estimated that half of all women aged 15–44 in the USA have had at least one unintended pregnancy.[68] It is important for GPs to realise that many of these pregnancies occur when a woman is using contraception. Within 1 year of starting to use a reversible method of contraception, 9% of women experience a contraceptive failure. This occurs in 7% of women using the pill, 9% using a male condom and in 19% practising withdrawal.[69]

These figures are very different from the contraceptive failure rates of <1% for combined oral contraception and <2–4% for progestogen-only pills that medical students are taught about in medical school. The reason for the differences in these figures relates to the differences between 'perfect users' and 'typical users.'

It is difficult enough for an adult to remember to take a pill every day, and in the case of the mini-pill within the same 3-hour window every 24 hours, but think about what you were like when you were a teenager and the lifestyle you led before you started working and had a reasonable daily routine. It then becomes easy to understand why contraceptive failures occur: because of sleeping in, going away,

CASE STUDY: She shouldn't have discontinued the pill.

Sally is 17 years old. She presents with an unplanned pregnancy of 9 weeks' gestation. Her history is one that is unfortunately commonly heard and not often addressed.

Sally had become sexually active about 10 months previously with her new boyfriend, James. At the commencement of sexual activity, she had conscientiously fronted up to her GP and requested contraception. She had used this successfully, but had not yet told her mother that she was on the pill. Some 2 years earlier, when Sally had suffered from moderately severe acne and been recommended the pill as a treatment modality, her mother had convinced her not to use it. Her mother had told her about all the side effects of the pill and how 'it could cause infertility later in life'. She had been convinced that she should avoid using it unless she was having sex.

Unfortunately, these messages stuck in Sally's mind. When her relationship with James broke up after 6 months, she did as her mother had advised and stopped taking the pill straight away.

The problem with Sally is that she is a teenager. Teenagers often engage in serial monogamy. As it came to pass, less than 1 month later, she met Pete and pretty soon became sexually active with him. While she restarted the pill soon after, the window of opportunity was there before the pill became active and the unplanned pregnancy resulted.

forgetting to restart the next packet after your period or hiding your pills so your mum will not find them and, then, because they are out of sight, they are out of mind and forgotten.

True contraceptive failure is rare. User failure usually occurs because of one of two reasons: either poor compliance or, as in Sally's case, discontinuation.

How common is non-compliance in users of the pill?

A study of compliance in oral contraceptive users using a questionnaire-based method found that 47% of users missed one or more pills per cycle and 22% missed two or more. [70] The same study found that women who lacked an established pill-taking routine, who had not read the information contained in the pill packet or who experienced spotting or heavy bleeding were more likely to miss pills. Interestingly, the authors record that 22% of users called their provider at least once because of pill-related side effects and some 9% visited their provider at least once for the same reason.

A more ingenious study measured non-compliance rates by using a microelectronic device that recorded whether each pill was removed from the packet. [71] The researchers compared this electronic data with information gathered directly from the women in the study, who kept a diary of their pill compliance over the same period of time. In 3 months of pill use, the electronic and self-reported data agreed on the number of days when pills were missed only 45% of the time; the level of agreement dropped from 55% in the first month to 38% in the third month. In each month, the proportion of no missed pills reported by the women was much higher than the proportion recorded electronically (53–59% versus 19–33%), and the proportion of at least three pills missed according to the electronic data was triple that derived from the women's reports (30–51% versus 10–14%). In addition, the electronic data recorded substantially more episodes in which women missed pills on two or more consecutive days (88 versus 30). These figures are staggeringly high and make one wonder how oral contraception is effective at all.

Is non-compliance an issue with injectable contraception?

Compliance rates are also relatively poor in users of injectable contraception such as Depo-Provera®. An injection of Depo-Provera® must be given routinely every 12 weeks, with a leeway of 2 weeks on either side of the due date. Yet often GPs find that the woman returns several weeks late for the injection. In a study conducted in South Africa, 30.4% of injectable contraception users and 18.4% of oral contraceptive users had stopped using their method temporarily before returning to the same method (called the non-use segment). [72] These women had not used any other form of contraception during this time. Almost one-third of injectable users (31.2%) had been late for their next injection at least once. Although nearly all women using injectables had experienced some menstrual disturbances, over one-third (38.5%) had not been informed by their providers about the possibility of these changes. Many women gave the disruption of their menstrual cycle as the reason for the non-use segment.

Are users of barrier methods often non-compliant?

In a review of factors affecting the consistent use of barrier methods of contraception, reasons for poor compliance are divided into method characteristics and user characteristics. [73] Method characteristics include the extent of interference with sexual spontaneity and enjoyment, the extent of partner cooperation required and the ability of the method to protect against human immunodeficiency virus and other sexually transmitted diseases. User characteristics include motivation to avoid unintended pregnancy, ability to plan, comfort with sexuality, and previous contraceptive use. Stage of sexual career, relationship characteristics, and physical and sexual abuse are important situational influences. These factors have a certain degree of universality for all methods of contraception.

Why and when do women discontinue contraceptive use?

Factors that are related to women discontinuing contraception are similar to those discussed above when looking at compliance. One of the main factors is the woman's beliefs about contraception. This is particularly important in the case of hormonal contraception. The old myths are still prevalent: it causes cancer, it makes you infertile later on, you need to have a break from it every now and then, it makes you put on weight and it will ruin your skin. Anecdotally, another important factor seems to be the desire in some women to assess if they really are fertile and can conceive.

How fast discontinuation occurs in some women is surprising for GPs, who will usually give a script for the pill for 12 months and therefore do not follow up very often. Trussell and Vaughan[69] found that overall, 31% of women discontinue the use of a reversible contraceptive for a method-related reason within 6 months of starting use and 44% do so within 12 months. However, 68% of discontinuers recommence use of a method within 1 month and 76% do so within 3 months.

What can GPs do to improve contraceptive compliance, reduce discontinuation rates and therefore reduce the number of unplanned pregnancies?

The answer is to provide good contraceptive counselling. First, the patient should choose the form of contraception that she feels she can manage best and that suits her and her individual circumstances. In practice, this means that a GP should ask two critical questions when engaging in contraceptive counselling:

1. How important is it for you not to be pregnant at this point in time?
2. How important is it for you to have predictable, well-controlled periods?

The answers to these two questions will determine which type of contraceptive method is best suited to a particular woman.

Two important questions that guide contraceptive options:
1. How important is it for you not to be pregnant at this point in time?
2. How important is it for you to have predictable, well-controlled periods?

Next, GPs have to be well informed about the methods they prescribe and give accurate information to patients about the side effects and potential pitfalls they may experience. This information should include whether or not side effects will persist and what the woman can do about them. One of the most important messages to give is that the user should not stop the contraception until she has spoken to you, as this may give you an opportunity to prevent discontinuation and offer help if any problems have occurred or the patient has any concerns.

Counselling tricks include asking the woman if she has heard anything bad about that particular form of contraception. This will give you the opportunity to dispel any myths. If it is a young woman, ask her whether or not she has discussed contraception with her mother and what her mother has advised her. Then you can educate not only your patient but her mother as well.

Non-compliance is a real problem and is often due to common myths about various forms of contraception.

You should also use the consultation as an opportunity to foreshadow any issue that might give rise to non-compliance. Ask the woman what time of day she will take her pill and give her some cues to think about. One idea is that she could keep the pill packet by her toothbrush so that she can see it every morning and remember to take her pill when she brushes her teeth. Another useful tip is to advise the patient to always keep an extra packet of pills in her handbag, so that if she remembers at work that she forgot to take the pill that morning, she has one to take on the spot. If she is a condom user, then make sure she knows that she should have a couple of condoms in her handbag too … just in case!

Most importantly, the GP should have at hand some good patient education material to give to patients when they commence contraception. This is widely available and can complement the sometimes confusing and frightening information that is included in the packets. Your local drug representative should also have a good collection of question-and-answer booklets about the pill that can be handed out.

The last thing to make sure of is that you have at least informed the woman about the availability of emergency contraception and given her an information sheet about it. Best practice takes this one step further and is to prescribe her emergency contraception to keep at home and to explain to her how to use it as a last resort.

By taking all these steps you will have done your best to ensure that, at least in your patients, non-compliance and discontinuation rates are low and that the contraception you prescribe has the best chance of success.

Summary of key points

- Contraceptive compliance rates are poor.
- Women may discontinue contraception because of false beliefs regarding contraception or because of method-related problems.
- GPs can improve compliance by:
  - allowing patients to choose the type of contraception that suits them
  - providing accurate information about each contraceptive method, including side effects and potential pitfalls
  - encouraging women not to stop use of their contraceptive method before speaking to the GP about it
  - providing take-home patient education material.

NATURAL FAMILY PLANNING

The concept of natural family planning is one to which most women are attracted. Natural family planning is the method used by many Catholics and those of other religions in which the use of contraception is prohibited. Before recommending it, however, GPs should be aware of the fact that, to use natural family planning successfully, both partners need to accept the limitations that it will have on sexual activity, and the relationship between the man and the woman needs to be an equal and respectful one.

The successful use of natural family planning requires a man and woman to be in a relationship where there is equality and where abstinence at some points of the menstrual cycle can be agreed upon by both parties.

There are several methods available to couples who want to use natural family planning; the most effective of these is the symptothermal method. All women should have a basic understanding of their own reproductive physiology and anatomy, regardless of whether or not they use this knowledge to assist with contraception. Unfortunately, this knowledge is not really addressed in sex education in schools and yet it is probably among the most critical information a woman can have in order to control her own fertility.

How do I explain the concepts involved in natural family planning to a patient and her partner?

During a normal monthly menstrual cycle, hormonal fluctuations result in a temperature rise at the time of ovulation, cervical mucus changes and changes in the cervix (texture, position in vagina and os size). Natural family planning involves developing an awareness of these changes (fertility awareness) and then working out when sexual intercourse is safe.

When is it safe to have intercourse?

The best way to decide when ovulation is occurring is the symptothermal method, otherwise known as the Billings method. This involves an awareness of the cervical mucus changes, with confirmation by observation of the rise in temperature.

A few days before ovulation, oestrogen causes the cervical mucus secretions to become thin and watery (much like raw egg white in appearance). The consistency changes after ovulation, induced by progesterone, to a thick, sticky, yellowy film impenetrable to sperm. Women learn to feel this mucus change and avoid sexual intercourse when the mucus is thin. (See also Ch 8 and Fig 8.5.)

In order to observe cervical mucus changes accurately, a couple can have intercourse only every second day. This is so that the woman can be confident that the mucus is cervical, rather than a mixture of semen and cervical mucus that results from intercourse.

Feeling the cervix can also help to determine the start of ovulation. The cervix becomes softer prior to ovulation and the os become wider; after ovulation, the cervix feels harder and the os closed to the fingertip.

At ovulation, the rise in progesterone causes the body temperature to rise (0.2–0.6 °C). If a woman relies only on measuring her temperature as an indicator of ovulation, she may have sex the night before she observes the rise and therefore conceive.

What is the calendar method?

In the calendar method, first the shortest and longest menstrual cycles over the previous six cycles are recorded. By subtracting 20 from the length of the shortest cycle, the first day of the fertile period is obtained. Likewise, by subtracting 11 from the length of the longest cycle, the last day of the fertile period can be identified.

How successful is natural family planning?

The failure rates for natural methods vary from 3% to 20%, but if more than one indicator method is used, and the couple is committed to its use, the lower rates can be achieved.

How can Persona be used to prevent pregnancy?

The Persona microcomputer plots a woman's luteinising and oestrone-3-glucuronide hormone levels using urine dipsticks. The computer indicates by red and green lights the unsafe and safe days to have sexual intercourse. The failure rate is about 5/100 woman-years.

Summary of key points

- All women should be aware of bodily changes that herald the fertile time of their menstrual cycle.
- The effective use of the natural family planning method for contraception can take place only in a relationship characterised by equality and respect, where both partners accept the limitations the method places on sexual activity.
- The symptothermal, or Billings, method is the most efficacious natural family planning method.
- The symptothermal method uses the recognition of fertile cervical mucus and temperature rise as markers of impending ovulation.

EMERGENCY CONTRACEPTION

What is the probability of conception occurring?

Patients are very poorly informed about the risk of conception occurring after a single act of intercourse. Many believe that pregnancy is a dead certainty, especially if sex occurred several days after the woman's period. The reality is that the probability of conception after a single act of intercourse has been calculated to be 33% if intercourse occurs on average every other day.[74,75] If sex occurs only once a week, the risk of pregnancy is only 15%. Most women who have intercourse on one single occasion will therefore not conceive. Conception occurs only around the time of ovulation. The exact number of days when a woman is fertile is difficult to calculate, because, while sperm remain active in the genital tract and are capable of fertilisation for up to 5 days, the egg is capable of being fertilised only for 24 hours. Fertilisation is most likely in the 6 days leading up to ovulation and most unlikely when intercourse occurs after ovulation.

So what is emergency contraception?

Emergency contraception used to be called 'the morning-after pill'. This name was found to misrepresent the true window of opportunity for use of emergency contraception, so it has been discarded. Emergency contraception is the only form of contraception that can be taken after unprotected intercourse to prevent pregnancy.

When is it needed?

Emergency contraception is called for in several situations, the most obvious being when no form of contraception was used during an episode of intercourse. However, women often present to GPs when a condom slipped off or broke during intercourse, or when she forgot to take one or more of her oral contraceptive pills. The other time of need is after a sexual assault.

All of these situations necessitate further advice. Broken condoms do occur and if that is the case the GP should advise the use of extra lubrication and more care when applying the condom. A condom will slip off when the male partner fails to withdraw his penis when still erect and even then the condom must be held at the base of the penis until he is well away from the woman's genital area. Only then should the condom be removed.

In the situation of missed pills, the GP must explore the following:

- In which section of the pill packet were the pills missed?
- Did intercourse occur and, if so, how many times and when?

CASE STUDY: 'I'm too young to be a grandfather.'

A GP colleague of mine rang me the other day. His 20-year-old daughter had recently arrived from another city where she was living for a holiday. Somehow he had come to learn that with the packing and travelling she had forgotten to recommence her oral contraception and had missed the first two active pills in the packet. 'I'm too young to be a grandfather', he confided as he asked me if she needed emergency contraception and how successful it might be at preventing an unplanned pregnancy.

Using the flow chart in Figure 3.1, the GP can then determine whether emergency contraception is necessary.

Types and use of emergency contraception

What kind of emergency contraception (EC) is available and when and how do you take it?

Progestogen-only EC is now the preferred method. The levonorgestrel EC method is preferred because of its greater efficacy and superior side-effect profile. For maximal effect, it should be started as soon as possible and within 72 hours of unprotected intercourse. Indeed, a randomised trial showed that the proportion of expected pregnancies prevented was 95% if the EC was used within the first 24 hours after unprotected sex. This dropped to 85% if the EC was taken at 25–48 hours and to 58% at 49–72 hours.[76]

Levonorgestrel should be given as a single 1.5 mg dose as soon as possible after unprotected intercourse and within 72 hours.

A single dose[77] of 1.5 mg of levonorgestrel is just as effective as two doses of 0.75 mg and, while it can also provide some protection when used on the fourth or even fifth day after unprotected intercourse, an IUD might be preferable in this circumstance.

The Yuzpe method was the most commonly used form of EC for many years. It consists of:

- 100 mg of ethinyloestradiol, together with 500 mg of levonorgestrel, commenced within 72 hours of unprotected intercourse and repeated 12 hours later.
- A Maxalon or Stemetil tablet taken with each dose of hormones. Some 50% of women taking EC experience nausea and 20% actually vomit.

Four tablets of Nordette 30 or Microgynon 30 taken twice, 12 hours apart, can be used as a substitute. Triphasic pills can be used in the same way if the eight tablets between days 12 and 21 of the pack are used.

The Yuzpe method of EC is somewhat less efficacious than using levonorgestrel, but remains an option.

An IUD can be inserted and used as EC. The benefit of this is that it can be inserted up to 5 days after intercourse. However, GPs need to be aware of the risks of STDs when unprotected intercourse has occurred.

Sixteen-year-old Mandy presented to see if she could get 'the morning-after pill', which her girlfriend had told her about. She didn't know what it was and she didn't know if she could still take it because it was now the afternoon and not the morning after and anyway she had had unprotected sex more than once in the last couple of days.

This was Mandy's second sexual partner after having become sexually active 6 months beforehand. She had been with this partner for 3 months. After they had had sex several times and she knew that they were 'together', she decided to start the pill. She had tried to mention condoms to him a couple of times, but he had only mumbled something back about the fact that he hated wearing them. Fearing that he might leave her for someone else because 'he only has to click his fingers and girls come running', she decided that she would act responsibly and start the pill. It made her feel more grown-up and adult-like being on the pill anyway. The current problem had arisen when she had realised that in this, her second month of taking Nordette, she had forgotten to restart the pill and had missed the first two tablets of the packet.

As in any other consultation in sexual and reproductive health, a request for emergency contraception raises several important issues that need to be addressed in order to implement best management. Why has this contraceptive method failed? Why weren't they using barrier methods? Why did the partner not want to use condoms? Why was this young couple unable to discuss this issue in an open and honest way? Why is Mandy here by herself? Is she at risk of an STD? Has she in fact thought about the risk of contracting an STD above and beyond her risk of pregnancy?

The International Planned Parenthood Federation (IPPF) recommendations for the type and timing of EC are given in Box 3.12.

How does emergency contraception work?

The regimens of EC currently available do not act as abortifacients. The mechanism of action of hormonal emergency contraception may be different according to whether or not ovulation has occurred when the pills are taken. If taken before ovulation, it is likely that emergency contraception actually inhibits ovulation. In other situations it may work by:

- trapping sperm in thickened cervical mucus
- inhibiting tubal transport of the egg or sperm
- interfering with fertilisation, early cell division, or transport of embryo
- preventing implantation by disrupting the uterine lining.

How safe is it?

While detractors of EC claim that GPs are subjecting women to 'mega doses' of hormones, EC is extremely safe. The Yuzpe method has been marketed by Schering as PC4 in the UK for many years and used in that country on more than four million occasions. During this time, there have been 115 reports of 159 reactions, 61 of which were pregnancies. There were only three cases of DVT and three of CVA, but none had clear correlations with the time that PC4 was used.[78] Research has shown there to be no effect on clotting factors and the International Planned Parenthood Federation has declared there to be no absolute contraindications to EC. With regard to progestogen-only EC, there are no contraindications to its use.

There are no contraindications to the use of progestogen-only emergency contraception.

What are the side effects?

The most common side effects of the Yuzpe method of EC are nausea and vomiting. About 50% of women experience nausea and 20% vomit. Hence, modern regimens of the Yuzpe method include the use of Maxalon or Stemetil, as described above.

With regard to side effects, the levonorgestrel EC method is favourable compared with the Yuzpe method: only mild nausea is sometimes experienced.

When should the woman recommence her normal contraceptive measures?

A common mistake in the prescription of EC is to advise the woman to wait until her next period before recommencing her oral contraception. What then often occurs is that the EC delays the woman's ovulation and then another episode of unprotected intercourse occurs, and the woman falls pregnant as a result of the second time she has unprotected sex.

There is no need to delay the commencement of contraception after EC is used. The best advice is to take the EC and 24 hours later to commence with the corresponding active hormone pill in the packet or another effective form of contraception. The woman must be advised to use condoms or abstain from sex for 7 days, but this is often a shorter delay than waiting for her next period.

Can EC be used more than once in a cycle?

The UK Faculty of Family Planning and Reproductive Health Care supports repeated use of EC in a cycle if repeated unprotected intercourse has occurred. If the unprotected intercourse has occurred within 12 hours of a EC dose, it is the consensus view of the faculty that further EC is not necessary.[79]

Repeated use of emergency contraception in a cycle is recommended if repeated unprotected intercourse has occurred.

What is recommended for women using liver-enzyme-inducing drugs?

Women using liver-enzyme-inducing drugs should be advised that an IUD is the preferred option for EC; however, where oral EC is desired they should be advised to take a total of 3 mg (two tablets) as a single dose, as soon as possible and within the 72 hours of unprotected sexual intercourse.[52]

What follow-up is needed?

Of those women who do not immediately start hormonal contraception after taking a dose of EC, more than 80% before, or within 2 days after, their expected date of menstruation; and 95% menstruate within 7 days after their expected date.[77] Generally speaking, EC users should be advised to have a pregnancy test if menstruation is delayed by more than 7 days, or is lighter than usual.[52] GPs may, however, recommend a routine follow-up to screen for STDs and to ensure that the woman has commenced or is continuing with a reliable contraceptive method.

Users of emergency contraception should be advised to have a pregnancy test if menstruation is delayed by more than 7 days, or is lighter than usual.

Does providing EC encourage risk-taking in women?

It is estimated that half of unintended pregnancies could be averted if EC were easily accessible and used. In trying to facilitate this, advance provision has been advocated. A Scottish study randomised women either to receive counselling and EC on demand or to receive EC in advance for later use should the need arise.[80] The results of this study showed that women who received EC in advance:

- were more likely to use EC (47% versus 27% of women who received counselling only [$p = 0.001$])
- were not more likely to use EC repeatedly
- used other methods of contraception equally well
- had fewer unintended pregnancies (3.3% versus 4.8% of women who received only counselling [$p = 0.14$]).

Given that there are no contraindications to EC use, another tactic has been to promote pharmacy access to EC (i.e. avoiding the need for a woman to have to seek a doctor's appointment for a prescription). A recent study compared advance provision, direct pharmacy access and doctor's provision of EC[81] and found that:

- women in the pharmacy access group were no more likely to use EC
- women in the advance-provision group were almost twice as likely to use EC than controls (even though the frequency of unprotected intercourse was similar)
- no matter to which group the women were assigned, only half of the study participants who had unprotected intercourse used EC over the study period
- women in the pharmacy access and advance-provision groups did not experience a significant reduction in pregnancy rate or increase in STIs
- there were no differences in the study group's patterns of contraceptive or condom use or sexual behaviours.

The authors concluded that, while removing the requirement to go through pharmacists or clinics to obtain EC increases use, the public health impact may be negligible because of high rates of unprotected intercourse and relative under-utilisation of the method. Given that there is clear evidence that neither pharmacy access nor advance provision compromises contraceptive or sexual behavior, it seems unreasonable to restrict access to EC to clinics.

What measures can the GP institute to increase awareness of EC among patients?

Good contraceptive counselling involves letting each woman of reproductive age who comes to your surgery know about the availability of EC. This can be achieved through the use of posters and brochures in the waiting room and by giving out information to each woman (or couple) you see who is either starting or using contraception. The evidence from the Scottish study described above[80] suggests that GPs should also be prescribing EC to women to keep at home so that it can be commenced on the woman's own initiative, instead of making her go through the embarrassment of presenting when she has need of it.

Are there any legal issues to consider?

Recently, several cases have been settled out of court in which women have sued their doctors for failing to diagnose pregnancy and therefore not giving them the opportunity to have an abortion. Since EC is the only treatment available to prevent unintended pregnancy after unprotected intercourse, it follows that soon GPs may be considered liable for failure to provide EC.

Is access to EC a right?

While some health professionals may have religious objections to the provision of EC, the argument has been made for the right of women to access EC, along with other contraceptive methods, and for the availability of EC over the counter with no minimum age for access.[82] These arguments are made on the basis that the principles of autonomy, non-maleficence and beneficence all weigh in favour of the rights of a woman faced with the possibility of an unintended pregnancy to unrestricted access to EC against providers whose religious views are opposed to this.[82]

Where can I get further information?

Princeton University is host to an excellent website (http://ec.princeton.edu/) on emergency contraception.

Conclusions

EC is a saviour for many women, especially young women who often have not started on the pill and find themselves having unprotected intercourse. The risk of pregnancy suddenly seems very real and they are very grateful to be able to fall back on EC while they decide what method of long-term contraception will best meet their future needs.

The challenge for health professionals and educators is how to let young people know about the availability of EC essentially before they seek advice regarding their long-term contraceptive needs. Part of the answer may be in incorporating information about EC into school-based sexuality and contraception education. Another suggestion is to make EC available over the counter at pharmacies. GPs should also be using any opportunity they have where there is contact between people of reproductive age and a health professional to provide this information. Health professionals also need to be made more aware of EC, how it works, its efficacy and possible side effects. They must act as the front line in promoting it and making sure that their patients or clients know about its existence. This can be done during a consultation by the provision of handouts or with pamphlets or posters in waiting rooms, as well as by making it known that EC is a service provided by incorporating this in practice or pharmacy information brochures.

Another way of making EC more available would be to provide the pills in advance of the event so that women can have them ready at home to take in an emergency situation. Having EC at home may also give a woman extra confidence in her primary method of contraception. A routine family planning or health maintenance visit is an ideal opportunity to discuss emergency options and review medical history and examination findings in order to identify the need for emergency contraceptive use and to review instructions for deciding about and using the treatment. If the woman is able to understand the instruction sheet and is certain that she does not want to be pregnant, then providing an emergency contraceptive kit to have on hand is an excellent idea.

Summary of key points

- The most efficacious form of EC is the levonorgestrel method, which involves one dose of 1.5 mg taken as soon as possible and within 72 hours of intercourse.
- An IUD can be used as EC up to 5 days after unprotected intercourse.
- There are no contraindications to the use of progestogen-only EC.
- Follow-up should involve a pregnancy test, STD screen and review of current contraception.
- Women need to be made aware of the availability of EC.
- EC should and can be made more available by providing it proactively either through GPs or over the counter at pharmacies.

STERILISATION

CASE STUDY: Vasectomy or tubal sterilisation?

Margaret is a 34-year-old G3 P2. Her youngest child is now 6 months old and she presents requesting advice about future contraception. She would like her husband to have a vasectomy but his mumbled response has been, 'I don't like the idea of being cut down there'. She therefore wants to find out about tubal sterilisation.

A familiar scenario? Frustratingly, it is common for the woman to present alone to this type of consultation. This means men rarely get to hear about vasectomy firsthand. The decision as to who in a couple undertakes a sterilisation procedure is therefore rarely made with both partners fully informed.

What issues need to be addressed when a patient asks to be sterilised?

GPs are often consulted for advice about sterilisation. Several issues need to be addressed when counselling couples before they go on to have the procedure:

- Why has the couple decided on sterilisation?
- Who initiated the idea?
- Are they aware of how the procedures are carried out and the risks and possible side effects, including the increased risk of ectopic pregnancy following tubal sterilisation if it fails?
- Have they considered how they might feel if their marriage ended or if a child might happen to die? Although it may be possible to reverse the procedure the success rates of this vary and it is unlikely to be done on a public waiting list.
- Does either partner feel ambivalent or coerced?
- What role does fertility have in the way the woman feels about her femininity and the man his masculinity?

TABLE 3.9 A comparison between vasectomy and tubal sterilisation (From Errey[92])

	Vasectomy	Tubal sterilisation
Efficacy	Very effective	Very effective
Time to be effective	Effective 3–6 months after surgery—requires confirmation	Effective immediately
Complications	Almost no risk of internal injuries or other life-threatening complications Very slight possibility of serious infection No anaesthetic-related deaths	Slight risk of internal injuries or other life-threatening complications Slight possibility of serious infection Few anaesthetic-related deaths
Acceptability	Minute scar Less expensive Slightly more reversible	Small scar More expensive Slightly less reversible
Procedure	Usually performed under local anaesthetic Back-up facilities needed	Systemic sedation as well as local anaesthesia required No back-up facilities needed
Possible long-term side effects	None demonstrated	Slight risk of ectopic pregnancy

- Are they aware of the availability of long-acting reversible forms of contraception as an alternative to sterilisation?

What are the chances that someone will ask to have a reversal of their sterilisation?

Essentially, if a person undergoes a sterilisation procedure voluntarily because they do not want to conceive and parent a new child, subsequent requests for reversal are low. Like other procedures such as abortion, coercion by other parties leads to feelings of regret afterwards. Thankfully, in most countries there is no legal necessity for a woman or a man to obtain their spouse's permission to be sterilised. Problems are also more likely to occur if the couple is experiencing marital conflict or have recently been involved in a crisis situation such as an unplanned pregnancy and abortion. Similarly, sterilisation is also commonly requested immediately after the birth of a new baby, sometimes at the time of a caesarean section. Even though perinatal mortality is very low in developed countries, couples are better off waiting at least 6 months after the birth of a new baby before proceeding with a sterilisation procedure, although patient autonomy should be respected.

Reversals of sterilisation procedures are difficult and not always successful, so couples should think very carefully before embarking on sterilisation, be it for the man or the woman. The younger the patient, the greater the regret, and the cumulative risk of pregnancy rises in the 10 years from the age that the procedure is carried out, so patients are best advised to opt for alternative forms of contraception until they reach 35+.

Which should I recommend, a vasectomy or tubal sterilisation?

When comparing vasectomy and tubal sterilisation, medical practitioners should point out that vasectomy is clearly a less risky procedure as it is a superficial operation, while tubal sterilisation is an intra-abdominal procedure. Vasectomy also carries a lower failure rate in terms of post-procedure pregnancies. The advantages and disadvantages of each procedure are listed in Table 3.9.

Does a vasectomy have any side effects or long-term implications?

Men have three main fears about vasectomy: the impact of the procedure on sexual functioning, pain likely to be encountered and long-term adverse effects.[83] It is important to dispel these fears with an accurate explanation about the anatomy of the male reproductive tract. Point out that ligation of the vas does not affect hormone production (which is responsible for libido) and that there is no compromise in the ability to attain and maintain an erection, nor a decrease in the amount of ejaculate emitted. Men may have heard that vasectomy has been linked to cancers of the reproductive tract (especially prostate cancer) and cardiovascular disease, and it is important to point out that newer, more rigorous studies have contradicted these findings and are more accurate.[84] It may also be reassuring to point out that peak bodies such as the American National Institute of Health and the World Health Organization continue to recommend vasectomy as a safe form of permanent contraception.

Vasectomy is not associated with any long-term adverse outcomes.

Do women have a higher risk of menstrual problems after tubal sterilisation?

Women may have heard from friends who have had a tubal sterilisation that their chances of menstrual problems and having a hysterectomy are greater after the procedure—the so-called 'post-tubal-sterilisation syndrome'. This issue has been debated in the literature, as early studies reported on increased menstrual and intermenstrual bleeding and increased rates of hysterectomy.[85]

Unfortunately, these early studies were not controlled for use of oral contraceptive pills. It is thought that many women who have a tubal sterilisation procedure have up to that point been on the pill. The COCP reduces the total amount of blood loss during menstruation and therefore women who stop the pill on having a tubal ligation may perceive normal blood loss to be heavy. Another confounding factor may be the fact that women usually have the procedure carried out during their 30s. As women enter their 40s, blood loss may increase anyway. The reports about increased rates of hysterectomy can also be explained by the fact that women who have chosen to end their fertility by a permanent surgical method of contraception are more likely to opt for a permanent cure to their menstrual problems by means of hysterectomy rather than rely on medical methods.

A recent review of the literature in this area[86] and a recent large prospective cohort study[87] have concluded that there is little or no support for the existence of a post-tubal-sterilisation syndrome.

Tubal sterilisation is not associated with an increased risk of menorrhagia or hysterectomy.

Is tubal sterilisation 100% effective?

One issue that is not often addressed in counselling is the information that has been available since 1996 concerning the efficacy of tubal sterilisation. This arose from a multicentre, prospective cohort study that followed 10,685 women for between 8 and 14 years.[88] It found the failure rates of most methods used for tubal sterilisation to be higher than those in previously published reports. More importantly, this

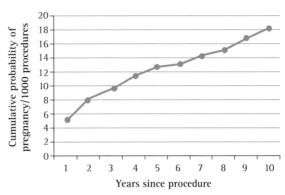

FIGURE 3.11 Cumulative probability of pregnancy among women undergoing tubal sterilisation for all methods (From Peterson et al[88])

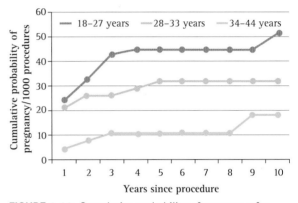

FIGURE 3.12 Cumulative probability of pregnancy for women undergoing tubal sterilisation by spring clip application, by age (From Peterson et al[88])

study established that doctors cannot quote a single figure as a failure rate for sterilisation, as there is a cumulative risk of pregnancy that rises as time passes (Fig 3.11). The study also found that the cumulative risk of pregnancy after tubal sterilisation varied with the age of the woman (Fig 3.12). Those women who had the procedure carried out at a younger age were more likely to have a sterilisation failure. It is also important to advise women that about a third of all sterilisation failures will be ectopic pregnancies.

The cumulative risk of pregnancy after tubal sterilisation increases with time.

Does a vasectomy result in instant sterilisation?

A vasectomy needs to be planned, with alternative forms of contraception used until two specimens of semen are free of sperm. Few couples realise that this may take between 3 and 6 months after the procedure is carried out (it usually occurs soon after 20 ejaculations have occurred).

How does vasectomy compare with tubal ligation in terms of risk of pregnancy?

Pregnancy can occur several years after either form of sterilisation. The risk of pregnancy with tubal sterilisation is higher than the risk with vasectomy[89] (Box 3.13).

How are tubal sterilisations carried out?

Until recently tubal sterilisations were carried out exclusively intra-abdominally, usually laparascopically using a variety of methods (Table 3.10 and Fig 3.13). A new method has now become available: hysteroscopic sterilisation (one brand of this method is called Essure). It uses a hysteroscopic method to place a coil inside the tubes, generating an inflammatory response that blocks the tubes. An early trial shows high efficacy if the device is correctly inserted[90] but prior to assuring women of contraceptive efficacy investigations must be carried out to ensure that the tubes are indeed blocked. These tests are usually undertaken 3 months after the procedure.

How are vasectomies carried out?

Two methods are now used to perform a vasectomy: the traditional method and the newer 'no scalpel' vasectomy method developed in China in the 1970s. The benefits of the latter method include lower rates of haematoma and wound infection and quicker recovery times. Sperm granulomas are still thought to occur in up to 25% of cases. The efficacy of the procedure seems to be more reliant on the methods used to occlude the vas, with electrocautery being more effective than ligation.

Summary of key points

- A vasectomy is a safer procedure than a tubal sterilisation.
- It is important to try to counsel couples together about sterilisation when they are trying to decide who will have the procedure.

BOX 3.13 Risk of pregnancy with form of sterilisation (From RCOG[12])

Tubal ligation
- The lifetime risk of pregnancy for tubal ligation is one in 200.
- Ten years after Filshie clip application, risk of pregnancy is two to three per 1000 procedures.

Vasectomy
After clearance, the risk of pregnancy is one in 2000.

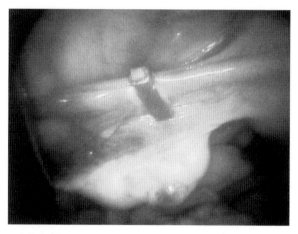

FIGURE 3.13 Sterilisation clip (From Rymer et al[95])

TABLE 3.10 Methods of occluding the fallopian tubes

Ligation with partial salpingectomy	The fallopian tubes are cut and tied with suture material. The modified Pomeroy method, which is common, involves tying a small loop in the tube and then cutting off the top segment of the loop.
Unipolar coagulation	Electrical current is used to block the fallopian tubes. This can be performed through the laparoscope and causes extensive damage to the tubes, making reversal harder to carry out if needed.
Bipolar coagulation	Usually causes less damage to the tubes than unipolar coagulation. This characteristic may, however, lead to the method's lower rate of effectiveness.
Silicone bands	A small round elastic band is stretched and then slipped over a loop of the fallopian tube. This can be carried out through a laparoscope and causes minimal damage to the tubes.
Spring clips (e.g. the Hulka clip and Filshie clips)	This method places a clip across each fallopian tube using a laparoscope and out of all methods causes the least damage to the tubes.

- Vasectomy does not lead to an increased risk of prostate cancer.
- Tubal sterilisation does not lead to increased rates of menstrual problems and hysterectomy.
- The cumulative risk of pregnancy following tubal sterilisation rises as time passes: women who have the procedure at a younger age are more likely to have a sterilisation failure.
- Post-vasectomy, a man needs to have two semen analyses carried out to ensure that the ejaculate is free of sperm and that the vasectomy has been successful.

TIPS FOR PRACTITIONERS

- Instead of starting a 20-minute tirade on important points about taking the pill, incorporate a short quiz into the counselling in order to get the young woman more involved.
- In assessing whether an adolescent is a mature minor, the GP can ask the young woman what she thinks will happen if she can't start on the pill and whether or not she feels able to inform her parents about being sexually active and commencing on contraception.
- Stress to women taking the COCP that those who are later-restarters are at high risk of pill failure because they lengthen the pill-free interval beyond 7 days.
- Most patients are embarrassed when asked if they know how to use a condom, but allowing them to practice placing and removing a condom on a plastic model will give them more confidence to use condoms in real-life situations.
- Users of the mini-pill should be instructed to take it 12 hours before the usual time that they engage in sexual activity in order to gain maximum effectiveness: for example if a woman usually has sex at night, she should take her mini-pill in the morning.
- Women who get regular periods on the mini-pill are at greatest risk of falling pregnant while taking it.
- Women suffering from oestrogen withdrawal headaches when using the COCP can either use a low-dose of HRT in the pill-free week or can shorten the pill-free interval or eradicate it altogether.
- Sometimes IUD strings get drawn up into the endocervix and are easily brought down by inserting a 'cytobrush' or a small pair of alligator forceps into the endocervix and looking for the strings.

- When removing an IUD, a GP should use sponge forceps and pull downwards with a smooth and strong action similar to that used when removing a placenta.
- In cases of BTB on the pill where a woman has taken the pills correctly, the woman should first be encouraged to continue for at least 3 months before changing pills.
- In this day and age, one of the few indications for using a COCP containing 50 mg of oestrogen is when the woman is on anti-epileptics that interact with the pill.

REFERENCES

1. World Health Organization Scientific Group. Cardiovascular disease and steroid hormone contraception (Technical Report Series 877). Geneva: WHO; 1998.
2. Beral V, Hermon C, Kay C, et al. Mortality associated with oral contraceptive use: 25 year follow up of cohort of 46,000 women from Royal College of General Practitioners' oral contraception study. BMJ 1999; 318: 96–100.
3. Derman RJ. An overview of the noncontraceptive benefits and risks of oral contraception. Int J Fertil 1992; 37(Suppl 1): 19–26.
4. Vessey M, Painter R. Oral contraceptive use and cancer. Findings in a large cohort study, 1968–2004. Br J Cancer 2006; 95(3):385–389.
5. Fernandez E, La Vecchia C, Franceschi S, et al. Oral contraceptive use and risk of colorectal cancer. Epidemiology 1998; 9(3):295–300.
6. International Planned Parenthood Federation. IMAP statement on hormonal contraception. IPPF Med Bull 2002; 36. Online. Available: http://www.ippf.org/medical/bulletin/pdf/oct_02_en.pdf [accessed 26.1.03].
7. Tuckey J. Combined oral contraception and cancer. Br J Fam Plann 2000; 26:237–240.
8. Ye Z, Thomas DB, Ray RM. Combined oral contraceptives and risk of cervical carcinoma in situ. WHO Collaborative Study of Neoplasia and Steroid Contraceptives. Int J Epidemiol 1995; 24:19–26.
9. Guillebaud J. Contraception your questions answered. 5th edn. Edinburgh: Churchill Livingstone; 2009.
10. Gallo MF, Lopez LM, Grimes DA, et al. Combination contraceptives: effects on weight. Cochrane Database Syst Rev 2006; 1:CD003987.
11. World Health Organization. Improving access to quality care in family planning. Medical eligibility criteria for contraceptive use. Geneva: WHO; 1996.
12. RCOG (Royal College of Obstetricians and Gynaecologists). Male and female sterilisation, guideline summary. Evidence-based clinical guideline number 4. 2004. Online. Available: http://www.rcog.org.uk/files/rcog-corp/uploaded-files/NEBSterilisationSummary.pdf [accessed 05.07.09].
13. Westhoff C, Kerns J, Morroni C, et al. Quick start: novel oral contraceptive initiation method. Contraception 2002; 66(3):141–145.
14. Faculty of Family Planning and Reproductive Health Care Clinical Effectiveness Unit. Faculty statement from the CEU on a new publication: WHO Selected Practice Recommendations for Contraceptive Use Update. Missed pills: new recommendations. J Fam Plann Reprod Health Care 2005; 31(2):153–155.

15. Faculty of Family Planning and Reproductive Health Care Clinical Effectiveness Unit. FFPRHC Guidance (October 2003): first prescription of combined oral contraception. J Fam Plann Reprod Health Care 2003; 29(4):209–222.

16. Faculty of Family Planning and Reproductive Health Care Clinical Effectiveness Unit. FFPRHC Guidance (April 2005). Drug interactions with hormonal contraception. J Fam Plann Reprod Health Care 2005; 31(2):139–151.

17. Endrikat J, Jaques MA, Mayerhofer M, et al. A twelve-month comparative clinical investigation of two low-dose oral contraceptives containing 20 micrograms ethinylestradiol/75 micrograms gestodene and 20 micrograms ethinylestradiol/150 micrograms desogestrel, with respect to efficacy, cycle control and tolerance. Contraception 1995; 52(4):229–235.

18. Rosenberg MJ, Waugh MS. Oral contraceptive discontinuation: a prospective evaluation of frequency and reasons. Am J Obstet Gynecol 1998; 179(3 Pt 1):577–582.

19. Faculty of Sexual and Reproductive Healthcare Clinical Effectiveness Unit in collaboration with the Royal College of Obstetricians and Gynaecologists. FSRH Guidance (May 2009) Management of Unscheduled Bleeding in Women Using Hormonal Contraception. 2009. Online. Available: http://www.ffprhc.org.uk/admin/uploads/UnscheduledBleedingMay09.pdf [accessed 05.07.09].

20. Lohr PA, Creinin MD. Oral contraceptives and breakthrough bleeding: what patients need to know. J Fam Pract 2006; 55(10):872–880.

21. Kjerulff KH, Erikson B, Langenburg PW. Chronic gynecological conditions reported by US women: findings from the National Health Interview Survey, 1984 to 1992. Am J Public Health 1996; 86:195–199.

22. Grant EC. Dangers of suppressing menstruation. Lancet 2000; 356:513–514.

23. Guillebaud J. Reducing withdrawal bleeds. Lancet 2000; 355:2168–2169.

24. McGurgan P, O'Donovan P, Duffy S, et al. Should menstruation be optional for women? Lancet 2000; 355:1730.

25. Thomas SL, Ellertson C. Nuisance or natural and healthy: should monthly menstruation be optional for women? Lancet 2000; 355:922–924.

26. Demacker PN, Schade RW, Stalenhoes AS. Influence of contraceptive pill and menstrual cycle on serum lipids and high-density lipoprotein cholesterol concentrations. Br Med J (Clin Res edn) 1982; 284:1213–1215.

27. Merki-Feld GS, Hund M. Clinical experience with NuvaRing in daily practice in Switzerland: cycle control and acceptability among women of all reproductive ages. Eur J Contracept Reprod Health Care 2007; 12(3):240–247.

28. Milsom I, Lete I, Bjertnaes A, et al. Effects on cycle control and bodyweight of the combined contraceptive ring, NuvaRing, versus an oral contraceptive containing 30 microg ethinyl estradiol and 3 mg drospirenone. Hum Reprod 2006; 21(9):2304–2311.

29. Oddsson K, Leifels-Fischer B, de Melo NR, et al. Efficacy and safety of a contraceptive vaginal ring (NuvaRing) compared with a combined oral contraceptive: a 1-year randomized trial. Contraception 2005; 71(3):176–182.

30. Kennedy KI, Rivera R, McNeilly AS. Consensus statement on the use of breastfeeding as a family planning method. Contraception 1989; 39:477–496.

31. Guillebaud J. Contraception: your questions answered. 3rd edn. London: Churchill Livingstone; 1999; 344, 267.

32. Korver T. A double-blind study comparing the contraceptive efficacy, acceptability and safety of two progestogen-only pills containing desogestrel 75 µg/day or levonorgestrel 30 µg/day: Collaborative Study Group on the Desogestrel-containing Progestogen-only Pill. Eur J Contracept Reprod Health Care 1998; 3(4):169–178.

33. Faculty of Sexual and Reproductive Healthcare Clinical Effectiveness Unit. FSRH Guidance (November 2008, updated June 2009). Progestogen-only pills. 2008. Online. Available: http://www.ffprhc.org.uk/admin/uploads/CEUGuidanceProgestogenOnlyPill09.pdf [accessed 08.04.10].

34. World Health Organization. Injectable contraceptives: their role in family planning. Monograph. Geneva: WHO; 1990.

35. National Collaborating Centre for Women's and Children's Health. Long acting reversible contraception. National Institute for Health and Clinical Excellence clinical guideline 30; 2005. Online. Available: http://guidance.nice.org.uk/CG30/Guidance/pdf/English [accessed 03.07.09].

36. Croxatto HB, Makarainen L. The pharmacodynamics and efficacy of Implanon: an overview of the data. Contraception 1998; 58(Suppl): 91–99.

37. Affandi B. An integrated analysis of vaginal bleeding patterns in clinical trials of Implanon. Contraception 1998; 58(Suppl):99–101.

38. Cherry S. Implanon: the new alternative. Aust Fam Physician 2002; 31:897–900.

39. Faculty of Sexual and Reproductive Healthcare Clinical Effectiveness Unit. FSRH Guidance (April 2008) Progestogen-only implants; 2008. Online. Available: http://www.ffprhc.org.uk/admin/uploads/CEUGuidanceProgestogenOnlyImplants April08.pdf [accessed 05.07.09].

40. Weisberg E, Hickey M, Palmer D, et al. A pilot study to assess the effect of three short-term treatments on frequent and/or prolonged bleeding compared to placebo in women using Implanon. Hum Reprod 2006; 21(1):295–302.

41. Yusuf F, Siedlecky S. Contraceptive use in Australia: evidence from the 1995 National Health Survey. Aust NZ J Obstet Gynaecol 1999; 39: 58–62.

42. Hagenfeldt K. Intrauterine contraception with the copper-T device: effect on trace elements in the endometrium, cervical mucus and plasma. Contraception 1972; 6: 37–54.

43. Ullmann G, Hammerstein J. Inhibition of sperm motility in vitro by copper wire. Contraception 1972; 6:71–76.

44. Tredway DR, Umezaki CU, Mishell DR Jr, et al. Effect of intrauterine devices on sperm transport in the human being: preliminary report. Am J Obstet Gynecol 1975; 123: 734–735.

45. Sivin I. IUDs are contraceptives, not abortifacients: a comment on research and belief. Stud Fam Plann 1989; 20:355–359.

46. Alvarez F, Brache V, Fernandez E, et al. New insights on the mode of action of intrauterine contraceptive devices in women. Fertil Steril 1988; 49:768–773.

47. Segal SJ, Alvarez-Sanchez F, Adejuwon CA, et al. Absence of chorionic gonadotropin in sera of women who use intrauterine devices. Fertil Steril 1985; 44:214.

48. Grimes DA. Intrauterine device and upper-genital-tract infection. Lancet 2000; 356:1013–1019.

49. Farley TM, Rosenberg MJ, Rowe PJ, et al. Intrauterine devices and pelvic inflammatory disease: an international perspective. Lancet 1992; 339:785–788.

50. Stanwood NL, Garrett JM, Konrad TR. Obstetrician-gynecologists and the intrauterine device: a survey of attitudes and practice. Obstet Gynecol 2002; 99:275–280.

51. Gupta S, Miller JE. A survey of GP views in intra-uterine contraception. Br J Fam Plann 2000; 26:81–84.

52. Faculty of Family Planning and Reproductive Health Care. UK medical eligibility criteria for contraceptive use (UKMEC 2009). 2009. Online. Available: http://www.ffprhc.org.uk/admin/uploads/UKMEC2009.pdf [accessed 08.04.10].

53. Wildemeersch D, Schacht E, Thiery M, et al. Intrauterine contraception in the year 2001: can intrauterine device use be revived with new improved contraceptive technology? Eur J Contracept Reprod Health Care 2000; 5:295–304.

54. Stewart A, Cummins C, Gold L, et al. The effectiveness of the levonorgestrel-releasing intrauterine system in menorrhagia: a systematic review. BJOG 2001; 108:74–86.
55. Wildemeersch D, Schacht E, Wildemeersch P. Treatment of primary and secondary dysmenorrhea with a novel 'frameless' intrauterine levonorgestrel-releasing drug delivery system: a pilot study. Eur J Contracept Reprod Health Care 2001; 6: 192–198.
56. Varila E, Wahlstrom T, Rauramo I. A 5-year follow-up study on the use of a levonorgestrel intrauterine system in women receiving hormone replacement therapy. Fertil Steril 2001; 76:969–973.
57. Faculty of Sexual and Reproductive Healthcare Clinical Effectiveness Unit. FSRH Guidance (November 2007) Intrauterine Contraception. 2007. Online. Available: http://www.ffprhc.org.uk/admin/uploads/CEUGuidanceIntrauterineContraceptionNov07.pdf [accessed 05.07.09].
58. Free MJ. Condoms: the rubber remedy. In: Corson SC, Derman RJ, Tyrer LB, eds. Fertility control. Boston, MA: Little, Brown; 1985.
59. Liskin L, Wharton C, Blackburn R, et al. Condoms: now more than ever. Popul Rep 1990; 8:Series H.
60. Lindberg LD, Sonenstein FL, Ku L, et al. Young men's experience with condom breakage. Fam Plann Perspect 1997; 29:128–131, 140.
61. Messiah A, Dart T, Spencer BE, et al. Condom breakage and slippage during heterosexual intercourse: a French national survey. French National Survey on Sexual Behavior Group (ACSF). Am J Public Health 1997; 87:421–424.
62. Golombok S, Harding R, Sheldon J. An evaluation of a thicker versus a standard condom with gay men. AIDS 2001; 15(2):245–250.
63. Faculty of Family Planning and Reproductive Health Care Clinical Effectiveness Unit. FFPRHC Guidance (January 2007) Male and Female Condoms. 2007. Online. Available: http://www.ffprhc.org.uk/admin/uploads/999_CEUguidanceMaleFemaleCondomsJan07.pdf [accessed 05.07.09].
64. Schirm AL, Trussell J, Menken J, et al. Contraceptive failure in the United States: the impact of social, economic and demographic factors. Fam Plann Perspect 1982; 14: 68–75.
65. Bounds W, Guillebaud J, Dominik R, et al. The diaphragm with and without spermicide. A randomized, comparative efficacy trial. J Reprod Med 1995; 40:764–774.
66. Fihn SD, Latham RH, Roberts P, et al. Association between diaphragm use and urinary tract infection. JAMA 1985; 254:240–245.
67. Fihn SD, Johnson C, Pinkstaff C, et al. Diaphragm use and urinary tract infections: analysis of urodynamic and microbiological factors. J Urol 1986; 136:853–856.
68. Henshaw SK. Unintended pregnancy in the United States. Fam Plann Perspect 1998; 30:24–29, 46.
69. Trussell J, Vaughan B. Contraceptive failure, method-related discontinuation and resumption of use: results from the 1995 National survey of family growth. Fam Plann Perspect 1999; 31:64–72, 93.
70. Rosenberg MJ, Waugh MS, Burnhill MS. Compliance, counseling and satisfaction with oral contraceptives: a prospective evaluation. Fam Plann Perspect 1998; 30:89–92, 104.
71. Potter L, Oakley D, de Leon-Wong E, et al. Measuring compliance among oral contraceptive users. Fam Plann Perspect 1996; 28:154–158.
72. Beksinska ME, Rees VH, Nkonyane T, et al. Compliance and use behaviour, an issue in injectable as well as oral contraceptive use? A study of injectable and oral contraceptive use in Johannesburg. Br J Fam Plann 1998; 24:21–23.
73. Beckman LJ, Harvey SM. Factors affecting the consistent use of barrier methods of contraception. Obstet Gynecol 1996; 88(Suppl 3):65S–71S.
74. Brown SS, Eisenberg L, eds. The best intentions: unintended pregnancy and the well being of children and families. Washington DC: National Academy Press; 1995.
75. Delbanco SF, Mauldon J, Smith MD. Little knowledge and limited practice: emergency contraceptive pills, the public and the obstetrician-gynaecologist. Obstet Gynaecol 1997; 89:1006–1011.
76. Task Force on Postovulatory Methods of Fertility Regulation. Randomised controlled trial of levonorgestrel versus the Yuzpe regimen of combined oral contraceptives for emergency contraception. Lancet 1998; 352:428–433.
77. Von Hertzen H, Piaggio G, Ding J, et al. Low dose mifepristone and two regimens of levonorgestrel for emergency contraception: a WHO multicentre randomised trial. Lancet 2002; 360:1803–1810.
78. Glasier A. Emergency postcoital contraception. N Engl J Med 1997; 337:1058–1064.
79. Faculty of Family Planning and Reproductive Health Care Clinical Effectiveness Unit. FFPRHC Guidance (April 2006). Emergency contraception. J Fam Plann Reprod Health Care 2006; 32(2):121–128; quiz 8.
80. Glasier A, Baird D. The effects of self-administering emergency contraception. N Engl J Med 1998; 339:1–4.
81. Raine TR, Harper CC, Rocca CH, et al. Direct access to emergency contraception through pharmacies and effect on unintended pregnancy and STIs: a randomized controlled trial. JAMA 2005; 293(1):54–62.
82. Weisberg E, Fraser IS. Rights to emergency contraception. Int J Gynaecol Obstet 2009. [Epub ahead of print].
83. Mumford SD. Vasectomy—the decision making process. San Francisco: San Francisco Press; 1977.
84. Cox B, Sneyd MJ, Paul C, et al. Vasectomy and the risk of prostate cancer. JAMA 2002; 287:3110–3115.
85. Williams EL, Jones HE, Merrill RE. Subsequent course of patients sterilised by tubal ligation. Am J Obstet Gynecol 1951; 61:423–426.
86. Gentile GP, Kaufman SC, Helbig DW. Is there any evidence for a post tubal sterilization syndrome? Fertil Steril 1998; 69: 179–186.
87. Peterson HB, Jeng G, Folger SG, et al. The risk of menstrual abnormalities after tubal sterilization. N Engl J Med 2000; 343:1681–1687.
88. Peterson HB, Xia Z, Hughes JM, et al. The risk of pregnancy after tubal sterilisation: findings from the US Collaborative Review of Sterilization. Am J Obstet Gynecol 1996; 174:1161–1168.
89. RCOG (Royal College of Obstetricians and Gynaecologists): Faculty of Family Planning and Reproductive Health Care. First prescription of combined oral contraception: recommendations for clinical practice. Br J Fam Plann 1999; 26:27–38.
90. Kerin JF, Carignan CS, Cher D. The safety and effectiveness of a new hysteroscopic method for permanent birth control: results of the first Essure pbc clinical study. Aust N Z J Obstet Gynaecol 2001; 41(Suppl):364–370.
91. Shimoni N, Westhoff C. Review of the vaginal contraceptive ring (NuvaRing). J Fam Plann Reprod Health Care 2008; 34(4):247–250.
92. Errey B. Vasectomy in review. Aust Fam Physician 1990; 19:841.
93. Greer IA, Cameron IT, Kitchner HC, et al. Mosby's colour atlas and text of obstetrics and gynaecology. London: Mosby; 2001; 66, 68.
94. International Planned Parenthood Federation. IMAP recommendation on single-dose levonorgestrel for emergency contraception. IPPF Med Bull 2003; 37(3).

95. Rymer J, Fish ANJ, Chapman M. Gynecology colour guide, 2nd edn. Edinburgh: Churchill Livingstone; 1999.

96. Trussell J, Hatcher RA, Cates W, et al. Contraceptive failure in the United States: an update. Stud Fam Plann 1990; 21:51–54.

97. Sundquist K. Contraception and safe sex: barriers are back. Mod Med 1997; 56–63.

98. Collaborative Group on Hormonal Factors in Breast Cancer. Breast cancer and hormonal contraceptives. Lancet 1996; 347:1713–1727.

99. FSRH (Faculty of Sexual and Reproductive Healthcare Clinical Effectiveness Unit). FSRH Guidance (November 2008, updated June 2009) Progestogen-only injectable contraception. 2009. Online. Available: http://www.fsrh.org/admin/uploads/ CEUGuidanceProgestogenOnlyInjectables09.pdf [accessed 03.07.09].

4

Unplanned pregnancy

OBJECTIVES

- To know why access to safe abortion is necessary.
- To understand the relationship between public policy and rates of abortion.
- To undertake effective pregnancy counselling.
- To accurately advise women about the nature of surgical abortion, what myths exist in the community and among health professionals and what risks are associated with surgical abortion.
- To compare and contrast medical and surgical abortion.
- To be aware of legal issues regarding abortion that are of concern to GPs.
- To appreciate the current threats to abortion services.

REPRODUCTIVE RIGHTS AND ABORTION

There are three incontrovertible facts about abortion:

1. Unsafely performed abortions are a major cause of morbidity and mortality among women.
2. The need for induced abortion is a prevalent and persistent reality.
3. Women need not die or suffer from the consequences of abortion because, when properly carried out, it is an extremely safe procedure.[1]

Complications from unsafe abortions account for approximately 40% of maternal deaths worldwide.[2] Indeed in Australia we have only to look back to 1970 to find that abortion was then the most common cause of maternal death in this country.[3] Increasing legal access to abortion is associated with improvement in sexual and reproductive health.[4] Conversely, unsafe abortion and related mortality are both highest in countries with narrow grounds for legal abortion[5]

Prior to its legalisation, abortion was the major cause of maternal death.

No society has been able to eliminate induced abortion as an element of fertility control. Induced abortion is the oldest and, according to some health experts, the most widely used method of fertility control.[2] It has been estimated that almost two in every five pregnancies (as many as 80 million pregnancies) worldwide are unplanned.[6] Some of these are carried to term, while others end in spontaneous or induced abortion. Estimates indicate that 46 million pregnancies are voluntarily terminated each year— 27 million legally and 19 million outside the legal system.[6] In the latter case, the abortions are often performed by unskilled providers or under unhygienic conditions or both, mainly in developing countries.

Approximately one in ten pregnancies end in an unsafe abortion, giving a ratio of one unsafe abortion to about seven live births.

Worldwide, an estimated 68,000 women die each year as a consequence of unsafe abortion. Where contraception is inaccessible or of poor quality, many women will seek to terminate unintended pregnancies, despite restrictive laws and lack of adequate abortion services. Prevention of unplanned pregnancies by improving access to quality family planning services must therefore be the highest priority, followed by improving the quality of abortion services and of post-abortion care.[7]

In most European countries, about two-thirds of women have at least one unintended pregnancy.[8] Typically, abortions performed after 12 weeks' gestation account for fewer than 10% of all pregnancy terminations and are usually done for reasons of fetal abnormality, deteriorating maternal health or, as is more likely to be the case with teenagers, delay in seeking help.[9]

Countries with open attitudes to teenage sexuality and sex education and where contraception is widely available have the lowest abortion rates.

At what age do women have abortions?

While unplanned pregnancy and abortion occurs more typically in younger women, interestingly over a third of women seeking a termination of pregnancy (TOP) are aged 30 years or over.[10] Between 1996 and 2006, there was a 29% increase in the number of women aged 30–50 years having a TOP.[11] A lack of effective contraceptive use and inaccurate perceptions of fertility may be an underlying reason for this.[12]

Many induced abortions are performed on adolescents and young adults. Access to surgical terminations is often limited for these women because of sociocultural barriers. Countries with an open attitude towards teenage sexuality and easy availability of oral contraception have lower abortion rates. Abortion rates are highest in those countries where information and services in family planning are weak and where women's sexual and reproductive rights are severely contained. In most developed countries, abortion rates vary from about 10 to 30 per 1000 women aged 15–44. The lowest rate is in the Netherlands (5/1000), which has one of the world's most liberal abortion laws.[9] This contrasts with the former USSR, which had officially reported rates of 112/1000 in the mid-1980s.[13] In Western countries, abortion rates peak at about age 20. Women under 25 years of age obtain 56% of abortions in England and Wales and 61% of abortions in the USA.[9] It is interesting to note that, while the rate of premarital sex is similar in North America and Western Europe, the rate of abortions in the Netherlands is one-fifth of the US rate.[9] In the Netherlands, family planning services for unmarried people are non-controversial and sex education and contraception are widely taught in schools to teenagers.

PREGNANCY COUNSELLING

What is pregnancy counselling?

GPs are often faced with the difficult situation of diagnosing pregnancy in a woman for whom such a diagnosis is not anticipated with joy or happiness. In these situations or when women present seeking advice about what to do in a situation of unplanned pregnancy, GPs need to engage in pregnancy counselling. While doctors and other health professionals are not compelled to take part in counseling or to arrange or perform an abortion if they have religious or other objections to it, they should not seek to impose this view on their patients and should inform them where they can seek advice from another practitioner who is prepared to discuss abortion. Indeed, recent changes to legislation in Victoria mandate this.[14]

CASE STUDY: Feeling alone and frightened

Nancy is an 18-year-old young woman who presented at 10 weeks' gestation requesting a referral for an abortion. Nancy was very distressed. She was a first-year university student who had become sexually active only in the last 6 months. She had not told her boyfriend she was pregnant nor her parents, as they are all Catholic and have mentioned before that they are anti-abortion. She wanted to continue her studies and develop a career before getting married and having children and in her heart she felt that having an abortion was the right thing for her to do in this situation, but she felt very alone and frightened of what her parents and boyfriend would do if they found out.

Pregnancy counselling involves giving women (and their partners) the information and support they require to make well-informed decisions and choices about the pregnancy. Key features of pregnancy counselling involve confidentiality, objectivity and being non-directive and non-judgmental while at the same time empathic and accepting.

The goal of pregnancy counselling is to assist a woman to come to her own decision as to how to proceed with an unplanned pregnancy.

How do I go about counselling a woman with an unplanned pregnancy?

Effective counselling requires sufficient time, something GPs do not often have a lot of. It can therefore be useful to provide some initial information to a woman who has been newly diagnosed with an unplanned pregnancy and ask her to return for a longer discussion when 40 minutes to an hour can be set aside.

Key features of pregnancy counselling involve confidentiality, objectivity and being non-directive and non-judgmental, while at the same time empathic and accepting.

At the counselling session, a GP should:

- Provide an atmosphere where the woman can fully express her feelings about the pregnancy.
- Help the woman to see her situation objectively. Often the partner's family or friends attempt to coerce the woman into following a course of action with which she does not feel comfortable. It is important that she recognises these influences and acknowledges how they are affecting her decision.
- Encourage her to consider all her options, namely abortion, adoption or continuing with the pregnancy and raising the child herself. The woman should spell out the positives and negatives of each of these courses of action in order to help her determine the right course of action in her particular situation.
- Provide information about the various supports available to her, financial or otherwise, as well as information about the abortion procedure or continuing with the pregnancy and the possible complications of each of these.
- Help the woman to understand why the pregnancy occurred. Besides exploring the reasons for contraceptive failure, it is important to identify more subtle reasons that may be underlying the entire situation. For example, sometimes pregnancy occurs because women want to prove their femininity or fertility or are testing their partner's affection. Pregnancy may also come about in an effort to 'cure' a failing relationship.
- Help the woman arrive at a decision with which she feels comfortable.
- Offer the woman an opportunity to talk after the decision is made (e.g. after the abortion or when the decision is made to continue the pregnancy), so that there is ongoing support.
- Discuss future contraception.

CASE STUDY: 'I'm concerned that something might be wrong.'

Susan is 26 years old. This was the first time I had met her. She came in with a very nervous demeanour, complaining of some watery pink vaginal discharge. She explained that she had had an abortion at 7 weeks' gestation some 4 months ago and had not returned for review to the abortion provider. She was concerned that 'something might be wrong'.

On further history, the discharge had been present for 24 hours and was not associated with any itch, pain or odour. She was otherwise well and had had two normal periods since the procedure. Her cycles were about 35 days long, however, and her last period was 2.5 weeks ago. I asked her if she had had a smear and swabs done when she had the abortion and she said no, that she had become sexually active at the age of 24 and had never had a smear.

I broached the subject of her abortion and she grew even more distressed than she had been. I asked her how she was feeling emotionally about the procedure and she explained that she regretted her decision and, if faced with the same decision now, she would not have gone through with it. When I asked why, she explained that she had felt pressured by those close to her to have an abortion, despite her religious reservations. She had then gone to a hospital some distance from her home, as she had gone to stay with a friend while it was carried out, not wishing to inform her family. At the hospital, misoprostol was applied PV several hours before the procedure was due and about an hour later she passed what appeared to be a sac in the toilet, followed soon after by some tissue that she presumed was the placenta. Susan had been quite unprepared for this and had become quite distressed. Despite this she proceeded to have a suction curette.

Some weeks later, after continuing to feel uncomfortable about the whole chain of events, Susan sought counselling. Like most women who are unaware of the religious and political climate concerning abortion issues, Susan did not know that the 'pregnancy advisory service' that she found in the telephone book was a counselling service subsidised by the Right-to-Life movement. It was only once she had been to see them a couple of times that they acknowledged this. They then referred her to an organisation called 'Women Who have been Hurt by Abortion'. Susan told me that she continues to see this second counsellor on a regular basis. Despite this I did not feel that Susan was resolving her issues. She visibly trembled as she spoke about the event.

I carried out a vaginal examination and found 'ovulation-type' mucus that was developing some pink staining as it moved over a rather 'angry' looking erosion. The vaginal walls looked normal and there was no obvious pathology visible. I carried out a smear, vaginal swab and smear from the posterior fornix, a cervical swab for M&C and a cervical swab for a PCR test for chlamydia. Her uterus and adnexae felt normal and I assured her that all had returned to normal after the abortion and that we needed to wait for the smear and swab results.

I then suggested that she did not seem to have resolved the issues that having the abortion had raised for her and that she may need to seek counselling from a person who she could be sure was objective.

In retrospect, several lessons can be learnt from Susan's case. The first is that the decision to have an abortion is a difficult one for any woman. Research shows that women who are coerced into either having an abortion or continuing with pregnancy are more likely to have a poor outcome and feel regretful. Those who have an opportunity to come to a decision by themselves have the best outcome. It is therefore incumbent on GPs who are often the first point of contact for women with an unplanned pregnancy to be aware of local pregnancy counsellors who are skilled, non-judgmental and objective.

The second issue is that if a woman has an unplanned pregnancy it means that she has had unprotected sex; therefore, if she is not with a long-term partner, she needs to be investigated for sexually transmitted diseases. Abortion providers have varying practices in terms of testing for STDs routinely, so as a woman's GP, it is always important to check this.

The third issue is that many women fail to return for a check-up after abortion. Despite the fact that many feel the need to reassure themselves that their anatomy is normal and that they are not diseased, they do not necessarily feel they want to return to the place where the abortion was carried out and so put it off.

The role of the GP is an important one post-abortion. The GP can offer reassurance that all is well from a physical perspective, follow up on the woman's emotional wellbeing and perhaps debrief, check that the woman has been appropriately investigated for STDs and, most importantly, ensure that effective contraception is in use.

Countering the myths about abortion

A new 'woman-centred' anti-choice strategy opposing abortion has become increasingly apparent in the media. The strategy contends that women do not really choose abortion but are pressured into it by others and then experience a range of negative effects afterwards, including an increased risk of breast cancer, infertility and post-abortion grief.[15] GPs need to be very aware of the evidence contradicting these complaints and be clear about rebutting them when counselling patients.

Does abortion lead to future infertility?

Studies have shown that first-trimester termination of pregnancy is not associated with either later infertility, increased risk of ectopic pregnancy or subsequent non-viable outcome.[16–18]

Does abortion lead to breast cancer?

The issue of whether or not having an abortion puts you at increased risk of developing breast cancer is an important one, given the already high prevalence of breast cancer in the community.

The science behind a possible association is plausible. The current widely accepted theory about the development of breast cancer holds that mutations that lead to breast cancer come about in cells that are proliferating rather than in cells that are quiescent.[19] It follows that any factor that may increase the period of time that cells spend proliferating may increase the risk of developing cancerous change. In breast tissue, cell proliferation is affected by hormonal factors, hence the research into the risk of developing breast cancer associated with the use of exogenous hormones such as hormone replacement therapy and the contraceptive pill.

One epidemiological association that has been found in relation to breast cancer is the protective effect endowed by having a full-term pregnancy.[20] This may be explained by the fact that in late pregnancy breast epithelial cells differentiate (i.e. they cease to proliferate). Conversely in early pregnancy the cells proliferate. Some researchers have therefore postulated that having an abortion (induced) or a miscarriage (spontaneous) for that matter may not only eliminate the long-term protection gained by having a full-term pregnancy, but may even increase the risk of breast cancer by altering the overall balance of cellular activity towards that of proliferation.[21]

This theory was first proposed in 1980. What followed was 15 years of epidemiological studies seeking to determine the truth. If you were a researcher setting out to determine whether or not the hypothesis was correct you would need to carry out a randomised, controlled trial in which half the women had an abortion and the other half didn't and follow them up prospectively to determine which group developed more breast cancer. You would have to control for the other factors associated with breast cancer such as age, parity, use of exogenous hormones and family history. This kind of trial is unethical and impossible to carry out. Thus, the trials that have been published to date are mainly case-controlled trials, starting at the other end of the timeline, looking at women who have developed breast cancer and trying to find out which of them have had abortions.

A large study to advance knowledge in this area actually tackled this issue by analysing data from two registries in Denmark: the National Registry of Induced Abortions and the Danish Cancer Registry. Published in 1997 in the *New England Journal of Medicine*,[22] this study examined the relationship between induced abortion and breast cancer by looking at the experiences of 1.5 million Danish women. This study had the largest data set of all previously published work and, while no registry can be perfect, the study did not rely on reporting by the women themselves. The authors adjusted for parity and for timing and number of abortions, as well as examining the effect of gestational age at the time of the abortion. They found that having an induced abortion had no overall effect on breast cancer risk.

These findings were confirmed by the Collaborative Group on Hormonal Factors in Breast Cancer,[23] which brought together the worldwide epidemiological evidence on the possible relationship between breast cancer and previous spontaneous and induced abortions. They concluded that pregnancies that end as a spontaneous or induced abortion do not increase a woman's risk of developing breast cancer, suggesting that the studies of breast cancer with retrospective recording of induced abortion yield misleading results, possibly because women who had developed breast cancer were, on average, more likely than other women to disclose previous induced abortions.

Abortion does not lead to future infertility, ectopic pregnancy or pregnancy problems, nor is it associated with an increased risk of breast cancer.

Is there such a thing as the 'post-abortion syndrome'?

Advocates of the right-to-life movement have put forth the concept of a 'post-abortion syndrome' and likened it to a post-traumatic stress disorder.

In the early 1990s, the US Surgeon General (Koop) undertook a review of the literature on the medical and psychological sequelae of abortion. The aim was to help overturn the 'Roe vs Wade' landmark US Supreme Court decision that legalised abortion in the USA during the first two trimesters of pregnancy, while Koop himself was publicly opposed to abortion.[9] His report, which was never officially released, could not find evidence of significant adverse consequences for women undergoing abortion and expressed doubts about the existence of a post-abortion syndrome.[24]

These findings are confirmed by a systematic review that looked at studies published in the last 10 years.[25]

There is no evidence for a post-abortion syndrome.

What the evidence does show is that, while adverse sequelae do occur in a minority of women, abortion in general does not cause deleterious psychological effects.[26,27] There is no evidence that, overall, abortion causes psychiatric illness.[28] The incidence of serious psychiatric illness is much higher following full-term delivery than following abortion.[27] Whether abortion causes psychological distress, and the degree and course of any distress, largely depend on the baseline psychological and social condition of the patient and the circumstances under which conception occurs, whether abortion is decided upon and whether abortion is carried out.[29] As the British Royal College of Obstetricians and Gynaecologist (RCOG) concludes,[30] 'some studies suggest that rates of psychiatric illness or self-harm are higher among women who have had an abortion, compared with women who give birth and to nonpregnant women of similar age. It must be borne in mind that these findings do not imply a causal association and may reflect continuation of pre-existing conditions'.

Abortion-related stress is usually maximal before the termination and decreases rapidly thereafter, this finding being consistent with other life events where resolution leads to relief of stress. Women most likely to show subsequent problems are those who were:

- pressured into the operation against their own wishes, either by relatives or because their pregnancy had medical or fetal contraindications
- exposed to unsympathetic attitudes from family and from clinic staff
- in a sociocultural environment in which the procedure was defined as criminal activity
- nulliparous women with a past history of interpersonal problems and negative religious or cultural attitudes to abortion.

It is important to note in this debate the facts that women who are denied an abortion are at increased risk of anxiety and other mental health problems[27]

and that the emotional and social costs of carrying an unwanted pregnancy to term appear to extend to the offspring.[31]

Most women feel relief after an abortion is carried out. Those with poor outcomes have usually been coerced into having an abortion or had significant moral and religious objections to abortion prior to having the abortion carried out.

Summary of key points
- The goal of pregnancy counselling is for the woman to achieve self-determination, i.e. for her to come to a decision with which she feels comfortable.
- Induced abortion does not lead to later infertility, ectopic pregnancy or subsequent pregnancy problems.
- Induced abortion has no overall effect on breast cancer risk.
- Abortion in general does not cause psychological problems and there is no evidence for a 'post-abortion syndrome'.
- Women most likely to show subsequent emotional problems as a result of abortion are those who are pressured into the procedure against their wishes or nulliparous women with a past history of interpersonal problems and negative religious attitudes towards abortion.

METHODS OF ABORTION

Surgical abortion

How safe is it to have an abortion?

First-trimester abortion carried out by well-trained practitioners in adequate facilities is one of the safest and easiest of gynaecological procedures to carry out, with a very low risk of complications. Beyond 10 weeks' gestation the health risks of abortion rise with each week of the pregnancy, the risks of late second-trimester abortion being three to four times higher than those in the first trimester (Fig 4.1). In countries such as Australia,[32] the overwhelming majority of surgical terminations of pregnancy (96%) are carried out in the first trimester of pregnancy. In the USA, 4% are obtained at 16–20 weeks, and 1.4% at >21 weeks.[33]

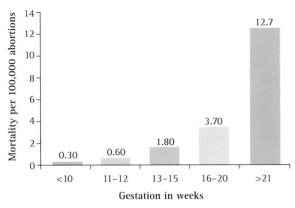

FIGURE 4.1 Mortality associated with abortion (From Gold[68])

TABLE 4.1 Medical indications for termination of pregnancy

Maternal indications	Fetal indications
• Maternal malignancy such as cervical cancer • Severe medical illness that may worsen with pregnancy (e.g. severe ischaemic heart disease, primary pulmonary hypertension, end-stage renal failure) • Severe psychiatric illness that may worsen with pregnancy	• Ingestion of a teratogen (e.g. warfarin, danazol, retinoic acid, methotrexate, cyclophosphamide and fluorouracil) • Severe fetal abnormality • Maternal infection that puts the fetus at risk of severe abnormality

Abortions carried out in the first trimester have very low rates of morbidity and mortality.

When women ask about the safety of abortion it is also worth pointing out that in developed countries, mortality associated with childbirth is 11 times higher than that for safely performed abortion procedures and 30 times higher than for abortions of up to 8 weeks' gestation.[9]

Mortality associated with pregnancy is 30 times higher than that associated with abortion carried out prior to 8 weeks' gestation.

What are the indications for the procedure?

Most abortions are carried out for psychosocial reasons when an unplanned pregnancy has ensued. Many countries do insist, however, on there being a medical indication for the procedure to be carried out. Possible medical indications for abortion are listed in Table 4.1.

Is any preoperative 'work-up' necessary?

When a woman presents requesting a termination of pregnancy, there are several issues that GPs should address preoperatively. The first of these is to date the pregnancy accurately to ensure that the woman is referred in a timely fashion for the procedure—ideally before 10 weeks' gestation. If women can accurately recall the date of commencement of their last normal menstrual period, their current gestation

TABLE 4.2 Equating uterine size with gestation

Uterine size	Gestation
Golf ball	Nulliparous
Large apricot	4–6 weeks
Small orange	6–8 weeks
Large orange	8–10 weeks
Grapefruit	10–12 weeks
Palpable abdominally	≥12 weeks

can be calculated and the uterine size used to double-check the date. A helpful way of correlating the uterine size with gestation during a pelvic examination is by equating the size of the uterus with the size of various fruit. This correlation is described in Table 4.2. If the uterus is palpable abdominally, the pregnancy is of ≥12 weeks' gestation.

Preoperatively, GPs should accurately determine the gestation of the pregnancy, check the woman's blood group and screen for chlamydia.

On many occasions the woman is unsure of the exact date of her last normal menstrual period (LNMP) or the pelvic examination reveals that the uterine size is inconsistent with the presumed gestation. In these situations, an ultrasound should be undertaken to date the pregnancy correctly. It is important to warn the patient that these ultrasounds are usually carried out transvaginally and involve the probe being placed inside the vagina. Most women will otherwise expect to have an abdominal ultrasound carried out. It is also important when writing the request for the ultrasound (or indeed if carrying out the ultrasound yourself) to note that the woman has requested an abortion, so that she is not shown the screen with pictures of the fetus and caused additional distress.

The second major issue to be dealt with preoperatively involves finding out the patient's blood group. If the woman is Rhesus-negative, she will require anti-D prophylaxis at the time of the abortion.

The third and equally important aspect of the preoperative work-up involves screening for *Chlamydia* (see Chapters 12 and 13). If the woman has fallen pregnant, she must have had unprotected intercourse and is at increased risk of *Chlamydia* (particularly if she is under 25). Screening can involve either a cervical swab or a first-catch urine for PCR testing. GPs may also want to take the opportunity to take a Pap smear (if the patient is due for one) during the pelvic examination.

Should contraceptive issues be addressed by the GP prior to the procedure?

While failure of contraception (if any was used) is the reason that women present with an unplanned pregnancy, many GPs feel reluctant to discuss this issue at the time women request a termination of pregnancy. This is because the woman is often distressed and embarrassed and is completely focused on her immediate concern, which is to obtain an abortion, rather than worrying about future contraception. For this reason, contraceptive advice given at this time may well fall on 'deaf ears'. The concern, however, is that if contraception is not addressed at this initial consultation it never will be, as few women return for a follow-up consultation after an abortion and most will resume sexual activity before seeing their doctor.

Two options are therefore available to the GP. If the woman can focus on the issue, it is useful to discuss what contraception was used and why it failed, and to offer alternative contraception that can be started after the procedure. If the COCP has failed because the patient has difficulty remembering to take it, options such as Depo-Provera®, Implanon or an IUD are worth considering, particularly as these can be injected, implanted or inserted at the clinic where the abortion is carried out, giving immediate contraceptive coverage. Alternatively, if the COCP is decided upon, the woman should be given a packet and advised to start the day following the

abortion with an active pill. This should also ensure contraceptive coverage by the time sexual activity resumes.

The second option is to delay contraceptive counselling until the follow-up appointment after the abortion and to stress the importance of attending for follow-up. Condom use can be advised if the patient resumes sexual activity prior to the usual 4-week check-up after the procedure. The problem with this approach is that many women fail to attend for follow-up after an abortion and the opportunity to ensure she has effective contraception is lost.

How is an abortion carried out if it is done during the first trimester?

Before 6 weeks, aspiration can be done with a hand-held vacuum syringe, without anaesthetic and/or cervical dilation. The procedure may be performed on an outpatient basis. In many developing countries the procedure is known by the term 'menstrual regulation'.

Surgical first-trimester abortion is carried out via vacuum aspiration.

During the first trimester, the most common surgical procedure to terminate a pregnancy is vacuum aspiration under either local (paracervical block with/without light sedation) or general anaesthesia. It is not carried out prior to 6 weeks' gestation because of a higher failure rate. Cervical dilation may be necessary, depending on the gestation of the pregnancy. The RCOG recommends routine use of cervical priming in women under 18 years of age and after 10 weeks' gestation.[30] A variety of agents can be used to dilate the cervix (Box 4.1) or the operator can undertake mechanical dilation using Hegar dilators, which are made of metal and come in a variety of sizes.

The procedure for a first-trimester termination of pregnancy involves the following steps:

1. The patient is anaesthetised and placed in stirrups.
2. The patient's genital area is washed and draped.
3. A vaginal examination is carried out and the degree of cervical dilation assessed.
4. Cervical dilation up to about 10 mm is carried out.
5. An oxytocic drug is given at the completion of cervical dilation to help to contract the uterus and prevent bleeding.

6. Suction curettage is carried out using a clear plastic curette that allows for visualisation of the products of conception as they are removed from the uterus. The procedure is completed when a 'gritty' feeling is present on further curettage and there is minimal bleeding. Many providers now perform the procedure under ultrasound guidance.

7. Rh prophylaxis should be administered to all those women who are Rh-negative prior to discharge.

A suction curettage takes about 5–10 minutes.

What advice should be given to the patient about symptoms and signs after the procedure?

Most women are discharged from the abortion facility within a few hours of the procedure. The woman should be accompanied home by a friend or family member, as she may still feel groggy after the procedure and should not drive.

Simple analgesia may be required, as normally there is some cramping pain, and there may be some bleeding that diminishes rapidly over the ensuing days. Tampons should not be used and the woman should not have sexual intercourse until the bleeding stops.

Normally patients feel well enough to return to work the following day. Emotionally the woman may feel 'topsy turvy' for a week or so until the symptoms of pregnancy subside (along with the pregnancy hormones).

Patients should be warned that if they develop fever, increasing pain or bleeding in the days following the procedure they should seek medical attention, as these symptoms may be signs of infection. Rarely, symptoms of pregnancy continue, indicating that the pregnancy may have continued despite the abortion procedure.

How is an abortion carried out if it is done during the second trimester?

There are three approaches to carrying out a mid-trimester abortion:[34]

1. dilation and evacuation (D&E)
2. instillation of saline, urea or a medication into the amniotic cavity
3. administration of intravaginal prostaglandins.

The choice of approach depends on the operator's experience and the patient's preference. Most later terminations are for reasons of fetal abnormality and are performed medically. D&E requires the cervix to be dilated more widely than for suction curettage, followed by piecemeal removal of the fetus using sponge forceps. The risks associated with D&E are similar to those of first-trimester abortion, but rates of complication may differ. Cervical injury is more common with second-trimester D&E than with earlier abortion, as is haemorrhage requiring transfusion.[30]

More recently, medical abortion using misoprostol has been practised, but at this gestation it is associated with a greater risk of complications than dilation and evacuation.[35]

What follow-up is required?

All patients should be urged to return for a check-up within 4–6 weeks of the procedure. At the check-up the doctor should ask about the patient's emotional wellbeing and how she feels about having had the procedure. This questioning will allow the patient to vent her feelings and debrief after her experience.

A history should be taken of bleeding and pain following the procedure, when this resolved and if there are any current physical symptoms. The patient should be asked if she has had a period.

Contraception as well as prevention against STDs should be discussed and, as mentioned previously, reasons for contraceptive failure explored and addressed.

There is no particular reason to undertake a vaginal examination unless something is uncovered in the history suggestive of pathology.

What complications can occur?

As mentioned earlier, complications arising from abortion occurring in the first trimester are rare (Table 4.3, p 98).

Summary of key points
- Ninety-six per cent of surgical terminations of pregnancy are carried out in the first trimester of pregnancy.

TABLE 4.3 Complications arising from surgical abortion

Early complications	Late complications
• Uterine perforation (2%)	• Retained products of conception (0.2–0.6%)
• Haemorrhage	• Sepsis (0.5%)
• Cervical lacerations	• Anaemia
• Failure to abort (usually due to undertaking the procedure too early)	• Thromboembolism
• Anaesthetic complications	• Cervical stenosis (0.02%)

TABLE 4.4 A comparison between medical and surgical methods of abortion (From Breitbart[67])

Medical abortion	Surgical abortion
• Some contraindications appropriate	• Rare contraindications, given the setting and requisite skills
• Available early in gestation	• May not be available during very early pregnancy
• Surgical aspiration needed in 2–10% at 7 weeks	• Surgical respiration needed in approximately 1% at 7 weeks
• Process occurs over a few days to a few weeks	• Procedure most commonly completed in 1 day
• Avoids anaesthesia and surgery	• Requires anaesthesia and surgery; more 'invasive'
• Bleeding commonly perceived as heavy	• Bleeding commonly perceived as light
• Possible drug side-effects	• Possible surgical complications, including uterine injury (rare)
• Patient has more control	• Care provider has more control

- Mortality associated with childbirth is 30 times that for abortions carried out up to 8 weeks' gestation.
- Preoperatively, a GP should determine the correct gestation, the patient's blood group and screen for *Chlamydia* infection.
- Contraceptive issues that led to the unintended pregnancy need to be addressed by the GP either at the initial consultation or at follow-up.
- First-trimester abortion is carried out by suction curettage.
- Postoperatively, the woman may feel some mild cramping and bleeding, which should cease within a day or two.
- Patients should be instructed to seek assistance if they develop fever, increasing pain or bleeding in the days following the procedure.

Medical abortion

In Europe and China, a clinically useful medical alternative to surgical abortion has been available since 1988. Mifepristone in combination with a prostaglandin analogue has been used in France, Sweden, the UK and China by >3 million women for abortion as late as 63 days' gestation.[36] A comparison between medical and surgical abortion is given in Table 4.4.

Why is medical abortion an important alternative to surgical abortion?

Medical abortion can be offered much more widely and by a much wider range of practitioners than surgical abortion, which requires specialised facilities and skills. Secondly, in countries where abortion is restricted by political constraints, medical abortion has the potential to increase access by moving the treatment into routine practice and decreasing the visibility attached to abortion providers.[37]

What is the mechanism for inducing a medical abortion?

Mifepristone (RU486) is a synthetic antiprogesterone. It is an effective abortifacient when combined with a prostaglandin (such as misoprostol) administered 2 days later. When administered, it saturates the progesterone receptors in the lining of the uterus. The early placental tissue separates from the uterine wall and abortion ensues.[38] Mifepristone also increases production of prostaglandins[39] and, by 24–36 hours after administration of the drug, uterine contractions begin and the sensitivity and responsiveness of the uterus to exogenous prostaglandins is about fivefold.[40] It is now used across the world to bring about medical abortion (see Table 4.5 for a list of countries where mifepristone is registered). In Australia misoprostol is only available for use by practitioners who seek special registration (authorised prescribers) from the federal government. This restriction means that accessibility remains extremely limited.

Although early work with mifepristone and prostaglandin regimens focused on gestations initially up to 7 weeks and then up to 9 weeks, there is now good evidence that this combination may be used to induce abortion throughout the first and second trimesters.[30]

TABLE 4.5 Countries where mifepristone is registered (Adapted from Gynuity Health Projects[70])

Date of registration	Countries where registered
1988	China, France
1991	UK
1992	Sweden
1999	Austria, Belgium, Denmark, Finland, Germany, Greece, Israel, Luxembourg, Netherlands, Spain, Switzerland
2000	Norway, Russia, Taiwan, Tunisia, Ukraine, USA
2001	New Zealand, South Africa
2002	Azerbaijan, Belarus, Georgia, India, Latvia, Serbia, Uzbekistan, Vietnam
2003	Estonia, Guyana, Moldova
2005	Albania, Hungary, Mongolia,
2007	Armenia, Portugal
2008	Romania, Nepal
2009	Italy

BOX 4.2 Schedule for medical abortion (From Clark et al[37])

First visit

1. Assess a woman's eligibility for medical abortion treatment:
   - gestation not more than 9 weeks
   - not an ectopic pregnancy
   - no contraindications.
2. Dispense the initial medication, mifepristone.

Second visit

Administer misoprostol, usually about 2 days after use of mifepristone. (This visit has been replaced by home use in the USA and UK, although it is still required in other jurisdictions, such as France).

Third visit (follow-up)

1. Determine if the abortion has been successful (uncommonly further treatment may be required).
2. Rule out any unusual complication (e.g. previously unrecognised ectopic pregnancy or gestational trophoblastic disease)

The most common medical abortion regimens involve a single oral dose of mifepristone, followed 48 hours later by a prostaglandin, usually misoprostol, given orally or vaginally and repeated doses of prostaglandin at intervals of around 4 hours if required.[41] There is no difference in outcome (a maximum of 80% of women experience complete abortion) when giving mifepristone in doses ranging from 50 to 400 mg singly or in divided doses over 4 days. Adding a small dose of misoprostol improves the efficacy to almost 100%.[36]

Up to 50% of women will have some bleeding and a few women (around 3%) will miscarry with mifepristone before the prostaglandin is administered. The majority will begin to bleed and pass products of conception within a few hours of prostaglandin administration. The experience for the woman may be much like a spontaneous miscarriage, with some pain and bleeding to be expected.[41] A schedule for medical abortion is given in Box 4.2.

Various regimens exist for mifepristone/prostaglandin medical abortions. The FDA-approved protocol involves the administration of 600 mg of mifepristone, followed two days later by 400 mg of oral misoprostol administered at a medical facility.[42] Other protocols are listed in Table 4.6 (p 100).

Alternatives to regimens with mifepristone and a prostaglandin analogue for medical abortion emerged because of the need for accessible, effective and safe options in areas of the world where mifepristone was unavailable. Methotrexate is an antineoplastic agent used in the treatment of severe rheumatoid arthritis, lupus, Crohn's disease and psoriasis. More recently it has been used in the treatment of gestational trophoblastic disease and in the treatment of early, unruptured ectopic pregnancies, with an efficacy rate of approximately 95%.[43,44] Trials using a combination of methotrexate and misoprostol for the termination of first-trimester pregnancy result in a success rate of up to 97%.[45,46] Protocols involve subjects receiving an injection of intramuscular methotrexate (50 mg/m^2 of body surface area) followed by 800 mg of misoprostol on either day 3–4 or day 5–7. The misoprostol can be taken orally or as a vaginal suppository. The regime works best when carried out before 6.5 weeks of amenorrhoea.[47] After treatment with prostaglandin, uterine emptying with a 4–5 mm catheter and manual vacuum aspiration is straightforward. The 1 in 20 or so aspiration procedures that seem to be needed with methotrexate abortions can be carried out, as for any other minor operation, by a trained person who need not be a gynaecologist or a specialist abortion provider.[48] In general, however, regimens involving methotrexate and misoprostol generally take longer to effect abortion than do those with mifepristone and a prostaglandin analogue.[36]

TABLE 4.6 Regimens licensed, recommended or used for medical abortion (From Fiala and Danielsson[64])

Licensed, used or recommended	Mifepristone dose	Prostaglandin	Dose and route of administration	Gestational age limit
Approved: France, 1991; most other European countries and the US, 2000	600 mg	Misoprostol	400 µg p.o.	49
Approved: UK, 1991; Sweden, 1992; Norway, 2000	600 mg	Misoprostol Gemeprost	400 µg p.o. 1 mg	49 63
Widely used	200 mg	Misoprostol	800 µg vaginally	63
Guidelines: RCOG, UK, 2004[30]	200 mg	Misoprostol	800 µg vaginally 800 µg vaginally; 400 µg repeated orally or vaginally after 4 hours, if no expulsion	63 50–63
Guidelines: WHO, 2003[65]	200 mg	Misoprostol	800 µg vaginally 400 µg p.o.	63 49

What issues should be covered when counselling women about medical methods of abortion?

Where medical abortion is available, counselling should include the comparative advantages and disadvantages of medical and surgical abortions. Women should be informed that medical abortion is accompanied by bleeding and pain similar to that of a miscarriage and that the total amount of blood loss is no greater than that of a surgical abortion. If medical abortion is chosen, it should be given with clear instructions on the schedule for use of the two drugs and be provided under medical supervision; an appropriate follow-up must be arranged to ensure that the termination is complete and uncomplicated. Should it result in an incomplete abortion, surgical measures are required.

Three large studies have been conducted using a combination of mifepristone and a prostaglandin, with overall success rates of between 94% and 96%.[49–51] This means that around 4–6% of women choosing to have medical abortions will require suction curettage because of an incomplete abortion.

The half-life of methotrexate is 8–15 hours. While use before conception has been associated with spina bifida, use after conception has not been shown to have any harmful affects.[52] However, because of the potential for teratogenicity, methotrexate/misoprostol termination of first-trimester pregnancy should probably remain a second-line option to RU 486. The advantages of methotrexate/misoprostol-induced abortions are that both of these compounds are widely available as generic, or 'off-patent', inexpensive drugs. This means that this form of medical abortion has the potential to increase choices for women and access to early abortion.

Do women find medical abortions acceptable?

Previous research on abortion has identified some factors that are important to acceptability.[53,54] These attributes include efficacy, safety, freedom from side effects and pain, ease or convenience, gentleness and non-invasiveness, privacy, autonomy and affordability. Many women are attracted to the idea of surgical abortion because they can receive sedation or a general anaesthetic, have the procedure and be back at work or at school the next day. The quickness of the procedure is appealing, even if the process to get to the abortion provider is difficult. The medical method, when compared with surgical termination of pregnancy, offers a lower success rate, takes longer from initiation to completion, involves the patient being aware and conscious of the bleeding and expulsion of products of the pregnancy, and hinders the provision of other methods of fertility control such as IUD insertion or sterilisation. It is therefore interesting to find that when women are offered a choice between medical and surgical methods of abortion, 60–70% choose the medical method.[55] Some of the reasons put forth by women who choose medical over surgical abortion is fear of surgery, convenience for work, less injury to the body, the fact that the surgery happens 'too fast' and their fear of general anaesthesia.[56,57]

Most women who undergo a medical method of termination say they are satisfied with it, would recommend it to friends and would use it again if they needed another abortion.[45] Medical abortion is seen as providing greater privacy and autonomy.[58] Women find that taking pills and using suppositories are more natural and less invasive than surgery.[45,59] In the studies of acceptability of medical termination, the drawbacks are well recognised. They include pain, the duration of bleeding, the number of visits required and the waiting time to know if the treatment has been successful.[45]

Are there any other reasons to prefer medical over surgical abortion?

There are significant economic benefits to the use of medical abortion over surgical abortion. The cost to the Australian community, for example, of surgical abortion for 72,000 abortions in Australia in 1991 was A$28 million. It has been estimated that the introduction of medical methods of abortion using antiprogestins and prostaglandin would save around A$10 million dollars for the Australian health budget.[60]

Conclusion

Provision of medical abortion services requires appropriate training. Clinicians must be prepared to counsel patients about what to expect with medical abortion, to handle questions and to assist patients in managing pain and bleeding. Knowing when to intervene in cases of heavy or prolonged bleeding is of primary concern, because most women who choose medical abortion do so out of a strong desire to avoid surgery. With appropriately trained clinicians and well-informed patients, medical abortion can provide a safe and effective method of early pregnancy termination that can result in increased access and options for reproductive healthcare throughout the world.

Summary of key points

- Medical abortion is used widely in Europe, China, Sweden and the USA.
- Established protocols for medical abortion utilise mifepristone (RU486), followed usually two days later by the prostaglandin misoprostol.
- In general, medical abortion is most effective when undertaken prior to 49 days' gestation.
- The overall abortion process takes longer with methotrexate than it does with mifepristone.
- Women find medical abortion acceptable and feel that it offers them a greater sense of control.

ABORTION AND THE LAW

Abortion laws vary considerably worldwide.[61] They have developed over time from different belief systems and conflicting moral, ethical and religious views. In some countries, they are based on the belief in the fundamental 'right to life' of the unborn child. Other countries approach abortion as a natural consequence of reproductive rights, with the belief that women have the right to control their own reproduction, not only for their own benefit but also for that of their family. In other situations, the critical issue is the control of a rapidly expanding population or else lack of access to contraceptive technology due to the country's poverty and lack of development. Figure 4.2 shows the current status of world abortion laws.

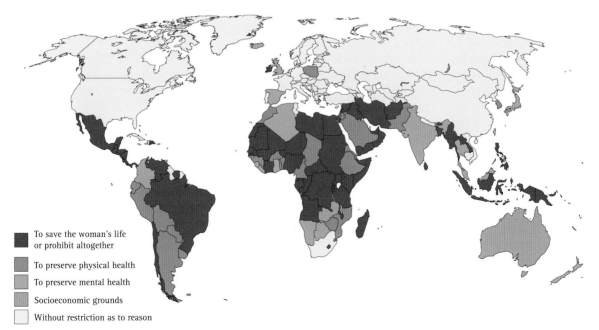

Legend:
- To save the woman's life or prohibit altogether
- To preserve physical health
- To preserve mental health
- Socioeconomic grounds
- Without restriction as to reason

FIGURE 4.2 World abortion laws, 2007, and the grounds upon which abortion is permitted (From Center for Reproductive Rights[69])

What is the current legal situation in the UK and Australia?

Abortion in Australia remains a subject of state law rather than national law, with the grounds on which abortion is permitted varying from state to state. In every state, abortion is legal to protect the life and health of the woman; however, most states operate on legal precedents, with abortion remaining in the criminal code (except for the ACT and Victoria). Because much of Australia's law is based on English legislation, the evolution of legislative change regarding abortion as it occurred in Britain in the 21st century is given below.[62]

- **1929:** The *Infant Life (Preservation) Act 1929* introduced the offence of 'child destruction' from the time when an embryo was viable at 28 weeks onwards, this being permissible only to save the mother's life. The maximum penalty was life imprisonment.
- **1938:** Bourne, a London obstetrician/gynaecologist, terminated the pregnancy of a 14-year-old girl who had been brutally raped by four soldiers, having both the girl's and her parents' consent. He reported his actions to the authorities to make it a test case. The Bourne case established that an abortion might lawfully be procured in order to protect the life of the mother (and that there was no clear distinction between a threat to life and a threat to health) and also outlined the rights, practices and duties of the medical profession.
- **1958:** The case of *R v. Newton and Stungo* made clear that in preserving the life or health of the mother, 'health' included mental health.
- **1967:** The *Abortion Act 1967* is a permissive law, i.e. abortion is permitted and prosecution will not follow if the following conditions are fulfilled:
  - Two medical practitioners agree on the need for an abortion to take place.
  - Continuation of pregnancy would involve risk to the life of the pregnant woman, injury to the physical or mental health of the woman or any existing children greater than if the pregnancy was terminated.
  - There is substantial risk that the child would be born with and suffer from such physical or mental abnormalities as to be seriously handicapped for life.
- **1991 onwards:** The current situation in the UK is based on amendments made in 1991 to the *Abortion Act 1967* and allows abortion in the following circumstances:
  - The continuance of the pregnancy would involve risk to the life of the pregnant woman greater than if the pregnancy were terminated.
  - The termination is necessary to prevent grave permanent injury to the physical or mental health of the pregnant woman.
  - The pregnancy has not exceeded its 24th week and the continuance of the pregnancy would involve risk, greater than if the pregnancy were terminated, of injury to the physical or mental health of the pregnant woman.
  - The pregnancy has not exceeded its 24th week and the continuance of the pregnancy would involve risk, greater than if the pregnancy were terminated, of injury to the physical or mental health of the existing child(ren) of the family of the pregnant woman.
  - There is a substantial risk that if the child were born it would suffer from such physical or mental abnormalities as to be seriously handicapped.

Do fathers have the right to stop an abortion from being performed?

In a case that came to the courts in Britain in 1997, a man took out an injunction trying to prevent his ex-lover from aborting the pregnancy which he had fathered. The case went to the highest court in the land before the woman's appeal was successful. The time taken for the process to go through the courts meant that the woman was forced to undergo an abortion at approximately 15 weeks instead of the safer one she had planned before 12 weeks' gestation.

In Australia the consent of the person thought to be the father (the putative father) is not needed, nor can he prevent the abortion happening. Paternity rights only arise on the birth of his child.

Does the fetus have any legal rights?

A fetus has no specific legal rights at present in Australia, although this issue is being examined on many fronts. In Britain, legislation was passed in 1997 to protect women from forced caesarean section. There have been several documented cases of this in the USA and UK.

CASE STUDY: Terrified her parents might throw her out

A young woman aged 15 presents to your surgery with a girlfriend to give her support. A home pregnancy test she did yesterday is positive, and she is very upset. She has not told anyone of the result except her friend and is terrified that her parents might throw her out of the house if they find out she is pregnant. She requests an abortion. She had become sexually active some 3 months previously and had not used any contraception. She is unsure of when her last normal menstrual period was.

What are the legal ramifications of a minor requesting a termination of pregnancy?

The major legal precedent regarding minors is the Gillick case outlined at the beginning of Chapter 3. It holds not only for the provision of contraception to minors but also for doctors undertaking a termination of pregnancy on a minor.

Abortions can be carried out on minors without parental consent, provided the 'mature minor' rule applies.

Is the legal situation different when a woman requests a later termination of pregnancy?

Because of the lack of definition of when a fetus is viable outside the womb and the ever-advancing ability of the medical profession to sustain a baby born prematurely, the law concerning the gestational limit for legal abortion is not clear in all cases. Viability is now usually defined as 24 weeks, although as in Australia abortion is illegal under statute law in most states there is no legal difference between termination at any gestation. In practice, most state departments of health have guidelines that require additional discussion (e.g. in a multidisciplinary team or the consent of two different doctors) before undertaking terminations at a very late stage.

What are the record-keeping obligations of GPs when a women requests an abortion?

In the area of abortion, dependent on case and not statute law, it is imperative that GPs maintain accurate and adequate records of the consultation. It is not sufficient merely to record that the patient requested a termination of pregnancy and that a referral was written. The records should reflect the fact that the case falls within the conditions laid down by the law in that state or jurisdiction and, where necessary, GPs should include details regarding the patients' state of mind, concerns, financial circumstances, health, marital status and so on—in short, all the facts upon which the GP bases his/her honest belief about the necessity of the abortion to prevent danger to the person's physical and or mental health.

Other factors, such as whether the pregnancy was the result of rape or whether the patient is consenting under duress, need to be recorded, in the latter instance because consent under these circumstances is not valid.

Summary of key points
- Abortion laws vary considerably worldwide.
- Fathers do not have the right to stop an abortion from occurring.
- A fetus currently has no specific legal rights.
- A termination of pregnancy can be carried out on a minor without parental consent if the situation falls within the parameters of the 'mature minor' rule.
- The legal situation when a woman requests a termination of pregnancy on a viable fetus is unclear.
- GPs should keep accurate records of consultations involving the issue of termination of pregnancy.

THREATS TO ABORTION SERVICES

Despite many women being able to undergo an abortion when they feel it is necessary, abortion remains within the criminal code in many countries. Even when it is not, there are many other threats to the safe provision of abortion services for women.

The first of these is that the opportunities for doctors to train in the area of abortion are diminishing. In the USA in 1995, only 12% of obstetric and gynaecological training programs offered training in first-trimester abortions and only 7% in second-trimester abortions.[63] Harassment of abortion providers reached a new pitch with the murder of five clinic workers in 1993–94. The risk of an individual abortion provider being killed in the course of work is now greater than the chance a provider will see a death among his or her abortion patients.[9] In Australia, a security guard working for an abortion clinic was shot dead in 2002. Other issues include poor payment, professional isolation secondary to low peer approval, few well-trained mainstream specialists acting as role models and teachers, and declining motivation to provide abortion services as the generations of doctors who remember the wards filled with women who had complications from illegal abortions retire or die.

The medical profession should consider abortion not as a *favour to bestow* but as an *obligation to perform*. The provision of abortion services is *an unavoidable responsibility of physicians and hospitals in rendering health care to women*.

Abortion needs to remain a part of a comprehensive fertility control strategy that should include sex education to young people, availability of postcoital contraception and ongoing research into the factors that influence sexual behaviour and the use or not of contraceptive techniques, research that can then inform all of our practices.

TIPS FOR PRACTITIONERS

- When undertaking pregnancy counselling:
  - let the woman define her situation identifying the nature of the problem
  - use reflection to clarify her thoughts and feelings
  - find out what she has been considering and explore any options that she has not considered
  - help her verbalise the pros and cons of each alternative and list them on paper
  - ask her how each choice would affect her future
  - ask her who else's life each choice would affect
  - provide information about the abortion procedure including: cost, method, what happens at the clinic, how long it takes, how long it takes to recover and complication rates
  - provide information about adoption
  - provide information about how much welfare is available for a mother and a child.
  - confirm that she is a person who can take control of her own life and is responsible for herself.
- It is important to point out to patients that abortion clinics and pregnancy counselling and advice services listed in the phone book may not be objective and may be a 'front' for those with political or religious agendas.
- If requesting an ultrasound scan to confirm gestation in a woman requesting an abortion, be sure to advise the ultrasonographer to turn the screen away from the woman so she is not distressed by seeing the picture of the fetus.
- When examining women to determine gestation, it is helpful to think of the size of the uterus in terms of the size of fruit.
- Screening for *Chlamydia* is necessary in women requesting abortion, because of the high prevalence of *Chlamydia* infection in this group and because, if *Chlamydia* is detected, treatment can avoid unnecessary complications.

REFERENCES

1. Coyteaux FM, Leonard AH, Bloomer CM. Abortion. In: Koblinsky M, Timyan J, Gay J, eds. The health of women: a global perspective. Boulder: Westview Press; 1993.
2. Roston E, Armstrong S. Preventing maternal deaths. Geneva: World Health Organization; 1989.
3. Shearman RP. Trends in maternal mortality in Australia: relevance in current practice. Aust NZ J Obstet Gynaecol 1990; 30:15–17.
4. Grimes DA, Benson J, Singh S, et al. Unsafe abortion: the preventable pandemic. Lancet 2006; 368(9550):1908–1919.
5. Berer M. National laws and unsafe abortion: the parameters of change. Reprod Health Matters 2004; 12(suppl 24):1–8.
6. Department for Economic and Social Information and Policy Analysis. World population prospects: the 2000 revision. New York: United Nations; 2001.
7. World Health Organization Department of Reproductive Health and Research. Unsafe abortion: global and regional estimates of incidence of unsafe abortion and associated mortality in 2000. 4th edn. 2004. Online. Available: http://whqlibdoc.who.int/publications/2004/9241591803.pdf [accessed 5 Jan 2010].
8. David HP. Abortion in Europe 1920–91: a public health perspective. Stud Fam Plann 1992; 23:1–22.
9. Kulczycki A, Potts M, Rosenfield A. Abortion and fertility regulation. Lancet 1996; 347:1663–1668.
10. Rowe HJ, Kirkman M, Hardiman EA, et al. Considering abortion: a 12-month audit of records of women contacting a pregnancy advisory service. Med J Aust 2009; 190(2): 69–72.
11. Abigail W, Power C, Belan I. Changing patterns in women seeking terminations of pregnancy: a trend analysis of data from one service provider 1996–2006. Aust NZ J Public Health 2008; 32(3):230–237.
12. Lee W, Mazza D. Reasons for termination of pregnancy in women aged 35 and over. Med J Aust 2009; 191(3):188–189.
13. Popov AA. Family planning and induced abortion in the USSR: basic health and demographic characteristics. Stud Fam Plann 1991; 22:368–377.
14. Parliament of Victoria. Abortion Law Reform Bill 2008. 2008. Online. Available: http://www.austlii.edu.au/au/legis/vic/bill/alrb2008219/ [accessed 5 Jan 2010].
15. Cannold L. Understanding and responding to anti-choice women-centred strategies. Reprod Health Matters 2002; 10:171–179.
16. Frank PI, Kay CR, Scott LM, et al. Pregnancy following induced abortion: maternal morbidity, congenital abnormalities and neonatal death. Royal College of General Practitioners/Royal College of Obstetricians and Gynaecologists Joint Study. Br J Obstet Gynaecol 1987; 94:836–842.
17. Frank PI, McNamee R, Hannaford PC, et al. The effect of induced abortion on subsequent pregnancy outcome. Br J Obstet Gynaecol 1991; 98:1015–1024.
18. Frank P, McNamee R, Hannaford PC, et al. The effect of induced abortion on subsequent fertility. Br J Obstet Gynaecol 1993; 100:575–580.
19. Preston-Martin S, Pike MC, Ross RK, et al. Increased cell division as a cause of human cancer. Cancer Res 1990; 50:7415–7421.
20. Kelsey JL, Gammon MD, John EM. Reproductive factors and breast cancer. Epidemiol Rev 1993; 15:36–47.
21. Russo J, Russo IH. Susceptibility of the mammary gland to carcinogenesis II. Pregnancy interruption as a risk factor in tumour incidence. Am J Pathol 1980; 100:497–508.
22. Melbye M, Wohlfahrt J, Olsen JH, et al. Induced abortion and breast cancer. N Engl J Med 1997; 336:81–85.
23. Collaborative Group on Hormonal Factors in Breast Cancer. Breast cancer and abortion: collaborative reanalysis of data from 53 epidemiological studies, including 83,000 women with breast cancer from 16 countries. Lancet 2004; 363(9414):1007–1016.
24. Human Resources and Intergovernmental Sub-committee. The federal role in determining the medical and psychological impact of abortion on women (excerpt). Fam Plann Perspect 1990; 22:36–39.
25. Charles VE, Polis CB, Sridhara SK, et al. Abortion and long-term mental health outcomes: a systematic review of the evidence. Contraception 2008; 78(6):436–450.
26. Romans-Clarkson SE. Psychological sequelae of induced abortion. Aust NZ J Psychiatry 1989; 23:555–565.

27. Dagg PK. The psychological sequelae of therapeutic abortion—denied and completed. Am J Psychiatry 1991; 148:578–585.

28. Stotland NL. The myth of the abortion trauma syndrome. JAMA 1992; 268:2078–2079.

29. Cozzarelli C, Cooper ML, Major B, et al. Psychological responses of women after first-trimester abortion. Arch Gen Psychiatry 2000; 57:777–784.

30. Royal College of Obstetricians and Gynaecologists. The care of women requesting induced abortion. Report no.7. London: 2004.

31. Lemkau JP. Emotional sequelae of abortion: implications for clinical practice. Psychol Women Q 1988; 12:461–472.

32. Adelson PL, Frommer MS, Weisberg E. A survey of women seeking termination of pregnancy in New South Wales. Med J Aust 1995; 163:419–422.

33. Herndon J, Strauss LT, Whitehead S, et al. Abortion surveillance—United States 1998. MMWR Surveill Summ 2002; 51:1–32.

34. Rosenfield A. The difficult issue of second-trimester abortion. N Engl J Med 1994; 331:324–325.

35. Autry AM, Hayes EC, Jacobson GF, et al. A comparison of medical induction and dilation and evacuation for second-trimester abortion. Am J Obstet Gynecol 2002; 187:393–397.

36. Creinin MD. Medical abortion regimens: historical context and overview. Am J Obstet Gynaecol 2000; 183(Suppl):S3–S9.

37. Clark WH, Gold M, Grossman D, et al. Can mifepristone medical abortion be simplified? A review of the evidence and questions for future research. Contraception 2007; 75(4):245–250.

38. Baulieu EE. RU486 as an antiprogesterone steroid: from receptor to contragestion and beyond. JAMA 1989; 262:1808–1814.

39. Smith SK, Kelly RW. The effect of the antiprogestin RU486 and ZK98734 on the synthesis and metabolism of prostaglandins F2a and E2 in separated cells from early human decidua. J Clin Endocrinol Metab 1987; 65:527–534.

40. Swahn ML, Brydgeman M. The effect of the antiprogestin RU486 on uterine contractility and sensitivity to prostaglandin and oxytocin. Br J Obstet Gynaecol 1988; 95:126–134.

41. Royal Australian and New Zealand College of Obstetricians and Gynaecologists. Termination of pregnancy: a resource for health professionals. 2005. Online. Available: http://www.ranzcog.edu.au/womenshealth/pdfs/Termination-of-pregnancy.pdf [accessed 24.08.09].

42. Jones RK, Henshaw SK. Mifepristone for early medical abortion: experiences in France, Great Britain and Sweden. Perspect Sex Reprod Health 2002; 34:154–161.

43. Lindblom B. Ectopic pregnancy: laparoscopic and medical treatment. Curr Opin Obstet Gynecol 1992; 4:400–405.

44. Stoval TG, Ling FW. Single-dose methotrexate: an expanded clinical trial. Am J Obstet Gynecol 1993; 168:1759–1762.

45. Schaff EA, Eisinger SH, Franks P, et al. Methotrexate and misoprostol for early abortion. Fam Med 1996; 28:198–203.

46. Hausknecht RU. Methotrexate and misoprostol to terminate early pregnancy. N Engl J Med 1995; 333:537–540.

47. Grimes DA. Mifepristone (RU 486) for induced abortion. Women's Health Issues 1993; 3:171–175.

48. Potts M. Non-surgical abortion: who's for methotrexate? Lancet 1995; 346:655–656.

49. Silvestre L, Dubois C, Renault M, et al. Voluntary interruption of pregnancy with mifepristone (RU 486) and a prostaglandin analogue: a large-scale French experience. N Engl J Med 1990; 322:645–648.

50. UK Multicentre Trial. The efficacy and tolerance of mifepristone and prostaglandin in first-trimester termination of pregnancy. Br J Obstet Gynaecol 1990; 97:480–486.

51. Ulmann A, Silvestre L, Chemama L, et al. Medical termination of early pregnancy with mifepristone (RU 486) followed by a PG analogue: study in 16369 women. Acta Obstet Gynecol Scand 1992; 71:278–283.

52. Ross GT. Congenital anomalies among children born to mothers receiving chemotherapy for gestational trophoblast neoplasms. Cancer 1976; 37:1043–1047.

53. David HP. Acceptability of mifepristone for early pregnancy interruption. Law Med Health Care 1992; 20:188–194.

54. Winikoff B, Coyaji K, Cabezas E, et al. Studying the acceptability and feasibility of medical abortion. Law Med Health Care 1992; 20:195–198.

55. Winikoff B. Acceptability of medical abortion in early pregnancy. Fam Plann Perspect 1995; 27:142–148, 185.

56. Henshaw RC, Naji SA, Russell IT, et al. Comparison of medical abortion with surgical vacuum aspiration: Women's preferences and acceptability of treatment. BMJ 1993; 307:714–717.

57. Tang GW, Lau WK, Yip P. Further acceptability evaluation of RU 486 and ONO 802 as abortifacient agents in a Chinese population. Contraception 1993; 48:267–276.

58. Thong KJ, Dewar MH, Baird DT. What do women want during medical abortion? Contraception 1992; 46:435–442.

59. Creinin MD, Park M. Acceptability of medical abortion with methotrexate and misoprostol. Contraception 1995; 52:41–44.

60. Healy DL. Prostaglandins and progesterone receptor antagonists in human fertility regulation. Aust NZ J Obstet Gynaecol 1994; 34:357–360.

61. Henshaw SK. Induced abortion: a world review, 1990. Int Fam Plann Perspect 1990; 16:59–65, 76.

62. Kenyon E. The dilemma of abortion. London: Faber & Faber; 1986.

63. Mackay HT, Mackay AP. Abortion training in obstetrics and gynecology residency programs in the United States, 1991–1992. Fam Plann Perspect 1995; 27:112–115.

64. Fiala C, Danielsson K-G. Review of medical abortion using mifepristone in combination with a prostaglandin analogue. Contraception 2006; 74(1):66–86.

65. World Health Organization. Safe abortion: technical and policy guidance for health systems. Geneva: World Health Organization; 2003.

66. El-Refaey H, Rajasekar D, Abdalla M, et al. Induction of abortion with mifepristone (RU 486) and oral or vaginal misoprostol. N Engl J Med 1995; 332:983–987.

67. Breitbart V. Counselling for medical abortion. Am J Obstet Gynecol 200; 183(Suppl 2):S26–S33.

68. Gold RB. Abortion and women's health a turning point for America? New York: Alan Guttmacher Institute; 1990.

69. Center for Reproductive Rights. The world's abortion laws. 2007. Online. Available: http://reproductiverights.org/sites/crr.civicactions.net/files/documents/Abortion%20Map_FA.pdf [accessed 24.08.2009].

70. Gynuity Health Projects. Mifepristone Approval. 2009. Online. Available: http://gynuity.org/downloads/mife_approval_2009_list.pdf [accessed 10.04.10].

5

Pelvic pain

OBJECTIVES

- To develop an approach to diagnosing the aetiology of chronic pelvic pain in an individual woman
- To be able to implement an integrated approach to the management of chronic pelvic pain
- To describe the current understanding of the pathophysiology of endometriosis
- To recognise the symptoms and signs of endometriosis
- To be able to institute management for endometriosis in the primary-care setting
- To understand the limitations of current evidence regarding the management of endometriosis

CHRONIC PELVIC PAIN

CASE STUDY: 'I've had the pain for 20 years.'

Laura was 42 years old. She presented saying her friend had recommended me to her and that she needed help with her pain. Over the course of the consultation, she told me that she had had pain in her lower abdomen for more than 20 years and that sometimes it was so bad that she didn't know what to do. No-one had been able to help her. She had seen dozens of different doctors over the last 20 years and had had countless tests and procedures carried out. Her appendix and gall bladder had been removed, and she had had three laparoscopies. The last gynaecologist she had seen had told her to have her womb taken out, but before she went ahead she said she wanted a second opinion. Could I help?

Why do patients with chronic pelvic pain often cause 'heartsink' in their GPs?

Chronic pelvic pain (CPP) can be defined as recurrent or constant pelvic pain of at least 6 months' duration, unrelated to periods, intercourse or pregnancy. A more detailed definition is given in Box 5.1. It is one of those enigmatic presentations that frustrate GPs because of the difficulties they have in both diagnosing the problem and then implementing effective treatment.

One reason that CPP is so difficult to deal with is because there is a wide range of possible causes and most of these have overlapping symptoms. The most contradictory aspect of CPP, however, is the fact that often there is little correlation between the severity of the pain and evidence of a physiological cause for the pain. This highlights the need for an integrated approach to the management of CPP and the implementation of a biopsychosocial approach.

How common a problem is chronic pelvic pain?

It is a very common presentation. The annual prevalence in the primary-care setting in women aged between 15 and 73 years is 38/1000. This is almost the same as the prevalence of migraine,

---

BOX 5.1 The American College of Obstetricians and Gynecologists' (ACOG) definition of chronic pelvic pain (From ACOG[1])

- Non-cyclic pain of 6 or more months duration
- Localised to the anatomic pelvis, anterior abdominal wall at or below the umbilicus, the lumbosacral back or the buttocks
- Of sufficient severity to cause functional disability or lead to medical care

---

asthma and back pain.[2] A community-based study undertaken in the USA has found a prevalence of 15% for pelvic pain of >1 year's duration.[3] It is the indication for about one-third of laparoscopies and 10–15% of hysterectomies performed in the USA.[4] A recent Australian study reported on pelvic pain experienced by women over the last 12 months, documenting the relationships between dyspareunia, dysmenorrhoea and chronic pelvic pain.[52] This is well illustrated in Figure 5.1.

How should chronic pelvic pain be approached?

Traditional medical models of pain assume a direct relationship between tissue damage and pain. While this model explains acute pain fairly well, it leads to the categorisation of chronic pain into 'real' (i.e. that for which there is an identifiable cause of tissue damage) and 'not real' (when no tissue injury can be observed). However, CPP should be approached in the same way as other chronic pain syndromes. Like other chronic pain syndromes (such as back pain) this split is unhelpful and judgmental. Instead, it is more constructive to consider that the onset and the persistence of CPP are influenced by a number of factors. These can include:

- chronic pathological processes in somatic structures or viscera
- prolonged or permanent dysfunction of the peripheral or central nervous system
- psychological mechanisms used by the patient to deal with the pain
- socioenvironmental factors.

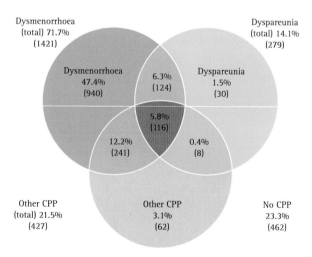

FIGURE 5.1 Prevalence of dysmenorrhoea, dyspareunia and other chronic pelvic pain among 1983 women aged 16–49 years who were currently menstruating and sexually active over a 12-month period (From Pitts et al[52])

While there are no differences in the prevalence across social class or with marital or employment status,[5] psychosocial factors that may impact on the development of CPP include:[6]

- familial pain models
- mood/anxiety states
- marital adjustment
- spouse's responses
- abuse history
- the use of somatisation

How a woman deals with her pain and social isolation can also exacerbate the situation.[7]

Numerous studies have documented the higher prevalence of both childhood and adult physical and sexual abuse in women who complain of CPP when compared with pain-free populations.[8–11]

Unfortunately, several adverse outcomes can arise from unresolved CPP. The severity of the pain can increase, often leading to the implementation of unproven surgical or medical intervention. Disability, or at least impaired health status, may come about. Depression and substance abuse can also ensue. Women with CPP may also have inappropriate healthcare utilisation. One study found that women with CPP had undergone five times as much previous surgery and sought treatment for four times as many somatic complaints when compared with women without pain.[10]

Women with chronic pelvic pain have often had multiple investigations, procedures and operations without any improvement in their condition.

What conditions can cause pelvic pain?

Several conditions can result in CPP. They may be gynaecological, gastrointestinal or genitourinary in nature (Table 5.1) and symptoms can arise from any of these systems. For example, one community-based study[12] has shown that about half of women with CPP have additional symptoms: 39% had irritable bowel syndrome and 24% had genitourinary symptoms. Furthermore, the prevalence of dysmenorrhoea and dyspareunia is higher in women with CPP than in those without CPP (81% and 41% respectively versus 58% and 14%). These results are concordant with other studies.[3,13]

GPs should be aware that while conditions such as endometriosis and pelvic adhesions can be found in women with CPP, they do not necessarily cause

TABLE 5.1 Major causes of chronic pelvic pain

Gynaecological	Gastrointestinal	Genitourinary
• Endometriosis	• Irritable bowel syndrome	Interstitial cystitis
• Adenomyosis	• Urethral syndrome	
• Pelvic inflammatory disease		
• Adhesions		

the pain. There is a poor correlation between the severity of endometriosis and pain. Indeed the majority of patients with mild, moderate and severe disease are asymptomatic.[14] Similar rates of both macroscopic and microscopic endometriosis have been found in women suffering from infertility and pelvic pain when compared with a pain-free group of women who had laparoscopic tubal ligation.[15] There is also no difference in the prevalence of pelvic adhesions in patients with CPP compared with pain-free women,[16] nor is there any benefit from lysis of the adhesions.[17]

Is there such a thing as pelvic congestion?

It has been suggested that other conditions are involved in the aetiology of CPP. These incidental or spurious conditions include uterine retroversion, peritoneal defects and pelvic venous congestion. The last of these is particularly controversial. Pelvic venous congestion is said to occur as a result of varices of the ovarian veins.[18] Some say it is a common finding in women with CPP, but the pathophysiology of this condition is poorly understood[19] and it is not clear whether 'pelvic congestion' is a normal or abnormal finding in women. A study of asymptomatic kidney donors showed a 9.9% prevalence of ovarian varices in the general population.[20] While interventional radiology has been used to 'treat' pelvic congestion, other authors state that there is no objective evidence to suggest that it is a significant factor in CPP in women.[21]

What aspects of the history are important?

Because patients attending a GP have often seen many doctors beforehand for the same problem, they may or may not have been investigated and they may or may not have been given a diagnosis or several diagnoses. It is therefore important to obtain a timeline of the development of the pain, asking all the questions necessary when taking a history of someone with pain regarding:

- onset
- duration

- intensity
- nature
- radiation
- relationship to menstrual cycle
- associated symptoms:
  - headache
  - nausea
  - bladder symptoms
  - bowel symptoms
  - dyspareunia
  - menstrual disturbances
  - back pain.

It is also important to find out about the patient's past history of medical and surgical problems, in particular:

- pelvic infection
- pelvic surgery
- appendicitis
- endometriosis.

Questions concerning a history of physical and/ or sexual abuse as a child, as well as a history of adult sexual assault or domestic violence should be sensitively posed. One way of pursuing this history is by saying something like 'When I've seen women with these kinds of problems before, I've found that many of them have experienced either child abuse or domestic violence or rape. Has that happened to you?'

The more recent history of the condition should also be sought, by asking whom the patient has already seen about this condition and what tests and/ or treatments have been carried out. It is worthwhile finding out exactly how disabling the condition is and whether or not it is interfering with the woman's daily activities. Often disability has developed gradually and it may be useful to identify inflection points in the curve of disability brought about by external life events or events within the family.[22]

What aspects of the examination are important?

Examination of the abdomen and the pelvis should be undertaken. A pelvic mass may be found, whether uterine or ovarian in origin. The exact site of the pain and any tenderness or guarding should also be noted. A vaginal examination may elicit pain on rocking the cervix. This stretches the uterosacral ligaments and may suggest pathology such as endometriosis or pelvic infection. A retroverted uterus is a common and is often an incidental finding. If the uterus is fixed, however, this may indicate the presence of dense adhesions.

What investigative pathway should be used?

Some suggest that undertaking a history and physical examination should be sufficient for the evaluation of a woman with CPP, unless specific abnormalities are detected.[6,23] Routine use of ultrasonography and laparoscopy is generally unrewarding and not indicated.[24] However, in an effort to find a cause and appease the patient, many women will be sent for an ultrasound to look for ovarian cysts, fibroids and large hydrosalpinges or pyosalpinges. A laparoscopy then follows, seeking signs of endometriosis or pelvic adhesions.

More than 40% of laparoscopies are performed for the diagnosis of CPP. Although laparoscopic evaluation is sometimes considered a routine part of the evaluation, ideally the decision to perform a laparoscopy should be based on the patient's history, physical examination and the findings of non-invasive tests. About 65% of women with CPP have at least one diagnosis detectable by laparoscopy and it is common to attribute causality to this diagnosis. Endometriosis is diagnosed in one-third of laparoscopies for CPP. Endometriosis requires histological confirmation to assure an accurate diagnosis. Adhesions are diagnosed in about one-quarter of laparoscopies. Ovarian cysts, hernias, pelvic congestion syndrome, ovarian remnant syndrome, ovarian retention syndrome, postoperative peritoneal cysts and endosalpingiosis are other diagnoses that are made laparoscopically in some cases.[25]

More than 40% of laparoscopies are performed in an attempt to determine the aetiology of chronic pelvic pain.

What non-drug management can I offer patients with chronic pelvic pain?

Management of CPP should involve an integrated approach and be therapeutic, as well as supportive and sympathetic.

Cognitive behavioural therapy may be helpful, not only by assisting the patient to control the pain but also in reducing disability and promoting wellbeing. By teaching muscle relaxation, controlled breathing and the use of imagery, GPs can help their patients decrease their general level of arousal and divert their attention from the physical signals that preoccupy them. Cognitive techniques that address maladaptive and negative thinking, such as fear of cancer, should also be introduced and rehearsed with the patient. Cognitive behavioural pain management should also focus on stress management and, in particular, on methods that can be used by the patient to identify the cause of her stress and how to address these issues in a constructive way (e.g. through problem solving, assertiveness and time management).

Another strategy is to encourage the patient to involve herself in recreational activities and to return to work if she has stopped. Physical exercise is recommended as a means of encouraging general wellbeing and patients should be educated about the benefits of good nutrition, sleep, relaxation and avoidance of substance abuse.

Focused psychotherapy may be necessary to address the long-term outcomes of child abuse or more recent sexual assault. Specific mental health disorders such as depression and anxiety, eating disorders and post-traumatic stress disorders should also be treated. If the woman is involved in an abusive relationship, this problem needs to be recognised and addressed. Substance abuse counselling and treatment may also be required. Couple counselling may be helpful where there is an inappropriate spousal response to the pelvic pain—for example, when the partner is either punitive or overly solicitous. Sexual counselling should also be offered if sexual dysfunction is an issue.

Are any forms of medication helpful?

By the time they present to you women will have tried many forms of medication. It is therefore important to review what treatment has already been tried and how it has been implemented.

Oral analgesics should be optimised. An NSAID can be given on a regular basis, rather than as required. This strategy is used in an attempt to decrease the continual 'self-monitoring' that encourages the patient to focus on the pain. Narcotics should be avoided because of their potential for addiction and abuse.

Some recommend the use of tricyclic antidepressants or selective serotonin reuptake inhibitors (SSRIs), as this therapeutic approach is often used in other forms of chronic pain. The use of psychotropic medication, however, does run the risk of reinforcing to the patient that their symptoms are 'all in their head' and not being taken seriously. Also, it neither addresses the specific reasons why chronic pain has developed in that particular patient nor gives her the skills to overcome the problem should it recur. SSRIs should therefore be used in conjunction with cognitive behavioural therapy and/ or psychotherapy.

Another approach is to try ovarian cycle suppression. This may be helpful when the pain is cyclical in nature. Three alternatives are available. First, a monophasic combined oral contraceptive can be used. Second, progestogens can be used. These can be administered either as continuous oral medication or as Implanon or Depo-Provera® (injectable). The last option—not often used by general practitioners—is the use of a gonadotrophin-releasing hormone agonist (GnRH-A).

The most recent Cochrane review has found that progestogen (medroxyprogesterone acetate) is associated with a reduction of pain during treatment, while goserelin gives a longer duration of benefit.[26] Counselling, supported by ultrasound scanning, is associated with reduced pain and improvement in mood. A multidisciplinary approach is beneficial for some outcome measures. Benefits are not demonstrated for:

- adhesiolysis (apart from where adhesions were severe)
- uterine nerve ablation
- sertraline
- or photographic reinforcement after laparoscopy.

The authors of this review warn, however, that the range of proven effective interventions for chronic pelvic pain remains limited and their recommendations are based largely on single studies.

Is there any role for surgery?

Many GPs will have seen women who have had recurrent surgical intervention for chronic abdominal or pelvic pain, despite no firm identification of any pathological process. Often the health of these women deteriorates over time as a result of complications arising from the surgery and increasing dependence on narcotics due in part to their frequent hospital admissions.

Current laparoscopic practice involves the removal of visible areas of endometriosis and, in some cases, the destruction of the nerve pathways thought to be responsible for carrying pain fibres from the pelvis (uterine nerve ablation and presacral neurectomy). The surgery may include excision and laser or diathermy ablation with or without adhesiolysis. Despite the wide use of this form of therapy for endometriosis, there have been few randomised controlled trials carried out to prove its efficacy.

Another Cochrane review looked at this issue and found that a combined surgical approach of laparoscopic laser ablation, adhesiolysis and uterine nerve ablation is likely to be a beneficial treatment for pelvic pain associated with minimal, mild and moderate endometriosis.[27] However, as only one trial was included in the analysis, this conclusion should be interpreted with caution.

As a last resort, many doctors offer women a hysterectomy for treatment of their CPP. It forms the principal indication for 10–15% of hysterectomies in the USA. Studies of this surgical option have shown, however, that despite a 74% initial resolution of the pain there was a recurrence rate of 40% in those women who did not have an identifiable pathology.[28] Furthermore, more than 60% of uteri and adnexa removed from women with CPP have been found to be histologically normal.[29]

Summary of key points
- CPP is common and the indication for up to 40% of laparoscopies and 10–15% of hysterectomies that are undertaken.
- GPs should approach CPP as a syndrome brought about by a combination of factors:
  - chronic pathological processes
  - prolonged dysfunction of the peripheral or central nervous system
  - psychological mechanisms used by the patient to deal with pain
  - socioenvironmental factors.
- There is a well-documented relationship between childhood and adult physical and sexual abuse and the development of CPP.
- Many conditions (such as endometriosis) found in women with CPP are not necessarily causative of the pain.
- The existence of 'pelvic congestion syndrome' is controversial.
- Cognitive behavioural therapy and physical exercise are recommended aspects of management for women with CPP.
- Surgical management is not always successful, with many women suffering a recurrence of their pain.

ENDOMETRIOSIS

What exactly is endometriosis?

Endometriosis is the presence of endometrial tissue outside of the lining of the uterine cavity, which induces a chronic, inflammatory reaction. The endometrial tissue is responsive to hormones and so causes cyclical bleeding. This causes local inflammation and subsequent fibrosis, peritoneal

---

CASE STUDY: Dysmenorrhoea with dyspareunia

Melinda, 27 year of age, presents to you with increasingly severe dysmenorrhoea. She has been using condoms for contraception and is no longer able to control the pain with the anti-inflammatory tablets you suggested at the last consultation 6 months ago. She also complains of the recent development of deep dyspareunia. She has been in her current relationship for the last 5 years.

Examination illicits similar pain and tenderness to that which she feels during intercourse. You refer her to a gynaecologist who undertakes a laparoscopy on Melinda. Ovarian adhesions are seen secondary to endometriosis.

---

damage and adhesions between organs in the pelvis. Ovarian implants lead to the formation of 'chocolate cysts', or endometriomas.

What are the latest theories about the causes of endometriosis?

In 1927, Sampson postulated that endometriosis was caused by retrograde flow of endometrial tissue during menstruation. This theory is supported by such findings as seeing blood flow from the fimbriated end of the tube in virtually all menstruating women having a laparoscopy.[30] More recently, it has been postulated that endometriosis is caused by the transformation of coelomic epithelium into endometrial-type glands as a result of unspecified stimuli. This theory may explain the reports of endometriosis in women who have never menstruated.[31] Blood-borne spread of endometrial tissue may also be a mechanism of causation, because, curiously, endometriosis has been described in sites far away from the pelvis. Such sites include the pleura and lungs, umbilicus, rectus abdominis muscle, omentum, liver, pancreas, gall bladder, and surgical scars such as episiotomy scars, laparoscopic trocar sites and amniocentesis tracts.

Research has shown that there is a genetic component to the disease, with one study reporting that 6.9% of first-degree relatives of patients with endometriosis also had the disease, compared with 1.0% of first-degree relatives of controls.[32] Immunological responses may also play an important part in the development of the disease.

How common is endometriosis?

The prevalence of endometriosis is thought to be between 3% and 10% in women in the reproductive age group,[33] but can range from 2% to 50%, depending on the diagnostic criteria used and the populations studied.[34] The rates are much higher in women having laparoscopies for investigation of infertility. In general, the risk of endometriosis increases where there is greater exposure to menstruation (e.g. reduced parity). The risk decreases in association with factors that decrease oestrogen levels (e.g. smoking and exercise).[35]

What symptoms and signs does endometriosis produce?

The classic symptoms of endometriosis are:

- pelvic pain
- dysmenorrhoea
- dyspareunia
- infertility.

In women with dysmenorrhoea the incidence of endometriosis ranges from 40% to 60%.

Characteristic of the pain of endometriosis is its cyclical nature and relation to menstruation. Patients may also experience painful bowel movements, back pain and abdominal symptoms. Classically, symptoms are exacerbated at the time of menstruation. The classical signs of endometriosis are listed in Box 5.2.

BOX 5.2 Classical signs of endometriosis

- Local tenderness in the cul de sac or uterosacral ligaments
- Adnexal enlargement or tenderness
- Pelvic masses
- A fixed, retroverted uterus
- Thickening or nodularity of the cul de sac/uterosacral ligaments

---

BOX 5.3 Relationship between pain and endometriosis

- Pain of acute onset is more likely to be due to infection or a haemorrhagic corpus luteum than to endometriosis.
- Consistently localised pain may indicate a deeply fibrotic endometrioma.
- Dyspareunia suggests rectovaginal endometriosis.

As previously noted, the severity of the symptoms (such as pain) is not necessarily related to the extent of the disease.[36] However, the suggestions offered in Box 5.3 may be helpful when considering the relationship between pain and endometriosis.[37]

The severity of the symptoms of endometriosis and the probability of its diagnosis increase with age.

How does one diagnose endometriosis?

No set of signs, symptoms or investigations give an absolute diagnosis of endometriosis. As far as the symptoms and signs are concerned, these may be caused by other disease processes. In most situations, a clinical diagnosis is made through the history and examination. Specific diagnosis probably requires visualisation and biopsy through laparoscopy: two examples of laparoscopic findings of endometriosis are shown in Figures 5.2 and 5.3. Visual inspection is usually adequate, but histological confirmation of at least one lesion is ideal. In cases of ovarian

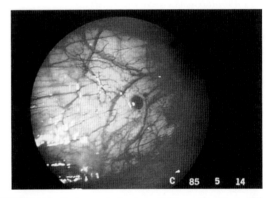

FIGURE 5.2 Endometriotic deposit (From James et al[53])

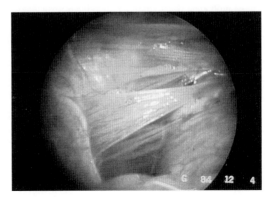

FIGURE 5.3 Adhesions secondary to endometriosis (From James et al[53])

endometrioma (greater than 3 cm in diameter) and in deeply infiltrating disease, histology should be obtained to identify endometriosis and to exclude rare instances of malignancy.[38] Some, however, advocate empirical drug treatment prior to laparoscopy.[39]

In endometriosis, symptoms and laparoscopic appearance do not always correlate.

Ultrasound is of limited value in the diagnosis of endometriosis, despite the fact that it is helpful when ovarian cysts are present. Guidelines state that CA125 has limited value as either a screening or diagnostic test and affirm that laparoscopy is the only diagnostic test that can reliably rule out endometriosis.[38] Because of this and its accuracy in detecting endometriosis, laparoscopy is regarded as the standard investigation.[38]

However, it is worthwhile considering the fact that the mean time between the onset of pain symptoms and the surgical diagnosis of endometriosis is 12 years in the USA and 8 years in the UK.[40] This has enormous implications in terms of the suffering that women experience and also the ability of the disease to progress during this time.

Does endometriosis cause infertility?

Whether or not endometriosis actually causes infertility is still controversial. In women with subfertility, the incidence of endometriosis ranges from 20 to 30%. It is interesting to reflect that a large percentage of the female population has some degree of endometriosis, yet <10% are infertile.[41] However, trials comparing success rates of donor insemination in women with and without endometriosis have shown that women without endometriosis were more likely to conceive.

Women with even small amounts of endometriosis have lower conception rates.[42]

Despite this, a systematic review of medical treatment for women with infertility and endometriosis did not find evidence that is provided any benefit,[43] and guidelines do not recommend treatment of endometriosis in women trying to conceive.[38] Although medical treatment of endometriosis has no benefit for infertility, ablation of endometriotic lesions plus adhesiolysis to improve fertility in minimal–mild endometriosis is effective compared with diagnostic laparoscopy alone.[38]

What treatment options are available?

When considering management, GPs should think about the predominant outcome they are seeking: whether it is a decrease in pain or an improvement in fertility, or both. They should also consider the woman's reproductive desires and whether any treatment at all is appropriate at that point in time.

With regard to medical management, the simplest form of therapy for women with mild pelvic pain is with NSAIDs. Evidence of their effectiveness is hard to find, however, and there is no evidence to suggest that any individual NSAID is more effective than another.[44] The next strategy is to aim for suppression of ovulation. A recent systematic review suggests that oral contraceptive pills are likely to be of benefit.[45] They are also one of the easiest regimens to implement through the use of a low-dose monophasic pill in a continuous fashion for 6–12 months.

The medical treatment of endometriosis usually involves suppression of the ovarian cycle.

Depo-Provera® can also be used to depress oestradiol levels, suppress ovulation and prevent menstruation. Danazol was for many years the treatment of choice but is no more effective than other hormonal measures and may have troublesome side effects related to the androgenic environment that it causes (Box 5.4). GnRH agonists administered intramuscularly, subcutaneously or intranasally can create a 'hypogonadic' state, or 'medical oophorectomy'. Results of treatment with GnRH agonists are similar to those found with the use of danazol. However, there are concerns regarding the long-term consequences on calcium metabolism and possible bone loss. Some therefore utilise HRT as an add-back treatment to control hypo-oestrogenic symptoms and prevent the development of osteoporosis.

BOX 5.4 The side effects of danazol

- Weight gain
- Oily skin
- Acne
- Hirsutism
- Reduction in breast size
- Unfavourable alteration in lipids
- Hepatic dysfunction
- Alteration in voice

The levonorgestrel intrauterine system (LNG-IUS) can also be used to manage dysmenorrhoea and endometriosis.[46] Its efficacy is similar to that of GnRH analogues[47] and, when used after surgery, it produces additional benefits when compared with surgery alone.[48]

Medical management is summarised in Table 5.2.

In women with pain attributable to endometriosis, hormonal treatments that suppress ovulation are beneficial.

There are no randomised controlled trials comparing medical versus surgical treatments for the management of endometriosis, and at the time of diagnosis the decision about medical or surgical treatment will depend on several factors, including the patient's choice, the availability of laparoscopic surgery, the desire for fertility and concerns about long-term medical therapy.[49] Surgical options for management range from conservative laparoscopic surgery to uterine nerve ablation, total hysterectomy and bilateral oophorectomy. Unfortunately, the evidence about the efficacy of these various forms of surgery is lacking.

What is the recurrence rate of endometriosis?

The recurrence rate is approximately 5–20% per year (reaching a cumulative rate at 5 years of as much as 40%). In women treated for pelvic pain, symptoms tend to recur once treatment has ceased,[50] although the intensity of the symptoms may be less severe.[51] Recurrence may occur in part because large lesions respond poorly to medical treatment. It is generally accepted that endometriomata are not amenable to medical treatment, although temporary clinical relief may be achieved.[49]

Summary of key points
- Endometriosis affects approximately 10% of women, with a higher prevalence in those with infertility.
- The classic symptoms of endometriosis are pelvic pain, dysmenorrhoea, dyspareunia and infertility.
- The severity of the pain is not necessarily related to the extent of the disease.
- The mean time between onset of symptoms and diagnosis is 8–12 years.

TABLE 5.2 Medical treatments for endometriosis[a] (From Farquhar[49])

Drug	Mechanism of action	Length of treatment recommended	Adverse events	Notes
Medroxyprogesterone acetate/ progestagens	Ovarian suppression	Long term	Weight gain, bloating, acne, irregular bleeding	May be given orally or by intramuscular or subcutaneous depot injection
Danazol	Ovarian suppression	3–6 months	Weight gain, bloating, acne, hirsutism, skin rashes	Adverse effects on lipid profiles
Oral contraceptive	Ovarian suppression	Long term	Nausea, headaches	Can be used to avoid menstruation by skipping the placebo pills
GnRH analogue	Ovarian suppression by competitive inhibitive action of GnRH analogue	6 months	Hot flushes, other symptoms of hypo-oestrogenism	By injection or nasal spray only
Levonorgestrel intrauterine system	Endometrial suppression, ovarian suppression in some women	Long-term use, but change every 5 years in women <40 years	Irregular bleeding	Also reduces menstrual blood loss

GnRH=gonadotrophin releasing hormone
[a]Decisions about medical therapy will depend on pattern's choice, available resources, plans for fertility and ongoing symptoms. Side-effect profile may influence choice.

- Management is dependent on whether the primary aim is pain control or treatment of infertility.
- Recurrence rates of endometriosis after treatment are substantial.

TIPS FOR PRACTITIONERS

- GPs should not get caught in the trap of categorising CPP as 'not real' because no pathology can be identified, as this is counterproductive to resolution of the problem.
- It is important to try to make the patient with CPP aware that her pain, like all forms of chronic pain, is attributable to physical factors as well as the psychological mechanisms she uses to cope with pain and socioenvironmental factors.
- Women with CPP may benefit from being taught muscle relaxation, controlled breathing and visualisation techniques to help them manage their pain.
- It is important to identify a history of child sexual abuse, rape or domestic violence in women suffering from CPP so that these issues can be addressed.
- Regular exercise to improve wellbeing should be encouraged in all patients with chronic pain.
- GPs should suspect endometriosis in patients when they find the following signs on examination:
  - local tenderness in the cul de sac
  - adnexal enlargement or tenderness
  - pelvic masses
  - a fixed, retroverted uterus.
- Avoid prescribing medical treatment for endometriosis in women who are trying to conceive.[49]
- The simpler treatments for endometriosis—such as the combined oral contraceptive pill, oral or depot medroxyprogesterone acetate, and the levonorgestrel intrauterine system—are as effective as the gonadotrophin releasing hormone analogues and can be used long term.[49]

REFERENCES

1. American College of Obstetricians and Gynecologists, Committee on Practice Bulletins. ACOG Practice Bulletin no. 51. Chronic pelvic pain. Obstet Gynecol 2004; 103:589–605.
2. Zondervan KT, Yudkin PL, Vessey MP, et al. Prevalence and incidence of chronic pelvic pain in primary care: evidence from a national general practice database. Br J Obstet Gynaecol 1999; 106:1149–1155.
3. Mathias SD, Kuppermann M, Liberman RF, et al. Chronic pelvic pain: prevalence, health-related quality of life, and economic correlates. Obstet Gynecol 1996; 87:321–327.
4. Reiter RC. A profile of women with chronic pelvic pain. Clin Obstet Gynaecol 1990; 33:130–136.
5. Zondervan K, Barlow DH. Epidemiology of chronic pelvic pain. Baillière's Best Pract Res Clin Obstet Gynaecol 2000; 14:403–414.
6. Reiter RC. Evidence-based management of chronic pelvic pain. Clin Obstet Gynaecol 1998; 41:422–435.
7. Vincent K. Chronic pelvic pain in women. Postgrad Med J 2009; 85(999):24–29.
8. Walker E, Katon W, Harrop-Griffiths J, et al. Relationship of chronic pelvic pain to psychiatric diagnoses and childhood sexual abuse. Am J Psychiatry 1988; 145:75–80.
9. Walling MK, Reiter RC, O'Hara MW, et al. Abuse history and chronic pain in women: I. Prevalences of sexual abuse and physical abuse. Obstet Gynecol 1994; 84:193–199.
10. Reiter RC, Gambone JC. Demographic and historical variables in women with chronic pelvic pain. Obstet Gynecol 1990; 75:428–432.
11. Paras ML, Murad MH, Chen LP, et al. Sexual abuse and lifetime diagnosis of somatic disorders: a systematic review and meta-analysis. JAMA 2009; 302(5):550–561.
12. Zondervan KT, Yudkin PL, Vessey MP, et al. Chronic pelvic pain in the community—symptoms, investigations, and diagnoses. Am J Obstet Gynecol 2001; 184:1149–1155.
13. Walker EA, Katon WJ, Jemelka R, et al. The prevalence of chronic pelvic pain and irritable bowel syndrome in two university clinics. J Psychosom Obstet Gynaecol 1991; 12: 65–75.
14. Buttram VC, Reiter RC. Endometriosis. In: Buttram VC, Reiter RC (eds). Surgical treatment of the infertile female. Baltimore: Williams & Wilkins; 1985:95.
15. Balasch J, Creus M, Fabregues F, et al. Visible and non-visible endometriosis at laparoscopy in fertile and infertile women and in patients with chronic pelvic pain: a prospective study. Hum Reprod 1996; 11:387–391.
16. Rapkin AJ. Adhesions and pelvic pain: a retrospective study. Obstet Gynaecol 1986; 68:13–15.
17. Peters AAW, Trimbos-Kemper GCM, Admirral C, et al. A randomised clinical trial on the benefit of adhesiolysis in patients with intraperitoneal adhesions and chronic pelvic pain. Br J Obstet Gynaecol 1992; 99:59–63.
18. Beard RW, Highman JH, Pearce S, et al. Diagnosis of pelvic varicosities in women with chronic pelvic pain. Lancet 1984; ii:946–949.
19. Foong LC, Gamble J, Sutherland IA, et al. Microvascular changes in the peripheral microcirculation of women with chronic pelvic pain due to congestion. Br J Obstet Gynaecol 2002; 109:867–873.
20. Belenky A, Bartal G, Atar E, et al. Ovarian varices in healthy female kidney donors: incidence, morbidity, and clinical outcome. AJR Am J Roentgenol 2002; 179(3):625–627.
21. Stenchever MA. Symptomatic retrodisplacement, pelvic congestion, universal joint, and peritoneal defects: fact or fiction? Clin Obstet Gynaecol 1990; 33:161–167.
22. Steege JF, Stout AL. Chronic gynecologic pain. In: Stewart DE, Stotland NL (eds). Psychological aspects of women's health care. Washington DC: American Psychiatric Press; 1993.
23. Ryder RM. Chronic pelvic pain. Am Fam Physician 1996; 54:2225–2237.
24. Steege JF, Stout AL, Somkuti SG. Chronic pelvic pain in women: toward an integrative model. Obstet Gynecol Surv 1993; 48:95–110.
25. Howard FM. The role of laparoscopy as a diagnostic tool in chronic pelvic pain. Baillière's Best Pract Res Clin Obstet Gynaecol 2000; 14:467–494.
26. Stones W, Cheong YC, Howard FM. Interventions for treating chronic pelvic pain in women. Cochrane Database Syst Rev 2005; 1:CD000387.

27. Jacobson TZ, Duffy JM, Barlow D, et al. Laparoscopic surgery for pelvic pain associated with endometriosis. Cochrane Database Syst Rev 2001; 4:CD001300.

28. Hillis SD, Marchbanks PA, Peterson HB. The effectiveness of hysterectomy for chronic pelvic pain. Obstet Gynecol 1995; 86:941–945.

29. Lee NC, Dicker RC, Rubin GL, et al. Confirmation of the preoperative diagnoses for hysterectomy. Am J Obstet Gynecol 1984; 150:283–287.

30. Liu DTY, Hitchcock A. Endometriosis: its association with retrograde menstruation, dysmenorrhoea and tubal pathology. Br J Obstet Gynaecol 1986; 93:859.

31. El-Mahgoub S, Yaseen S. A positive proof for the theory of coelomic metaplasia. Am J Obstet Gynaecol 1980; 137: 137–140.

32. Simpson JL, Elias J, Malinek LR, et al. Heritable aspects of endometriosis. I. Genetic Studies. Am J Obstet Gynaecol 1980; 137:327–331.

33. Olive DL, Schwartz LB. Endometriosis. N Engl J Med 1993; 328:1759–1769.

34. Fauconnier A, Chapron C. Endometriosis and pelvic pain: epidemiological evidence of the relationship and implications. Hum Reprod Update 2005; 11(6):595–606.

35. Eskanazi B, Warner ML. Epidemiology of endometriosis. Obstet Gynecol Clin North Am 1997; 24:235–238.

36. Marana R, Muzii L, Caruana P, et al. Evaluation of the correlation between endometriosis extent, age of the patients and associated symptomatology. Acta Eur Fertil 1991; 22: 209–212.

37. Martin DC, Ling FW. Endometriosis and pain. Clin Obstet Gynecol 1999; 42:664–686.

38. Royal College of Obstetricians and Gynaecologists. The investigation and management of endometriosis 2006 (Green Top Guideline no. 24). Online. Available: http://www.rcog.org.uk/files/rcog-corp/uploaded-files/GT24InvestigationEndometriosis2006.pdf [accessed 9 Aug 2009].

39. Valle RF. Endometriosis: current concepts and therapy. Int J Gynaecol Obstet 2002; 78:107–119.

40. Hadfield R, Mardon H, Barlow D, et al. Delay in diagnosis of endometriosis: a survey of women from the USA and the UK. Hum Reprod 1996; 11:878–880.

41. Burns WN, Schenken RS. Pathophysiology of endometriosis-associated infertility. Clin Obstet Gynecol 1999; 42:586–610.

42. Jansen RP. Minimal endometriosis and reduced fecundability: prospective evidence from an artificial insemination by donor program. Fertil Steril 1986; 46:141–143.

43. Hughes E, Brown J, Collins JJ, et al. Ovulation suppression for endometriosis. Cochrane Database Syst Rev 2007; 3:CD000155.

44. Allen C, Hopewell S, Prentice A, et al. Nonsteroidal anti-inflammatory drugs for pain in women with endometriosis. Cochrane Database Syst Rev 2009; 2:CD004753.

45. Davis L, Kennedy SS, Moore J, et al. Modern combined oral contraceptives for pain associated with endometriosis. Cochrane Database Syst Rev 2007; 3:CD001019.

46. Yap C, Furness S, Farquhar C. Pre and post operative medical therapy for endometriosis surgery. Cochrane Database Syst Rev 2004; 3:CD003678.

47. Petta CA, Ferriani RA, Abrao MS, et al. Randomized clinical trial of a levonorgestrel-releasing intrauterine system and a depot GnRH analogue for the treatment of chronic pelvic pain in women with endometriosis. Hum Reprod 2005; 20(7): 1993–1998.

48. Vercellini P, Frontino G, De Giorgi O, et al. Comparison of a levonorgestrel-releasing intrauterine device versus expectant management after conservative surgery for symptomatic endometriosis: a pilot study. Fertil Steril 2003; 80(2):305–309.

49. Farquhar C. Endometriosis [see comment]. BMJ 2007; 334(7587):249–253.

50. Vercellini P, Trespidi L, Colombo A, et al. A gonadotropin-releasing hormone agonist versus a low dose oral contraceptive for pelvic pain associated with endometriosis. Fertil Steril 1993; 60: 75–79.

51. Fedele L, Bianchi S, Bocciolone L, et al. Buserilin acetate in the treatment of pelvic pain associated with minimal and mild endometriosis; a controlled study. Fertil Steril 1993; 59: 516–521.

52. Pitts MK, Ferris JA, Smith AM, et al. Prevalence and correlates of three types of pelvic pain in a nationally representative sample of Australian women. Med J Aust 2008; 189(3): 138–143.

53. James D, Pilai M, Rymer J, et al. Obstetrics, Gynaecology, Neonatology interactive colour guides, CD-ROM. Edinburgh: Churchill Livingstone; 2002.

6

Polycystic ovary syndrome

OBJECTIVES

- To develop an understanding of the metabolic factors involved in polycystic ovary syndrome (PCOS)
- To describe the manifestations of PCOS
- To understand the principles of management of PCOS
- To describe the long-term consequences of PCOS

UNDERSTANDING PCOS

> ### CASE STUDY: 'Polycystic ovaries'
>
> Twenty-year-old Marie had come in for a routine Pap smear and check-up. I noticed that she had a laparoscopy scar and asked her what she had had done. She replied that she had had her ovaries 'golf-balled' some two years previously. When I asked why, she answered that she had been told that she had 'polycystic ovaries' but was unsure about why she had actually had the procedure.

What is polycystic ovary syndrome (PCOS)?

Stein and Leventhal first described PCOS in 1935 as a symptom complex associated with anovulation. It was said to be present in women who had oligomenorrhoea, hirsutism and obesity, together with a demonstration of enlarged polycystic ovaries. More recently, a consensus definition for PCOS has been reached (Box 6.1).[1]

Other conditions can also be present as part of PCOS, but these are not among the diagnostic criteria; they include obesity, insulin resistance, impaired glucose tolerance and type 2 diabetes mellitus, dyslipidaemia, cardiovascular disease, obstructive sleep apnoea and infertility.[2]

How many women have polycystic ovaries?

As many GPs practising in women's health know, the ultrasonographic description of polycystic ovaries is commonly found in asymptomatic women. In fact, studies have found that approximately 25% of normal women demonstrate the classic features of polycystic ovaries described in Box 6.2. A 'necklace-like' appearance or 'string-of-pearls' pattern of follicular cysts is said to be 'typical' of polycystic ovaries.[3,4] These findings have become even more common with the use of high-resolution transvaginal ultrasounds. Around 14% of women on oral contraceptive pills have also been found to have polycystic ovaries.[4]

How many women have polycystic ovary syndrome?

General estimates for the prevalence of PCOS based on old definitions range between 5% and 10% in women of reproductive age.[5,6] Estimates

---

> ### BOX 6.1 The Rotterdam Consensus Group criteria for the definition of polycystic ovary syndrome (From Rotterdam ESHRE/ASRM-sponsored POCS Consensus workshop group[1])
>
> The diagnosis of PCOS requires that at least two of the following three criteria are met:
>
> 1. Oligo-ovulation and/or anovulation.
> 2. Clinical and/or biochemical signs of hyper-androgenism. Clinical hyperandrogenism includes hirsutism, acne, or androgenic alopecia. Biochemical hyperandrogenism (or hyperandrogenaemia) includes a raised level of circulating androgens such as total testosterone, free testosterone or free androgen index (FAI), or dehydroepiandrosterone-sulphate (DHEAS).
> 3. Polycystic ovaries on ultrasound (defined as the presence of 12 or more follicles in either ovary measuring 2–9 mm in diameter, and/or increased ovarian volume greater than 10 mL). If a follicle >10 mm in diameter is present, the scan should be repeated at a time of ovarian quiescence in order to calculate the ovarian volume.
>
> Other causes for hyperandrogenism that mimic PCOS (e.g. congenital adrenal hyperplasia, Cushing's syndrome or androgen-secreting tumours) should be excluded

> ### BOX 6.2 The range of clinical manifestations of PCOS (Adapted from Balen[35])
>
> **Signs and symptoms**
> - Obesity
> - Menstrual disturbance
> - Oligomenorrhoea:
>   - amenorrhoea
>   - regular cycle
> - Hyperandrogenism
> - Infertility
>
> **Hormone systems that might be disturbed**
> - Insulin ↑
> - Sex-hormone-binding globulin ↓
> - Androgens (testosterone and androstenedione) ↑
> - Luteinising hormone ↑
> - Prolactin ↑
> - Oestradiol, oestrone ↑
>
> **Possible late sequelae**
> - Dyslipidaemia:
>   - LDL ↑
>   - HDL ↑
>   - triglycerides ↑
> - Diabetes mellitus
> - Cardiovascular disease and hypertension
> - Endometrial cancer

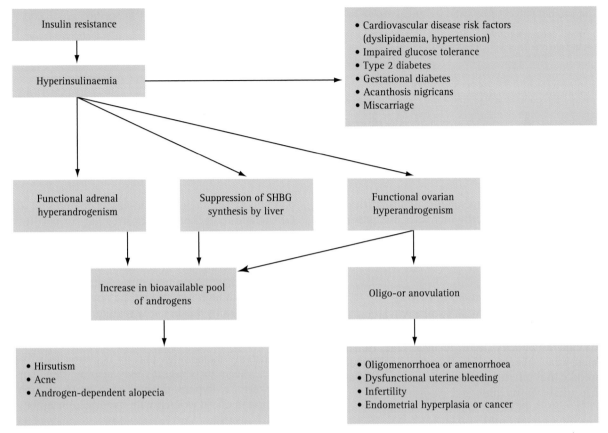

FIGURE 6.1 The central role of insulin resistance in the promotion of reproductive and metabolic sequelae of PCOS (From Costello[14])

using the Rotterdam Consensus definitions indicate that the prevalence is as high as 20–25%, although symptoms are often mild[7] and about 20% of women with polycystic ovaries have no symptoms.[8] Another way of viewing the prevalence is that 70–90% of women with oligomenorrhoea or anovulation have PCOS.[9]

How does PCOS come about?

PCOS is a heterogeneous condition, with both genetic and environmental factors influencing its development. The familial nature of PCOS is well established,[10] with about 35% of mothers and 40% of sisters of PCOS patients affected by the disorder.[11]

Over time, focus on causation of PCOS has shifted from the ovary to the hypothalamic–pituitary axis and then to some primary defects of insulin activity as the primary pathological cause of the syndrome. Insulin resistance is a key pathophysiological feature of PCOS,[12] and the association between increased insulin resistance and PCOS is a consistent finding in all ethnic groups.[13] Insulin resistance results in hyperinsulinaemia, functional adrenal hyperandrogenism, suppression of serum human binding globulin (SHBG) synthesis by the liver and functional ovarian hyperandrogenism[14] (Fig 6.1), which in turn give rise to symptoms such as hirsutism, acne and oligomenorrhoea. More serious sequelae include infertility, impaired glucose tolerance, a fourfold to sevenfold increase risk of diabetes and a potentially increased risk of cardiovascular disease.[15] However, insulin resistance is seen in only 10–15% of slim women and 20–40% of obese women with PCOS,[16] so clearly work remains to be done in clarifying the aetiology and nature of this puzzling condition.

The proportion of overweight and obese women with PCOS appears to be the same as in the general population.[17] While obesity does not cause PCOS, weight gain is an important contributor (both genetic and environmental) to phenotype in many women with PCOS and may be enough to unmask the condition, which may otherwise have remained asymptomatic. Indeed, obesity increases the degree of insulin resistance typically found in PCOS women;[18] thus, obese women often have more

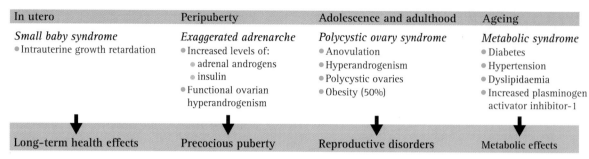

In utero	Peripuberty	Adolescence and adulthood	Ageing

Small baby syndrome
 • Intrauterine growth retardation
	Exaggerated adrenarche
	 • Increased levels of:
	   • adrenal androgens
	   • insulin
	 • Functional ovarian hyperandrogenism
		Polycystic ovary syndrome
		 • Anovulation
		 • Hyperandrogenism
		 • Polycystic ovaries
		 • Obesity (50%)
			Metabolic syndrome
			 • Diabetes
			 • Hypertension
			 • Dyslipidaemia
			 • Increased plasminogen activator inhibitor-1

Long-term health effects	Precocious puberty	Reproductive disorders	Metabolic effects

FIGURE 6.2 Manifestations of PCOS at different ages (From Norman, Wu, Stankiewicz[21])

severe hormonal and metabolic abnormalities.[19] As obesity in the community increases, the prevalence of the PCOS phenotype and its associated glucose intolerance — including diabetes — are expected to rise significantly.[20]

What are the manifestations of PCOS?

The clinical manifestations of PCOS (shown in Box 6.2, see p 120) affect all ages, ranging from childhood (premature puberty) to the teenage years (hirsutism, menstrual abnormalities), early adulthood and middle life (infertility, glucose intolerance), and later life (diabetes mellitus and cardiovascular disease) (Fig 6.2).[21] PCOS is the most common cause of anovulatory infertility and hirsutism.[10]

Seventy to ninety per cent of women with oligomenorrhoea have PCOS.

There exists a theoretical risk for endometrial cancer, because of chronic anovulation and unopposed oestrogen exposure, as well as for breast cancer related to obesity, hyperandrogenism and infertility.

Summary of key points
- PCOS is the most common cause of anovulatory infertility and hirsutism.
- PCOS manifests with oligomenorrhoea, hirsutism and obesity.
- While 25% of women will have polycystic ovaries on ultrasound examination only 6% have the syndrome.
- PCOS is familial in nature.
- Hyperinsulinaemia is thought to be the key to pathogenesis.

DIAGNOSING PCOS

How does PCOS present to GPs?

The symptoms, signs and biochemical features vary greatly in women with PCOS and can change over time in individual women.[22] Many women,

particularly in their late adolescence, present to GPs with oligomenorrhoea or irregular periods. It is important to remember the prevalence of PCOS in these situations and to take a history and examination prior to ordering any investigations. Women with PCOS may have accompanying acne and/or hirsutism and some, though not all, will be obese. There may also be a family history of irregular cycles, type 2 diabetes, obesity, and endometrial cancer or breast cancer. The examination may reveal acne, hirsutism, a high body mass index and on occasion palpable ovaries. Acanthosis nigrans may also be seen. This hyperkertotic, hyperpigmented skin lesion is more common in obese women with hyperinsulinaemia.

What is the differential diagnosis of PCOS?

The differential diagnosis includes other hormonal conditions such as Cushing's syndrome, late-onset congenital adrenal hyperplasia, androgen-secreting tumour, hypothyroidism and hyperprolactinaemia.

What investigations should be undertaken to confirm the diagnosis?

The investigations to be undertaken include the following:

- LH:FSH ratio
- testosterone
- sex-hormone-binding globulin
- free androgen index
- progesterone on day 21 to check for ovulation.

Screening tests for impaired glucose tolerance (IGT) and type 2 diabetes (T2DM) in women with PCOS are controversial. The incidence of these conditions is high (diabetes 4% and IGT 15.6%) in women with PCOS[23] (especially in older women and those with abdominal obesity and a family history of diabetes) and is much higher than in the general population.[24] Some recommend that all women with PCOS have a 2-hour 75 g oral glucose tolerance test (OGTT) and lipid profile testing at diagnosis.[23] The

Rotterdam Consensus Group recommends that only obese women (with a BMI >28) have an OGTT, as a fasting plasma glucose is a poor predictor of both IGT and T2DM.[1] If and when an ultrasound is conducted, it is a good idea to check for endometrial hyperplasia at the same time.

The incidence of impaired glucose tolerance and type 2 diabetes is much higher in women with PCOS, particularly women who are older, obese and with a family history of diabetes, than in the general population.

A GENERAL PRACTICE APPROACH TO MANAGEMENT

Lifestyle modification

Lifestyle modification, including a weight-reducing diet and exercise, is recommended as first-line therapy for all obese women with PCOS.[25] GPs should encourage women to have realistic goals (aiming initially for about 5% weight loss) and to achieve sustainable lifestyle changes.[20] Even a small degree of weight loss of 5–10% of total body weight is effective in inducing ovulation in many women and is successful in reducing insulin resistance and restoring ovulation, regular cycles and fertility.[26–28] This is so even where women remain overweight despite their weight loss and lifestyle changes.

Pharmacologic therapy should ideally be considered only if lifestyle modifications fail to resolve spontaneous ovulatory cycles after 3–6 months.[29] In combination with lifestyle changes, insulin sensitisers such as metformin have a role in those at highest risk, especially where impaired fasting glucose or impaired glucose tolerance is already established.[20] While there is no evidence to say that metformin brings about weight loss, it does have theoretical benefits including reduction of insulin resistance and prevention of type 2 diabetes and cardiovascular disease, and leads to the restoration of regular periods in over half of predominately obese PCOS women with oligomenorrhoea or amenorrhoea.

Achieving pregnancy

For women who want to get pregnant, clomiphene citrate is the initial medication of choice to bring about ovulation (Box 6.3).

After some debate as to whether rates of pregnancy can be improved by adding metformin to clomiphene, recent research involving direct comparison of metformin and clomiphenes[30] has resulted in metformin no longer being recommended in the routine management of infertility brought about by anovulatory PCOS.[8]

A significant proportion of women with anovulatory PCOS are resistant to clomiphene therapy and require gonadotrophin therapy (FSH injections) ± surgery (laparoscopic ovarian diathermy).

Irregular and heavy periods

Cycle control in women who do not wish to conceive can be achieved with an oral contraceptive pill, preferably one with cyproterone acetate (CPA) or drosperinone (which will both have a more specific anti-acne effect). The COCP reduces the circulating levels of testosterone by increasing levels of SHBG and decreasing androgen secretion.

Hirsutism

As well as cosmetic measures, treatment with an anti-androgen may be required to control hirsutism. It is important to warn patients that any anti-androgen therapy will take about 6 months to produce any noticeable improvement. Anti-androgens inhibit the binding of dihydrotestosterone to receptors at the hair follicle. Cyproterone acetate is the most commonly administered anti-androgen, and is prescribed in combination with ethinyloestradiol, as an OCP such as Diane or Brenda. Liver dysfunction is an extremely rare but serious complication, and liver function tests should be monitored after about 2 years of therapy with high-dose CPA. Liver side effects have not been reported with lower doses of CPA, such as those used in a COCP or hormone replacement therapy.

Where contraception is not needed, spironolactone can be used. It will inhibit ovarian and adrenal synthesis of androgens. Spironolactone is a mineralo-corticoid antagonist with anti-androgenic actions and

> **BOX 6.3 Instructions for the use of clomiphene citrate**
>
> - Take for 5 days, starting on the third or fifth day of the menstrual cycle, following either a spontaneous or induced bleed with progesterone withdrawal.
> - The starting dose is 50 mg daily for 5 days. If ovulation does not occur in the first cycle of treatment, the dose is increased to 100 mg and, subsequently, to a maximum of 150 mg.

is an alternative to CPA. It can be given at a dose of 50–150 mg/day and can also be used in conjunction with an oral contraceptive pill, which in itself may improve hirsutism by increasing the level of serum hormone binding globulin. When used alone, it is commonly associated with irregular and annoying vaginal bleeding, and thus is also best administered in combination with low-dose oestrogen therapy.

Pure anti-androgens such as flutamide and finasteride have been less effective than anticipated in the treatment of women with PCOS and hyperandrogenism.

GnRH analogues have been used to treat hirsutism with good results, but cannot be used for a long period of time because of the significant long-term risks of persistent hypo-oestrogenism.

Eflornithine cream (Vaniqa®) is a relatively new product licensed for the treatment of facial hirsutism in women. It irreversibly inhibits an enzyme (ornithine decarboxylase) involved in controlling hair growth and proliferation. When discussing this product with women, it is important to advise them that treatment does not remove hairs but slows down hair growth such that users require less frequent hair removal by other methods. Once treatment stops, however, hair re-grows to pre-treatment levels within 8 weeks.

SURGERY

Should surgery be recommended to patients with PCOS?

Many surgical methods have been used in an attempt to induce ovulation and conception in women with PCOS. These methods include wedge resection of enlarged ovaries, cyst puncture and ovarian tissue puncture. Laparoscopic ovarian 'drilling' using diathermy has been used in the treatment of PCOS for more than 15 years. The major concern with this form of therapy is the high rate of postoperative adhesions.[31] Another issue is that it does not seem to be directed at any of the aetiological factors involved in the development or expression of PCOS.

In cases of PCOS, surgery to the ovaries provides only temporary results and does not address underlying metabolic disturbance.

Surgery is an option, however, for women who want to conceive. Compared with the use of gonadotrophins to induce ovulation, laparoscopic surgery has a lower cost per pregnancy, low risk of multiple pregnancy and lower abortion rates, but, on the downside, there is a risk of adhesions and ovarian failure. Surgery is also more logical where women require laparoscopic assessment of the pelvis in order to determine and treat causes of infertility other than PCOS (e.g. endometriosis, which is more common in women with PCOS because of the existence of prolonged unopposed oestrogen).[32]

CONSEQUENCES

Are there any long-term consequences of PCOS?

Increasingly, the long-term consequences of PCOS are becoming recognised. Women with PCOS have a sevenfold increased risk of developing type 2 diabetes mellitus.[33] They may also be at risk of developing later cardiovascular disease[34] and endometrial cancer, the latter because of the presence of unopposed oestrogen.

Women with PCOS have a sevenfold increased risk of developing type 2 diabetes mellitus.

In conclusion, Marie's 'golf-balling' procedure, undertaken at the age of 20 when she was not desirous of an immediate pregnancy, was probably premature. It would have been important to try to explain to her the multifactorial origins of her condition and to help her understand the issues and therapies so that she could maintain some control over the management of her condition.

Summary of key points
- Management of PCOS is symptom oriented.
- Sustainable lifestyle change and associated weight reduction are first line management for obese women with PCOS.
- Women with PCOS are at higher risk of non-insulin-dependent diabetes mellitus, cardiovascular disease and endometrial cancer.

TIPS FOR PRACTITIONERS
- In women presenting with irregular cycles, it is worth checking for a family history of PCOS, diabetes and cardiovascular disease.
- While metformin is less useful than oral contraceptives (OCs) to regulate the menstrual cycle, it should be considered as initial intervention

in overweight or obese PCOS patients in whom OCs are contraindicated or who have an initial metabolic derangement.[36] In order to reduce the side effects of metformin, start with 500 mg daily (slow release) and increase over several weeks to 1.5–2 g daily.

- Even a small degree of weight loss is beneficial in managing the symptoms and consequences of PCOS.

REFERENCES

1. Rotterdam ESHRE/ASRM-sponsored POCS Consensus Workshop Group. Revised 2003 consensus on diagnostic criteria and long-term health risks related to polycystic ovary syndrome (PCOS). Hum Reprod 2004; 19(1):41–47.
2. Stankiewicz M, Norman R. Diagnosis and management of polycystic ovary syndrome: a practical guide. Drugs 2006; 66(7):903–912.
3. Polson DW, Adams J, Wadsworth J, et al. Polycystic ovaries—a common finding in normal women. Lancet 1988; 1(8590):870–872.
4. Clayton RN, Ogden V, Hodgkinson J, et al. How common are polycystic ovaries in normal women and what is their significance for the fertility of the population? Clin Endocrinol 1992; 37:127–134.
5. Knochenhauer ES, Key TJ, Kahsar-Miller M, et al. Prevalence of the polycystic ovary syndrome in unselected black and white women of the southeastern United States: a prospective study. J Clin Endocrinol Metab 1998; 83:3078–3082.
6. Diamanti-Kandarakis E, Kouli CR, Bergiele AT, et al. A survey of the polycystic ovary syndrome in the Greek island of Lesbos: hormonal and metabolic profile. J Clin Endocrinol Metab 1999; 84:4006–4011.
7. Michelmore KF, Balen AH, Dunger DB, et al. Polycystic ovaries and associated clinical and biochemical features in young women. Clin Endocrinol (Oxf) 1999; 51:779–786.
8. Balen AH, Rutherford AJ. Managing anovulatory infertility and polycystic ovary syndrome. BMJ 2007; 335(7621):663–666.
9. Hull MG. Epidemiology of infertility and polycystic ovarian disease: endocrinological and demographic studies. Gynaecol Endocrinol 1987; 1:235–245.
10. Franks S, Gharani N, Waterworth D, et al. The genetic basis of polycystic ovary syndrome. Hum Reprod 1997; 12:2641–2648.
11. Azziz R, Kashar-Miller MD. Family history as a risk factor for the polycystic ovary syndrome. J Pediatr Endocrinol Metab 2000; 13:1303–1306.
12. Dunaif A. Insulin resistance and the polycystic ovarian syndrome: mechanisms and implication for pathogenesis. Endocrinol Rev 1997; 18:774–800.
13. Carmina E, Koyama T, Chang L, et al. Does ethnicity influence the prevalence of adrenal hyperandrogenism and insulin resistance in PCOS? Am J Obstet Gynecol 1992; 167:1807–1812.
14. Costello MF. Polycystic ovary syndrome–a management update. Aust Fam Physician 2005; 34(3):127–133.
15. Teede H, Zoungas S, Hutchison S, et al. Insulin resistance, metabolic syndrome, diabetes and cardiovascular disease in polycystic ovary syndrome. Endocrine 2006; 30: 45–53.
16. Legro RS, Castracane VD, Kauffman RP. Detecting insulin resistance in polycystic ovary syndrome: purposes and pitfalls. Obstet Gynecol Surv 2004; 59:141–154.
17. Azziz R, Woods KS, Reyna R, et al. The prevalence and features of the polycystic ovary syndrome in an unselected population. J Clin Endocrinol Metab 2004; 89(6):2745–2749.
18. Legro RS, Bentley-Lewis R, Driscoll D, et al. Insulin resistance in the sisters of women with polycystic ovary syndrome: association with hyperandrogenemia rather than menstrual irregularity. J Clin Endocrinol Metab 2002; 87:2128–2133.
19. Apridonidze T, Essah PA, Iuorno MJ, et al. Prevalence and characteristics of the metabolic syndrome in women with polycystic ovary syndrome. J Clin Endocrinol Metab 2005; 90(4):1929–1935.
20. Teede HJ, Stuckey BG. Polycystic ovary syndrome and abnormal glucose tolerance. Med J Aust 2007; 187(6):324–325.
21. Norman RJ, Wu R, Stankiewicz MT. 4: Polycystic ovary syndrome. Med J Aust 2004; 180(3):132–137.
22. Balen AH, Conway GS, Kaltsas G, et al. Polycystic ovary syndrome: the spectrum of the disorder in 1741 patients. Hum Reprod 1995; 10:2107–2111.
23. Dabadghao P, Roberts BJ, Wang J, et al. Glucose tolerance abnormalities in Australian women with polycystic ovary syndrome. Med J Aust 2007; 187(6):328–331.
24. Dunstan DW, Zimmet PZ, Welborn TA, et al. The rising prevalence of diabetes and impaired glucose tolerance: the Australian Diabetes, Obesity and Lifestyle Study. Diabetes Care 2002; 25(5):829–834.
25. Brassard M, AinMelk Y, Baillargeon JP. Basic infertility including polycystic ovary syndrome. Med Clin North Am 2008; 92(5):1163–1192, xi.
26. Clark AM, Ledger W, Galletly C, et al. Weight loss results in significant improvement in pregnancy and ovulation rates in anovulatory obese women. Hum Reprod 1995; 10(10):2705–2712.
27. Huber-Buchholz MM, Carey DG, Norman RJ. Restoration of reproductive potential by lifestyle modification in obese polycystic ovary syndrome: role of insulin sensitivity and luteinizing hormone. J Clin Endocrinol Metab 1999; 84(4):1470–1474.
28. Norman RJ, Davies MJ, Lord J, et al. The role of lifestyle modification in polycystic ovary syndrome. Trends Endocrinol Metab 2002; 13(6):251–257.
29. Baillargeon JP, Iuorno MJ, Nestler JE. Insulin sensitizers for polycystic ovary syndrome. Clin Obstet Gynecol 2003; 46(2):325–340.
30. Legro RS, Barnhart HX, Schlaff WD, et al. Clomiphene, metformin, or both for infertility in the polycystic ovary syndrome. N Engl J Med 2007; 356(6):551–566.
31. Campo S. Ovulatory cycles, pregnancy outcome and complications after surgical treatment of polycystic ovary syndrome. Obstet Gynecol Surv 1998; 53:297–308.
32. Kovacs G, Wood C. The current status of polycystic ovary syndrome. Aust N Z J Obstet Gynaecol 2001; 41:65–68.
33. Dahlgren E, Johansson S, Lindstedt G, et al. Women with polycystic ovary syndrome wedge resected in 1956 to 1965: a long-term follow-up focusing on natural history and circulating hormones. Fertil Steril 1992; 57:505–513.
34. Rajkhowa M, Glass MR, Rutherford AJ, et al. Polycystic ovary syndrome: a risk factor for cardiovascular disease? BJOG 2000; 107:11–18.
35. Balen AH. Secondary amenorrhoea. In: Edmonds DK, ed. Dewhurst's textbook of obstetrics and gynaecology for postgraduates. 6th edn. Oxford: Blackwell Science; 1999.
36. Palomba S, Falbo A, Zullo F, et al. Evidence-based and potential benefits of metformin in the polycystic ovary syndrome: a comprehensive review. Endocr Rev 2009; 30(1): 1–50. Epub 04.12.08.

7

Initial management of infertility

OBJECTIVES

- To describe the prevalence and causation of infertility
- To understand which factors are important in the history and examination of an infertile couple
- To know how to initiate investigation of the infertile couple
- To understand the benefits and limitations of different tests used to investigate infertility
- To appreciate the emotional implications of embarking on investigation and management of infertility

INCIDENCE AND CAUSES OF INFERTILITY

CASE STUDY: Concerned about fertility

Suzy is 33 years old. She presents requesting a medical certificate for an upper respiratory tract infection that has prevented her from attending work that day. In passing, she asks how long she should wait before seeing a doctor for 'infertility'. Suzy has pursued a highly successful career in public relations following her university education. At the age of 22 she had an unplanned pregnancy, which was aborted. She recently married her partner of 5 years and now feels ready to have a child. She is concerned that she hasn't fallen pregnant despite 'trying' for the last 3 months and is worried that her previous abortion may have rendered her infertile.

Natural human fertility is surprisingly rather low. While it may seem to GPs that it is always those women who do not want to get pregnant who do so and those that want a child who are not able to fall pregnant, it is important to get a true perspective on rates of human fertility. Peak human fertility (the chance of pregnancy per menstrual cycle in the most fertile of couples) is no higher than 33%.[1]

Eighty-four per cent of couples in the general population will conceive within 1 year if they do not use contraception and have regular sexual intercourse. Of those who do not conceive in the first year, about half will do so in the second year (cumulative pregnancy rate 92%).[2]

Infertility appears to have increased over the last few decades. This may be because:

- the voluntary delay in childbearing has uncovered the age-related decline in fertility
- the use of the combined oral contraceptive pill has hidden the fact that many women are oligomenorrhoeic or amenorrhoeic
- increased numbers of sexual partners leads to increased levels of PID in the community
- couples are aware of the availability of reproductive technology to assist them and so delay childbearing.

What are the most common causes of infertility?

There are several mandatory preconditions for fertility:

- Sexual intercourse has to occur, placing the sperm in the vagina.
- Ovulation must occur, making an egg available for fertilisation.

- Sperm must be able to fertilise the ovum.
- The fallopian tube must be patent and functioning.

The causes of infertility and their approximate frequency are given in Table 7.1.

Sperm dysfunction is the most common cause of infertility, accounting for 30% of cases. Problems are often detected in motility, morphology and ability to penetrate mucus. Complete absence of sperm is rare.

Women complaining of infertility should be advised to give up smoking. Men who smoke should be advised to stop, in order to remove one variable that may affect their fertility.

The next most common problem is related to ovulatory failure, with women experiencing either amenorrhoea or oligomenorrhoea. The latter condition is most commonly due to polycystic ovary syndrome (PCOS). Fallopian tube blockage or damage is most commonly due to a past history of *Chlamydia* infection that may or may not have been detected earlier on.

Other factors that may be playing a significant role in a couple's subfertility include:

- the relationship between increasing age and infertility
- extremes of weight
- smoking.

TABLE 7.1 Causes of infertility and their approximate frequency (From Hull et al[16])

Cause	Frequency* (%)
Sperm defects or dysfunction	30
Ovulation failure (amenorrhoea or oligomenorrhoea)	25
Unexplained infertility	25
Tubal infective damage	20
Endometriosis (causing damage)	5
Coital failure or infrequency	5
Cervical mucus defects or dysfunction	3
Uterine abnormalities (such as fibroids or abnormalities of shape)	1

*Total exceeds 100%, as 15% of couples have more than one cause of subfertility.

The longer the duration of infertility, the less likely it is that a couple will fall pregnant, especially if it is longer than 3 years.[3] Equally, a previous full-term pregnancy is associated with a better chance of conception.[3] In 25% of cases, no definite cause of infertility is found.[1]

Summary of key points
- Peak human fertility is no higher than 33% per menstrual cycle.
- 84% of couples will attain a pregnancy within 12 months of unprotected intercourse.
- Sperm dysfunction is the commonest cause of infertility, followed by ovulatory failure.
- In 25% of couples no cause is found for their infertility.

INITIAL GP INVESTIGATION AND MANAGEMENT

When should a GP commence investigation in a couple claiming to be infertile?

The answer to this question is dependent on many factors, the most important of which is probably the woman's age.

If a couple in their 20s present earlier than 6 months after trying to conceive, it is reasonable to offer some general fertility advice and preconception care. This might include asking about the regularity of the menstrual cycle and the frequency of intercourse in relation to peak time of fertility in the menstrual cycle, as well as counselling about weight and smoking. If they are still not successful after a year, the couple can then return for a more thorough history and examination.

It is important to be aware that once a couple presents to a doctor with subfertility, they are getting on to a 'treadmill' that it is difficult to leave. They have to deal with the fact that either the man or the woman may be infertile or that there is no explanation for their infertility. They may feel guilty or blame their partner for causing the problem. Sexual relations become pressured because of the need to have intercourse 'at the right time', and women build up their expectations of conceiving, often to be disappointed by finding that they are menstruating again. They will often describe being on an 'emotional rollercoaster'. Hence some recommend that in a younger couple medical involvement in this intimate area should be delayed for as long as possible.

In older couples, with regular unprotected sexual intercourse, 94% of fertile women aged 35 years,

TABLE 7.2 Chance of live birth per treatment cycle (From NICE Guidelines[6])

Age of woman	Chance of live birth per treatment cycle
23–35 years	Greater than 20%
36–38 years	15%
39 years	10%
40 years or older	6%

and 77% of those aged 38 years, will conceive after 3 years of trying,[4] demonstrating the decline in female fertility with age (the effect of age on male fertility is less clear). Because of this decline, guidelines recommend earlier investigation. This is also because the success of assisted conception techniques is also highly related to maternal age (Table 7.2). In particular if the woman is over 35 there is a substantial fall in the chance of success with in vitro fertilisation.[5]

GPs should be aware that many patients will present with difficulties in falling pregnant, having not received any preconception care. It is therefore imperative GPs take the opportunity to go through the checklist of preconception care advice (see Chapter 8) with patients and ensure that the woman has adequate knowledge to identify her peak fertile time, has immunity against rubella and varicella, and is taking the appropriate dose of folate.

If a couple present concerned about their fertility, the GP should use the consultation as an opportunity to provide preconception care.

Are there any tests that patients can perform at home?

Home-based tests can be useful in several situations. First, they are appropriate for those couples who are concerned about fertility (before attempting to conceive for 1 year) and who do not warrant immediate investigation. Another group are those who are undergoing medical investigation, who may welcome involvement in the process and who might feel empowered by gathering information about their own cycle. Patients should not undertake these tests indefinitely because of the stress they may generate. Three months is probably sufficient time to

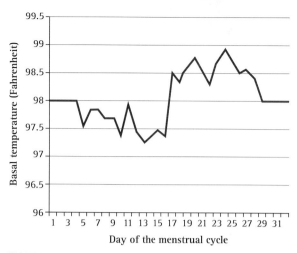

FIGURE 7.1 An example of a basal body temperature chart showing ovulation

gather the maximum amount of information that can be garnered from such tests. The two tests that are available to women who are concerned about their fertility are tests that involve charting their basal body temperature and using an ovulation predictor kit.

1. **Basal body temperature charting** Patients may choose to purchase a basal body temperature thermometer, on which the range of temperatures displayed is narrower than those on the ordinary household thermometer. A woman should take her temperature before getting out of bed each morning and chart it on graph paper. (An example of an ovulatory basal body temperature chart is given in Fig 7.1.) The temperature drops at the time of the menses, then rises by 0.5 of a degree Fahrenheit 2 days after the peak of the LH surge. Ovum release probably occurs one day before the first temperature elevation. The temperature remains elevated for 13–14 days, then drops again with the menses. A temperature elevation for longer than 16 days is suggestive of pregnancy. Interestingly, UK guidelines state that 'The use of basal body temperature charts to confirm ovulation does not reliably predict ovulation and is not recommended', quoting level B evidence to support their statement.[6]

2. **Ovulation predictor kits** Some kits, such as Persona, test urine for luteinising hormone (LH), which rises temporarily prior to ovulation. This is indicated by a change of colour in the indicator stick. The kit is used every morning, until the stick changes colour just before the egg is released. In order to conceive, intercourse should occur on

that day or the following day, or both. Other kits such as Maybe Baby are saliva based and look for ferning related to oestrogen rises at the time of ovulation.

What medical history is relevant in a subfertile couple?

Ideally, a couple should be seen together by their GP when either one of them initially voices concern about their lack of ability to conceive. Seeing a couple together places everything out in the open and means that both partners receive the same information with the same emphasis. Often, however, it is the woman who initially presents to the GP. Her partner may not be familiar with seeing doctors or may be frightened or embarrassed about the prospect of being questioned about his fertility, undergoing an examination and perhaps needing to produce a semen sample.

Both partners should be involved in the management of their infertility.

The nature of the medical history that should be taken from the couple is given in Boxes 7.1 and 7.2.

It is important to ensure that there are no underlying issues related to sexual intercourse that the couple may be too embarrassed to ask about. Some direct questions can be asked,[7] such as:

- (To the man) 'Any difficulty with erections and being able to maintain these to have adequate intercourse on demand?'
- (To the woman) 'Do you have any difficulty with penetration, such as pain or discomfort?'
- (To the man) 'Do you usually reach orgasm, and ejaculate during intercourse?'

What examination should be undertaken?

In a woman, the purpose of the examination is to look for clues to an underlying endocrine disorder that affects ovulation, such as PCOS. The GP should therefore calculate body mass index, look for signs of androgen excess, such as acne and facial hair, and galactorrhoea. Pelvic examination should focus on looking for any structural abnormalities and for signs of pelvic infection or endometriosis, such as localised tenderness.

In a man, the examination focuses on the genitalia, assessing testicular size and the presence of a varicocoele. Varicocoeles are present in 15% of the male population and in approximately 40% of men presenting with infertility.[8] While the exact pathophysiology of varicocoele-induced testicular dysfunction is not well understood, varicocoele repair may be considered as the primary treatment option when a man with a varicocoele has suboptimal semen quality and a normal female partner. On the other hand, IVF with or without intracytoplasmic sperm injection (ICSI) may be considered the primary treatment option when there is an independent need for such techniques to treat a female factor, regardless of the presence of varicocoele and suboptimal semen quality.[9]

In what order should investigations be carried out?

As with all investigative pathways, the least invasive and cheapest investigations should be carried out first. Initially semen analysis should be undertaken, while at the same time assessing that ovulation is occurring.

What should a GP know about semen analyses?

Semen analysis is the primary investigation carried out on men with infertility. Despite this, it is a poor predictor of sperm function and male fertility. Men should be instructed to collect a masturbated sample after abstaining from ejaculation for 36–48 hours. The sample should be kept at ambient temperature (in a pocket and not in the fridge) and should be delivered to the laboratory within 1–2 hours of issue.

Semen analysis should be undertaken where possible by a laboratory associated with a treatment facility for infertility. Various entities have published suggested normal values for sperm count, motility and morphology (the World Health Organization criteria are listed in Table 7.3). However, these values have been questioned for their evidence basis and reliability for predicting infertility.

Because of the long development cycle of sperm, which can be influenced by various factors such as an intercurrent illness or fever, semen samples can vary widely from ejaculate to ejaculate. If the result of the first semen analysis is abnormal, a repeat confirmatory test should be offered and ideally undertaken 3 months after the initial analysis to allow time for the cycle of spermatozoa formation to be completed.[6] However, if a gross spermatozoa deficiency (azoospermia or severe oligozoospermia) has been detected, the repeat test should be undertaken as soon as possible.[6]

BOX 7.1 Important factors in the history of a woman complaining of subfertility

- Age
- Duration of infertility (For how long has the couple had regular, unprotected intercourse?)
- Menstrual regularity and presence of premenstrual symptoms
- Ability to recognise preovulatory cervical mucus
- Coital frequency and timing, presence of any sexual problems
- Gynaecological problems such as menorrhagia, dysmenorrhoea, dyspareunia, intermenstrual or postcoital bleeding
- Hirsutism
- Galactorrhoea
- Current medical illness—in particular, any systemic disease such as diabetes or thyroid disease
- Past medical or surgical history with particular attention to conditions that may have caused pelvic adhesions or tubal scarring (e.g. STDs, pelvic inflammatory disease, Crohn's disease, endometriosis, ovarian cysts, appendicectomy)
- Past obstetric and gynaecological history, including menarche, previous contraception, previous pregnancies and outcomes, cervical smear history, past cone biopsy
- Drug treatment, both prescribed and recreational
- Smoking, consumption of alcohol and caffeine
- Diet, including recent weight gain or loss

BOX 7.2 Important factors in the history of a man complaining of subfertility

- Erectile or ejaculatory difficulty
- History of undescended testes
- Past medical history, focusing on STDs and mumps
- Past surgical history, focusing on hernia repairs and orchidopexy
- Occupational history, asking about exposure to excessive heat or toxins such as cellulose thinners
- Current medical illness
- Prescribed drugs, in particular those that can interfere with male fertility, such as sulfasalazine, cimetidine, high-dose nitrofurantoin and chemotherapeutic agents
- Drug misuse (such as anabolic steroids)
- Smoking, consumption of alcohol and caffeine
- Fathered a child in the past

TABLE 7.3 World Health Organization reference values for semen analysis, 2000 (From Rowe et al[14])

Criterion	Reference value
Volume	2.0 mL or more
Liquefaction time	Within 60 minutes
pH	7.2 or more
Sperm concentration	20 million spermatozoa per millilitre or more
Total sperm number	40 million spermatozoa per ejaculate or more
Motility	50% or more motile (grades a and b[a]), or 25% or more with progressive motility (grade a) within 60 minutes of ejaculation
Morphology	15% or 30%[b]
Vitality	75% or more live
White blood cells	Fewer than 1 million per millilitre

[a]Grade a: rapid progressive motility (sperm moving swiftly, usually in a straight line) Grade b: slow or sluggish progressive motility (sperm may be less linear in their progression).

[b]Currently being reassessed by the WHO; in the interim, the proportion of normal forms accepted by laboratories is either the earlier WHO lower limit of 30% or 15% based on strict morphological criteria.

Screening for antisperm antibodies should not be offered because there is no evidence of effective treatment to improve fertility.[6]

The male partner should normally have semen analysis performed during the initial investigation.

What tests are done to confirm ovulation?

While ovulation can be presumed if women develop breast tenderness and other symptoms premenstrually (indicating the presence of progesterone in the second half of the cycle), ovulation should be confirmed by undertaking a mid-luteal-phase progesterone assay. This blood test is usually taken on day 21 of a 28-day cycle—but may need to be conducted later in the cycle (for example day 28 of a 35-day cycle)—and repeated weekly thereafter until the next menstrual cycle starts. The progesterone level should be >30 nmol/L.

Ovulation should be confirmed by the measurement of serum progesterone in the mid-luteal phase.

If the cycle is irregular, it is worth checking luteinising hormone (LH), follicle-stimulating hormone (FSH) and testosterone levels for the presence of endocrine disorders, most commonly PCOS. FSH and LH should be measured from day 2 to day 5 of the menstrual cycle. A raised LH (with a normal FSH) is suggestive of PCOS.

Women who are concerned about their fertility should not be offered a blood test to measure prolactin. This test should be offered only to women who have an ovulatory disorder, galactorrhoea or a pituitary tumour.[6] Nor should they undergo thyroid testing, as women with possible fertility problems are no more likely than the general population to have thyroid disease.[6]

Are there any tests that can be done to determine ovarian reserve?

Many women seek to delay childbearing for as long as possible and ask whether there are any tests that can tell them how much time they have left before they can no longer have children. For some women this is especially important: carriers of fragile X are known to be more likely to undergo premature menopause and for women undergoing IVF ovarian reserve is an important predictor of success.

Age, antral follicle count, basal FSH, FSH/LH ratio, mean ovarian volume, infertility duration, number of previous cycle cancellations and body mass index are all, in decreasing significance, independent factors that determine low ovarian reserve.[10]

Tests of ovarian reserve currently have limited sensitivity and specificity in predicting fertility, but an FSH and ovarian ultrasound done in a specialist ultrasound practice may be useful. Women who have high levels of gonadotrophins should be informed that they are likely to have reduced fertility.[6] The value of assessing ovarian reserve using inhibin B is uncertain and is therefore not recommended.[6]

What tests are done to confirm fallopian tube function?

Confirmation of tubal patency can be by laparoscopy and dye insufflation of the fallopian tubes or by hysterosalpingogram.

Laparoscopy allows for better diagnosis of the cause of tubal problems, if there are any, because the pelvis can be seen and diseases such as pelvic

The female partner should have a test of tubal patency during the initial investigation. Hysterosalpingogram may be used to screen for tubal patency in low-risk couples. For evaluation of the pelvis, a diagnostic laparoscopy with dye transit is preferable.

inflammatory disease (PID) and endometriosis can be excluded and avascular peritubal adhesions can be divided on the spot.

Many gynaecologists would delay these investigations if there was evidence that the woman was not ovulating and offer ovulation induction first, only checking the tubes if the woman was not pregnant after 3–6 cycles (assuming a low risk for tubal problems) If the woman was ovulating, however, and there was a normal sperm count, investigation of tubal patency would be a higher priority.

Are any other tests necessary or useful?

Abnormalities of cervical mucus production or sperm–mucus interaction are rarely identified as the sole or principal cause of infertility. Previously, a routine postcoital test was recommended for all couples. It involved examining a specimen of cervical mucus (obtained before expected ovulation) for the presence of motile sperm hours after intercourse. The test is unreliable, however, and contemporary treatments for unexplained infertility effectively negate any unrecognised cervical factors. Routine postcoital testing is therefore unnecessary.[11]

Endometrial biopsy was another test done until recently in women with infertility. It aimed to assess the histological stage of the endometrium and to compare it with the chronological stage of the woman's menstrual cycle. Asynchronous endometrial development was said to be associated with impaired fertility. Recent guidelines now advise against routine endometrial biopsy to evaluate the luteal phase as part of the investigation of the infertile couple.[6]

Hysteroscopy should not be considered as a routine investigation in the infertile couple, because there is no evidence linking the treatment of uterine abnormalities with enhanced fertility. Equally, an ultrasound examination of the endometrium is unnecessary in the initial investigation of infertility. However, ultrasound evaluation of the ovaries may be useful.[6]

Sperm function tests are specialised tests and should not be used in the routine investigation of the infertile couple, and routine testing for antisperm antibodies in semen is not recommended.[6]

What are the indications for early referral to a specialist fertility clinic?

Couples that are older, not ovulating and have abnormal semen or evidence of tubal damage should be offered early referral to a specialist fertility clinic.

What management for subfertility can GPs initiate?

Besides delivering preconception care, GPs should educate patients about the menstrual cycle, ovulation and the timing of intercourse. While recent guidelines advise that 'timing intercourse to coincide with ovulation causes stress and is not recommended',[6] I believe this stance is paternalistic and that understanding how to optimise chances of conception is a reproductive right.[12]

A GP's role in the management of infertility, apart from providing information to the couple and support, varies according to the cause of the infertility.

Where there is a disorder of ovulation, PCOS is responsible in most cases of oligomenorrhoea and in up to a third of cases where there is amenorrhoea. First-line treatment for PCOS has to be weight loss. GPs can take an active role in helping women achieve this.

The body mass index of the female partner should be assessed and, whether ovulatory or not, the woman should be advised and assisted to lose weight if her BMI is >30.

Over recent years, there has been much debate as to whether metformin or clomid is more effective at promoting fertility in women with PCOS. It seems likely that clomid remains the most appropriate first-line treatment for anovulation in PCOS, while initial promising results for metformin have not been confirmed. Prescription of clomid is usually limited to specialist obstetricians/gynaecologists. Clomiphene is an anti-oestrogen that works by blocking oestrogen receptors in the pituitary, thereby promoting the release of additional FSH and LH, which stimulate follicular development. The risk of multiple pregnancies with the use of clomiphene is approximately 8%. Clomiphene can give rise to ovarian hyperstimulation syndrome, which, while extremely rare, can be fatal. A reported link with ovarian cancer is unproven and applies only if the woman does not succeed in getting pregnant.

What advice can GPs give about infertility treatments and their success rates?

GPs often provide an objective voice for an infertile couple who embark on the treadmill of reproductive technology. GPs can provide patients with a realistic prognosis (with and without treatment) and provide information, support and counselling. They can also advise couples about treatment options and valid alternatives such as adoption, fostering or indeed childlessness.

Basically there are three forms of assisted reproduction available to infertile couples:

1. **In vitro fertilisation (IVF)** is indicated for tubal disease, unexplained infertility, endometriosis, male factor infertility, failed donor insemination or cervical hostility. Donor oocytes may be used where there are failed ovaries (e.g. premature menopause). Superovulation is used in order to harvest oocytes, and spermatozoa are prepared and added to the oocytes in vitro. A fine plastic canula is then used to place a maximum of two embryos 1 cm from the uterine fundus. Surplus embryos can be cryopreserved.
2. **Gamete intrafallopian transfer (GIFT)** is suitable for all the indications of IVF, except where there are blocked or absent fallopian tubes. In GIFT the oocytes are collected laparoscopically, mixed with sperm and transferred to the fimbrial end of the fallopian tube. Currently GIFT is not commonly utilised.
3. **Intracytoplasmic sperm injection (ICSI)** is used where there is sperm dysfunction. Sperm are harvested from the epididimis or testis and injected into the ovum, bringing about fertilisation. The embryo is then transferred into the uterus.

In general terms, a GP can advise that the 'take-home-baby rate' for GIFT and IVF is up to 30% in women under 35 and varies depending on the quality of the assisted reproduction clinic. Couples should be cautioned, however, about possible complications that arise from assisted reproductive technology. Comparative figures between IVF and natural conception for singleton pregnancies are given in Table 7.4.

Summary of key points
- In women over 35 there is a substantial fall in the chance of success with IVF.
- Initial investigations include semen analysis and tests to confirm ovulation.
- Hysterosalpingogram or laparoscopy can be used to assess the fallopian tubes.

TABLE 7.4 Perinatal outcomes in singletons after in vitro fertilisation (IVF) and natural conception: results of a meta-analysis of clinical trials (Adapted from Jackson et al[15])

Outcome	IVF	Natural conception	Odds ratio (95% CI)
	\multicolumn{2}{c}{Approximate absolute risk (%)}		
Perinatal mortality	2	0.7	2.9 (1.61–2.98)
Preterm delivery	11.5	5.3	1.95 (1.73–2.20)
Birth weight <2500 g	9.5	3.8	1.77 (1.40–2.22)
Birth weight <1500 g	2.5	1.0	2.70 (2.31–3.14)
Small for gestational age	14.6	8.9	1.60 (1.25–2.04)

CI = confidence interval

- The take-home-baby rate for assisted reproduction techniques such as GIFT and IVF is approximately 20%.

TIPS FOR PRACTITIONERS

- General practitioners should send semen samples to the same laboratory used by the specialist infertility clinic to which the couple will be referred.
- Men should be advised that there is an association between elevated scrotal temperature and reduced semen quality, but that it is uncertain whether wearing loose-fitting underwear will improve fertility.
- In the absence of galactorrhoea or symptoms of thyroid disease, there is no value in measuring thyroid function or prolactin in women with subfertility.

REFERENCES

1. Cahill DJ, Wardle PG. Management of infertility. BMJ 2002; 325:28–32.
2. te Velde ER, Eijkemans R, Habbema HD. Variation in couple fecundity and time to pregnancy, an essential concept in human reproduction. Lancet 2000; 355(9219):1928–1929.
3. Snick HKA, Snick TS, Evers JLH, et al. The spontaneous pregnancy prognosis in untreated subfertile couples: the Walcheren primary care study. Hum Reprod 1997; 12:1582–1588.

4. van Noord-Zaadstra BM, Looman CW, Alsbach H, et al. Delaying childbearing: effect of age on fecundity and outcome of pregnancy. BMJ 1991; 302(6789):1361–1365.
5. Templeton A, Morris JK, Parslow W. Factors that affect outcome of in vitro fertilisation treatment. Lancet 1996; 343:1402–1406.
6. NICE Guidelines. Clinical Guideline 11, Fertility: assessment and treatment for people with fertility problems. February 2004. Online. Available: http://www.nice.org.uk/nicemedia/pdf/CG011fullguideline.pdf [accessed 11.06.09].
7. McLachlan RI, Yazdani A, Kovacs G, et al. Management of the infertile couple. Aust Fam Physician 2005; 34(3):111–113, 115–117.
8. Nagler HM, Luntz RK, Martinis FG. Varicocoele. In: Lipshultz LI, Howard SS, eds. Infertility in the male. St Louis: Mosby Year Books; 1997:336–359.
9. Practice Committee of American Society for Reproductive Medicine. Report on varicocele and infertility. Fertil Steril 2008; 90(5, Suppl):S247–249.
10. Younis J, Jadaon J, Izhaki I, et al. A simple multivariate score could predict ovarian reserve, as well as pregnancy rate, in infertile women. Fertil Steril 2009. Epub 13.04.09.
11. Practice Committee of American Society for Reproductive Medicine. Optimal evaluation of the infertile female. Fertil Steril 2006; 86(5, Suppl 1):S264–267.
12. Royal College of Obstetricians and Gynaecologists. The initial investigation and management of the infertile couple. Royal College of Obstetricians and Gynaecologists Press; 1998.
13. Hampton K, Mazza D. Should spontaneous or timed intercourse guide couples trying to conceive? Hum Reprod 2009. 24(12):3236–3237. Epub 17.09.09.
14. Rowe PJ, Comhaire FH, Hargreave TB, et al. WHO manual for the standardized investigation, diagnosis and management of the infertile male. Cambridge: Cambridge University Press; 2000.
15. Jackson RA, Gibson KA, Wu YW, et al. Perinatal outcomes in singletons following in vitro fertilization: a meta-analysis. Obstet Gynecol 2004;103:551–563.
16. Hull M, Glazener C, Kelly NJ, et al. Population study of causes, treatment, and outcome of infertility. Br Med J 1985; 291:1693–1697.

8

Preconception care

OBJECTIVES

- To understand the importance of being proactive in the delivery of preconception care
- To develop a structured approach to the delivery of preconception care
- To be aware of the medical and genetic issues that need to be addressed and managed preconceptionally
- To be aware of lifestyle factors that may impact on pregnancy outcomes and to be able to counsel women effectively regarding these factors
- To counsel women effectively about how to optimise their chances of conception
- To understand the rationale for periconceptional folate supplementation
- To be able to prescribe periconceptional folate supplementation

PRECONCEPTION COUNSELLING

CASE STUDY: 'I'm thinking of getting pregnant soon.'

Jan was 27 years old. She had married 18 months ago and attended her GP saying, 'I'm thinking about getting pregnant in about 6 months, is there anything I need to do before I start trying?'

Jan's medical history was essentially normal. She had been on the COCP since the age of 16 with no particular problems. She did smoke, however. The GP pulled out a 'preconception care checklist' and went through each item with Jan. The GP gave her some advice about smoking cessation, ordered rubella and varicella serology to check Jan's immunity and advised her to continue taking the pill until the results came back. The GP then went over some reproductive physiology and explained to Jan when peak fertility occurred and how to recognise it by becoming aware of changes in mucus.

Together the GP and Jan decided she would discontinue the COCP in 3 months. She would commence taking folate supplementation straight away and would use condoms for the first month or two after discontinuing the pill in order to learn when and if she was ovulating. When the consultation was over the GP appreciated how Jan's presentation specifically for preconception advice had provided an opportunity to discuss preconception issues in a structured fashion. The GP made a note to let women attending her practice know about the need for and availability of preconception care by encouraging them to make an appointment before they stopped using their contraception.

What is preconception care and why is it important?

Preconception care is essentially 'risk management' and aims to identify and modify biomedical, behavioural and social risks to a woman's health or pregnancy outcome through prevention and management. It involves health promotion, screening, and interventions aimed at reducing risk factors that might affect future pregnancies. These steps should be taken before conception or early in pregnancy in order to have a maximal effect on health outcomes.[1]

The provision of preconception care can also increase pregnancy planning.[2] This is important because planned pregnancies typically have improved outcomes for both women and infants, and we know that approximately half of all pregnancies are unplanned.[3] In addition, 52%[4] of women who have a negative pregnancy test in the general practice setting have a medical risk factor that could adversely affect a future pregnancy.

What is the GP's role in preconception care?

Nearly all women realise the importance of optimising their health before pregnancy and know that the best time to receive information about pregnancy health is before conception. The vast majority of women prefer to receive information about preconception health from their primary care physician, yet in one survey only 39% of women could recall their physician ever discussing this topic.[5]

GPs can make a difference, however, by providing counselling to women before they get pregnant and even before they think about getting pregnant. They can do this by introducing the concept and availability of preconception care to women when they present for contraception, Pap smears or other reasons, and inviting them to return when they are ready to conceive but before ceasing contraception.

GPs should introduce the concept and availability of preconception care to women when they attend for contraception, Pap smears or other reasons, and invite them to return when they are ready to conceive but before ceasing contraception

What specific issues need to be addressed in preconception counselling?

There are a number of issues that GPs should address during preconception counseling (see the preconception care checklist in Box 8.1). GPs can go through the issues raised in the checklist with the woman and reinforce them with brochures and information to take home. Once a GP ascertains that preconception care is relevant for the patient, a convenient way to utilise the checklist and structure the care is to take the history and order the relevant screening tests at the initial consultation, and then to discuss the results, vaccinate if necessary and provide lifestyle and any medical advice that is required at the second consultation.

Reproductive life plan

Why should GPs have a discussion with their patients about a reproductive life plan?

Research suggests that many women have clear aspirations with regard to parenthood by their late teens or early 20s.[6] About 92% of women express a desire to have one or two children within the confines of a stable relationship by the age of 35,[7] with only 6–8% of Australian women aspiring to childlessness.[8]

BOX 8.1 Preconception care checklist

Medical issues

- **Reproductive life plan.** Assist your patient in developing a plan that includes whether they want to have children and, if so, the number, spacing and timing of the children.
- **Reproductive history.** Have there been any problems with previous pregnancies such as infant death, fetal loss, birth defects, low birth weight, preterm birth or gestational diabetes? Are there any ongoing risks that could lead to a recurrence in a future pregnancy?
- **Medical history.** Are there any medical conditions that may affect future pregnancies? Are chronic conditions such as diabetes, thyroid, hypertension, epilepsy and thrombophilias well managed, and do any medications need to be changed to accommodate pregnancy?
- **Medication use.** Review all current medications, including over-the-counter medications, vitamins and supplements. Avoid categories C and D medications
- **Genetic/family history.** Assess risk of chromosomal/genetic disorders, based on family history/ethnic background (e.g. neural tube defects (NTD), cystic fibrosis, fragile X, Tay–Sachs disease, thalassaemia, sickle cell anaemia).
- **General physical assessment.** Pap smear and breast examinations should be done before pregnancy. Assess body mass index, blood pressure and ask about periodontal disease.
- **Substance use.** Ask about tobacco, alcohol and illegal drug use.

Screening

- Blood type and antibody screen
- **STIs.** Screen as indicated for STIs such as syphilis, gonorrhoea, *Chlamydia* and HIV.
- **Psychosocial health.** Screen for depression, anxiety and domestic violence.
- **Cystic fibrosis and other carrier screening.** Screen as indicated by genetic/family history.
- **Rubella and varicella serology.** Screen as indicated.

Vaccinations (as indicated)

- Measles–mumps–rubella (MMR)
- Influenza
- Diphtheria/tetanus/pertussis (Boostrix)
- Varicella
- **Pneumococcal.** Indicated for women at high risk.
- **Hepatitis B.** Indicated for women at high risk.

Lifestyle issues

- **Family planning.** Based on the patient's reproductive life plan, discuss fertility awareness, chance of conception, and the risks of delayed childbearing, infertility and fetal abnormality. For patients not planning to become pregnant, discuss effective contraception and emergency contraceptive options.
- **Folic acid supplementation.** Women should take a daily 0.4–0.5 mg supplement of folic acid for at least 1 month prior to pregnancy and for the first 3 months after conception. In women at high risk (i.e. women with a reproductive or family history of NTD or type 1 diabetes, or on medication for epilepsy/seizures), the daily dose should be increased to 5 mg.
- **Healthy weight, nutrition and exercise.** Caution against being over- or underweight. Recommend regular moderate intensity exercise and assess the risk of nutritional deficiencies (e.g. vegan, lactose intolerance, calcium or iron deficiency).
- **Psychosocial health.** Provide support and identify coping strategies to improve emotional health and wellbeing.
- **Smoking, alcohol and illegal drug cessation** (as indicated). Smoking, alcohol and illegal drug use during pregnancy can have serious consequences for an unborn child and should be stopped prior to conception.
- **Healthy environments.** Repeated exposure to hazardous toxins in the household and workplace environments can affect fertility and the risk of miscarriage and birth defects. Discuss avoidance of 'TORCH' infections:
  - toxoplasmosis: avoidance of cat litter, garden soil and raw/undercooked meat
  - cytomegalovirus, parvovirus B19 (fifth disease): wash hands frequently and observe strict infection control for child and healthcare workers
  - listeriosis: avoidance of pâté, soft cheeses, pre-packaged salads, deli meats and chilled/smoked seafood

Sources: Royal Australian College of General Practitioners[53], Oh and Gilstrap[54], Lu[55], National Health and Medical Research Council[24].

There is, however, a significant gap between the number of children women tell researchers they want and those they achieve. It is this gap, between women's fertility aspirations and their fertility attainment, that explains much of our sustained low fertility rates and resulting predictions that a quarter of women will end their fertile years childless. In other words, while some of our low fertility rates can be explained either by infertility or by women making autonomous choices to remain childless, the remainder are the result of circumstances constraining women's freedom to choose motherhood, not choice.[6]

There is a significant gap between the number of children women tell researchers they want and those they achieve.

The average age of Australian first-time mothers has risen from 25 in 1991 to nearly 30 in 2003.[9] This trend, repeated in other Western countries, has been labelled the 'epidemic of pregnancy in middle age'.[10] Female fertility declines with increasing age. Age-related fertility problems increase after 35 and dramatically after 40.[10] For those who do fall pregnant later in life, there are associated adverse outcomes to deal with. Pregnancies in older women are more likely to result in adverse outcomes, with increased rates of stillbirth, miscarriage and ectopic pregnancy,[11] as well as multiple births and congenital malformations.[12] Pregnancies in women older than 40 years are associated with more non-severe complications, premature births and interventions at birth.[13] Levels of pregnancy disease are increased, and older mothers are more likely to experience severe morbidity.[14]

Pregnancies in older women are more likely to result in adverse outcomes.

Women are ill-informed about the relationship between age and infertility. In the USA, 88% of women overestimated by 5–10 years the age at which fertility begins to decline.[15] An Australian study of women aged over 35 seeking assisted reproductive technology (ART) found that 18% were unaware of the impact of age on infertility.[16]

Women are ill-informed about the relationship between age and infertility

In addition, women are misinformed about the efficacy of ART, overestimating their chance of having a baby using these techniques.[17] This belief in the ability of ART to overcome the 'biological clock' and achieve a pregnancy in most women and at almost any age is ill-founded.[18]

What advice should be given about age and fertility?

Fecundity declines gradually but significantly, beginning approximately at age 32 years, and decreases more rapidly after age 37 years, reflecting primarily a decrease in egg quality in association with a gradual increase in the circulating level of follicle-stimulating hormone.[19] There is a 50% decrease in apparent fecundability at the age of 35 years[20] (Fig 8.1). Another way of expressing this to patients is that while 71% of patients aged 30 will conceive within 3 months, only 41% of those aged 36 will conceive within 3 months.[21]

Women also have limited knowledge about the association between fetal abnormality and increasing maternal age.[22]

Questions to ask the woman regarding her reproductive life plan include:

- Does she want to have children? If so, how many and how far apart does she want them?
- Has she considered the age at which she desires to have her first child?

GPs should advise that from a medical point of view the ideal is to have the first child by 30, as fertility

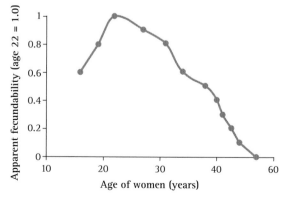

FIGURE 8.1 Age curve of apparent fecundability (From Wood[20])

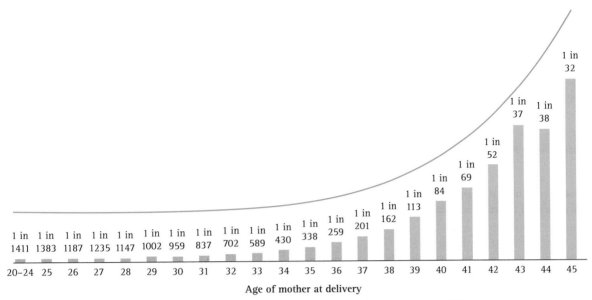

FIGURE 8.2 Maternal age and risk of live born baby with Down syndrome (From Morris et al[52])

TABLE 8.1 Genetic inheritance and examples of genetic diseases (From Delatycki and Massie[56])

Inheritance pattern	Explanation	Examples
Autosomal recessive	• A mutation in the same gene is inherited from each parent. • Each parent is a healthy carrier, as they have a second unaffected copy of the gene. • If both parents are carriers of an autosomal recessive condition, there is a 1:4 (25%) chance that each child will be affected. • It is estimated that all people carry 5–10 autosomal recessive mutations.	• Cystic fibrosis • Spinal muscular atrophy • Haemachromatosis • Alpha-thalassaemia • Beta-thalassaemia • Sickle cell disease • Tay-Sachs disease
Autosomal dominant	• Having a mutation in one pair of a particular gene is sufficient to result in the disease. • The child of a person with a dominant condition has a 1:2 (50%) chance of inheriting the condition.	• Neurofibromatosis type 1 • Huntington's disease
X-linked	• Because females have two X chromosomes, mutations in X chromosome genes cause mild or no manifestations in females but fully manifest in males who have only one X chromosome. • If a woman carries a mutation in a gene on one of her X chromosomes, there is a 1:2 (50%) chance that any son she has will be affected by the particular condition.	• Fragile X • Haemophilia A • Duchenne's muscular dystrophy

declines with age and the risk of fetal abnormality increases with age, as shown in Figure 8.2.

Assessing and managing risk

Why are ethnicity and family history important in preconception care?

Whereas most women are being made aware of the availability combined first-trimester screening for Down syndrome (regardless of age), women also need to know that their ethnicity and family history may mean that they could be a carrier of a genetic disease. GPs should explore with the patient and her partner whether there is a family history of birth defects or mental retardation, haemoglobinopathies (thalassaemia in those of Mediterranean heritage and sickle cell disease in African-Americans), cystic fibrosis, Tay-Sachs disease, phenylketonuria, cystic fibrosis or congenital hearing loss.

Table 8.1 explains the genetic inheritance associated with some genetic diseases and Table 8.2 gives the carrier frequency and incidence of some of the conditions for which genetic screening can be offered.

TABLE 8.2 Frequency of carrier status and disease in ethnic groups for conditions for which carrier screening is commonly offered (From Delatycki and Massie[56])

Disease	Ethnic group	Carrier frequency	Incidence in newborns
Cystic fibrosis	Caucasians	1:25	1:2500
Tay-Sachs disease	Ashkenazi Jews	1:28	1:3100
Sickle cell anaemia	Black Africans and African-Americans	Up to 1:5	Up to 1:100
Beta-thalassaemia	Mediterranean and Middle Eastern	Up to 1:5	Up to 1:100
Alpha-thalassaemia	South-east Asians and Chinese	1:10	1:400

What issues in a woman's reproductive history are pertinent to preconception care?

Complications that have occurred in previous pregnancies, such as those listed in Box 8.2, may recur in subsequent pregnancies. Identifying these issues and looking for causative or contributory factors may assist in preventing them from occurring in subsequent pregnancies or at least minimise their impact when prevention is not possible.

It is also important to consider whether there is a history of polycystic ovary syndrome, endometriosis, previous ectopic pregnancy or sexually transmissible infections (STIs), as these conditions might put the woman at risk of delayed fertility or infertility.

What medications and toxins should be avoided during pregnancy?

Another issue to make women aware of is that of environmental toxins and drug use during pregnancy. The fetus is very vulnerable to toxins and drugs, particularly in the first trimester when the development of the organs occurs. Often women will expose themselves to medications and toxins before they are aware that they are pregnant. Some women will be exposed to these toxins in their work environment and will need to change jobs prior to becoming pregnant. Agents that are toxic to the fetus are listed in Box 8.3. Women should also be advised to seek advice before taking medication during pregnancy to avoid ingesting substances that might be harmful to the fetus.

What chronic conditions can impact on pregnancy outcome?

The medical history of the woman needs review preconceptionally to identify any conditions that may put her or the fetus at risk of an adverse outcome. It is particularly important that the management of diabetic women is optimised prior to conception. Management of other common chronic conditions such as hypertension, epilepsy, thyroid disease, thromboembolism, depression and anxiety requires attention, as in some cases the medication for these conditions will need to be altered either preconceptionally or during the pregnancy itself.

Screening and vaccinations

What vaccinations are recommended prior to pregnancy?

The Australian immunisation handbook recommends that pertussis vaccination be offered to both partners prior to pregnancy and that women should consider influenza vaccination. Hepatitis B and pneumococcal vaccination should be considered in high-risk groups, and rubella and varicella vaccination in non-immune women.[24]

Rubella (German measles) is usually a mild febrile disease affecting children, but it can also

---

BOX 8.2 Pregnancy complications that may recur in subsequent pregnancies

- Miscarriages
- Stillbirths
- Birth defects
- Low birth weight
- Preterm birth
- Previous congenital malformation
- Preeclampsia
- Gestational diabetes
- Postnatal depression

BOX 8.3 Environmental toxins

- Metals such as lead and mercury
- Solvents such as benzene and toluene
- Plastics such as vinyl chloride
- Pesticides such as 245T and organophosphates
- Gases such as carbon monoxide and anaesthetic gases
- Radiation

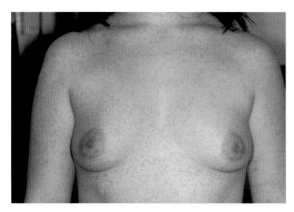

FIGURE 8.3 The characteristic rash of rubella: discrete and confluent erythematous maculopapular lesions are present. (From Black and Mackay[57])

affect adolescents and adults. Children usually present with few symptoms, but rubella can present with low-grade fever, swollen glands, joint pain, headache, mild coryza, conjunctivitis and a rash (Fig 8.3), which appears on the face and neck and lasts for 2–3 days. About 50% of cases will not have a recognisable rash. Complications of rubella include arthralgia and arthritis, mainly in females. Encephalitis is a rare complication, more frequent in adults than children.

The issue for women is that if rubella is contracted during the first trimester of pregnancy it has serious consequences for the developing fetus. Congenital rubella syndrome (CRS) occurs in up to 90% of infants born to women who contract rubella during this time. Early infection may also cause intrauterine death and spontaneous abortion. The incidence of congenital defects is rare if the disease is contracted after the twentieth week of pregnancy.

Rubella is a mild febrile disease in children and adults which causes congenital rubella syndrome in 90% of infants exposed during the first trimester.

How is rubella spread?

Rubella is spread through airborne droplets or direct contact with the nose or throat secretions of infected persons. The incubation period is 14–21 days, and the period of infectivity is from 1 week before until 4 days after the onset of the rash. The disease is highly contagious. It is also most prevalent during winter and spring.

How can it be prevented?

Most countries now vaccinate all children with MMR (trivalent vaccine consisting of measles, mumps and rubella vaccines). The vaccine is also available as monovalent rubella. Both vaccine formulations are attenuated live rubella virus prepared in cell culture and are highly effective in eliciting an immune response to rubella virus.

Most of the congenital rubella that now occurs in developed countries occurs in children born to mothers who recently emigrated from areas where the prevalence of this disease is higher. The decrease in the rates of congenital rubella has been the direct consequence of effective immunisation policies.[23]

In some women the immune response to rubella is not sustained and they may be lacking immunity by the time they fall pregnant. GPs should encourage women to measure their rubella antibodies well before conception to ensure that they are immune.

Australian immunisation guidelines[24] suggest that women born overseas (especially in Asia, Pacific islands, sub-Saharan Africa and South America) who have migrated after the age of routine vaccination, non-English-speaking women, women over the age of 35 and Muslim women are more likely to be seronegative to rubella. Vaccinated women should be tested for seroconversion 6–8 weeks after vaccination. Women who have negative or very low antibody levels after vaccination should be revaccinated. If their antibody levels remain low after a second vaccination, it is unlikely that further vaccinations will improve this. Although two doses of MMR vaccine are routinely recommended, if rubella immunity is demonstrated after receipt of one dose of a rubella-containing vaccine, no further dose is required unless indicated by subsequent serological testing.

Are there any special concerns about vaccinating a woman against rubella preconceptionally?

The rubella vaccine, whether MMR or the monovalent variety, is a live vaccine. There is therefore the theoretical risk of infecting a developing fetus. Previously, the advice to women has been to delay conception until at least 3 months after vaccination. More recently, immunisation guidelines have shortened this delay to 28 days.[24,25]

Should varicella vaccination be recommended too?

Congenital varicella syndrome has been reported after varicella infection in pregnancy and can result in skin scarring, limb defects, ocular anomalies and neurological malformations. There is a higher risk to the fetus if maternal infection occurs in the second trimester, compared with infection in the first trimester (1.4% versus 0.55%).[26] If the woman gives no clinical history of having had chicken pox and is not immune to varicella, two doses of vaccine are recommended 1 month apart.[24] Like rubella vaccination, the varicella vaccine contains live virus and so the woman should be advised to avoid pregnancy for 28 days after the last vaccine.

Rubella and varicella immune status should be known well before conception to allow for vaccination if necessary.

Summary of key points

- Since unintended pregnancy is common, GPs should be proactive about offering preconception care to women of reproductive age.
- There is an increasing trend towards delayed childbearing.
- Women are ill-informed about the relationship between age and fertility and between age and risk of fetal abnormality.
- Preconception care offers an opportunity to prevent recurrence of complications arising in previous pregnancies.
- Since the rubella and varicella vaccines contain live virus, women should delay conception till at least 28 days after receiving the vaccine.
- Varicella vaccination in a non-immune adult requires two doses 1 month apart.

Family planning

Depending on the patient's individual circumstances and reproductive life plan, fertility awareness, chance of conception and risks inherent in delayed childbearing such as infertility and fetal abnormality should be raised. For patients not planning to become pregnant GPs should ensure that the woman has effective contraception and is aware of the availability of emergency contraception.

Fertility awareness

Fertility awareness empowers women to have control over their reproductive health. It helps them to identify what is healthy and normal throughout their reproductive life, as well as to recognise signs and symptoms that may indicate a need to seek healthcare. Fertility awareness is a skill that all women should be taught to assist them either in contraception or conception at a time of their own choosing.

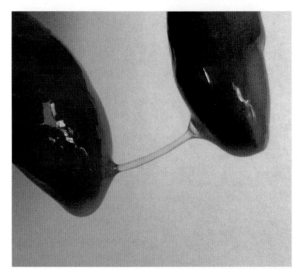

FIGURE 8.4 Ovulatory mucus

Fertility awareness should be regarded as a core 'competence' for women with regard to health education and literacy.

Many women, however—particularly those who have used hormonal contraception for a long time—have poor knowledge and awareness of when they ovulate. Low levels of fertility awareness may result in women miscalculating their peak fertile time and delay conception. It is therefore incumbent on GPs when delivering preconception care to teach women how to recognise the basic signs of ovulation.

Teaching the basic signs of ovulation should be integral to the delivery of preconception care.

The mucus method, as described by Billings and Billings,[27] involves women becoming aware of the changes to cervical mucus throughout the menstrual cycle. These are as follows:

1. Immediately following menstruation there are a variable number of days with no vaginal discharge.
2. Then the woman will start to become aware of mucus in increasing quantities, which appears to be 'cloudy' or 'sticky' (Fig 8.4).
3. Immediately prior to ovulation, the mucus becomes clear, copious and slippery with the characteristics of raw white of egg (spinnbarkeit). The woman

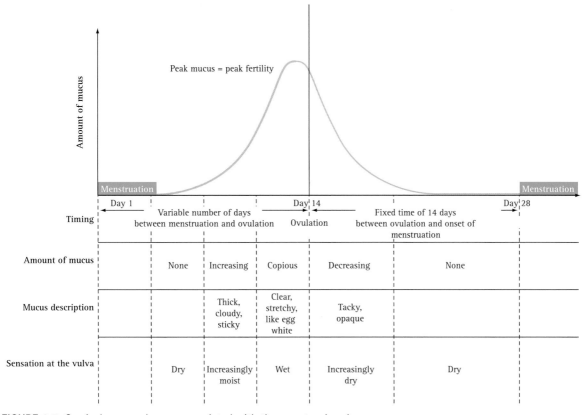

Figure on graph labels:

Amount of mucus

Peak mucus = peak fertility

Menstruation | Menstruation

Day 1   Day 14   Day 28

Timing | Variable number of days between menstruation and ovulation | Ovulation | Fixed time of 14 days between ovulation and onset of menstruation

Amount of mucus		None	Increasing	Copious	Decreasing	None	
Mucus description			Thick, cloudy, sticky	Clear, stretchy, like egg white	Tacky, opaque		
Sensation at the vulva		Dry	Increasingly moist	Wet	Increasingly dry	Dry	

FIGURE 8.5 Cervical mucus changes associated with the menstrual cycle

may feel 'damp' around the vulval area. These signs characterise the time of peak fertility.

4. Following ovulation, there is again a variable period of thick, opaque, diminished-volume discharge that can be 'tacky' and slightly yellow in colour, and often leaves a flaky stain on underwear. This is followed by dry days.

In addition to mucus changes women may be aware of increased libido at the time of ovulation and notice 'mittleshmerz' or ovulation pain, which can be sharp or dull pain in the lower back or pelvis and is usually one-sided.

It is important to point out that ovulation occurs 14 days before the onset of bleeding. If a woman has a 28-day cycle, she will be ovulating on day 14. However, if her cycle is 35 days long, she will be ovulating on day 21. A graph can be drawn out for the woman during a consultation to explain these changes (Fig 8.5).

In the menstrual cycle the time between ovulation and menstruation is always 14 days.

Research shows that the timing of sexual intercourse in relation to ovulation strongly influences the chance of conception.[28] Conception occurs only during a 6-day interval that ends on the estimated day of ovulation. The probability of conception ranges from 10% when intercourse occurs 5 days before ovulation to 33% when it occurs on the day of ovulation itself. The chance of conception falls to zero 24 hours after ovulation. There is no evident relationship between the age of sperm and the viability of the conceptus, although only 6% of pregnancies can be firmly attributed to sperm that are 3 or more days old. Cycles producing male and female babies have similar patterns of intercourse in relation to ovulation. For counselling purposes, the points in Box 8.4 are helpful to reiterate.

The maximum chance of conception each month is 33%.

Folic acid supplementation

Women of reproductive age should be taking folate supplements on a daily basis to help prevent neural tube defects (NTDs) (Fig 8.6) in the first few weeks of pregnancy. The evidence for folate supplementation has been present for many years. Randomised controlled trials show that an intake of at least 0.4 mg of folate prior to and during early pregnancy can reduce both the recurrence[29] as well as the first occurrence of NTDs.[30]

An adequate intake of folate in the periconceptional period has the capacity to prevent 70 per cent of all cases of NTD.

The prevalence of NTDs has been estimated at approximately 1 in 600.[31] The increased use of folate, the numbers of babies born with NTDs can be reduced.

Another reason for folate use during pregnancy is to reduce the prevalence of anaemia during the latter part of the pregnancy. Megaloblastic anaemia occurs as a result of plasma expansion, low levels of folate at the commencement of the pregnancy and increased excretion of folate throughout. Before prophylaxis with folate was introduced on a widespread basis in pregnancy, overt anaemia occurred in approximately one in 200 pregnancies and was found to be as high as a quarter of all pregnancies in some centres.[32]

Why aren't women using folate in the preconception period?

Despite the fact that research has shown that an adequate intake of folate in the periconceptional period has the capacity to prevent 70 per cent of all cases of NTD[33] and the issuing of guidelines supporting folate supplementation by women of reproductive age,[53] women have a low level of awareness of the benefits of folate supplementation[34]

BOX 8.4 Important points to raise when counselling about chance of conception

- The maximum chance of conception is 33% in each cycle.
- The egg lives for only 24 hours.
- Sperm live in the reproductive tract of women for a maximum of 3–5 days.
- Couples can optimise their chance of conception by having intercourse at the time of peak fertility (every second day is sufficient) and in that way have sperm waiting in the reproductive tract for the egg to be released.

---

and less than 50% of women supplement their diet with folate periconceptionally.[35] This proportion is lower in women from lower socioeconomic groups and indigenous, rural and younger women. It is also lower in multiparous women.[35] Another study has found that only 30% of women attending hospital antenatal clinics achieved full compliance with folate supplementation recommendations in terms of both timing and dose.[36]

Less than 50% of women supplement their diet with folate periconceptionally, with lower percentages among women from lower socioeconomic groups and indigenous, rural and younger women.

Women are more likely to respond to information given by a healthcare provider, but only 53% of women who had heard of folate reported that the information was given to them by a GP or an obstetrician.[37] Obstetricians and general practitioners are not adequately educating their female patients about the need for periconceptional folic acid supplementation.[34,35]

GPs and obstetricians do not adequately educate women about the need for periconceptual folate supplementation.

Which are the high-risk groups?

GPs should place special emphasis on those women in their practice who are at higher risk of NTDs. In these high-risk groups, the recommendation is to use 4.0–5.0 mg of folate (10 times the dose for the low-risk woman) per day for 2–3 months prior

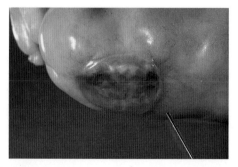

FIGURE 8.6 A neural tube defect in a fetus following termination of the pregnancy after ultrasound detection (From Greer et al[58])

to conception and for at least the first 3 months of pregnancy.[38]

Women at high risk of bearing a child with a neural tube defect require 4.0–5.0 mg of folate daily.

About 10% of NTDs are due to chromosomal anomalies, but other factors are also known to predispose to NTDs. These are largely thought to be multifactorial in origin[39] and include maternal diabetes and exposure to anticonvulsants such as sodium valproate and carbamazepine.[40]

Diabetes, exposure to antiepileptics and family history all increase risk of having a baby with a neural tube defect.

The recurrence risk for couples with a previous NTD-affected pregnancy is 3–4% and the risk for any first-degree relatives is 1%.[41]

While not in a high-risk group, oral contraceptive users may have reduced levels of folate.[42] Since, in practice, hormonal contraceptives have about a 4–5% failure rate, it is not unreasonable to recommend routine folate supplementation to all women who are on the pill.

Oral contraceptive users have reduced levels of folate.

How can folate levels in women be increased?

One solution is to fortify foods with folate so that women are unconsciously attaining preventive levels of folate in their normal diet. This has already taken place in the USA, where in January 1998 the Food and Drug Administration, after considerable debate, made fortification of cereals with folic acid mandatory,[43] and this is imminent in Australia. At issue is the ability of the public to recognise which foods are fortified and to what levels.

Why not just increase the intake of folate-rich foods?

While it is a good public health message to promote increased intake of food containing high levels of folate (Table 8.3), when folate is consumed as fresh food it has low levels of bioavailability and effectivity. The natural, reduced forms of folate

TABLE 8.3 Food sources of folate

Food type	Serve size	Folate levels
Vegetables		
Spinach (raw)	1 cup	Excellent
Asparagus (cooked)	half cup	Excellent
Lettuce (chopped)	1 cup	Very good
Broccoli (cooked)	half cup	Good
Green peas (cooked from frozen)	half cup	Good
Cereal foods		
Weetbix	2 biscuits	Excellent
Cornflakes	1 cup	Excellent
Wholemeal bread	2 slices	Good
Fruit (including juices)		
Orange juice (fresh)	1 cup	Very good
Orange	Medium	Good
Banana	Medium	Good
Legumes (cooked from dry, drained)		
Lentils	half cup	Excellent
Black-eyed beans	half cup	Excellent
Chickpeas	half cup	Excellent
Lima/Butter bean	half cup	Very good
Nuts		
Peanuts quarter	cup	Very good
Almonds	quarter cup	Good
Walnuts	quarter cup	Good

are very susceptible to oxidative destruction during harvesting, storage and cooking of food.[32] Natural forms of folate are therefore only one-quarter to a one-half as bioavailable as synthetic folic acid.[44] Synthetic folic acid is not as susceptible to such destruction. It is for this reason that folate supplementation is recommended.

In many countries food is fortified with folate, but this does not necessarily achieve the recommended dose for folate supplementation.

The real solution is therefore for women to buy folate supplements and to remember to take them of their own initiative. Again, there are problems with standards and cost. Many women are already taking multivitamins. Many of these products are marketed as being specifically for women and contain calcium and other ingredients thought to be beneficial to women. Levels of folate will be variable and it is important to stress that the minimum dose recommended for daily use is 0.4–0.5 mg.

BOX 8.5 Lifestyle advice

Exercise, weight and nutrition
- Regular aerobic exercise during pregnancy appears to improve (or maintain) physical fitness and body image. Available data are insufficient to infer important risks or benefits for the mother or infant.[45]
- Obesity or being underweight increase pregnancy risks.
- Obesity increases the risk of hypertension, preeclampsia, diabetes and a large infant.
- Assess risk of nutritional deficiencies (e.g. veganism, lactose intolerance, calcium or iron deficiency, Vitamin D).

Quitting smoking[46]
- Smoking doubles the risk of having a low-birthweight baby and significantly increases the rate of perinatal mortality and several other adverse pregnancy outcomes.
- The mean reduction in birthweight for babies of smoking mothers is 200 g.
- High-quality interventions to help pregnant women quit smoking produce an absolute difference of 8.1% in validated late-pregnancy quit rates.
- If abstinence is not achievable, it is likely that a 50% reduction in smoking would be the minimum necessary to benefit the health of mother and baby.

Alcohol[47]
- Heavy maternal alcohol consumption during early pregnancy is required for the development of fetal alcohol syndrome, but not all children exposed to alcohol in utero will be affected to the same degree, and some will not be affected at all.
- The amount of alcohol necessary for fetal damage is unclear. On this basis, GPs should advise that there is no safe limit of alcohol consumption during pregnancy.[48]

Illegal drugs
- Women using illegal drugs should be encouraged to abstain and those who use daily should be referred to drug-treatment programs prior to pregnancy.
- Cocaine use is associated with miscarriage, prematurity, growth retardation and congenital defects.
- Marijuana use can cause prematurity and neonatal jitteriness.
- Heroin use may lead to intrauterine growth retardation, hyperactivity and severe neonatal withdrawal syndrome.

In general women should take 0.4 mg of folate for at least 1 month prior to their pregnancy and for the first 3 months of their pregnancy.

Another way to aid in folate supplementation at the time of conception would be for pharmaceutical companies that manufacture oral contraception to fortify individual pills with 0.4 mg of folate. This is a big task, particularly because it would be an admission on their part that a percentage of women taking oral contraception still fall pregnant either because they miss pills or because the pill-free interval (the 7 days of sugar pills in most pill packs) is too long for some women to maintain ovarian suppression.

Who needs to hear the message?

It is relatively easy for GPs to remember to give the folate message to women who attend for pre-pregnancy counselling. These women are usually a very motivated, intelligent and conscientious group. They deliberately plan when they want to get pregnant and do all in their power to make sure that everything is correct and in position before they conceive. Therefore, the group that is missing out consists of the less well-educated women and those with unplanned pregnancies.

It is for this reason that GPs need to join other health professionals in promoting folate supplementation to all women of reproductive age, regardless of whether or not they use contraception.

Summary of key points
- The prevalence of neural tube defects is 1 in 600.
- Folate supplementation reduces neural tube defects by 70% and helps prevent anaemia in pregnancy.
- The recommended dose of folate supplementation is 0.4 mg taken daily for a period of 3 months prior to conception and the first trimester of the pregnancy.
- Women at high risk of having a child with a neural tube defect include those with diabetes and those exposed to anticonvulsants such as sodium valproate and carbamazepine, as well as those with a family history of NTD.
- Women at high risk should take 4.0–5.0 mg folate daily.

Lifestyle advice

Lifestyle advice should be given to women to optimise their chances of conception as well as in order to prevent pregnancy complications. Lifestyle advice concerning exercise, weight and nutrition, smoking, alcohol and illicit drug use is summarised in Box 8.5.

GPs should provide support and identify coping strategies to improve emotional health and wellbeing in women contemplating pregnancy, particularly in those with a history of depression or who are currently using antidepressants. In this latter group, a review of the benefits and disadvantages of antidepressant use is warranted, and the dose or type of medication used may need alteration.

Enquiry should be made about possible exposure to hazardous toxins in the household and workplace environment which may affect fertility and increase the risk of miscarriage and birth defects.

A progressive increase has been found in the time taken to become pregnant with increasing numbers of negative lifestyle factors[49] (Fig 8.7).

What infections should women be counselled about preconceptionally?

Before conception, women should consider being screened for human immunodeficiency virus and syphilis infection because, if detected, treatment can be offered to prevent the transmission of disease to the fetus.

While women can receive immunisation against rubella and varicella prior to the pregnancy, there are no immunisations against toxoplasmosis, cytomegalovirus (CMV), and parvovirus B19.

Toxoplasmosis is a parasite commonly found in raw meat or cat faeces. New owners of cats that go outside are most at risk. Women should be counselled to avoid contact with cat faeces in litter boxes, to wear gloves while gardening, and to avoid eating raw or undercooked meat.[50]

CMV exposure is a special risk for childcare and healthcare workers. Persons at risk should wash their hands frequently and use gloves to prevent transmission. Parvovirus B19 (slapped cheek syndrome) is transmitted by prolonged close contact with small children who have the disease in household or childcare settings. Serologic testing is possible to document previous immunity but is not routinely recommended for these organisms.[51]

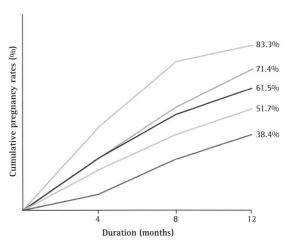

FIGURE 8.7 The effect of increasing numbers of negative lifestyle variables on the cumulative conception rates within 1 year for a pregnant population. These variables include:
- women smoking >15 cigarettes/day
- men smoking >15 cigarettes/day
- alcohol intake (men) >20U/week;
- coffee/tea intake (women) >7 cups/day
- women's weight >70 kg
- social deprivation score >60
- women's age >35 years and/or partner's age >45 years at the time of discontinuing contraception.

The lines represent the cumulative conception rates for subgroups with different numbers of negative lifestyle variables as follows:
--- no negative variables
— one negative variable
— two negative variables
— three negative variables
— four or more negative variables. (From Hassan and Killick[49])

Avoidance of paté, soft cheeses, pre-packaged salads, deli meats, and chilled/smoked seafood will help prevent listeriosis infection.

TIPS FOR PRACTITIONERS

- Natural forms of folate are not as bioavailable as synthetic folic acid. It is therefore preferable to use supplements, rather than just increase dietary intake of folate.
- A checklist that a patient can take home with her is useful during preconception counselling.
- It may be helpful to discuss preconception care over two consultations, the first taking a history and ordering relevant screening tests and the second involving vaccination and lifestyle advice.

- Women who are vaccinated against varicella and or rubella should not conceive for 28 days, because the vaccine contains live virus from which there is a small risk of contracting the disease itself.
- About 50% of cases of rubella do not exhibit a recognisable rash.

REFERENCES

1. Atrash HK, Johnson K, Adams M, et al. Preconception care for improving perinatal outcomes: the time to act. Matern Child Health J 2006; 10(5):S3–11.
2. Moos MK, Bangdiwala SI, Meibohm AR, et al. The impact of a preconceptional health promotion program on intendedness of pregnancy. Am J Perinatol 1996; 13:103–108.
3. Henshaw SK. Unintended pregnancy in the United States. Fam Plann Perspect 1998; 30(1):24–29, 46.
4. Jack BW, Campanile C, McQuade W, et al. The negative pregnancy test. An opportunity for preconception care. Arch Fam Med 1995; 4:340–345.
5. Frey KA, Files JA. Preconception healthcare: what women know and believe. Matern Child Health J 2006; 10(5 Suppl):S73–S77.
6. Cannold L. What, no baby?: Why women are losing the freedom to mother, and how they can get it back. Fremantle: Fremantle Arts Centre Press; 2005.
7. Wicks D, Mishra G. Young Australian women and their aspirations for work, education, and relationships. In: Carson E, Jamrozik A, Winefield T, eds. Unemployment: economic promise and political will. Brisbane: Australian Academic Press; 1998:89–100.
8. Weston R, Qu L, Parker R, et al. 'It's not for lack of wanting kids.' A report on the Fertility Decision Making Project. Australian Institute of Family Studies; 2004; Report No. 11.
9. Laws PJ, Sullivan EA. Australia's mothers and babies 2003. AIHW cat. no. PER 29. Perinatal Statistics Series no. 16. Sydney: AIHW National Perinatal Statistics Unit; 2005.
10. Bewley S, Davies M, Braude P. Which career first? BMJ 2005; 331(7517):588–589.
11. Andersen A-MN, Wohlfahrt J, Christens P, et al. Maternal age and fetal loss: population based register linkage study. BMJ 2000; 320(7251):1708–1712.
12. Stein Z, Susser M. The risks of having children in later life. BMJ 2000; 320(7251):1681–1682.
13. Baird DT, Collins J, Egozcue J, et al. Fertility and ageing. Hum Reprod Update 2005; 11(3):261–276.
14. Waterstone M, Bewley S, Wolfe C, et al. Incidence and predictors of severe obstetric morbidity: case-control study. Commentary: obstetric morbidity data and the need to evaluate thromboembolic disease. BMJ 2001; 322(7294):1089-1094.
15. Madsen P. Just the facts, ma'am. Coming clean about fertility. Fertil Steril 2003; 80(Suppl 4):27–29.
16. Hammarberg K, Clarke VE. Reasons for delaying childbearing–a survey of women aged over 35 years seeking assisted reproductive technology. Aust Fam Physician 2005; 34(3):187–188, 206.
17. Hammarberg K, Astbury J, Baker H. Women's experience of IVF: a follow-up study. Hum Reprod 2001; 16(2):374–383.
18. Chapman MG, Driscoll GL, Jones B. Missed conceptions: the need for education. Med J Aust 2006; 184(7):361–362.
19. American College of Obstetricians and Gynecologists. ACOG committee opinion. Age-related fertility decline. Obstet Gynecol 2008; 112(2 Pt 1):409–411.
20. Wood J. Oxford reviews of reproductive biology. New York: Oxford University Press; 1989.
21. Kaplan B, Nahum R, Yairi Y, et al. Use of various contraceptive methods and time of conception in a community-based population. Eur J Obstet Gynecol Reprod Biol 2005; 123:72–76.
22. Mulvey S, Wallace EM. Levels of knowledge of Down syndrome and Down syndrome testing in Australian women. Aust NZ J Obstet Gynaecol 2001; 41(2):167–169.
23. Reef SE, Frey TK, Theall K, et al. The changing epidemiology of rubella in the 1990s: on the verge of elimination and new challenges for control and prevention. JAMA 2002; 287:464–472.
24. National Health and Medical Research Council. The Australian immunisation handbook. 9th edn. Canberra: Australian Government Publishing Services; 2008.
25. ACIP. Revised ACIP recommendation for avoiding pregnancy after receiving a rubella-containing vaccine. JAMA 2002; 287:311–312.
26. Tan M, Koren G. Chickenpox in pregnancy: revisited. Reprod Toxicol 2006; 21:410–420.
27. Billings JJ, Billings E. The Billings ovulation method. An update. Aust Fam Physician 1988; 17(10):843–846.
28. Wilcox AJ, Weinberg CR, Baird DD. Timing of sexual intercourse in relation to ovulation. Effects on the probability of conception, survival of the pregnancy, and sex of the baby. N Engl J Med 1995; 333(23):1517–1521.
29. Medical Research Council Vitamin Study Research Group. Prevention of neural tube defects: results of the Medical Research Council Vitamin Study. Lancet 1991; 338:131–137.
30. Czeizel AE, Dudas I. Prevention of the first occurrence of neural-tube defects by periconceptional vitamin supplementation. N Engl J Med 1992; 327:1832–1835.
31. Owen TJ, Halliday JL, Stone CA. Neural tube defects in Victoria, Australia: potential contributing factors and public health implications. Aust NZ J Public Health 2000; 24:584–589.
32. Chanarin I. Megaloblastic anaemias. 2nd edn. Oxford: Blackwell; 1979.
33. Lumley J, Watson L, Watson M, et al. Periconceptional supplementation with folate and/or multivitamins for preventing neural tube defects. Cochrane Database Syst Rev 2001; (3):CD001056.
34. Marsack CR, Alsop CL, Kurinczuk JJ, et al. Pre-pregnancy counselling for the primary prevention of birth defects: rubella vaccination and folate intake. Med J Aust 1995; 162:403–406 [see comment; erratum appears in Med J Aust 1996; 165(3):130].
35. Watson LF, Brown SJ, Davey M-A. Use of periconceptional folic acid supplements in Victoria and New South Wales, Australia. Aust NZ J Public Health 2006; 30(1):42–49.
36. Conlin ML, MacLennan AH, Broadbent JL. Inadequate compliance with periconceptional folic acid supplementation in South Australia. Aust NZ J Obstet Gynaecol 2006; 46(6):528–533.
37. Perelman V, Singal N, Einarson A, et al. Knowledge and practice by Canadian family physicians regarding periconceptional folic acid supplementation for the prevention of neural tube defects. Can J Clin Pharmacol 1996; 3:145–148.
38. National Health and Medical Research Council. Revised statement on the relationship between dietary folic acid and neural tube defects such as spina bifida. Canberra: NHMRC; 1993.
39. Hall JG, Friedman JM, Kenna BA, et al. Clinical, genetic, and epidemiological factors in neural tube defects. Am J Hum Genet 1988; 43:827–837.
40. Holmes LB. Spina bifida: anticonvulsants and other maternal influences. Ciba Found Symp 1994; 181:232–238.

41. Harper PS. Practical genetic counselling. 4th edn. Oxford: Butterworth-Heinemann; 1993:177.
42. Sauberlich HE. Folate status of US population groups. In: Bailey LB, ed. Folate in health and disease. New York: Dekker; 1995:171–194.
43. Kennedy DS. Spina bifida. Med J Aust 1998; 169:182–183.
44. Cuskelly CJ, McNulty H, Scott JM. Effect of increasing dietary folate on red-cell folate: implications for prevention of neural tube defects. Lancet 1996; 347:657–659.
45. Kramer MS, McDonald SW. Aerobic exercise for women during pregnancy. Cochrane Database Syst Rev 2006; 3:CD000180.
46. Walsh RA, Lowe JB, Hopkins PJ. Quitting smoking in pregnancy. Med J Aust 2001; 175(6):320–323.
47. O'Leary CM, Heuzenroeder L, Elliott EJ, et al. A review of policies on alcohol use during pregnancy in Australia and other English-speaking countries, 2006. Med J Aust 2007; 186(9):466–471.
48. NHMRC. Australian alcohol guidelines for low-risk drinking Draft for public consultation October 2007. 2007. Online. Available: http://www.nhmrc.gov.au/guidelines/_files/draft_australian_alcohol_guidelines.pdf [accessed 9.12.08].
49. Hassan MA, Killick SR. Negative lifestyle is associated with a significant reduction in fecundity. Fertil Steril 2004; 81:384–392.
50. Piper JM, Wen TS. Perinatal cytomegalovirus and toxoplasmosis: challenges of antepartum therapy. Clin Obstet Gynecol 1999; 42:81–96.
51. American College of Obstetricians and Gynecologists. Perinatal viral and parasitic infections. ACOG Practice Bulletin Number 20, September 2000. Obstet Gynecol 2000; 96:1–13.
52. Morris J, Mutton D, Alberman E. Corrections to maternal age-specific live birth prevalence of Down's syndrome. J Med Screen 2005; 12(4):202.
53. Royal Australian College of General Practitioners. Guidelines for preventive activities in general practice (the red book). 7th edn. Melbourne: RACGP; 2009.
54. Oh W, Gilstrap L, eds. Guidelines for perinatal care. 5th edn. Elk Grove Village, IL: American Academy of Pediatrics, American College of Obstetricians and Gynecologists; 2002.
55. Lu MC. Recommendations for preconception care. American Family Physician 2007; 76(3):397–400.
56. Delatycki MB, Massie J. Antenatal and pre-pregnancy screening for genetic conditions. Australian Doctor 2006; 9 June:35–42.
57. Black M, Mackay M. Obstetric and gynaecologic dermatology. 2nd edn. London: Mosby; 2002:82.
58. Greer IA, Cameron IT, Kitchner HC, et al. Mosby's colour atlas and text of obstetrics and gynaecology. London: Mosby; 2001:106.

9

Early pregnancy loss

OBJECTIVES

- To diagnose the cause of early bleeding in pregnancy
- To manage women presenting with spontaneous miscarriage
- To be aware of the epidemiology and causes of spontaneous miscarriage and ectopic pregnancy
- To diagnose ectopic pregnancy
- To understand the rationale for the various treatment methods for ectopic pregnancy
- To be able to counsel women about their chances of a successful subsequent pregnancy

SPONTANEOUS MISCARRIAGE

While many pregnancies are lost before the woman even realises she is pregnant (and mistaken for a heavy or late period), a not uncommon presentation in general practice is bleeding in early pregnancy. For the family doctor, this distressing consultation often follows the joyous one at which pregnancy is confirmed and plans for antenatal care are made.

Women may present with abdominal pain and bleeding of varying severity. The GP has several roles:

- to ensure that the woman's life is not in danger from an undiagnosed ectopic pregnancy or haemorrhage
- to confirm the diagnosis
- to advise the patient about fetal viability and management of the current situation
- to address the psychological as well as physical needs of the patient.

Generally women and their partners are hesitant to disclose a newly diagnosed pregnancy to family and friends until 12–14 weeks have passed. This is not without reason, given that 12–16% of all clinically recognised pregnancies end in miscarriage.[1] In fact the rate of pregnancies lost is probably even higher, since many miscarriages occur before pregnancy is even diagnosed.

What symptoms point to an early pregnancy loss?

Women present to GPs with bleeding during the first few weeks of pregnancy quite commonly. Bleeding is most common between the ninth and twelfth weeks and pain is usually not a significant feature unless the cervix is starting to open.

Thankfully, the availability of ultrasound has made management of these women much easier, for the GP at any rate.

About one quarter of all pregnant women experience spotting or bleeding in the first few weeks of pregnancy, and one half of those who bleed will miscarry.[2]

What should a GP do?

After a history is taken (Box 9.1), an examination needs to be performed. It is important first to take note of the vital signs of the patient. A temperature may indicate sepsis, while rapid pulse and postural drop, or lowered blood pressure point to loss of a large amount of blood and the need for urgent attention and stabilisation.

CASE STUDY: Concerned she was miscarrying

Twenty-nine-year-old Cheryl presented to the surgery with a smile on her face. Her period was a week late and she wanted to confirm that she was pregnant. She'd married earlier that year and had been keen to start a family. She took the positive pregnancy test home with her to show her husband, beaming from ear to ear. Three weeks later she returned, this time looking quite anxious. She'd had a small amount of bleeding and was concerned she was miscarrying. Examination was unremarkable, with a normal pulse and blood pressure. Vaginal examination revealed a small amount of dark blood visible in the posterior fornix. The cervix was closed and non-tender, uterine size 'bulky' and no adnexal masses were palpable.

Key features of the general examination of a woman bleeding in early pregnancy are her vital signs, postural drop, abdominal tenderness and/or guarding.

Once these parameters are established, the GP should examine the abdomen, looking for signs of tenderness and guarding in either iliac fossa, as this may be indicative of a ruptured ectopic pregnancy. The next step is to carry out a pelvic examination. After positioning the speculum accurately, the blood loss present in the vagina should be noted and the cervix carefully examined. It is often handy to wipe away any blood or mucus covering the os so as to enable inspection and to confirm this with digital examination, as its shape may be the key to diagnosis. A closed os in a pregnant woman during the first trimester can mean that the presentation is one of a threatened miscarriage or a missed miscarriage (i.e. the pregnancy has been lost and the process

BOX 9.1 Questions to ask when a woman presents with the onset of bleeding in the first trimester of pregnancy

- Date of last normal menstrual period
- Obstetric history
- Duration of bleeding
- Amount of blood lost (i.e. how many pads or tampons have been used; were they soaked or just spotted?)
- Appearance of loss (bright, dark)
- Any clots passed?
- Any products of conception passed?
- Any pain associated with the bleeding?

is complete). An open os indicates an inevitable or incomplete miscarriage.

When a woman presents with bleeding in early pregnancy, a GP should assess vital signs, do a urinary pregnancy test (unless pregnancy is already confirmed), establish gestation based on the last menstrual period, palpate the abdomen, and undertake a speculum and bimanual assessment.

Occasionally, women present in early pregnancy either bleeding more heavily and/or in a great deal of pain. In these situations there may be some products of conception in the os itself which, when removed, cause the bleeding and pain to subside. Sometimes bulging membranes can also be seen through an open os in the case of an inevitable miscarriage.

If the patient is stable the usual course of action is to obtain a transvaginal ultrasound. There are two ways in which an ultrasound can assist patient management. First, it will confirm whether or not the pregnancy is intrauterine or ectopic. Second, if the pregnancy is intrauterine the sonographer may be able to confirm whether or not a fetal heart is present and, if not, whether or not products of conception remain in the uterus. Sometimes it is difficult to assess the contents of the uterus or indeed whether or not it is an ectopic pregnancy. Success is dependent on gestational age and the skill of the ultrasonographer. If cardiac activity is detected by ultrasound early in the pregnancy, the chance of miscarriage is reduced to 5.5%.[3]

The routine early use of ultrasound may, however, lead to a diagnosis of incomplete miscarriage, blighted ovum or missed miscarriage (Box 9.2), when the natural outcome may be spontaneous complete miscarriage; the ultrasound may therefore encourage unnecessary intervention.[4,5]

It is important to make the patient aware that the ultrasound will be performed vaginally and to ask her if she wishes to see the screen. If the pregnancy is unplanned and she is considering an abortion anyway, you may need to advise the sonographer to position the screen away from the view of the patient.

What are the causes of early fetal loss?

It can be reassuring for patients to be told that if a pregnancy ends in early miscarriage, 'the pregnancy would not have continued' and 'it is nature's way of dealing with problems in a fetus'. While historically, 50% of spontaneously expelled fetuses have been thought to be chromosomally abnormal,[6] this figure is probably an underestimate.

The major cause of miscarriage is genetic abnormalities in the fetus.

In spontaneous miscarriages, the majority of chromosomal anomalies (95%) are numerical. About 60% are trisomies, trisomy 16 being the most common. A further 20% are found to have 45,X (Turner's syndrome). Interestingly, approximately 99% of fetuses with 45,X are expelled spontaneously. Another 15% have polyploidy, especially triploidy. In the case of a numerical chromosomal anomaly in a fetus, parental chromosomes are usually normal, so karyotype analysis of the parents is not indicated.

How should the GP assist with the emotional consequences of spontaneous miscarriage?

When pregnancies are planned, and even when unplanned but wanted, an early miscarriage is very traumatic. Expectations, plans and hopes are dashed and patients can and do present very emotionally.

BOX 9.2 Ultrasound criteria for types of miscarriage

Complete miscarriage	Incomplete miscarriage	Missed miscarriage
• No intrauterine gestational sac	• No intrauterine gestational sac	• Intact intrauterine gestational sac
• No ovarian/fallopian mass	• No ovarian/fallopian mass	• Fetal pole seen
• Products of conception (POC) passed	• POC passed	• No fetal heart beat
• No evidence of POC in uterus	• More POC seen in uterus	• Crown–rump length (CRL) is >6 mm **OR**
• Endometrial thickness <15 mm in longitudinal section		• Intact intrauterine gestational sac measuring >20 mm
		• Fetal pole not seen

Current management of these situations often fails to provide adequate support for women and their partners,[7] who often feel that they might have contributed to the miscarriage in some way. It is therefore important to offer patients follow-up after a miscarriage, to ensure that they are not becoming depressed and that they have an opportunity to talk about their experiences and how the miscarriage has affected their personal lives and relationships (Box 9.3).

In dealing with women and their partners who are facing these difficult circumstances, it is also important not to use language that may cause additional distress. For this reason, 'miscarriage' is the preferred term, rather than abortion. Definitions of terms commonly used in relation to first-trimester bleeding are given in Table 9.1.

Do all women suffering from a spontaneous miscarriage require a D&C?

More than 80% of women with a first-trimester spontaneous miscarriage have complete natural passage of tissue within 2 to 6 weeks, with no higher complication rate than that from surgical intervention.[8] However, for the last 50 years, women experiencing an early miscarriage have been managed by surgical evacuation of the uterus through a D&C. While this procedure is a common one, it is not without some risks. Apart from anaesthetic risks, there are also the risks of early complications such as infection, bleeding and, less frequently, injury to the cervix or uterine perforation and later on Asherman syndrome (intrauterine scars resulting in adhesions that can obliterate the uterine cavity to varying degrees).

Before ultrasound was available, it was clinically difficult to determine whether or not a spontaneous

miscarriage was complete at the time of presentation. The reasons for recommending a D&C therefore seemed quite reasonable: the sooner products of conception are evacuated from the uterus, the smaller the risk of heavy bleeding or infection. With the growing momentum of the evidence-based movement, however, the routine use of D&C in situations of early miscarriage has come into question and two other approaches can be utilised: expectant management or medical management with agents such as misoprostol.

TABLE 9.1 Definitions of terms related to first-trimester bleeding

Term	Definition
Anembryonic pregnancy	Presence of a gestational sac larger than 18 mm without evidence of embryonic tissues (yolk sac or embryo); this term is preferable to the older and less accurate term 'blighted ovum'
Ectopic pregnancy	Pregnancy outside the uterine cavity (most commonly in the fallopian tube, but may occur in the broad ligament, ovary, cervix, or elsewhere in the abdomen)
Embryonic demise	An embryo larger than 5 mm without cardiac activity; this replaces the term 'missed abortion'
Gestational trophoblastic disease or hyda-tidiform mole	Complete mole: placental proliferation in the absence of a fetus; most have a 46,XX chromosomal composition; all derived from paternal source
Recurrent pregnancy loss	More than two consecutive pregnancy losses; 'habitual aborter' has also been used but is no longer appropriate
Spontaneous miscarriage	Spontaneous loss of a pregnancy before 20 weeks' gestation
Complete miscarriage	Complete passage of all products of conception
Incomplete miscarriage	Occurs when some, but not all, of the products of conception have passed
Inevitable miscarriage	Bleeding in the presence of a dilated cervix; indicates that passage of the conceptus is unavoidable
Septic miscarriage	Incomplete miscarriage associated with ascending infection of the endometrium, parametrium, adnexa, or peritoneum
Threatened miscarriage	Bleeding before 20 weeks' gestation in the presence of an embryo with cardiac activity and closed cervix

---

BOX 9.3 The role of the GP in managing the psychological consequences of spontaneous miscarriage

1. Dispel the woman's feelings of guilt that something she did brought about the miscarriage.
2. Make the woman aware of how common miscarriage actually is.
3. Acknowledge and legitimise the grief that a woman and her partner often feel following a miscarriage.
4. Provide accurate advice about future fertility and when they should attempt conception again.

Both expectant and medical management of spontaneous miscarriage may be appealing to some women, as both methods obviate the need for surgery and an anaesthetic and may be perceived as more natural. Both are highly successful (expectant management 86% and medical management 100%), but expectant management is more likely to fail where there is embryonic demise or anembryonic pregnancy.[9]

Expectant management is successful within 2–6 weeks without increased complications in 80–90% of women with first-trimester incomplete spontaneous miscarriage and in 65–75% of women with first-trimester missed miscarriage or anembryonic gestation (presenting with spotting or bleeding and ultrasound evidence of fetal demise).[8]

Another issue for women to consider is that expectant management involves more outpatient visits.[9]

Medical management involves the use of an agent such as misoprostol, given either vaginally or orally. Women managed in this way have more bleeding (the bleeding can extend up to three weeks) but less pain than those treated surgically (surgical management also involves greater risk of trauma and infectious complications).[10]

Surgical evacuation should be considered for women experiencing spontaneous miscarriage with unstable vital signs, uncontrolled bleeding or evidence of infection.[8]

What do women prefer to do when they have a spontaneous miscarriage: to take a wait-and-see approach, to seek medical management or to have a D&C?

Women have a strong preference for expectant treatment, but believe their doctor's recommendation is a significant factor in their final decision.[11] GPs therefore need to offer all options to patients and to consider individual patient preferences when making recommendations regarding the management of first-trimester incomplete spontaneous miscarriage. This is particularly important because patient choice is associated with positive quality-of-life outcomes.[12]

What about anti-D prophylaxis?

Anti-D prophylaxis should be administered to women who are Rh-negative in an effort to avoid the formation of antibodies in ectopic pregnancy

and any miscarriage, regardless of gestational age of the fetus or uterine evacuation method.[13] A dose of 250 IU (50 µg) Rh D immunoglobulin should be offered to every Rh-negative woman with no preformed anti-D, to ensure adequate protection against immunisation for the following indications up to and including 12 weeks' gestation[13]:

- miscarriage
- termination of pregnancy
- ectopic pregnancy
- chorionic villus sampling.

There is insufficient evidence to support the use of Rh D immunoglobulin in bleeding prior to 12 weeks' gestation in an ongoing pregnancy, although if the pregnancy then requires curettage Rh D immunoglobulin should be given. If miscarriage or termination occurs after 12 weeks' gestation, 625 IU (125 µg) Rh D immunoglobulin should be offered.[13]

For successful immunoprophylaxis, Rh D immunoglobulin should be administered as soon as possible after the sensitising event, but always within 72 hours (level 1 evidence). If Rh D immunoglobulin has not been offered within 72 hours, a dose offered within 9–10 days may provide protection.[14]

Is there anything I can recommend to women to prevent miscarriage?

Vitamins, bed rest and progestogens have been suggested as ways to prevent miscarriage in women. However, recent systematic reviews are not supportive of these suggestions. Vitamin supplements, alone or in combination with other vitamins, prior to pregnancy or in early pregnancy, do not prevent women experiencing miscarriage or stillbirth. In addition, while women taking vitamin supplements may be less likely to develop preeclampsia, they are more likely to have a multiple pregnancy.[15] Bed rest is also of no current proven value: there is insufficient high-quality evidence to support a recommendation of bed rest in order to prevent miscarriage in women with confirmed fetal viability and vaginal bleeding in the first half of pregnancy.[16] There is no evidence to support the routine use of progestogen to prevent miscarriage in early to mid-pregnancy. However, there seems to be evidence of benefit in women with a history of recurrent miscarriage.[17]

Do any groups of women with miscarriages require specialist investigation?

Women with recurrent miscarriages (>3) require investigation for underlying conditions. These women are best referred to obstetricians for investigation and further management to optimise their chances of carrying a pregnancy successfully to term. Another group of women who require advice prior to conception are those with late miscarriages, which may be due to cervical incompetence. This may be an issue for women who have had treatments for high-grade cervical dysplasia in the past.

Summary of key points

- 15–20% of all pregnancies end with early miscarriage.
- Bleeding in early pregnancy most commonly occurs between the ninth and twelfth weeks.
- A transvaginal ultrasound will assist in determining whether the pregnancy is intrauterine or ectopic and, if it is intrauterine, whether it is still viable.
- The single most common cause of spontaneous miscarriage is chromosomal abnormalities.
- GPs should recognise the emotional consequences of spontaneous miscarriage in their patients.
- Women should be offered a choice of the various forms of management for spontaneous miscarriage.
- Surgical management is the preferred option where there is heavy bleeding or infection.
- Vitamin use, bed rest and progestogens do not prevent miscarriage.

ECTOPIC PREGNANCY

GPs are often faced with scenarios such as the one described in this case study, where the differential diagnosis is between a threatened miscarriage and an ectopic pregnancy. Interestingly, the prevalence of ectopic pregnancies has increased by up to sixfold since 1970.[18] Possible reasons for this increase may be that there has been an increase in the prevalence of sexually transmissible diseases and tubal sterilisations or because women are conceiving later in life with a corresponding increase in the number of years in which tubal problems could occur. The more likely explanation, however, is that the diagnostic technique used today (i.e. vaginal versus abdominal ultrasound) is better able to determine the exact location of a pregnancy.

What is the prevalence of ectopic pregnancy?

Ectopic pregnancies occur in approximately 1–2% of all pregnancies, with 95% of all ectopics located in the fallopian tubes.[19] Thirty years ago, most ectopic pregnancies (>80%) were diagnosed once

---

CASE STUDY: She did not 'feel' pregnant.

Haslinda, 32 years old, presented to her GP rubbing the lower right aspect of her abdomen. She explained that she had a sharp, continuous pain that had woken her from her sleep. On further questioning, the GP found out that Haslinda had stopped her COCP some 4 months previously, hoping to conceive her second child. Her last normal menstrual period was some 7 weeks ago, but she was unsure if she was really pregnant because she had had four or five episodes of spotting over the last few weeks and did not 'feel' pregnant. A urine beta human chorionic gonadotrophin (βHCG) test was performed and was positive. Haslinda's blood pressure and pulse were stable and she had no postural drop. A speculum examination was performed and showed that there was no blood in the vagina and that the cervical os was closed. The uterus was estimated to be about 6 weeks' gestation and there was no adnexal tenderness or masses palpable.

The GP remained concerned about the possibility that Haslinda might have an ectopic pregnancy and arranged for a vaginal ultrasound to be performed without delay. The scan was not able to detect an intrauterine pregnancy and so Haslinda was referred to the local maternity hospital for further management of her presumed ectopic pregnancy.

---

they had already ruptured. Fortunately, today more than 80% are diagnosed before they rupture.[20] Nevertheless, a ruptured ectopic pregnancy remains a true medical emergency and is the leading cause of maternal mortality in the first trimester, accounting for 6% of all maternal deaths in the USA.[21] Women with a history of ectopic pregnancy also have a much poorer reproductive future. Only about 60% of women who receive a diagnosis of an ectopic pregnancy are subsequently able to have an intrauterine pregnancy.[22] Despite these figures, screening asymptomatic pregnant women for ectopic pregnancy is not warranted.[23]

What increases the risk of a woman having an ectopic pregnancy?

Impaired tubal function is the cause of ectopic pregnancies. A summary of the risk factors is given in Table 9.2. The strongest risk factor is tubal pathology brought about by previous surgery, pelvic infection and endometriosis. However, the majority of women presenting with an ectopic pregnancy have none of the risk factors that have been identified in the literature.[24] A previous ectopic pregnancy also increases a woman's chances of having another one. The risk of recurrence of ectopic pregnancy is up to approximately 10% among women with one previous ectopic pregnancy and at least 25% among women with two or more previous ectopic pregnancies.[22] Interestingly, ectopic pregnancy is not related to any genetic abnormality in the fetus or to a previous history of induced abortion or caesarean section. It is related to infertility treatment, however: 4–5% of pregnancies achieved via in vitro fertilisation are ectopic, a rate 2–3% higher than that found in the general population.[25]

Risk factors for ectopic pregnancy include a past history of STDs and pelvic pathology such as pelvic infection and endometriosis.

In women at high risk of an ectopic pregnancy (i.e. those with a history of a previous ectopic, a pregnancy that has occurred after tubal sterilisation, or with an IUD in situ or when the pregnancy has resulted from assisted reproductive techniques), it is wise to screen as soon as practicable for an intrauterine pregnancy using a transvaginal ultrasound.

A previous ectopic makes another more likely.

TABLE 9.2 Risk factors for ectopic pregnancy (From Pisarska et al[30])

Risk factor	Odds ratio
High risk	
• Tubal surgery	21.0
• Sterilisation	9.3
• Previous ectopic pregnancy	8.3
• In utero exposure to diethylstilboestrol	5.6
• Use of IUD	4.2–45.0
• Documented tubal pathology	3.8–21.0
Moderate risk	
• Infertility	2.5–21.0
• Previous genital infections	2.5–3.7
• Multiple sexual partners	2.1
Slight risk	
• Previous pelvic/abdominal surgery	0.9–3.8
• Cigarette smoking	2.3–2.5
• Vaginal douching	1.1–3.1
• Early age at first intercourse (<18 years)	1.6

While the overall risk of pregnancy, including ectopic pregnancy, is reduced with IUD use, the risk of ectopic pregnancy relative to intrauterine pregnancy is increased by the use of IUDs.

What symptoms should make a GP suspect an ectopic pregnancy?

In most situations, an ectopic pregnancy is not easy to diagnose clinically and a high index of suspicion should be maintained. The most common presenting symptoms are abdominal pain associated with amenorrhoea.[26] However, some 40–50% of patients will have had some vaginal bleeding, which is often mistaken for a normal menstrual period.[27] Table 9.3 shows the frequency of occurrence of symptoms related to ectopic pregnancy.

A high index of suspicion is necessary to diagnose ectopic pregnancies, which are still the leading cause of maternal mortality in the first trimester of pregnancy.

Most women with ectopic pregnancy have no risk factors, and the classic triad of symptoms of amenorrhoea, abdominal pain and irregular vaginal bleeding is absent in more than half of cases.[28]

What investigations should be undertaken?

A βHCG is necessary in the evaluation of any women of reproductive age with a history of abdominal pain and irregular vaginal bleeding or amenorrhoea. This is nearly always positive by the time an ectopic pregnancy becomes symptomatic, although cases have been reported of ruptured tubal ectopics where the βHCG was negative.[29] If the pregnancy test carried out in the GP's surgery is negative, other reasons for the patient's symptoms can be investigated. If positive, however, the next step is usually to carry out a transvaginal ultrasound to ensure the presence of an intrauterine pregnancy.

TABLE 9.3 Symptoms and signs associated with an ectopic pregnancy

Symptoms and signs	Frequency in ectopic pregnancy (%)
Abdominal tenderness	75
Cervical motion tenderness	67
Palpable adnexal mass	50
Haemodynamic compromise	20

Transvaginal ultrasound will reliably detect an intrauterine pregnancy if the βHCG is >1500 IU/L and the gestation is 5–6 weeks. When the initial ultrasound is not diagnostic, women should be followed up with serial βHCGs.

Serial quantitative βHCG levels may assist in differentiating between an ectopic and intrauterine pregnancy.

Quantitative levels of βHCG can be used as a biochemical marker to help distinguish between an ectopic pregnancy and an intrauterine pregnancy. Produced by the trophoblastic cells of the developing embryo, βHCG levels in normal pregnancies double every 1.5 days early in pregnancy and every 3.5 days by 7 weeks' gestation. In abnormal intrauterine pregnancies and in ectopic pregnancies, the doubling time is longer. Measurement can be carried out either initially or in a serial fashion, but the meaningfulness of serial βHCGs is compromised by the fact that abnormal results may represent either an abnormal intrauterine pregnancy or an ectopic.

Are any other investigations helpful?

Several other methods of diagnosing an ectopic pregnancy can also be used (Fig 9.1 summarises these diagnostic tests), although these have largely been superseded by the advent of readily available transvaginal ultrasound.

Progesterone measurements are useful as a single-time screening device.[30] The hormone is made by the corpus luteum when stimulated by a viable pregnancy. If the serum progesterone is >25 ng/mL, an ectopic pregnancy is unlikely, but if the level is <5 ng/mL, the pregnancy is non-viable and an ectopic is worth considering. The only caveat is that it is not a reliable test in those women at risk of ectopic pregnancy after hormonal infertility treatments.

Uterine curettage can be carried out to exclude an ectopic pregnancy, but only when a non-viable pregnancy has been documented by either a serum progesterone of <5 ng/mL or by an absence of an increase in βHCG after 48 hours. An ectopic pregnancy is diagnosed when there is an absence of chorionic villi found in the curettings and when there is not a decrease in the βHCG by 15% or more after 8–12 hours. Culdocentesis can also be carried out to diagnose an ectopic pregnancy. This procedure involves the aspiration from the perineal cul-de-sac through the vaginal fornix. If non-clotting, bloody fluid is found, a ruptured ectopic has occurred. It is rarely done these days, however, as an ultrasound can reveal the presence of any free fluid.

How are ectopic pregnancies currently managed?

Over the last decade the management of ectopic pregnancy has shifted from one where surgery was the only feasible option to the increasing use of medical management.

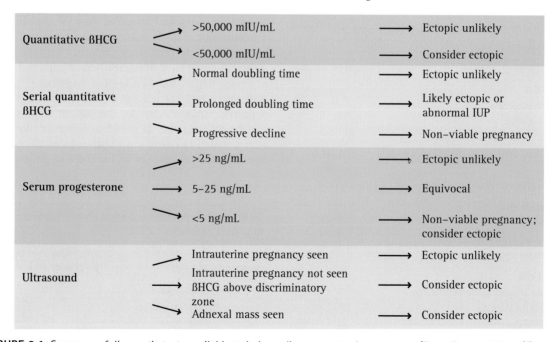

Quantitative βHCG	>50,000 mIU/mL	Ectopic unlikely
	<50,000 mIU/mL	Consider ectopic
Serial quantitative βHCG	Normal doubling time	Ectopic unlikely
	Prolonged doubling time	Likely ectopic or abnormal IUP
	Progressive decline	Non–viable pregnancy
Serum progesterone	>25 ng/mL	Ectopic unlikely
	5–25 ng/mL	Equivocal
	<5 ng/mL	Non–viable pregnancy; consider ectopic
Ultrasound	Intrauterine pregnancy seen	Ectopic unlikely
	Intrauterine pregnancy not seen βHCG above discriminatory zone	Consider ectopic
	Adnexal mass seen	Consider ectopic

FIGURE 9.1 Summary of diagnostic tests available to help to diagnose ectopic pregnancy (From Carr and Evans[31])

Medical management of ectopic pregnancy avoids surgery and its risks, may better preserve tubal patency and function and has a lower cost than surgery.

There are three forms of management available for ectopic pregnancy: surgical, medical and expectant. Which one is chosen depends on several factors, the most important of which are whether or not the ectopic has ruptured, desire for future fertility and the gestation/size of the ectopic.

If the patient is unstable, laparotomy is preferred to laparoscopy.

When patients are hypotensive, in severe pain or where there is evidence of rupture, and when the quantitative βHCG is >10,000 mIU/mL and the gestational sac measures greater than 3.5 cm surgical management is clearly favoured. Laparotomy is performed when the patient is unstable; otherwise the procedure is carried out laparascopically. Once the fallopian tube is visualised the ectopic pregnancy is located and removed (Fig 9.2). Salpingectomy is usually undertaken if the contralateral tube is normal; a salpingostomy (where the tube is preserved) can be undertaken, but ectopic pregnancy persists in >10% of patients treated with a salpingostomy. The persistence of tissue is more likely to occur with small ectopic pregnancies, when therapy is carried out early (<42 days after the LNMP) or when the βHCG remains high postoperatively.[32]

Salpingectomy is usually undertaken if the contralateral tube is normal.

In considering the management options for ectopic pregnancy the goal must be to minimise any morbidity associated with both the ectopic and the treatment of the ectopic while at the same time working towards maximising the woman's chances for a successful future pregnancy.

What is the role of methotrexate in the management of ectopic pregnancy?

Medical management with methotrexate is being used more commonly with earlier detection of

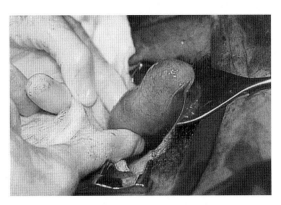

FIGURE 9.2 Ectopic gestation distending the fallopian tube (From James et al[33])

ectopic pregnancy. Methotrexate is a folic acid antagonist that interferes with DNA synthesis and cell multiplication and inhibits the rapidly growing trophoblastic cells in the ectopic pregnancy. Women most suitable for methotrexate therapy are those with a serum HCG below 3000 IU/L, minimal symptoms[34] and with no contraindications to methotrexate (see Box 9.4).

Methotrexate can be used to treat ectopic pregnancy in a single dose or multiple doses but is associated with side effects of nausea, dizziness and a transient increase in abdominal pain that requires monitoring.

Methotrexate is given as an intramuscular injection and the dose is calculated according to the patient's body surface area (50 mg/m^2).[34] With a single injection, the success rate is 87%. With variable (multiple) doses, the success rate is 93%.[35] The single-dose method is often preferred, as it is simpler to administer and can be repeated if βHCG levels do not drop by day 7. Systemic methotrexate can produce side effects of nausea, dizziness, oral

BOX 9.4 Contraindications to methotrexate

- Breastfeeding
- Immunodeficiency
- Liver disease
- Blood dyscrasias
- Active pulmonary disease
- Peptic ulcer disease
- Renal dysfunction
- Known sensitivity to methotrexate

irritation and transient transaminase elevations, but when using the single-dose method these side effects are experienced by <1%.[36] However, up to 60% of patients do suffer from a transient increase in abdominal pain.[37] It is unclear what the reason for this is. It may be due to degenerating trophoblast with some peritoneal irritation, or it may be a side effect of the methotrexate. It does raise fears, however, that the treatment has not been successful and that rupture is pending (this can occur in up to 5% of medically treated patients). It is best, therefore, to offer an NSAID and if pain persists to evaluate the patient and perhaps check her Hb level.

Expectant management can be offered when the ectopic pregnancy is very small, as many of these will resolve spontaneously. This usually occurs when the patient has decreasing levels of βHCG at the time of presentation and an initial level of <200 mIU/mL, and is asymptomatic. In this situation the rate of spontaneous resolution is 88%.

Rates of tubal patency and subsequent fertility are similar when comparing the treatment of ectopic pregnancy with methotrexate to conservative surgical management. However, the subsequent ectopic pregnancy rate is lower with methotrexate.[30]

Who is expectant management suitable for?

Expectant management is an option for clinically stable asymptomatic women with an ultrasound diagnosis of ectopic pregnancy and a decreasing serum HCG, initially less than serum 1000 IU/L.[34]

What is the incidence of recurrence after an ectopic pregnancy?

No matter which form of treatment is decided upon, the incidence of recurrence of the ectopic pregnancy is similar with all the methods and ranges from 6% to 12%.[36]

Summary of key points
- Between 1% and 2% of pregnancies are ectopic.
- Ectopic pregnancies account for 6% of all maternal deaths.
- Ectopic pregnancy is the leading cause of maternal mortality in the first trimester.
- A history of STDs and/or pelvic infection puts a woman at increased risk of ectopic pregnancy.
- The most common presenting symptom of an ectopic pregnancy is abdominal pain associated with amenorrhoea.
- Investigation of a woman with an ectopic pregnancy involves a quantitative βHCG and an ultrasound.

- Whether management is surgical or medical depends on whether or not the ectopic has ruptured, the desire for future fertility and the gestation/size of the ectopic.

TIPS FOR PRACTITIONERS

- The three features of significance in assessing bleeding during early pregnancy are:
  - the passage of products of conception
  - uterine size in relation to period of amenorrhoea
  - whether the cervix is open or closed.
- Routine use of early ultrasound may diagnose conditions that naturally end in spontaneous, complete miscarriage, thereby encouraging unnecessary intervention.
- Where the pregnancy is wanted, miscarriage is associated with disappointment and grief. GPs should offer support to patients who are distressed by their loss.
- Anti-D prophylaxis should be administered to Rh-negative women after ectopic pregnancy and a completed miscarriage.
- While both tubal sterilisations and IUDs decrease the rate of pregnancy overall, if a pregnancy does occur it is more likely to be ectopic.
- Only about 60% of women who have an ectopic pregnancy are subsequently able to have an intrauterine pregnancy.

REFERENCES

1. Everett C. Incidence and outcome of bleeding before the 20th week of pregnancy: prospective study from general practice. BMJ 1997; 315:32–34.
2. Nyberg DA, Laing FC, Filly RA. Threatened abortion: sonographic distribution of normal and abnormal gestation sacs. Radiology 1986; 158:397–400.
3. Pandya PP, Snijders RJ, Psara N, et al. The prevalence of non-viable pregnancy at 10–13 weeks of gestation. Ultrasound Obstet Gynecol 1996; 7:170–173.
4. Crowther CA, Kornman L, O'Callaghan S, et al. Is an ultrasound assessment of gestational age at the first antenatal visit of value? A randomised clinical trial. B J Obstet Gynaecol 1999; 106:1273–1279.
5. Hemminki E. Treatment of miscarriage: current practice and rationale. Obstet Gynecol 1998; 91:247–253.
6. Gardner RJM, Sutherland GR. Chromosome abnormalities and genetic counseling. 2nd edn. New York: Oxford University Press; 1996:59–190, 248, 313–317.
7. Friedman T. Women's experience of general practitioner management of miscarriage. J R Coll Gen Pract 1989; 39:456-458.
8. Butler C, Kelsberg G, St Anna L, et al. Clinical inquiries. How long is expectant management safe in first-trimester miscarriage? J Fam Pract 2005; 54(10):889–890.
9. Bagratee JS, Khullar V, Regan L, et al. A randomized controlled trial comparing medical and expectant management of first trimester miscarriage. Hum Reprod 2004; 19(2):266–271.

10. Weeks A, Alia G, Blum J, et al. A randomized trial of misoprostol compared with manual vacuum aspiration for incomplete abortion. Obstet Gynecol 2005; 106(3):540–547.

11. Molnar AM, Oliver LM, Geyman JP. Patient preferences for management of first-trimester spontaneous abortion. J Am Board Fam Pract 2000; 13:333–337.

12. Wieringa-De Waard M, Hartman EE, Ankum WM, et al. Expectant management versus surgical evacuation in first trimester miscarriage: health-related quality of life in randomized and non-randomized patients. Hum Reprod 2002; 17(6):1638–1642.

13. Women's Health Australasia. Management of early pregnancy loss. Clinical practice guideline Mar 2008. Online. Available: http://www.wcha.asn.au/docs_library/Mgt%20of%20Early%20 Pregnancy%20Loss%20CPG.pdf [accessed 02.08.2009].

14. National Blood Authority. Guidelines on the prophylactic use of Rh D immunoglobulin (anti-D) in obstetrics. 2003. Online. Available: http://www.nba.gov.au/pubs/pdf/glines-anti-d.pdf [accessed 02-08-2009].

15. Rumbold A, Middleton P, Crowther CA. Vitamin supplementation for preventing miscarriage. Cochrane Database Syst Rev 2005(2):CD004073.

16. Aleman A, Althabe F, Belizán J, et al. Bed rest during pregnancy for preventing miscarriage. Cochrane Database Syst Rev 2005(2):CD003576.

17. Haas DM, Ramsey PS. Progestogen for preventing miscarriage. Cochrane Database Syst Rev 2008(2):CD003511.

18. Centers for Disease Control. Ectopic pregnancy—United States, 1988–1989. MMWR Morb Mortal Wkly Rep 1992; 41:32.

19. Hankins GD, Clark SL, Cunningham FG, et al. Ectopic pregnancy. In: Operative obstetrics. Norwalk, CN: Appleton & Lange; 1995:437–456.

20. Saraj AJ, Wilcox JG, Najmabadi S, et al. Resolution of hormonal markers of ectopic gestation: a randomized trial comparing single-dose intramuscular methotrexate with salpingostomy. Obstet Gynecol 1998; 92:989–994.

21. Centers for Disease Control. Ectopic pregnancy–United States, 1990–1992. MMWR Morb Mortal Wkly Rep 1995; 44(3):46–48.

22. Seeber BE, Barnhart KT. Suspected ectopic pregnancy. Obstet Gynecol 2006; 107(2 Pt 1):399–413.

23. Mol BW, van der Veen F, Bossuyt PM. Symptom-free women at increased risk of ectopic pregnancy: should we screen? Acta Obstet Gynecol Scand 2002; 81(7):661–672.

24. Ankum W, Mol B, van der Veen F, et al. Risk factors for ectopic pregnancy: a meta-analysis. Fertil Steril 1996; 65:1093–1099.

25. American Fertility Society, Society for Assisted Reproductive Technology. Assisted reproductive technology in the United States and Canada: 1994 results generated from the American Society for Reproductive Medicine/Society for Assisted Reproductive Technology Registry. Fertil Steril 1996; 66:697–705.

26. Weckstein LN, Boucher AR, Tucker H, et al. Accurate diagnosis of early ectopic pregnancy. Obstet Gynecol 1985; 65:393–397.

27. Fylstra D. Tubal pregnancy: a review of current diagnosis and treatment. Obstet Gynecol Surv 1998; 53:320–328.

28. Ramakrishnan K, Scheid DC. Ectopic pregnancy: forget the 'classic presentation' if you want to catch it sooner. J Fam Pract 2006; 55(5):388–395.

29. Kooi S, Kock H. A review of the literature on nonsurgical treatment in tubal pregnancies. Obstet Gynecol Surv 1992; 47:743–749.

30. Pisarska MD, Carson SA, Buster JE. Ectopic pregnancy. Lancet 1998; 351:1115–1120.

31. Carr RJ, Evans PE. Ectopic pregnancy. Primary Care 2000: 27:169–183.

32. Rulin M. Is salpingostomy the surgical treatment of choice for unruptured tubal pregnancy? Obstet Gynecol 1995; 86:1010–1013.

33. James D, Pilai M, Rymer J, et al. Obstetrics, gynaecology, neonatology interactive colour guides. CD-ROM. Edinburgh: Churchill Livingstone; 2002.

34. Royal College of Obstetricians and Gynaecologists. The management of tubal pregnancy. Guideline no. 21. 2004. Online. Available: http://www.rcog.org.uk/files/rcog-corp/uploaded-files/ GT21ManagementTubalPregnancy2004.pdf [accessed 02.08.2009].

35. Nieuwkerk P, Hajenius P, van der Veen F, et al. Systemic methotrexate therapy versus laparoscopic salpingostomy in tubal pregnancy: part II. Patient preferences for systemic methotrexate. Fertil Steril 1998; 70:518–522.

36. Seifer D. Persistent ectopic pregnancy: an argument for heightened vigilance and patient compliance. Fertil Steril 1997; 68:402–404.

37. Stovall T. Medical management should be routinely used as a primary therapy for ectopic pregnancy. Clin Obstet Gynecol 1995; 38:346–352.

OBJECTIVES

- To review the purpose of the postnatal visit
- To be aware of the issues that require attention from the GP in the postpartum period
- To understand the aetiology of common breastfeeding problems
- To diagnose and manage common breastfeeding problems
- To understand the prevalence and epidemiology of postnatal depression
- To be aware of the reasons why postnatal depression remains difficult to diagnose
- To become familiar with the nature and use of the Edinburgh Postnatal Depression Scale
- To manage postnatal depression

POSTNATAL CARE — WHAT SHOULD IT ENTAIL?

What is the normal course of events for women in the postpartum period?

With the increasingly prevalent phenomenon of early discharge after childbirth, GPs must be cognisant of the normal physiological changes that occur in women in the first days/weeks postpartum. These are listed in Box 10.1.

BOX 10.1 What to expect in the first days/ weeks of the postpartum period

Uterus
- Reduces in size from 1 kg and 5000 mL immediately after delivery to its non-pregnant size of 70 g and 5 mL.
- Immediately after delivery the uterus should be halfway between the umbilicus and the symphysis pubis. By 2 weeks it should return to the pelvis and by 6 weeks it will have returned to its normal size.

Lochia
- There is fairly heavy discharge for the first 2–3 days, rapidly decreasing after that but on occasion lasting for several weeks.
- Breastfeeding assists in the resolution of the lochia, perhaps because of more rapid involution of the uterus caused by the uterine contractions associated with breastfeeding.
- In most women the endometrium is re-established by 3 weeks postpartum.

Cervix and vagina
- The cervix reforms within hours of delivery and by 1 week forms the normal patulous of a multiparous woman (admitting one finger).
- Vulvar and vaginal tissues return to normal within days, although they may become hypo-oestrogenic with breastfeeding.

Return of ovarian function
- May occur as early as 3–4 weeks postpartum in women who do not breastfeed.
- Lactational amenorrhoea is said to occur for up to 6 months in 98% of women who fully breastfeed.

Cardiovascular system
- Pregnancy-related cardiovascular changes return to normal within 2–3 weeks of delivery.
- Immediately after delivery approximately 5 kg of weight are lost as a result of diuresis and the loss of extravascular fluid.

Why has the traditional postnatal visit been set at 6 weeks?

Traditionally women have been instructed to return to see their obstetrician 6 weeks after their baby's birth.[1] At this appointment the practitioner usually inquires about breastfeeding, undertakes an abdominal and vaginal examination and advises the woman about contraception. The focus of this visit has been to ensure that 'things have returned to normal'. This form of postnatal care however, devotes time and resources to routine examinations that screen for morbidities that are no longer the major health burden for women[2] and does not necessarily address the needs of women at this time. The content and timing of postnatal care therefore needs to be reviewed.[3]

What postnatal problems commonly arise?

There are high levels of maternal morbidity after childbirth. One study has documented that 85% of women report at least one health problem 2 weeks after childbirth, and 12–18 months later 76% of women are still suffering from at least one problem.[4] The common problems encountered by women in the postnatal period[5] are listed in Box 10.2.

Despite the fact that more than 90% of women attend a postnatal check-up,[6] they are unlikely to raise problems such as back pain, urinary incontinence, depression, haemorrhoids and perineal pain with their doctor.[7] They are also unlikely to discuss sexual problems, which are common after childbirth. While only 15% of women report these problems to a health professional, some 83% experience sexual problems in the first 3 months after delivery. This declines to 64% at 6 months but does not reach the pre-pregnancy level of 38%.[8] Common problems include vaginal dryness, painful penetration, pain during intercourse, pain on orgasm, vaginal tightness, vaginal looseness, bleeding/irritation after sex and loss of sexual desire.

BOX 10.2 Common postnatal problems

- Tiredness and exhaustion
- Pain from caesarean wound
- Backache
- Painful perineum
- Sexual problems
- Haemorrhoids
- Depression
- Problems in the relationship with partner
- Mastitis if breastfeeding
- Bowel problems

What advice can a GP give to women about weight gain or weight loss in the postpartum period?

In the USA about 50% of women are either overweight or obese (body mass index >25).[9] For many of these women their weight gain occurred with each pregnancy. Advice may therefore be sought from a GP about weight loss in the postpartum period. While many women expect to lose weight while breastfeeding, the reality is that weight loss during lactation is very variable. On average women can expect to lose between 0.6–0.8 kg per month, but the range is between 5.6 kg loss and 5.5 kg gain per month.[10]

Some researchers are concerned that if women deliberately try to lose weight while they are lactating, the growth of their infant may be compromised.[11] However, a recent study has shown that maternal loss of 0.5 kg per week induced by dieting and exercise did not affect infant growth.[12]

The best advice that a GP can give is probably that women should be careful about weight gain throughout their pregnancy, instead of relying on losing weight in the postpartum period. Women who are of normal weight before pregnancy and who gain an amount that is within the range recommended usually return to their pre-pregnancy body mass index without any necessary intervention. However, those who find the weight they have gained during pregnancy hard to lose should not be too keen to achieve drastic weight loss too early during the postpartum period if they are lactating. Women should consider postponing rigorous diet and exercise programs until the baby is 6 months old and no longer entirely dependent on the mother for nutrition.

How should postnatal care be delivered?

How exactly postnatal care should be delivered in order to optimise maternal and child health remains debatable. Simply bringing the timing of the postnatal visit forward to 1–2 weeks postpartum does not bring about improved outcomes.[13] Midwife-led, flexible postnatal care tailored to the needs of the individual was shown in a study to help to improve women's mental health but not their physical health.[2]

Recent UK guidelines have identified the essential core (routine) care that every woman and her baby should receive in the first 6–8 weeks after birth.[14] Key priorities of these guidelines are:

- that women be advised at the first postnatal contact of the signs and symptoms of potentially life-threatening conditions (Table 10.1) so that they can seek medical assistance.

- the need for all maternity care providers (whether working in a hospital or in primary care) to encourage breastfeeding.

- to enquire at each postnatal contact about the woman's emotional wellbeing, what family and social support she has and her usual coping strategies for dealing with day-to-day matters. Women and their families/partners should be encouraged to tell their healthcare professional about any changes in mood, emotional state and behaviour that are different from the woman's normal pattern.

- To offer parents information and advice to enable them to assess their baby's general condition, identify signs and symptoms of common health problems and to contact a healthcare professional or emergency service if required.

From a GP's perspective, women should be advised during their pregnancy of their GP's availability to address postpartum issues. They should feel free to consult their GP at any time and not wait for scheduled visits. They should also feel that their GP is willing to talk and is sympathetic to their emotional needs.

When women do present to their GP in the postnatal period, the presenting complaint should be addressed first, but then the GP should focus on the following issues[14]:

- **Mental health.** While formal debriefing of the birth experience is not recommended, (it is important to check early (10–14 days after birth) for resolution of 'baby blues' (tearfulness, feelings of anxiety and low mood) and to encourage

TABLE 10.1 Signs and symptoms of potentially life-threatening conditions (From NICE[14])

Signs and symptoms	Condition
• Sudden and profuse blood loss or persistent increased blood loss • Faintness, dizziness or palpitations/tachycardia	Postpartum haemorrhage
• Fever, shivering, abdominal pain and/or offensive vaginal loss	Infection

• Headaches accompanied by one or more of the following symptoms within the first 72 hours after birth:
  – visual disturbances
  – nausea, vomiting
	Pre-eclampsia/eclampsia

• Unilateral calf pain, redness or swelling • Shortness of breath or chest pain	Thromboembolism

women to help to look after their mental health by looking after themselves. Good general advice includes taking gentle exercise, finding time to rest, getting help with caring for the baby, talking to someone about their feelings and ensuring they can access social support networks.

- **Perineal care and dyspareunia.** This is a common concern, particularly for those women who experienced an episiotomy or tear. Early in the postpartum period, women should be advised to change pads frequently and, after using cold packs initially for pain relief, to use paracetamol in the first instance and then NSAIDs if required. Between 2 and 6 weeks, women should be asked about resumption of sexual intercourse and any dyspareunia. A major causative factor for dyspareunia in breastfeeding women is lack of oestrogen, which can cause an inflamed, almost 'atrophic'-looking vagina. While liberally applied water-based lubricant may help, some women need topical vaginal oestrogen cream or pessaries.
- **Fatigue.** Persistent fatigue may come about as a result of physical issues, such as a low haemoglobin secondary to postpartum haemorrhage, or mental health issues.
- **Constipation, haemorrhoids and faecal incontinence.** These may occur in the postpartum period and require assessment and advice.
- **Urinary incontinence.** After childbirth women may experience incontinence for the first time in their lives and should receive advice about the importance of pelvic floor exercises to assist with this problem.
- **Contraception.** Methods and timing of resumption of contraception should be discussed within the first week of the birth. For breastfeeding women progestogen-only methods are ideal, but it is important to counsel women about expected bleeding changes with these products (see Chapter 3). While many women will be quite content to use condoms or withdrawal—especially as sex may not be as frequent in the postnatal period as it was previously—women need to be offered the choice of options that are available to them. If a woman wants to space her children, it is worthwhile suggesting that she has an IUD.
- **Immunisation.** GPs should check whether rubella vaccination is required and administer it if necessary. It is also important to note the hepatitis B and C status of the mother, as follow-up vaccinations/testing of the baby may be required.

- **Breastfeeding.** A GP should reviewing breastfeeding technique and the infant's growth, and examine the breasts and nipples.
- **Domestic violence.** GPs should be aware of the risks, signs and symptoms of domestic abuse and know what services to contact for advice and management.
- **Pap smear status.** If a pap smear is indicated, ideally it is best to wait until 8–12 weeks postpartum (although it can be done at the 6-week check-up).

Summary of key points
- The content and timing of the traditional 6-week check-up needs to be altered to address postpartum morbidity and assist in its prevention.
- High levels of maternal morbidity exist after childbirth and in the postpartum period.
- In the postpartum period women are unlikely to raise issues such as back pain, urinary incontinence, depression, haemorrhoids, perineal pain and sexual problems with their doctor.
- GPs should stress their availability in the postpartum period and their willingness to discuss emotional issues.
- Women who want to lose weight postpartum should postpone rigorous dieting and exercise if they are lactating until the baby is 6 months old and no longer dependent on the mother for nutrition.

COMMON BREASTFEEDING PROBLEMS AND ISSUES

How does a mother know if the baby is getting enough milk?

Because mothers cannot visualise how much milk a baby is receiving during breastfeeding (unlike in bottle-feeding, where it is obvious), they are often anxious that the baby is not receiving an adequate amount of milk or that their milk supply is poor.

Mothers should be advised that the baby is getting enough milk if:

- there are 6–8 wet cloth nappies per day (this is more difficult to assess when the baby wears disposable nappies)
- there is growth in length and head circumference
- the baby has soft bowel motions
- the baby is alert and reasonably content for some periods in a day
- there are weight gains of on average 500 g a month
- the baby has good skin colour and muscle tone.

What common breastfeeding problems present to the GP?

Most women have made the decision whether or not to breastfeed prior to the birth of their baby. While breastfeeding is initiated in hospital, many women are discharged before their milk 'comes in' (day 3–5 post-delivery). With the increasing trend towards early discharge, GPs are faced with the whole range of breastfeeding problems, which are summarised in Box 10.3.

What are the causes of nipple pain?

Most women can expect to get some nipple pain in the first week postpartum, but by day 7 it should have subsided. Persistence of pain is usually caused by a baby's incorrect latch-on technique. Less commonly, it can be due to nipple thrush. Cracked and sore nipples are caused either by poor positioning, poor latch-on technique or dermatological conditions such as eczema or psoriasis.

The best way to assess if a woman is feeding her baby correctly is to observe her latching the baby on and feeding (Figs 10.1 and 10.2).

GPs should observe feeding in order to determine if the correct technique is being used.

In advising a mother about correct technique, the following should be covered[15]:

1. The mother should be seated comfortably and well supported, neither leaning back nor hunched forward.
2. The baby's whole body should be turned towards the mother, supported behind the neck and

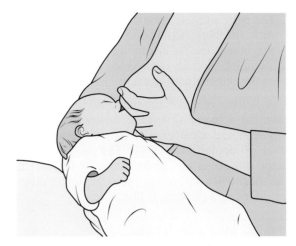

FIGURE 10.1 Poor positioning for breastfeeding

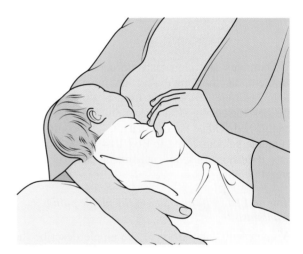

FIGURE 10.2 Good positioning for breastfeeding

shoulders (not head) and held at the level of the breast. The baby should be held close, chest-to-chest with his/her head tilted back slightly.
3. Gently touch the baby's mouth with breast to encourage the baby to open the mouth to a wide gape. The tongue needs to be forward over the lower gum and well down.
4. Move the baby to the breast (not the breast to the baby), making sure the baby takes a good mouthful of breast and areola. The lips should be flanged, creating a seal, and should not appear rolled in.
5. The baby's chin should be well in against the breast and the nose clear. The breast should not look or feel pulled out of shape.
6. When the baby is feeding well, jaws, facial muscles and tips of ears will all move. Swallowing will often be audible.

BOX 10.3 Common breastfeeding problems

Breast pain
- Engorgement
- Obstructed milk duct
- Mastitis

Nipple pain
- Poor technique
- Thrush

Other
- Flat or inverted nipples
- Weaning
- Suppression of lactation

7. The baby's cheeks should not hollow with each suck, and there should be no loud tongue clicks. If attachment deteriorates during the feed or feeding is painful, carefully detach baby by pushing down on the chin and start again.

A plethora of agents are suggested to ease nipple pain, but a recent systematic review showed that no one topical agent showed superior results in the relief of nipple discomfort.[16] The most important factor in decreasing the incidence of nipple pain was the provision of education in relation to proper breastfeeding technique and latch-on.

Incorrect latch-on technique is the main cause of nipple pain when feeding.

Dummies and teats may be contributing to the problem, as they encourage an incorrect sucking action (different from that used at the breast) and are best discouraged at least until breastfeeding is established. Other factors that may be contributing to nipple pain are listed in Box 10.4, while Box 10.5 lists indicators of good attachment and successful breastfeeding.

How do I know if the cause of the nipple pain is candidiasis?

Women with candidiasis of the nipple describe the pain as burning, with sharp shooting pain radiating

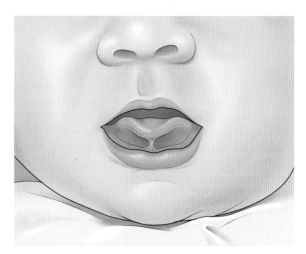

FIGURE 10.3 Tongue tie

through the nipple and areola and into the breast. The pain is present during feeds and between feeds and is described as excruciating.

Breastfeeding women with these symptoms have been shown to be significantly more likely than other breastfeeding women to grow *Candida* from their nipples.[17] A swab of the nipple, however, is not a useful diagnostic test for this condition, as the sensitivity of the test is very low. Other symptoms of thrush could include rash and pruritus of the nipple and areola.

BOX 10.4 Factors contributing to nipple pain

- Poor positioning
- Poor attachment
- Tongue tie (Fig 10.3)
- Nipple thrush
- Incorrect use of a breast pump
- Incorrect breaking of suction at the breast (This is best done by pushing down on the chin to break the suction or inserting the little finger into the corner of the mouth. A baby should not be dragged off the breast.)
- Incorrect use of a nipple shield
- Sensitivity to creams or ointments
- Prolonged contact with a wet breast pad
- Use of dummies or teats (These encourage an incorrect sucking action and should be discouraged until breastfeeding is established.)
- Contact dermatitis/eczema or psoriasis of the nipple

BOX 10.5 Indicators of good attachment and successful breastfeeding (From NICE[14])

Indicators of good attachment and positioning
- Mouth wide open
- Less areola visible underneath the chin than above the nipple
- Chin touching the breast, lower lip rolled down, and nose free
- No pain

Indicators of successful feeding in a baby
- Audible and visible swallowing
- Sustained rhythmic suck
- Relaxed arms and hands
- Moist mouth
- Regular soaked/heavy nappies

Indicators of successful breastfeeding in a woman
- Breast softening
- No compression of the nipple at the end of the feed
- Woman feels relaxed and sleepy

Nipple candidiasis can cause nipple pain but it is hard to diagnose.

The baby should be treated with one-quarter teaspoon miconazole gel or nystatin oral drops four times daily. Dummy use should be avoided. However, if the baby insists on a dummy, it should be sterilised by boiling it daily and replacing it with a new one weekly. The mother should be treated with miconazole gel or nystatin ointment applied to the nipples four times daily after feeds. Breast pads should be changed after every feed and bras every day. Bras should be washed in hot water. Treatment should be continued for 1 week after cessation of symptoms.

Unfortunately, it is not uncommon for patients with these symptoms not to respond to topical therapy. This is attributed to invasion of *Candida* into the ducts of the breast.[18] The mother could then be offered treatment with a systemic fungal agent such as fluconazole 150 mg daily for 5 days. Longer treatment may be necessary in some cases.

The management of nipple thrush involves treatment of both baby and mother.

What are the common causes of breast pain?

A recent UK survey has found painful breasts to be the second most common reason to stop breastfeeding within the first 2 weeks following birth.[19] The common causes of breast pain include breast engorgement, a blocked duct and mastitis. The signs and symptoms of these three conditions are compared and contrasted in Table 10.2 (p 172).

Why does breast engorgement happen?

In the first week after birth, as milk production increases women experience a sense of fullness, warmth and heaviness in their breasts. In a small proportion of women, the production of breast milk may initially exceed the infant's requirements. This results in the breasts feeling hot, tender, swollen and even painful. If left untreated, this overdistension exerts pressure on the surrounding tissue, which then leads to oedema and the clinical symptoms of breast engorgement. Engorgement can also occur when weaning or when breastfeeding ceases abruptly (e.g. because of illness).

TABLE 10.2 A comparison of the different causes of breast pain (From Lawrence & Lawrence[55])

Characteristics	Engorgement	Blocked duct	Mastitis
Onset	Gradual	Gradual	Sudden
Site	Bilateral	Unilateral	Usually unilateral
Swelling and heat	Generalised	Little or no heat	Localised, red, hot, swollen
Body temperature	<38.4°C	<38.4°C	>38.4°C
Systemic symptoms	Feels well	Feels well	Flu-like symptoms

Breast engorgement is due to milk production exceeding the baby's requirement and can be avoided by ensuring that there is no delay in initiating breastfeeding, positioning is effective and breastfeeding patterns are unrestricted.

What management should be recommended for engorgement?

Several treatments have in the past been suggested to alleviate breast engorgement. These include massage, local application of heat, ice packs, medication, the application of cold cabbage leaves and increased frequency of breastfeeding until the condition resolves. A Cochrane review[20] on the efficacy of these treatments has found that cabbage leaves and cold gel packs were equally effective in the treatment of engorgement. Since both cabbage extract and placebo cream were equally effective, the alleviation in symptoms may have been brought about by other factors, such as breast massage. The effectiveness of ultrasound treatment was thought to be due to radiant heat or massage. Pharmacologically, oxytocin was not an effective engorgement treatment, while Danzen, an anti-inflammatory and bromelain/trypsin complex—not commonly used in the general practice setting—significantly improved the symptoms of engorgement.

In conclusion, the initial prevention of breast engorgement should remain the key priority. When engorgement does occur, recent guidelines suggest that frequent unlimited breastfeeding, including prolonged feeding from the affected breast, should be undertaken along with breast massage and, if necessary, hand expression and analgesia.[14] Usually, engorgement peaks on the fifth to seventh day postpartum before resolving.

What is recommended for a blocked duct?

This condition usually presents as a unilateral lump with a well, afebrile mother. The lump should be treated with warm compresses and massage over the lump and towards the areola to encourage the blockage to dislodge and the lobule involved to drain. Breastfeeding should continue to drain the breast of milk.

A blocked duct can be differentiated from mastitis because the patient has no systemic symptoms.

How should a GP treat mastitis?

Mastitis is precipitated by stasis of milk and is usually caused by *Staphylococcus aureus*. The symptoms are a red, hot, swollen, painful wedge-shaped area of the breast associated with maternal fever. When women present with mastitis, the GP should prescribe a penicillinase-resistant antibiotic. Antibiotic options include:

- dicloxacillin or flucloxacillin 500 mg 6-hourly *or*
- cephalexin 500 mg 6-hourly *or*
- if there is a history of penicillin allergy, erythromycin 500 mg, 6 hourly.

All oral antibiotics should be continued for 10 days. If severe cellulitis has developed, antibiotics may need to be given intravenously.

Mastitis is best treated with a penicillinase-resistant antibiotic and by encouraging the woman to continue feeding from the affected breast to facilitate drainage.

Adequate rest, fluids and paracetamol should also be recommended. If the mother tries to wean or does not drain the affected breast adequately through feeding, an abscess may develop (Fig 10.4). Simple abscesses can be drained under ultrasound control, if necessary repeatedly. However, loculated abscesses will require formal surgical drainage.

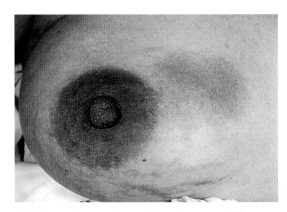

FIGURE 10.4 Breast abscess (From James et al[56])

What advice should be given to a woman who needs to express her milk so that she can return to work?

A breastfeeding mother who wishes to return to work will need to consider the implications of this for feeding. She has several options:

1. to express milk for the carer to feed the baby when she is at work
2. to use childcare at the workplace, so that she can go and breastfeed the baby on demand
3. to breastfeed only when at home and when at work to have the carer formula-feed the baby
4. to suppress lactation and switch over completely to formula.

While these options seem plausible on paper, it is often the infant who decides whether or not alternating between breast milk and formula is acceptable.

Expressing milk can be tiresome and the mother may feel that the volume she is able to express decreases over time. The GP can give the following tips regarding expressing breast milk:

- The mother should express whenever the baby is likely to breastfeed normally.
- About 150 mL/kg per 24 hours is the usual intake for a baby, so for example if a 6 kg baby has six feeds per day and is having three feeds while the mother is at work then 450 mL of expressed breast milk will be required.
- Expressing more frequently (e.g. every 1–2 hours) will result in smaller volumes with each effort; however, it will also serve to increase the supply of milk produced within the next 24–48 hours.
- Mothers can hand-express or use a hand pump or electric pump to express the milk. For an explanation of how to express breast milk, see Figure 10.5 (p 174).

Once breastfeeding is established, a let-down reflex will assist women to express breast milk and should result in a volume of between 600 and 700 mL of milk per day. However, anxiety and tiredness can prevent this from occurring.

Expressed breast milk (EBM) should be stored in a sterile, covered plastic or glass container. Freshly expressed EBM should be cooled before it is added to other cooled or frozen EBM. It can be stored in the:

- refrigerator for 3–5 days
- freezer compartment of refrigerator for 2 weeks (if the freezer is inside the fridge)
- freezer (if the freezer door is separate from that of the refrigerator) for 3 months
- deep freeze for 6–12 months.[21]

The carer should follow the instructions below when feeding with EBM:

- Keep EBM frozen until required.
- Thaw EBM using either cool or warm water.
- Shake EBM gently before using it if it has separated.
- Do not refreeze EBM.
- Discard any thawed EBM if not consumed within 24 hours.
- Do not use microwave to heat EBM.

CASE STUDY: Frazzled with a 4-month-old

Jillian, 34 years, was a beautician who ran her own 'day spa'. Looking frazzled, she attended her GP with her 4-month-old baby. Over the last month she had noticed that at the night feed (10 pm) the baby was not settling, whereas she had previously fallen asleep on the breast. The baby appeared to be looking for more, and the maternal and child health nurse had commented that her baby's weight gain had slowed over the same time period. She really wanted to breastfeed until the baby was at least 1 year old but felt that her milk supply was on the decline as her breasts didn't feel as full in the morning as they had previously. Jillian was feeling quite tired, having returned to part-time work in the past month. She was encouraged to try and get more rest and to keep up her levels of hydration, making sure that she had a big glass of water when she fed the baby and that she drank throughout the day. Ways of building supply were also discussed, such as breastfeeding more frequently (2–3 hourly, or a total of at least eight feeds in 24 hours), expressing after feeds and making sure not to miss feeds. Jillian was also offered the use of domperidone to build supply, with an explanation of the potential side effects and risks.

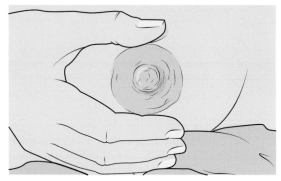

(a) Place thumb and forefinger on either side of the areola

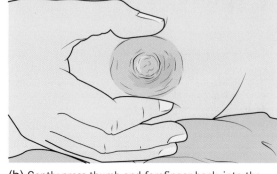

(b) Gently press thumb and forefinger back, into the breast tissue

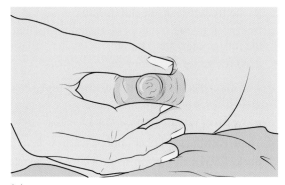

(c) Press thumb and forefinger towards each other and continue this compressing motion, in a rhythmical manner, until the let-down reflex is triggered

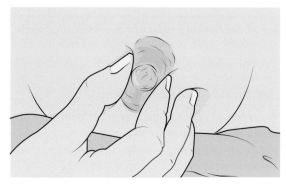

(d) When the flow ceases, move to another section, working your way around the areola.

FIGURE 10.5 How to hand-express breast milk

How can women build their supply if they feel the baby is still hungry after a feed?

Non-phamarmacological methods of increasing the supply of breast milk involve rest, hydration and increasing rates of drainage (i.e. by increasing the frequency of breastfeeding to 2–3-hourly, so that a total of at least eight feeds occurs in 24 hours: to achieve this, a mother may need to wake her baby for some feeds). Offering each breast twice at each feed and/or expressing after feeds are other techniques that may increase supply.

Domperidone is a dopamine antagonist. A prescription medication used for nausea and vomiting, unlike metoclopramide, it passes poorly into the brain and has few central nervous system (CNS) side effects. It increases levels of prolactin and therefore breast-milk production. It can be used when breast-milk supply is low and when non-medication methods alone are not enough to increase milk supply, and may be especially useful for mothers of preterm babies or very sick newborns, or adoptive mothers.

A woman can start by taking 10 mg three times a day and, after a few days, increase the dose to 20 mg three times a day. The maintenance dose is normally 20 mg (two tablets) three times a day until breast-milk supply is well established. This may take 2–4 weeks. Once supply is well established, the dose can be decreased to 10 mg (one tablet) three times a day for 1 week, before stopping the medication altogether.[22] Some reported side effects include headache (most common), abdominal pain, dry mouth, rash and trouble sleeping. Other side effects such as restlessness and muscle spasm may occur, but they are very rare. Very small amounts of domperidone are expected to pass into the breast milk.

The US Food and Drug Administration (FDA) issued a warning in June 2004 about the use of domperidone in inadequate lactation, due to concerns over cardiac problems following intravenous use.[23] Domperidone can prolong the QT interval. As discussed above, the amounts of the drug in breast milk are very low and lactation experts do not consider the warnings relevant to its use in inadequate lactation.[24] However, the possible cardiac risk should be borne in mind in 'at risk' mothers (e.g. those on potent CYP34A inhibitors such as ketoconazole and erythromycin and those who drink grapefruit juice).[25] The cardiac risk to nursing mothers cannot therefore be dismissed.[26]

A recent review of the use of galactogogues to augment lactation argues that the evidence to support pharmacological agents is poor and that if mothers are provided with education and practise techniques that support lactation physiology, galactagogues appear to have little or no added benefit.[26]

How can lactation be suppressed?

Suppression of lactation is necessary when breast-feeding is no longer required (for example, with perinatal death and infant adoption) or when the mother is too ill to breastfeed. Bromocriptine (Parlodel) works by suppressing prolactin production: 2.5 mg is given on the first day, increasing after 2–3 days to 2.5 mg twice daily for 14 days. It may cause postural hypotension, however. More recently carbergoline as a single dose (1 mg) has been used, as it has a lower side-effect profile.[27,28]

Carbergoline (1 mg as a single dose) is as effective as bromocriptine for suppression of lactation, with a lower side-effect profile.

What advice should be given to a woman who wants to wean her baby?

It is usually recommended that weaning takes place over a month. Every few days another feed should be substituted with formula until the baby no longer breastfeeds.

Weaning should not take place abruptly; otherwise engorgement or mastitis can ensue.

Summary of key points
- Mothers can feel confident about the amount of milk they are supplying if the baby is gaining on average 500 g a month.
- The main cause of nipple pain is incorrect latch-on technique.

- Candidiasis of the nipple causes sharp, shooting pain radiating through the nipple, areola and into the breast, as well as rash and pruritus.
- Breast pain can be secondary to breast engorgement, a blocked duct or mastitis.
- Weaning can be achieved by slowly increasing the number of feeds substituted.

POSTNATAL DEPRESSION

How common is postnatal depression?

A recent meta-analysis of studies of postnatal depression (PND) has found the prevalence within the first few postnatal months to be in the order of 13%.[29] Depression in the postnatal period is no more common than the prevalence at other times in a woman's life, but there is an increased rate of onset in pregnancy and the postpartum period.[30]

How does it manifest?

In the first few days after childbirth, many women suffer from the 'blues'. They may feel mildly depressed, tearful and irritable. This subclinical mood swing peaks at 4–5 days after delivery and usually resolves by day 10. There is some evidence that those women suffering from the 'blues' are at increased risk of subsequent PND.[31,32]

PND is that form of depression temporally associated with childbirth. However, it is not different from its non-puerperal counterpart, that is, the symptoms of postpartum depression and major depression are the same (Box 10.6). Indeed, the American Psychiatric Association's *Diagnostic and Statistical Manual of Mental Disorders* does

> **BOX 10.6 The symptoms of postnatal depression (From NICE[43])**
>
> - Depressed mood
> - Tearfulness
> - Anorexia and weight loss
> - Inability to feel joy or happiness or to take an interest in things
> - Decreased libido
> - Lethargy
> - Thoughts of death and suicide
> - Altered sleep pattern
> - Feelings of hopelessness, inability to cope and worthlessness
> - Poor concentration
> - Psychomotor retardation

not distinguish between postpartum and non-postpartum presentations of mood disorders, except for specifying a 'postpartum onset' within the first 4 weeks postpartum.[33] However, episodes occurring within the first postpartum year are also considered to have a postpartum onset.[34]

Why is PND difficult to diagnose?

The problem lies in distinguishing the symptoms of PND from the normal sequelae of childbirth. The postpartum period is associated with many physical and emotional challenges for a woman, such as sheer physical exhaustion, sleep deprivation, hormonal changes, changes in roles and increased responsibilities and demands. It is no wonder that most women experience some of the symptoms commonly associated with depression, such as lethargy, decreased libido and irritability.

Women and their families, however, (like doctors) fail to recognise when these symptoms fall outside the norm. Many GPs will seek to reassure the woman that her symptoms are part of the normal period of adjustment when they have actually crossed the boundary into the realms of depression.

Another reason why postpartum depression can remain undetected is that many women fail to attend a doctor, feeling shame at their inability to do what should come naturally and fearing that they will be labelled 'bad' mothers. Others fail to attend a GP because they are unsure who can help them.

PND can also either manifest abruptly or be insidious in its onset. In the latter case, detection and management is often delayed, if indeed help is ever sought.

What are the consequences of PND for mother and child?

PND can result in deleterious effects on the child, mother and family. These effects may include neglect of the child, family breakdown, self-harm and suicide. However, the more common consequences include emotional and behavioural problems, and cognitive delay in the children of depressed mothers.[35-38]

What else could PND be?

PND needs to be distinguished from puerperal psychosis. Psychosis occurs in 0.2% of women in the postpartum period[39] and is a medical emergency because of the risk the psychosis poses for both the mother and child. The psychosis usually develops within the first month of delivery and is characterised by inability to sleep, agitation and the development of delusions or hallucinations, often concerning the

baby.[33] These women require urgent admission to hospital for stabilisation.

The only other conditions that need to be included in a differential diagnosis of PND are anaemia and thyroid disease. If an excessive amount of blood has been lost during the delivery or there has been antenatal anaemia, the woman may be suffering from extreme lethargy as a result of the anaemia. About 5% of women suffer from thyroid disease in the postpartum period. Hypothyroidism may manifest as depression; equally hyperthyroidism may manifest with weight loss, agitation and panic attacks.

Are there any risk factors for postnatal depression?

One of the most recognised risks for PND is a prior history of psychiatric disease. The risk of PND in

---

CASE STUDY: 'I've never felt so bad in all my life.'

Jessica was a 30-year-old woman who had worked in a professional capacity prior to her pregnancy. Her baby was now 6 months old. She explained that for the first 3 months the baby had had continual 'colic'. A couple of months ago she had returned to work half time but over the last month had felt increasingly unwell. Early on the symptoms she described were very 'physical' in nature: nausea, dizziness and extreme lethargy. She had approached several doctors, who had tested her haemoglobin level, explained that she was probably overtired with breastfeeding and returning to work and had advised her to rest and take vitamin supplements. By the time she saw her third GP, she said she was 'desperate'. She said that she had never felt so bad in all her life. Over the last 2 weeks she had completely lost her appetite and felt unable to eat at all; she had consequently started to shed weight at an alarming rate. She felt anxious and panicky and did not want to be left alone with the baby. She was convinced she was going to die and wanted to write a long letter to her baby explaining how much she loved him. Her husband and family were at a complete loss and did not know what was wrong.

By the time Jessica was finally diagnosed with postnatal depression, her symptoms were classic. She had anorexia, weight loss, inability to concentrate, inability to feel joy or take an interest in her baby, depressed mood, lethargy, thoughts of death, anxiety and some mild panic attacks. Unfortunately it had taken 2–3 months from the initial onset of her symptoms to her diagnosis. During this time she had consulted several GPs and one neurologist.

Jessica was started on an SSRI and some minor tranquillisers. Within 2 weeks she no longer required the latter and had started to feel significantly better and within 6 weeks felt fully recovered. She remained on the antidepressants for 1 year.

these women is thought to be in the order 25–30%.[40] Other risk factors for postpartum depression include psychological distress in late pregnancy, perceived social isolation during pregnancy and high parity.[41] Contrary to popular belief, no association has been found between pregnancy or delivery complications and postpartum depression[41] nor between PND and sociodemographic variables.[42] Predictive factors for perinatal depression are listed in Box 10.7

What can GPs do to improve detection of postnatal depression?

Because of the high incidence of postpartum depression, the effects the illness has on mother and child and the fact that health workers often fail to make an early diagnosis, screening for postnatal depression is recommended.

Recent evidence-based guidelines[43] suggest that the following two questions can be used to identify possible depression (usually at 4–6 weeks and 3–4 months):

- During the past month, have you often been bothered by feeling down, depressed or hopeless?
- During the past month, have you often been bothered by having little interest or pleasure in doing things?

A third question should be considered if the woman answers 'Yes' to either of the initial questions:

- Is this something you feel you need or want help with?

As part of a subsequent assessment or for routine monitoring of outcomes, self-report measures such as the Edinburgh Postnatal Depression Scale (EPDS), Hospital Anxiety and Depression Scale (HADS) or Patient Health Questionnaire 9 (PHQ9) can be used.

BOX 10.7 Predictive factors for perinatal depression

- Past or present severe mental illness including:
  - schizophrenia
  - bipolar disorder
  - psychosis in the postnatal period
  - severe depression
- Previous treatment by a psychiatrist/specialist mental health team, including inpatient care
- Family history of perinatal mental illness

The Edinburgh Postnatal Depression Scale[44] was developed in the primary-care setting and is a simple, quick self-report questionnaire with a high degree of sensitivity and specificity.[44] The 10-item questionnaire asks the woman to assess how she is feeling and therefore serves not only as a screening tool but is also an indication that her doctor is interested in these issues and willing to discuss them.

The EPDS (Table 10.3, p 178) can be completed by the patient, usually under the supervision of a healthcare worker. It can be used throughout the antenatal and postnatal periods. A score of 12 or more indicates possible clinical depression.[45]

How is postnatal depression best managed?

In mild cases of PND, the choice of therapy, be it psychotherapeutic or pharmacological, can be left to the patient. In more severe cases, pharmacological therapies are warranted. All the standard antidepressants are effective in the management of postnatal depression. SSRIs can be especially helpful because they are non-sedating, anxiolytic and well tolerated. The choice of which antidepressant to use should be guided by the patient's response and the side-effect profile of the medication. GPs can put women in touch with support groups in the community that provide information and education about PND, and should also try to ensure that the woman has the full support of her family and friends during this difficult time. Interpersonal psychotherapy (which focuses on interpersonal relationships and the woman's changing roles) reduces depressive symptoms and improves social adjustment, and can be used as an alternative or an adjunct to pharmacotherapy.[46]

Postnatal depression is unlike other forms of depression, however, in that while the patient is undergoing treatment for her condition she usually has the ongoing responsibility, and hence the anxieties, of parenting her child. While standard treatments for depression will therefore decrease maternal symptoms, they appear to have less direct benefit on parenting stress and the mother–infant relationship, while the effect on the infant is unclear.[47] Best practice now demands that women who need inpatient care for a mental disorder within 12 months of childbirth should be admitted to a specialist mother and baby unit, unless there are specific reasons for not doing so.[43]

Table 10.4 (p 179) lists current recommendations for the treatment of perinatal depression.

TABLE 10.3 The Edinburgh Postnatal Depression Scale (EPDS) (From Cox et al[44]. ©1987 The Royal College of Psychiatrists.)

As you have recently had a baby, we would like to know how you are feeling. Please underline the answer which comes closest to how you have felt in the past 7 days, not just how you are feeling today.

In the past 7 days

1   *I have been able to laugh and see the funny side of things.*

As much as I always could	Not quite so much now	Definitely less than I used to	Not at all

2   *I have looked forward with enjoyment to things.*

As much as I ever did	Rather less than I used to	Definitely less than I used to	Hardly at all

3*   *I have blamed myself unnecessarily when things went wrong.*

Yes, most of the time	Yes, some of the time	Not very often	No, never

4   *I have been anxious or worried for no good reason.*

No, not at all	Hardly ever	Yes, sometimes	Yes, very often

5*   *I have felt scared or panicky for no very good reason.*

Yes, quite a lot	Yes, sometimes	No, not much	No, not at all

6*   *Things have been getting on top of me.*

Yes, most of the time I haven't been able to cope at all	Yes, sometimes I haven't been coping as well as usual	No, most of the time I have coped quite well	No, I have been coping as well as ever

7*   *I have been so unhappy that I have had difficulty sleeping.*

Yes, most of the time	Yes, sometimes	Not very often	No, not at all

8*   *I have felt sad or miserable.*

Yes, most of the time	Yes, quite often	Not very often	No, not at all

9*   *I have been so unhappy that I have been crying.*

Yes, most of the time	Yes, quite often	Only occasionally	No, never

10*   *The thought of harming myself has occurred to me.*

Yes, quite often	Sometimes	Hardly ever	Never

*Response categories are scored 0, 1, 2 and 3 according to increased severity of the symptom. Items marked with an asterisk are reverse scored 3, 2, 1 and 0. The total score is calculated by adding together the scores for each of the 10 items. A score of 12 or greater, or an affirmative answer on question 10 (the presence of suicidal thoughts) raises concern and indicates a need for more thorough evaluation.

Is it safe to take antidepressants when breastfeeding?

This question raises the most angst for patients and their doctors when trying to manage PND. Over recent years breastfeeding has been vigorously promoted to women as being 'best practice', providing the baby with the optimum nutrition and having multiple benefits for both mother and child. On the other hand, women are exhorted to be very vigilant during pregnancy and lactation about not ingesting any harmful substances or medications that may affect the baby.

Unfortunately, information available to women and their doctors regarding the safety of psychotropic drug use during breastfeeding is inadequate. There have been no controlled studies on the safety of psychotropic medications in nursing mothers, with case reports and small case series for each of the different psychotropic drugs serving as the basis for suggested treatment guidelines.[48] All psychiatric medications studied have been found to be excreted in breast milk.[49] The recommendations of current evidence-based guidelines for antidepressant use in pregnancy and breastfeeding are listed in Box 10.8.

What are the long-term outcomes for women suffering from postnatal depression?

As with other forms of depression, women who have had an initial episode of PND are more likely to go on to have non-puerperal and puerperal relapses.[50] Indeed, the risk of developing PND in a subsequent pregnancy is as high as 50%.[51]

TABLE 10.4 Management of perinatal depression (Adapted from NICE[43])

Type of depression	Planning a pregnancy	During pregnancy	Breastfeeding
Mild	• Withdraw antidepressant and consider watchful waiting. If intervention is needed, consider: (a) self-help approaches (guided self-help, C-CBT, exercise) (b) brief psychological treatments (counselling, CBT and IPT).	• Unplanned pregnancy: see *Planning a pregnancy* • New episode of mild depression: consider: (a) self-help approaches (guided self-help, C-CBT, exercise) (b) non-directive counselling at home (listening visits) (c) brief CBT/IPT. • New episode of mild depression with a history of severe depression: consider antidepressant if psychological treatments declined or not responded to.	See *During pregnancy*.
Moderate and severe depression	• If latest presentation was *moderate* depression, consider: (a) switching to CBT/IPT if taking an antidepressant (b) switching to an antidepressant with lower risk. • If latest presentation was *severe* depression, consider: (a) combining CBT/IPT and anti-depressant (switching to one with lower risk) (b) switching to CBT/IPT.	• Unplanned pregnancy: see *Planning a pregnancy*. • New episode of moderate depression: see mild depression (above). • Moderate depressive episode and a history of depression, or a severe depressive episode, consider: (a) CBT/IPT (b) antidepressant if preferred by the woman (c) combination treatment if there is no, or a limited, response to psychological or drug treatment alone.	See *During pregnancy*.

CBT = cognitive behavioural therapy; C-CBT = computerised CBT; IPT = interpersonal psychotherapy

---

BOX 10.8 Antidepressant use in pregnancy and breastfeeding (Adapted from NICE[43])

Risks to consider
- Lowest-known risks during pregnancy—tricyclic antidepressants (TCAs) such as amitriptyline, imipramine, nortriptyline—but if taken in overdose most are more likely to cause death than selective serotonin reuptake inhibitors (SSRIs)
- Lowest-known risk with an SSRI during pregnancy: fluoxetine
- Fetal heart defects with paroxetine taken in the first trimester
- Persistent pulmonary hypertension in the neonate with SSRIs taken after 20 weeks' gestation
- High blood pressure with venlafaxine at high doses, together with higher toxicity in overdose than SSRIs and some TCAs and increased difficulty of withdrawal

- Withdrawal or toxicity in the neonate with all antidepressants (in most cases the effects are mild and self-limiting)
- Lower than other antidepressants in breast milk: imipramine, nortriptyline and sertraline
- Higher levels in breast milk: citalopram and fluoxetine

Actions to take
Advise a woman taking paroxetine who is planning pregnancy or has an unplanned pregnancy to stop taking the drug.

What can GPs to do to prevent the recurrence of postnatal depression in women?

There are a number of steps that a GP can take to aid in the prevention of recurrent PND in a woman. It is important to provide family planning advice so that the woman can choose either not to become pregnant again or to delay her subsequent pregnancy to a time when she is ready and is not facing any other stressors likely to contribute to another bout of depression.

Second, GPs can either provide counselling themselves or refer the woman to a counsellor to deal with any relationship or other life issues that may have contributed to the onset of the depression. Supportive counselling, the development of problem-solving skills, basic cognitive restructuring, breathing exercises and stress management may be beneficial. Equally important is the provision of education and information about depression and anxiety, so that the woman and her family are fully informed about all its aspects. Prophylactic antidepressant medication has not been found consistently to reduce the risk of recurrent PND.[52]

GPs should also be on the lookout for signs of psychological distress antenatally, especially in women considered to be at higher risk of depression (Box 10.9). A recent study has found that developing depression antenatally is at least as likely, if not more likely, than developing depression postnatally.[53] Depression during pregnancy has been associated with increased obstetric complications such as intrauterine growth retardation, preterm labour and placental abruption, as well as altered neonatal behaviour.[54] If antenatal treatment with antidepressants is required, the minimum effective dosage should be used; if the mother does not plan to breastfeed, the dose should be halved in the week prior to delivery to minimise any potential withdrawal in the infant. The infant should be observed for withdrawal symptoms in the first few days postpartum. If the mother plans to breastfeed, the dose remains the same throughout and the breastfed infant will need to be monitored for adverse reactions.

Summary of key points

- The prevalence of PND is about 13%.
- PND can create emotional, behavioural and cognitive problems for the baby.
- There is no association between pregnancy or delivery complications and postpartum depression nor between PND and sociodemographic variables.
- Screening for postnatal depression, and probably for antenatal depression, should be carried out.
- Each case should be considered on an individual basis when determining whether a woman should use psychotropic medication during pregnancy and/or lactation.
- The risk of recurrence of PND is in the order of 50%.

TIPS FOR PRACTITIONERS

- Sometimes a change in position can help breast drainage. Suggest that the mother feeds with the baby's chin pointing towards the affected area.
- A swab of the nipple is not a useful diagnostic test for candidiasis, as the sensitivity of the test is very low.
- In order to facilitate breastfeeding, there is an old saying, 'Never rest the breast'. This means that even when there is a problem such as mastitis, it is crucial to continue to feed from that breast, or at least to express milk, in order to encourage drainage of the milk and resolution of the problem.
- Women who show evidence of psychological distress antenatally are more likely to suffer from PND.
- Prior to diagnosing postnatal depression, GPs should perform thyroid function tests and a full blood count, as thyroid disease and anaemia are differential diagnoses of PND.

BOX 10.9 Risk factors for depression during pregnancy and the postnatal period

- Past history of depression and anxiety disorder or other psychiatric condition
- Past history of child abuse or poor parental care
- Lack of current emotional or practical supports
- Poor quality of relationship with, or absence of, a partner
- Domestic violence (past or current)
- Current major stressors or losses
- Low self-esteem
- Drug and alcohol abuse
- Dysfunctional personality or coping style

REFERENCES

1. American Academy of Pediatricians (AAP) and American College of Obstetricians and Gynecologists. Guidelines for perinatal care. 4th edn. Elk Grove Village, IL: AAP; 1997: 176–182.
2. MacArthur C, Winter HR, Bick DE, et al. Effects of redesigned community postnatal care on women's health 4 months after birth: a cluster randomised controlled trial. Lancet 2002; 359:378–385.
3. Gunn J. The six-week postnatal check up. Should we forget it? Aust Fam Physician 1998; 27:399–403.
4. Glazener CM, Abdalla M, Stroud P, et al. Postnatal maternal morbidity: extent, causes, prevention and treatment. Br J Obstet Gynaecol 1995; 102:282–287.
5. Brown S, Lumley J. Maternal health after childbirth: results of an Australian population based survey. Br J Obstet Gynaecol 1998; 105:156–161.
6. Bick DE, MacArthur C. Attendance, content and relevance of the six-week postnatal examination. Midwifery 1995; 11: 69–73.
7. Glazener CMA, Macarthur C, Garcia J. Postnatal care: a time for change. Contemp Rev Obstet Gynaecol 1993; 5:130–136.
8. Barrett G, Pendry E, Peacock J, et al. Women's sexual health after childbirth. Br J Obstet Gynaecol 2000; 107:186–195.
9. Flegal KM, Carroll MD, Kuczmarski RJ, et al. Overweight and obesity in the United States: prevalence and trends, 1960–1994. Int J Obes Relat Metab Disord 1998; 22:39–47.
10. Butte NF, Hopkinson JM. Body composition changes during lactation are highly variable among women. J Nutr 1998; 128(2 Suppl):381S–385S.
11. Butte NF. Dieting and exercise in overweight, lactating women. N Engl J Med 2000; 342:502–503.
12. Lovelady CA, Garner KE, Moreno KL, et al. The effect of weight loss in overweight, lactating women on the growth of their infants. N Engl J Med 2000; 342:449–453.
13. Gunn J, Lumley J, Chondros P, et al. Does an early postnatal check-up improve maternal health: results from a randomised trial in Australian general practice. Br J Obstet Gynaecol 1998; 105:991–997.
14. NICE (National Institute of Clinical Excellence). NICE Clinical Guideline 37: Routine postnatal care for women and their babies. 2006; Online. Available from: http://www.nice.org.uk/nicemedia/pdf/CG037fullguideline.pdf [accessed 16.08.2009].
15. Commonwealth of Australia. Best practice guide to common breastfeeding problems. 1999. Online. Available: http://www.health.gov.au/pubhlth/publicat/document/brfeed/practice_guide.pdf [accessed 19.01.2003].
16. Morland-Schultz K, Hill PD. Prevention of and therapies for nipple pain: a systematic review. J Obstet Gynecol Neonat Nurs 2005; 34:428–437.
17. Amir LH, Garland SM, Dennerstein L, et al. Candida albicans: is it associated with nipple pain in lactating women? Gynecol Obstet Invest 1996; 41:30–34.
18. Amir LH, Pakula S. Nipple pain, mastalgia and candidiasis in the lactating breast. Aust NZ J Obstet Gynaecol 1991; 31:379–380.
19. Foster K, Lader D, Cheesbrough S. Infant feeding 1995: survey carried out by the ONS. London: The Stationery Office; 1997.
20. Snowden HM, Renfrew MJ, Woolridge MW. Treatments for breast engorgement during lactation (Cochrane Review). In: The Cochrane Library, Issue 4. Oxford: Update Software; 2002.
21. National Health and Medical Research Council. Infant feeding guidelines for health workers. Canberra: AGPS; 1996.
22. Royal Women's Hospital Melbourne. Domperidone for increasing breast milk supply. 2008. Online. Available: http://www.thewomens.org.au/Domperidoneforincreasingbreastmilksupply [accessed 05.01.2010].
23. Hampton T. FDA warns against breast milk drug. JAMA 2004; 292:322.
24. Betzold C. Is domperidone safe for breastfeeding mothers? [author response] J Midwifery Women's Health 2004; 49:461.
25. Medicines Control Council. Interaction between ketoconazole and domperidone and the risk of QT prolongation—important safety information. S Afr Med J 2006; 96:596.
26. Anderson PO, Valdes V. A critical review of pharmaceutical galactagogues. Breastfeed Med 2007; 2:229–242.
27. European Multicentre Study Group for Cabergoline in Lactation Inhibition. Single dose cabergoline versus bromocriptine in inhibition of puerperal lactation: randomised, double blind, multicentre study. European Multicentre Study Group for Cabergoline in Lactation Inhibition. BMJ 1991; 302:1367–1371.
28. Buhendwa L, Zachariah R, Teck R, et al. Cabergoline for suppression of puerperal lactation in a prevention of mother-to-child HIV-transmission programme in rural Malawi. Trop Doct 2008; 38:30–32.
29. O'Hara MW, Swain AM. Rates and risk of postpartum depression—a meta-analysis. Int Rev Psychiatry 1996; 8:37–54.
30. Regier DA, Boyd JH, Burke JD Jr, et al. One-month prevalence of mental disorders in the United States. Based on five epidemiological catchment area sites. Arch Gen Psychiatry 1988; 45:977–986.
31. Cox JL, Connor Y, Kendell RE. Prospective study of the psychiatric disorders of childbirth. Br J Psychiatry 1982; 140:111–117.
32. Hannah P, Adams D, Lee A, et al. Links between early post-partum mood and post-natal depression. Br J Psychiatry 1992; 160:777–780
33. American Psychiatric Association. Diagnostic and statistical manual of mental disorders. 4th edn. Washington, DC: American Psychiatric Association; 2000.
34. Nonacs R, Cohen LS. Postpartum mood disorders. Prim Psychiatry 1998; 5:51–62.
35. Murray L. The impact of postnatal depression on infant development. J Child Psychol Psychiatry 1992; 33:543–561.
36. Murray L, Cooper P. Postpartum depression and child development. Psychol Med 1997; 27:253–260.
37. Sinclair D, Murray L. Effects of postnatal depression on children's adjustment to school. Br J Psychiatry 1998; 172:58–63.
38. Murray L, Sinclair D, Cooper P, et al. The socioemotional development of 5 year olds with postnatally depressed mothers. J Child Psychol Psychiatry 1999; 40:1259–1271.
39. Epperson CN. Postpartum major depression: detection and treatment. Am Fam Physician 1999; 59:2247–2254, 2259–2260.
40. O'Hara MW. Postpartum depression: causes and consequences. New York: Springer-Verlag; 1995.
41. Nielsen Forman D, Videbech P, Hedegaard M, et al. Postpartum depression: identification of women at risk. Br J Obstet Gynaecol 2000; 107:1210–1217.
42. Josefsson A, Angelsioo L, Berg G, et al. Obstetric, somatic, and demographic risk factors for postpartum depressive symptoms. Obstet Gynecol 2002; 99:223–228.
43. NICE (National Institute for Health and Clinical Excellence). NICE Clinical Guideline 45, Antenatal and postnatal mental health: clinical management and service guidance. 2007. Online. Available: http://www.nice.org.uk/nicemedia/pdf/CG45 fullguideline.pdf [accessed 16.08.2009].
44. Cox JL, Holden JM, Sagovsky R. Detection of postnatal depression. Development of the 10-item Edinburgh Postnatal Depression Scale. Br J Psychiatry 1987; 150:782–786. Note: The Edinburgh Postnatal Depression Scale is © 1987 The Royal College of Psychiatrists. The Edinburgh Postnatal Depression Scale may be photocopied by individual researchers

or clinicians for their own use without seeking permission from the publishers. The scale must be copied in full and all copies must acknowledge the following source: Cox JL, Holden JM and Sagovsky R (1987). Detection of postnatal depression. Development of the 10-item Edinburgh Postnatal Depression Scale. British Journal of Psychiatry 150, pp 782–6. Written permission must be obtained from the Royal College of Psychiatrists for copying and distribution to others or for republication (in print, online or by any other medium). Translations of the scale, and guidance as to its use, may be found in Cox JL and Holden J Perinatal mental health: a guide to the Edinburgh Postnatal Depression Scale. London: Gaskell; 2003.

45. Buist AE, Barnett BEW, Milgrom J, et al. To screen or not to screen—that is the question in perinatal depression. Med J Aust 2002; 177:S101–S105.

46. O'Hara MW, Stuart S, Gorman LL, et al. Efficacy of interpersonal psychotherapy for postpartum depression. Arch Gen Psychiatry 2000; 57:1039–1045.

47. McLennan JD, Offord MD. Should postpartum depression be targeted to improve child mental health? J Am Acad Child Adolesc Psychiatry 2002; 41:28–35.

48. Burt VK, Suri R, Altshuler L, et al. The use of psychotropic medications during breast-feeding. Am J Psychiatry 2001; 158:1001–1009.

49. Llewellyn A, Stowe ZN. Psychotropic medications in lactation. J Clin Psychiatry 1998; 59:41–52.

50. Philipps LH, O'Hara MW. Prospective study of postpartum depression: 4 1/2-year follow-up of women and children. J Abnorm Psychol 1991; 100:151–155.

51. Cooper PJ, Murray L. The course and recurrence of post-natal depression. Br J Psychiatry 1995; 166:191–195.

52. Wisner KL, Perel JM, Peindl KS, et al. Prevention of recurrent postpartum depression: a randomized clinical trial. J Clin Psychiatry 2001; 62:82–86.

53. Evans J, Heron J, Francomb H, et al. Cohort study of depressed mood during pregnancy and after childbirth. BMJ 2001; 323:257–260.

54. Miller LJ, Shah A. Major mental illness during pregnancy. Primary Care Update for OB/GYNS 1999; 6(5): 163–168.

55. Lawrence RA, Lawrence RM. Breastfeeding: A guide for the medical profession. 5th edn. St Louis: Mosby; 1999.

56. James D, Pilai M, Rymer J, et al. Obstetrics, gynaecology, neonatology interactive colour guides. CD-ROM. Edinburgh: Churchill Livingstone; 2002.

11

Breast problems

OBJECTIVES

- To be aware of the epidemiology of breast lumps
- To understand the nature of the triple test and its uses
- To manage breast lumps, cysts and fibroadenomas
- To be able to diagnose and manage women who present with mastalgia and nipple discharge
- To be able to distinguish between physiological and pathological forms of nipple discharge
- To understand the nature of the genetic inheritance of breast cancer
- To be able to counsel women with a family history of breast cancer about what screening practices they should undertake

BREAST SYMPTOMS PRESENTING TO GPs

Nearly all women today know of someone, either a friend or relative, who has had breast cancer. This has led to enormous anxiety among women and a greater preparedness to present to doctors with their concerns about changes they notice in their breasts. There is strong evidence that most women first discover breast lumps or other abnormalities themselves[1] and that most patients with breast symptoms are seen first by their GP.[2] On average, a GP would see between 13[3] and 34 women with new breast problems in 1 year and, of these, one would have cancer.[1]

A recent Dutch study characterising breast symptoms occurring in primary care found that breast symptoms were reported in about 3% of all visits by female patients and that breast pain and breast mass were the most common breast-related complaints. Breast symptom complaints were highest among women aged 25 to 44 years (48 per 1000) and among women aged 65 years and older (33 per 1000). Of the women complaining of breast symptoms, only 3.2% had breast cancer diagnosed. A breast mass had a markedly elevated positive likelihood ratio for breast cancer (15.04; 95% confidence interval, 11.74–19.28).[4]

BREAST LUMPS

Is it normal breast tissue or something I should be concerned about?

Sometimes it is difficult for GPs to tell what is normal tissue and what is an abnormal breast mass that requires further attention. This is particularly true of premenopausal women, whose normal glandular tissue can feel very nodular, especially in the upper outer quadrant of the breast. There are some important differentiating factors worth remembering, however:

- Nodularity waxes and wanes during the menstrual cycle, whereas abnormal masses are characterised by persistence throughout the menstrual cycle.
- Abnormal masses can be discrete or poorly defined, but they differ in character from:
  - the surrounding breast tissue
  - the corresponding area in the contralateral breast.

What is the differential diagnosis of a breast lump?

The differential diagnosis of a dominant breast mass includes macrocyst (clinically evident cyst), fibroadenoma, prominent areas of fibrocystic change, fat necrosis and cancer.

What is it most likely to be?

When GPs see women of all different ages presenting with the same symptom (a breast lump) it is essential to remember the changing frequencies of different discrete breast lumps with age (Fig 11.1). Women in their 20s and 30s are much more likely to have a fibroadenoma. Breast

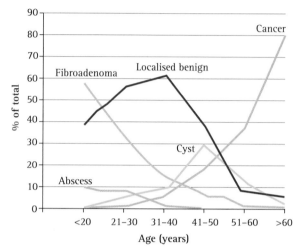

FIGURE 11.1 Changing frequencies of different discrete breast lumps with age (From Dixon & Mansel,[35] with permission from Anthea Carter)

CASE STUDY: 'My best friend has just been diagnosed with breast cancer.'

Rosie was 42 and had very large breasts. She presented to her GP one day saying that she thought she could feel a lump in the right breast. She had felt it in the shower that morning for the first time. Upon further enquiry, it transpired that Rosie's best friend had been diagnosed the previous week with breast cancer. This had made Rosie feel extremely anxious, even though her last breast check-up had been only 6 months previously. Rosie was still menstruating normally. She had had three children in her mid- to late-20s and had breastfed them all for about a year. She had no family history of breast cancer.

On examination, no discrete lump was palpable. Rosie had thought she felt something in the upper outer quadrant, in an area where the breast tissue was very dense and fibrous. She was reassured that it was probably nothing but that she should monitor the area over the next couple of months to see if there were any changes noticeable with the menstrual cycle. She was given an information brochure on breast cancer and its risk factors and advised that mammography was worthwhile only from the age of 50. She seemed slightly reassured but remained anxious.

cysts peak at the age of 50 and the incidence of cancer rises slowly before menopause and then more sharply after that, with the largest incidence >60 years.

Conversely, it is worthwhile remembering the differing frequencies of presenting symptoms of breast cancer (Table 11.1).

Seventy-six per cent of women with breast cancer present with a lump.

What questions should be asked on history?

When assessing a woman who presents with a breast lump, the GP should take special note of the following factors:

- site (Is it constant or changing?)
- duration
- any changes since the lump was first noticed
- relationship to menstrual cycle
- relationship to exogenous hormones
- associated symptoms.

The relevant past history includes:

- risk factors for breast cancer (see later)
- current medication or recent changes in medication, especially exogenous hormones
- hormonal status/menstrual history
- parity and age at first full-term pregnancy
- previous breast problems, including past investigations or biopsy results
- strong family history of breast or ovarian cancer
- most recent imaging.

TABLE 11.1 Relative frequencies of presenting symptoms of breast cancer* (From NBOCC[5])

Symptom	Frequency of presentation
Lump	76%
Pain alone	10%
Nipple changes	8%
Breast asymmetry or skin dimpling	4%
Nipple discharge	2%

*Based on the Presentation of Symptomatic Women to the Breast Unit of the Peter MacCallum Cancer Centre, Melbourne, in 2004.

How should a rigorous clinical breast examination be carried out?

After exposing the chest, the examination commences with inspection under a good light and with the woman in three positions:

1. with arms by her side
2. with arms raised above her head
3. pressing on hips and leaning forward in order to contract the pectoral muscles.

During inspection the GP should pay attention to:

- the contours of the breast, looking for:
  - skin changes such as erythema, dimpling, puckering, peau d'orange
  - visible lumps
- the nipples, looking for:
  - difference in height
  - any inversion
  - erythema, eczema, nodules or ulcers.

Palpation should follow with the patient lying flat, with the ipsilateral arm under her head. Using the flat of the fingers palpate all quadrants of the breast, the axillary tail, and around and behind the nipple. If the breasts are large a pillow can be placed under the shoulder to assist in examining the outer quadrants of the breast. Alternatively, the non-examining hand may be used to immobilise the breast in order to better examine it.

After both breasts have been examined, the patient should sit or stand and the GP should palpate the supraclavicular and axillary fossae for lymph nodes.

When making notes, the GP should record details of any lumps found including size, shape, consistency, mobility, tenderness, fixation and the exact position.

What are the critical issues in the evaluation of a woman with a breast lump?

If a lump is found, the next question is to determine the likelihood of cancer. This can be assessed using the triple test (clinical breast examination, mammography and fine-needle aspiration cytology); a positive triple test is found in 99.6% of breast cancers. Negative results in all components of the triple test provide good evidence that a cancer is unlikely (<1%).[5] The accuracy of the triple test and each of its components is given in Table 11.2 (p 186).

The likelihood of cancer is determined with the triple test, which consists of clinical breast examination, mammography and fine-needle aspiration cytology.

TABLE 11.2 The accuracy of the triple test and each of its components (From NBOCC[5])

	Triple test	Clinical examination	Mammography	Fine–needle aspiration cytology
TPR (%)	>99.6	85	90	91
FPR (%)	<38	20	27	7
Specificity (%)	>62	80	73	93

The triple test is defined as positive if any one of its components is suspicious or malignant.
TPR, true positive rate = sensitivity; FPR, false positive rate = (100–specificity).

The problem with the triple test, however, is the varying degree of sensitivity and specificity of the different components of the test. For example, a clinical breast examination may be more sensitive in the hands of an experienced practitioner. Mammography is less effective in younger women,[6] in whom ultrasound has a lower false positive rate and is more sensitive.

When should I order an ultrasound and when should I order a mammogram?

In women under the age of 25 and those who are pregnant or lactating, an ultrasound is recommended as the first imaging modality. Mammography is only justified if the clinical findings or the ultrasound results are suspicious of malignancy.

In those 25–35 years, ultrasound is again the preferred imaging modality, although mammography is acceptable if the woman is in the upper range of this age group. It should be used in conjunction with an ultrasound when:

- the clinical and/or ultrasound findings are suspicious or show signs of malignancy
- the ultrasound findings are indeterminate
- the ultrasound findings are not consistent with the clinical findings
- there is a strong family history of breast cancer.

In those over 35, mammography is the preferred imaging modality. Ultrasound should also be used if the lump is consistent with a simple cyst and where the mammogram results are inconsistent with the clinical findings. For this age group GPs can therefore request a mammogram ± ultrasound when they refer the patient for imaging.

When ordering a mammogram is there anything special I need to do?

It is important to note on the referral form that this is not a screening mammography but a diagnostic one. The usual screening study, consisting of two standard views of the breast (craniocaudal and mediolateral oblique), is therefore inappropriate. The radiologist should be notified of the area of clinical concern so that it can be defined with a radiopaque marker to ensure that any noted mammographic abnormalities correspond to the clinical finding. Extra views can then be obtained to ensure that the lesion is adequately visualised.

When do breast cysts occur?

While breast cysts can occur at any age, they are more common in those over 40, accounting for <10% of breast masses in those under 40.[6]

Breast cysts are most common in women over 40, but are uncommon postmenopausally.

What do they feel like?

Cysts are firm and mobile and may be tender. They fluctuate with the menstrual cycle and tend to occur during periods of hormonal irregularity.

What should a GP do when confronted with an obvious breast cyst?

If an ultrasound or mammogram reveals a simple cyst, the next step is to aspirate the cyst using a fine-bore needle (Fig 11.2). Routine cytologic examination of cyst fluid is not indicated if it appears normal (straw to dark-green colour) and no lump remains,[5] because of the low likelihood of cancer and the fact that cytologic identification of atypical cells in cyst fluid is not uncommon. This results in the clinical dilemma of a patient whose cyst resolves with aspiration and whose mammogram is normal, but whose cytology report indicates the need for biopsy.[7]

Breast cysts are treated by aspiration. If the fluid is bloody or there is a residual mass, biopsy is required.

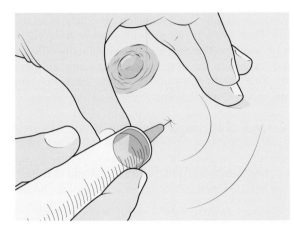

FIGURE 11.2 Breast cyst aspiration: palpable breast cyst steadied and needle passed into the centre

Women should be advised to return for review if the cyst refills; if there is persistent refilling, the patient should be referred to a surgeon.[5] One follow-up study of 389 women who underwent cyst aspiration found that 44 women had a recurrent cyst and 20 had a solid mass at the aspiration site. In biopsies of the 20 solid masses, two cancers were found.[8] If there is bloody fluid or a lump remains after aspiration of what appears to be a simple cyst on imaging, the fluid should be sent for cytological testing and the patient referred to a surgeon.

What if non-palpable cysts are found on mammography?

If they are confirmed as simple cysts on ultrasound examination, they require no treatment.

What are fibroadenomas?

Fibroadenomas used to be considered benign tumours of the breast. They are now considered to be aberrations of normal breast development, histologically resembling a hyperplastic breast lobule.[9] They are also known as the 'breast mouse', because they appear to be very mobile.

Fibroadenomas are relatively common, accounting for 12% of all palpable breast masses,[10] 60% of which are in women <20 years.[11]

Is there a relationship between fibroadenomas and breast cancer?

The general consensus is that having a fibroadenoma does not bring about an increased risk of breast cancer.[10,12]

What do fibroadenomas feel like?

They are discrete lumps usually round or oval in shape, firm, rubbery, smooth and very mobile. They range in size from very small to >5 cm. They are usually located in the upper outer quadrant.

While fibroadenomas are often very characteristic, the diagnosis is correct only in half to two-thirds of cases.[13,14] Therefore, a clinical diagnosis is not sufficient to exclude cancer, even in young women, and all women with discrete masses should have a triple test.

How are fibroadenomas managed?

If cancer is excluded using the triple test, the patient has a choice between conservative management or surgical excision. If conservative management is chosen, the limitations of the triple test should be explained to the patient (approximately 1% of cancers can be misdiagnosed), the patient should be followed up on a regular basis, with repeat ultrasonography every 6–12 months, and be reassessed if there is any change.[9]

When should I refer the patient to a surgeon?

Indications for referral are described in Box 11.1. Referrals should be directed towards surgeons with expertise in breast disease.[5]

Summary of key points
- Abnormal masses persist throughout the menstrual cycle and differ in character from the surrounding breast tissue and the contralateral breast.
- The frequencies of different discrete breast lumps change with age.

BOX 11.1 Indications for surgical referral in the presence of a breast change

The patient should be referred to a surgeon:
- if any one component of the triple test is positive, i.e:
  - clinical examination is suspicious or malignant
  - imaging is indeterminate, suspicious or malignant
  - fine-needle aspirate cytology or core biopsy is indeterminate, suspicious or malignant
- where a cyst aspiration is incomplete or results in bloody aspirate (not traumatic), or when a lump remains post-aspiration
- if there is spontaneous unilateral discharge from a single duct, especially in women 60 years and over
- if any test result is inconsistent and requires additional investigation.

- The likelihood of a breast lump being cancer is best determined using the triple test: clinical examination, mammography and fine-needle aspiration cytology.
- Mammography is less effective in younger women, in whom ultrasound has a lower false positive rate and is more sensitive.
- Simple breast cysts are managed by aspirating the fluid and following up.
- Fibroadenomas are more common in younger women and are not associated with an increase in breast cancer risk. However, the diagnosis should be confirmed using the triple test.

MASTALGIA

What is mastalgia?

The clinical name given to painful breasts is mastalgia or mastodynia and it is one of the most common breast complaints that women present with to a general practitioner.

Do all women have painful breasts from time to time?

Mastalgia, like premenstrual symptoms, is suffered by most women at some stage of their lives and is part of a 'normal' state of affairs. It is only when the symptoms start to interfere with daily life and persist over a long time that it becomes a 'disease' state.

Are there different types of mastalgia?

Mastalgia can be divided into three groups. The first is cyclical mastalgia, which affects about two-thirds of all sufferers of mastalgia. This occurs in premenstrual women, usually commencing in the woman's 20s. Pain starts premenstrually and is relieved by menstruation. The pain is characteristically bilateral and located in the upper outer quadrants, although one side might predominate. Sometimes the pain can radiate down the arm.

The second and less common group is that of non-cyclical mastalgia. The women suffering from this complaint are usually about 10 years older than those with cyclical mastalgia. In this group, the pain can be unilateral or bilateral and is usually concentrated in the inner, lower aspects of the breast.

Mastalgia is very subjective and is suffered by most women at some stage. It can be cyclical or non-cyclical and the aetiology is unclear.

A small group of patients actually have chest wall pain and not true mastalgia at all. The pain in these women is well localised, usually unilateral and may be in the chostocondral joint (Tietze's syndrome).

What is the cause of mastalgia?

Like many diseases suffered by women, mastalgia was thought, in the twentieth century, to be due to a 'nervous and irritable temperament'. The aetiology of this condition has not progressed much further since then, except to acknowledge that most women will have some degree of breast tenderness or pain premenstrually at some point in their lives. Broadly the condition is thought to be hormonal in origin, particularly because for many women symptoms cease at the time of menopause.

The research carried out focusing on the aetiology of mastalgia is interesting. From a hormonal perspective, an increase in prolactin response to thyrotrophin-releasing hormone has been associated with breast pain.[15] Another published theory centres on the fatty acid profiles of women suffering mastalgia. Studies have found that these women have increased saturated fatty acids and reduced proportions of essential fatty acids.[16]

How should GPs approach a patient complaining of mastalgia?

In patients who present with breast pain, the following approach is recommended:

History
- Duration and nature of pain
- Location of pain

CASE STUDY: Premenstrual breast soreness

Joanne, a 19-year-old university student, came in complaining of breast pain. She was sexually active and on a triphasic pill. She told me that she had developed some breast soreness just before her period since commencing the pill but that this month her nipples had felt particularly tender and her breasts were too uncomfortable to touch. My first thought was 'she must be pregnant'. I examined her and found nothing abnormal. A urine HCG was negative. I reassured her by saying that cancer usually presented as a non-painful lump and that she was too young to be likely to develop breast cancer anyway, but she (like her mother and me) was mostly concerned that she might be pregnant. I sent off a bHCG just to make sure and it came back as negative. She was reassured by this result and did not seek further treatment.

- Variation with menstruation
- Menstrual history
- Family history
- Past history
- Medication use—particularly focused on hormones and contraception

Examination
- Thorough breast examination
- Pelvic examination to rule out an oestrogen-secreting ovarian tumour

Investigations
- Pregnancy test if pregnancy is possible
- Mammography in patients older than 35 or those with localised pain but no palpable lesion

Is breast pain associated with breast cancer?

Most women presenting with breast symptoms of any sort are terrified that they may have breast cancer. This anxiety is not so ill-placed, given the very high lifetime prevalence of breast cancer in most developed countries (approximately 1 in 11). However, women with breast pain can be reassured that only 2% of all breast pain cases result in a breast cancer diagnosis and less than 7% of all painful lumps are cancerous.[17]

Breast pain is rarely associated with breast cancer.

What is the management of mastalgia?

Many women with mastalgia have spontaneous resolution of their symptoms after 2 or 3 months. There are women, however, whose pain compromises their ability to undertake day-to-day tasks. This group requires treatment that varies according to the type of mastalgia they have and whether or not they want to become pregnant.

Eight-five per cent of patients with mastalgia will be content with reassurance.[18]

While there is overlap between the initial therapeutic approaches for patients with cyclic and non-cyclic mastalgia, hormonally active medications are more effective for patients with cyclic mastalgia and are indicated only for patients with severe,

---

BOX 11.2 Agents shown to have no effect on mastalgia

- Diuretics
- Non-steroidal anti-inflammatory drugs (NSAIDs)
- Narcotics
- Vitamin E
- Vitamin B^6
- Medroxyprogesterone acetate
- Evening primrose oil

---

prolonged symptoms.[19] Current guidelines[20] suggest that first-line treatment should involve education, reassurance and advice to wear a well-fitting bra that provides good support. There is no evidence to support reducing caffeine intake, use of vitamin E or the commonly suggested evening primrose oil.[21] There is some evidence to support the use of flaxseed as a first-line treatment for cyclical mastalgia, as well as the use of topical non-steroidal anti-inflammatory gels. Box 11.2 lists agents that have been shown to have no effect on mastalgia.

A recent meta-analysis reviewed the effectiveness of bromocriptine, danazol, evening primrose oil and tamoxifen in the therapy of mastalgia.[21] The authors concluded that while bromocriptine, danazol and tamoxifen all offer significant relief from mastalgia, tamoxifen is associated with the least number of side effects and should be the drug of first choice. Dosage is 10 mg daily, given between days 15 and 25 of the cycle. However, tamoxifen has a risk of potentially serious adverse effects, with the principal concerns being deep venous thrombosis and endometrial cancer. It should therefore be reserved for women with severe mastalgia refractory to other measures.[19]

Summary of key points
- Mastalgia is more common premenopausally than postmenopausally.
- Mastalgia is rarely a presenting symptom of breast cancer.
- Breast pain has a high spontaneous remission rate.

NIPPLE DISCHARGE

How common is nipple discharge?

Nipple discharge is a fairly common symptom in women and the third most common breast complaint after breast pain and breast mass.[22] Discharge can be expressed manually in about 10% of women[23] and if a pump is used in over half of women.[24] It is relatively uncommon for a GP to be confronted with this complaint, however.

What causes it?

Nipple discharge can either be physiological or pathological in origin. Physiological nipple discharge is usually idiopathic. The frequencies of causes of physiological nipple discharge in primary care are given in Table 11.3. The most common cause of pathological nipple discharge is an intraductal papilloma (44%), followed by duct ectasia (23%), mastitis and breast abscess, and breast carcinoma. Only 11% of such pathological discharges are due to carcinoma, and only 1–5% of carcinomas present in this way.[25]

The three most common causes of persistent, unilateral single-duct nipple discharge are intraductal papilloma, duct ectasia and carcinoma.

An intraductal papilloma is a benign condition caused by epithelial hyperplasia and occurs most frequently in women 45–50 years of age. In 20–50% of patients, it is characterised by a bloody or serosanguinous nipple discharge. It appears as a small, fragile, wart-like or finger-like growth within the lumen of the mammary duct near the nipple and in 95% of cases involves a single duct and is unilateral.[22] When occurring peripherally, however, intraductal paillomas may be multifocal and associated with atypical hyperplastic cells and an increased risk of breast cancer.[26]

CASE STUDY: Continuing discharge after breastfeeding

32-year-old Helen presented with her youngest child of 2 years, who had a bad cough. After sorting out the child she said, 'I just have one more question'. She explained that since stopping breastfeeding over a year ago she noticed that she had some continuing nipple discharge. The discharge was a yellow-green colour and milky in consistency. It was never spontaneous and only appeared in small quantities when she squeezed her nipple. It appeared to be emerging from several ducts and from both nipples, though one nipple had slightly more discharge than the other. The GP examined her breasts and found no abnormality. Helen was reassured that the kind of discharge she had was probably physiological and that no other measures were necessary.

TABLE 11.3 Frequency of causes of physiologic nipple discharge in primary care (From Schwartz[38])

Cause	Frequency	Presentation
Idiopathic	40–50%	Bilateral milky/watery discharge
Galactorrhoea (prolonged lactation)	25–30%	Bilateral milky
Medication	10–15%	Bilateral milky/watery discharge
Anovulatory syndromes	1–2%	Bilateral milky/watery discharge/irregular periods
Sella turcica lesions	1–2%	Bilateral milky/watery discharge/irregular periods

Intraductal papilloma is the most common cause of bloody nipple discharge in the absence of a mass.

Duct ectasia is found in 15–20% of patients with nipple discharge,[27] with peak incidence in women older than 50 years. It is caused by glandular involution, with terminal ducts becoming obstructed by fibrotic tissue strands leading to accumulation of secretory material. Dilation of subareolar ducts with accumulation of stagnant secretions causes obstruction and subsequent discharge.[28] Mammary duct ectasia may be asymptomatic and subclinical, or may present as breast pain, a breast mass, nipple discharge, nipple retraction, non-puerperal breast abscess or a mammary fistula.[29]

Of the three major causes of nipple discharge, breast carcinoma is the least likely cause.

The likelihood of cancer is greatly increased when a palpable mass is present in association with the discharge (especially unilateral), positive mammographic or galactographic findings, and age over 50 years.[22] An associated carcinoma may be found in up to 10–15% of patients with nipple discharge.[30]

Should galactorrhoea be considered differently from nipple discharge?

Non-puerperal galactorrhoea and pathologic nipple discharges are evaluated differently. This is because galactorrhoea is not a symptom of breast cancer or primary breast pathology. With galactorrhoea, if all pharmacological and physiological causes have been excluded, a prolactin level and a TSH should be obtained to rule out hyperprolactinaemia and hypothyroidism. If the prolactin level is elevated, imaging of the brain is warranted to look for a pituitary tumour.

How can a GP differentiate between physiological and pathological discharge?

Nipple discharges are classified as pathological if they are spontaneous (i.e. they stain bras or sheets), bloody or associated with a mass. Pathological discharges are usually unilateral and confined to one duct (Fig 11.3a). In comparison, physiological discharges usually occur only with compression and are characterised by multiple duct involvement (Fig 11.3b). These discharges are frequently bilateral. With either type, the discharge fluid may be clear, yellow, white or dark-green. Table 11.4 highlights the differences between the two forms of discharge.

The GP should ask about all of these factors, as well as about recent or current pregnancy, breast trauma, surgery and menopausal status. It is important in premenopausal women to ask about symptoms of amenorrhoea, headache, visual disturbance, change in appetite or temperature tolerance, as these may be signs of an underlying pituitary or hypothalamic problem.

Various medications can also elevate prolactin levels and may be implicated in the development of galactorrhoea. These medications and other causes of elevated prolactin levels are listed in Table 11.5.

The GP should then undertake a careful breast examination, looking for all the classic signs of breast cancer such as skin dimpling, retraction and a palpable mass. The nipple should be carefully inspected looking for the signs of Paget's disease (Box 11.3 p 192). This commences as a raw area on the middle of the nipple and over time involves the entire nipple area causing itching and irritation. An attempt should also be made to ascertain whether the discharge is confined to a single duct or to multiple ducts.

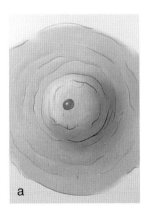
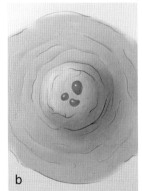

FIGURE 11.3 (a) Single duct discharge (b) Multiple duct discharge

TABLE 11.4 A comparison between physiological and pathological nipple discharge

Physiologic	Pathologic
Occurs with nipple compression	Spontaneous
Multiple duct involvement	Single duct involvement
Bilateral	Unilateral
No associated mass	Associated mass
Colour may be clear, white, yellow or green	Colour may be clear, white, yellow, green or bloody

TABLE 11.5 Causes of elevated prolactin

Physiological Such as nipple stimulation, pregnancy, postpartum and sexual orgasm	
Endocrine • Polycystic ovaries • Chest wall trauma • Hypothalamic and pituitary lesions • Hypothyroidism	
Pharmacological (Adapted from Torre and Falorni[39])	
Antipsychotics • Typical	Haloperidol, chlorpromazine, thioridazine, thiothixene
• Atypical	Risperidone, amisulpride, molindone, zotepine
Antidepressants • Tricyclics	Amitriptyline, desipramine, clomipramine, amoxapine
• SSRI	Sertraline, fluoxetine, paroxetine
• MAO-I	Pargyline, clorgyline
Other psychotropics	Buspirone, alprazolam
Prokinetics	Metoclopramide, domperidone
Antihypertensive	Alpha-methyldopa, reserpine, verapamil
Opiates	Morphine
H2 antagonists	Cimetidine, ranitidine
Others	Fenfluramine, physostigmine, chemotherapics

Are any investigations necessary?

There are varying recommendations regarding the investigation of a new nipple discharge. When the examination is entirely normal and the history points to a physiological discharge, some say reassurance is all that is necessary, with a mammogram in women over the age of 35.[7] Others argue that the key issue is whether or not the nipple discharge contains blood and whether the woman is over 60. This is because in women with a nipple discharge, most cancers occur in women who have a bloody discharge or who are 60 years of age or older (see Table 11.6).

In order to see if the discharge contains blood, it can be tested using any haem-sensitive test strip. If it is positive, surgical referral is necessary. If negative, the woman should be advised to avoid checking for discharge because stimulation of the nipple (i.e. squeezing to check for discharge) actually promotes discharge. A physiological discharge often resolves when the nipple is left alone.

What further management is required in cases of pathological nipple discharge?

All patients should be referred for surgical evaluation when the GP considers the discharge to be pathological. The surgeon will probably order a diagnostic mammogram to look for non-palpable masses or calcifications.

Cytology of the nipple discharge is not recommended because although it is highly specific it has a low sensitivity (45%); therefore, while a positive cytology result is helpful, a negative result cannot be used to rule out cancer.

Galactography (contrast mammography or ductography) requires a skilled radiologist to pass a catheter into the duct and then inject a small amount of radiocontrast material into the involved duct in order to demonstrate a filling defect during mammography. It is most often used when trying to identify a lesion for biopsy when a woman has a significant discharge from a single duct, but its use remains controversial,[31] as a negative galactogram does not reliably exclude the presence of breast cancer and is not a replacement for surgery.

A terminal duct excision is both diagnostic and, for discharges that turn out to have a benign cause, therapeutic.

Summary of key points

- Nipple discharge is quite common in women.
- It is a rare presentation to general practitioners.
- Nipple discharge is more likely to be physiological when it is bilateral, due to expression, and involves multiple ducts.
- Nipple discharge is more likely to be pathological when it is spontaneous, unilateral and only involves a single duct.
- Discharge containing blood and discharge occurring in a woman >60 years is more likely to be due to cancer.
- Physiological discharge will resolve spontaneously if it is not encouraged.
- Pathological discharge requires referral for surgical evaluation.

WOMEN WITH A FAMILY HISTORY OF BREAST OR OVARIAN CANCER

Underlying any discussion about an individual woman's breast and ovarian cancer risk should be awareness of the background risk for the general population. Approximately 1 in 11 women will develop breast cancer at some time during their life and about 1 in 100 women will develop ovarian cancer.[32]

BOX 11.3 The features of Paget's disease

- Redness
- Crusting
- Drying
- Excoriation
- An eczematous appearance

TABLE 11.6 Percentage probability of cancer by age and nature of discharge (From NBOCC[5])

Discharge	Age <60 years	Age >60 years
Serous	<1%	3%
Bloody	3%	9%

CASE STUDY: 'My mother has had breast cancer…'

Peggy presented requesting advice. She was 35 years old and had three children. Her mother had had breast cancer diagnosed at the age of 48. She also had a great aunt who had died of breast cancer but she was not sure at what age. Neither of her two older sisters had breast cancer but she was concerned about her risk. She wanted advice about how to prevent breast cancer from occurring.

What does it mean to have a family history of breast cancer?

A family history of breast or ovarian cancer can involve one or more blood relatives on either the father's or mother's side of the family. While a family history may be due to chance (given the high rates of breast and ovarian cancer in our community), it could also point to a genetic origin for the cancer/s. The stronger the family history, the more likely the involvement of a faulty gene. Key factors associated with a family history of breast or ovarian cancer are given in Box 11.4.

How significant is family history in the development of breast cancer?

Up to 10% of breast cancer in Western countries is due to genetic predisposition.[33] Cancer susceptibility generally has an autosomal dominant inheritance with limited penetrance, meaning that it can be transmitted through either sex and that some family members may transmit the abnormal gene without developing cancer themselves.

What genes are involved in the development of breast cancer?

While it is not yet known how many breast cancer genes there may be, two breast cancer genes (BRCA1 and BRCA2) account for approximately 5% of all breast and ovarian cancers. Some 2% of Ashkenazi Jewish women carry one of these affected genes.

Many families affected by breast cancer show an excess of ovarian, colon, prostatic and other cancers attributable to the same inherited mutation. Those more likely to be carrying the mutation are those:

- who develop bilateral breast cancer
- who develop a combination of breast cancer and another epithelial cancer
- women who get the disease at an early age.

According to estimates of lifetime risk, about 12% of women (120 out of 1000) in the general population will develop breast cancer at some time during their lives, compared with about 60% of women (600 out of 1000) who have inherited a harmful mutation in BRCA1 or BRCA2.[21,34] In other words, a woman who has inherited a harmful mutation in BRCA1 or BRCA2 is about five times more likely to develop breast cancer than a woman who does not have such a mutation.

Lifetime risk estimates for ovarian cancer among women in the general population indicate that 1.4% (14 out of 1000) will be diagnosed with ovarian cancer compared with 15–40% of women (150–400 out of 1000) who have a harmful BRCA1 or BRCA2 mutation.[35,36]

Most breast cancers that are due to a genetic mutation occur before the age of 65; hence a woman with a strong family history of breast cancer of early onset who is still unaffected at 65 has probably not inherited the genetic mutation.

How can a GP quantify the degree of risk involved to a patient with a family history of breast cancer?

In simple terms one could say that a woman's risk of breast cancer is two or more times greater if she has a first-degree relative (mother, sister or daughter) who developed the disease before the age of 50, and the younger the relative when she developed breast cancer the greater the risk.

The information in Box 11.5 (p 194), put together by the Australian National Breast Cancer Centre, describes categories of risk and gives a lifetime risk for each category.[32] What follows is the recommended management of women with these risks.[32]

What is the management of women at or slightly above average risk?

These women should be reassured that over 90% of women in this group will not get breast cancer.

Women 50–69 years should undertake screening mammograms every two years. A firm recommendation regarding clinical breast examination (CBE) is not possible, as there is no evidence to either encourage or discourage the use of CBE as a screening method in women of any age. The routine recommendation of breast self-examination is controversial because of the increased morbidity related to it and the fact that there is no decrease in mortality.[37] However a woman should maintain a general awareness of her breasts and report to her GP any changes she notices in her breasts.

What is the management of women at moderately increased risk?

These women should be advised that between 75% and 90% will not get breast cancer. No clear

---

BOX 11.4 Key factors associated with increased risk of breast cancer (From NBOCC[32])

- Multiple relatives affected by breast cancer (male or female) or ovarian cancer
- Younger age at cancer diagnosis in relatives
- Relatives affected by both breast and ovarian cancer
- Relatives affected with bilateral breast cancer
- Ashkenazi Jewish ancestry

BOX 11.5 Categories of risk of breast cancer (From NBOCC[32])

Women at average risk or slightly above average risk of breast cancer

Lifetime risk = 1 in 14 to 1 in 8
- Covers more than 95% of the female population
- No confirmed family history of breast cancer
- One 1° relative diagnosed with breast cancer at age 50 or older
- One 2° relative diagnosed with breast cancer at any age
- Two 2° relatives on the same side of the family diagnosed with breast cancer at age 50 or older
- Two 1° or 2° relatives diagnosed with breast cancer, at age 50 or older, but on different sides of the family (i.e. one on each side of the family)

Women at moderately increased risk of breast cancer

Lifetime risk: 1 in 8 to 1 in 4
- Covers less than 4% of the female population
- One 1° relative diagnosed with breast cancer before the age of 50 (without the additional features of the potentially high-risk group)
- Two 1° relatives, on the same side of the family, diagnosed with breast cancer (without the additional features of the potentially high-risk roup)
- Two 2° relatives, on the same side of the family, diagnosed with breast cancer, at least one before

the age of 50, (without the additional features of the potentially high-risk group)

Women at potentially high risk of breast cancer

Lifetime risk: 1 in 4 to 1 in 2 or higher if shown to have a high-risk breast cancer gene mutation
- Covers less than 1% of the female population
- Women who are at potentially high risk of ovarian cancer
- Two 1° or 2° relatives on one side of the family diagnosed with breast or ovarian cancer **plus** one or more of the following features on the same side of the family:
  - additional relative(s) with breast or ovarian cancer
  - breast cancer diagnosed before the age of 40
  - bilateral breast cancer
  - breast **and** ovarian cancer in the same woman
  - Ashkenazi Jewish ancestry
  - breast cancer in a male relative
- One 1° or 2° relative diagnosed with breast cancer at age 45 or younger **plus** another 1° or 2° relative on the same side of the family with sarcoma (bone/soft tissue) at age 45 or younger
- Member of a family in which the presence of a high-risk breast cancer gene mutation has been established

---

guidelines exist in this group with regards optimal management; however, women in this group should at the very least attend for screening mammograms, and mammography from a younger age, or more frequently, should be considered on an individual basis. Further advice may be available after assessment by a specialist cancer or genetics service. Again, a firm recommendation regarding CBE is not possible, as there is no evidence to either encourage or discourage the use of CBE as a screening method in women of any age. A woman should maintain a general awareness of her breasts and report to her GP any changes she notices in her breasts.

What is the management of women at potentially high risk?

Of these women 50–75% will not get breast cancer. However, it is important to emphasise the importance of early detection. These women should see a cancer

specialist and plan an individualised surveillance program that may include:

- attending for regular clinical breast examination
- annual mammography with or without other imaging techniques
- surveillance for ovarian cancer.

The age at which screening commences may be influenced by aspects of family history. Although this should be determined on an individual basis, it is generally accepted practice to begin screening at least five years prior to the age of diagnosis of the closest relative. Women should of course immediately notify their GP of any breast changes, should they occur.

Summary of key points
- 10% of breast cancer in Western countries is due to genetic predisposition.

- Two breast cancer genes, BRCA1 and BRCA2, account for about 1–2% of all breast cancers.
- Those more likely to be carrying the mutation are those who develop bilateral breast cancer or a combination of breast cancer and another epithelial cancer, or women who get the disease at an early age.
- A woman's risk of breast cancer is two or more times greater if she has a first-degree relative (mother, sister or daughter) who developed the disease before the age of 50, and the younger the relative when she developed breast cancer the greater the risk.

TIPS FOR PRACTITIONERS

- When examining a woman with a large breast, a pillow under the shoulder will help spread out the breast and assist in the examination of the upper outer quadrant.
- When ordering a mammogram for a suspicious breast lump, it is important to alert the radiographer to the fact that it is a diagnostic mammogram not a screening one.
- The fluid obtained from aspirating a breast cyst can be discarded, provided that it is not blood-stained.
- In women with nipple discharge, most cancers occur in those who are over 60 and have a bloody discharge.
- Some women complaining of mastalgia will in fact have chest wall pain, or Tietze's syndrome (pain in the costochondral joint).
- Many women with mastalgia have spontaneous resolution of their symptoms over 2–3 months.
- Discharge from the nipple can be expressed in about 10% of women.
- The critical issue when confronted with a woman with a nipple discharge is to decide whether it is physiological or pathological in nature.
- Many families affected by breast cancer show an excess of ovarian, colon and prostatic cancer attributable to the same inherited mutation.

REFERENCES

1. Nichols S, Walters WE, Wheeler MJ. Management of female breast disease by Southampton general practitioners. Br Med J 1980; 281:1450–1453.
2. Bywaters JL. The incidence and management of female breast disease in general practice. J R Coll Gen Pract 1977; 27:353–357.
3. Roberts MM, Elton RA, Robinson SE, et al. Consultations for breast disease in general practice and hospital referral patterns. Br J Surg 1987; 74:1020–1022.
4. Eberl MM, Phillips RL, Jr, Lamberts H, et al. Characterizing breast symptoms in family practice. Ann Fam Med 2008; 6(6):528–533.
5. NBOCC (National Breast and Ovarian Cancer Centre). The investigation of a new breast symptom: A guide for general practitioners. February 2006. Online. Available: http://www.nbocc.org.au/bestpractice/resources/IBS172_theinvestigationofan.pdf [accessed 12.08.09].
6. Morrow M, Wong S, Venta L. The evaluation of breast masses in women younger than forty years of age. Surgery 1998; 124:634–640.
7. Morrow M. The evaluation of common breast problems. Am Fam Physician 2000; 61:2371–2385.
8. Hamed S, Coady A, Chaudary MA, et al. Follow-up of patients with aspirated breast cysts is necessary. Arch Surg 1989; 124:253–255.
9. Houssami N, Cheung MNK, Dixon JM. Fibroadenoma of the breast. Med J Aust 2001; 174:185–188.
10. Dixon JM. Cystic disease and fibroadenoma of the breast: natural history and relation to breast cancer risk. Br Med Bull 1991; 47:258–271.
11. Dixon JM, Morrow M. Breast disease: a problem based approach. New York: WB Saunders; 1999; 47–53.
12. Dent DM, Cant PJ. Fibroadenoma. World J Surg 1989; 13:706–710.
13. Cant PJ, Madden MV, Close PM, et al. Case for conservative management of selected fibroadenomas of the breast. Br J Surg 1987; 74:857–859.
14. Wilkinson S, Forrest AP. Fibroadenoma of the breast. Br J Surg 1985; 72:838–840.
15. Ayers JW, Gidwani GP. The 'luteal breast': hormonal and sonographic investigation of benign breast disease in patients with cyclic mastalgia. Fertil Steril 1983; 40:779–784.
16. Horrobin DF, Manku MS. Premenstrual syndrome and premenstrual breast pain (cyclical mastalgia): Disorders of essential fatty acid (EFA) metabolism. Prostaglandins Leukot Essent Fatty Acids 1989; 37:255–261.
17. Barton MB, Elmore JG, Fletcher SW. Breast symptoms among women enrolled in a health maintenance organization: frequency, evaluation, and outcome. Ann Intern Med 1999; 130:651–657.
18. Holland PA, Gateley CA. Drug therapy of mastalgia. What are the options? Drugs 1994; 48:709–716.
19. Smith RL, Pruthi S, Fitzpatrick LA. Evaluation and management of breast pain. Mayo Clinic Proc 2004; 79(3):353–372.
20. Rosolowich V, Saettler E, Szuck B, et al. Mastalgia. J Obstet Gynaecol Can 2006; 28(1):49–57.
21. Srivastava A, Mansel RE, Arvind N, et al. Evidence-based management of mastalgia: a meta-analysis of randomised trials. Breast 2007; 16(5):503–512.
22. Hussain AN, Policarpio C, Vincent MT. Evaluating nipple discharge. Obstet Gynecol Surv 2006; 61(4):278–283.
23. Newman HF, Klein M, Northrup JD, et al. Nipple discharge: frequency and pathogenesis in an ambulatory population. NY State J Med 1983; 83:928.

24. Lobe SM, Schnitt SJ, Connolly JL, et al. Benign breast disorders. In: Harris JR, Hellman S, Henderson IC (eds), et al. Breast diseases. Philadelphia, PA: Lippincott; 1987; 15.

25. Jardines L. Management of nipple discharge. Am Surg 1996; 62:119–122.

26. Raju U, Vertes D. Breast papillomas with atypical ductal hyperplasia: a clinicopathologic study. Hum Pathol 1991; 27:1231–1238.

27. Dixon JM. Periductal mastitis/duct ectasia. World J Surg 1989; 13(6):715–720.

28. Smith MA, Boyd L, Osuch JR, et al. Breast disorders. In: Smith MA, Shimp LA (eds). 20 common problems in women's health care. New York: McGraw Hill; 2000.

29. Devitt JE. Benign breast disease in the postmenopausal woman. World J Surg 1989; 13(6):731–735.

30. King TA, Carter KM, Bolton JS, et al. A simple approach to nipple discharge. Am Surg 2000; 66(10):960–965, discussion 965–966.

31. Dawes LG, Bowen C, Venta LA, et al. Ductography for nipple discharge: no replacement for ductal excision. Surgery 1998; 21:685–691.

32. NBOCC (National Breast and Ovarian Cancer Centre). Advice about familial aspects of breast cancer and epithelial ovarian cancer: a guide for health professionals. 2006. Online. Available: http://www.nbocc.org.au/bestpractice/resources/BOG182_adviceaboutfamiliala.pdf [accessed 16.08.2009].

33. McPherson K, Steel CM, Dixon JM. ABC of breast diseases: breast cancer epidemiology, risk factors, and genetics. BMJ 2000; 321:624–628.

34. PDQ® Cancer Information Summary. National Cancer Institute, Bethesda, MD. Genetics of breast and ovarian cancer (PDQ®)—health professional. Date last modified 04/24/2009. Online. Available: http://www.cancer.gov/cancertopics/pdq/genetics/breast-and-ovarian/healthprofessional [accessed 15.05.2009].

35. National Cancer Institute. SEER Cancer Statistics Review, 1975–2005. Online. Available. http://seer.cancer.gov/csr/1975_2005/index.html [accessed 20.04.2009].

36. Dixon JM, Mansel RE. Congenital problems and aberrations of normal breast development and involution. In: Dixon JM (ed). ABC of breast diseases. London: British Medical Journal Publishing Group; 1995.

37. Thomas DB, Gao DL, Ray RM, et al. Randomized trial of breast self-examination in Shanghai: final results. J Natl Cancer Inst 2002; 94:1445–1457.

38. Schwartz K. Breast problems. In: Sloane PD, Slatt LM, Curtis P (eds), et al. Essentials of family medicine. 3rd edn. Baltimore: Williams and Wilkins; 1998; 337.

39. Torre, DL, Falorni A. Pharmacological causes of hyperprolactinemia. Ther Clin Risk Manag 2007; 3(5):929–951.

12

Screening women

OBJECTIVES

- To have an understanding of the principles behind screening and the criteria for a successful screening program
- To know the epidemiology of breast and cervical cancer
- To be aware of the controversies concerning breast cancer screening using mammography, clinical breast examination and breast self-examination
- To counsel women effectively about the benefits and harms of breast cancer screening
- To be able to counsel women effectively about cervical cancer prevention
- To understand the rationale behind Pap smear screening policies
- To manage reported Pap smear abnormalities
- To undertake screening for sexually transmissible infections (STIs)
- To know when it is appropriate to perform a pelvic examination
- To be able to respond appropriately to requests for ovarian cancer screening

THE PRINCIPLES OF SCREENING

What is screening?

Screening involves the systematic, population-wide recruitment and application of a test to symptom-free individuals considered to be at sufficient risk of a specified disorder to benefit from further investigation or direct preventive action.[1] In other words, screening can be defined as the application of diagnostic tests or procedures to asymptomatic people for the purpose of dividing them into two groups: those who have a condition that would benefit from early intervention and those who do not.[2]

What constitutes an ideal screening program?

Internationally recognised screening principles published under the auspices of the World Health Organization provide guidelines by which to evaluate screening programs. These are listed in Box 12.1.

The most crucial aspect of a screening program, however, is that early detection must enable early intervention in order to reduce morbidity

---

> **BOX 12.1 Criteria for the implementation of a screening program (From Hart[106])**
>
> **The disease**
> - It must be an important health problem.
> - The natural history of the disease must be understood (including development from latent to symptomatic stage).
> - There should be a recognisable or early symptomatic stage.
>
> **The screening test**
> - There must be a suitable test or examination of reasonable specificity and sensitivity.
> - Screening must be continuous.
> - The test must be acceptable by the population being screened.
>
> **Follow-up (intervention)**
> - Facilities must exist for assessment and treatment.
> - There must be an accepted form of effective treatment.
> - There must be an agreed policy on who to treat.
>
> **Economy**
> - The cost of screening patients (including diagnosis and treatment of patients diagnosed) must be economically balanced in relation to possible expenditure on medical care as a whole.

---

and mortality. If improved outcomes cannot be demonstrated, the rationale for screening is lost. Early diagnosis by itself does not justify a screening program. The only justification for a screening program is early diagnosis that leads to a measurable improvement in outcome.

BREAST CANCER SCREENING

Why should we bother screening for breast cancer?

Breast cancer is the most common malignancy in women, comprising 18% of all female cancers worldwide.[3] Approximately one million new cases are diagnosed in the world each year, with the average lifetime risk of breast cancer in the USA at birth being 12%, or one in eight.[4]

The risk of developing breast cancer increases with age, beginning in the fourth decade of life. The probability of developing invasive breast cancer over the following 10 years is 0.4% for women aged 30–39, 1.5% for women aged 40–49, 2.8% for women aged 50–59, and 3.6% for women aged 60–69.[5] This high prevalence, together with studies showing that most women with symptomatic breast cancer could not be cured by local surgery,[6,7] prompted the search for a mechanism to screen women for early disease.

While breast cancer mortality is clearly higher in the developed world, it is still the most common cancer in women in developing countries. The epidemiology of breast cancer is complex. Major risk factors include age, geographical variation, age at menarche and menopause, age at first pregnancy, family history, previous benign breast disease and radiation, fat intake and hormone use.[4]

Most mammographic screening programs recommend 2-yearly screening for women between the ages of 50 and 70 years.

As the evidence from research became apparent in the 1970s and 1980s, many countries established breast cancer screening guidelines and programs. The UK government initiated screening for breast cancer in 1987 by a single, medial–lateral oblique view of each breast every 3 years for all women aged 50–64 years. The breast screening program in Australia—BreastScreen—began in 1991 and provides two-view mammographic screening at 2-year intervals, mainly for women aged 50–69 years. The US Preventive

Services Task Force revised its recommendations in November 2009[8] and now recommends that:

- biennial screening mammography be carried out for women aged 50–74 years.
- the decision to start regular, biennial screening mammography before the age of 50 years should be an individual one and take patient context into account, including the patient's values regarding specific benefits and harms
- the current evidence is insufficient to assess the additional benefits and harms of screening mammography in women 75 years of age or older.

An example of a screening mammogram showing breast cancer is given in Figure 12.1.

Mammography is not routinely recommended in women between the ages of 40 and 49 because the breasts are more dense and the mammogram less effective at finding abnormalities in this age group.

What is so controversial about breast cancer screening?

Breast cancer screening remains one of the most controversial areas in medicine, despite significant research having been carried out in the last 40 years. This is particularly so because of the large amounts of government money being spent on wide-scale screening programs all over the world and because breast cancer is the most common female malignancy.

CASE STUDY: 'Like getting her breast slammed in a car door'

Judith was 53 years old. She attended her GP for a repeat prescription of her antihypertensive that she had been taking for 4 years. The GP, checking the history, noted that while Judith had had a routine smear the previous year there was no record of any mammogram results. She asked Judith if she had commenced breast cancer screening. Judith shook her head, answering that her friend who had had a mammogram told her it was like getting her breast slammed in a car door. The GP explained that a mammogram was slightly uncomfortable, as the X-ray required the breast to be compressed between two plates. She also told Judith that current government policy was to recommend mammographic screening to all women between the ages of 50 and 70 and went on to explain the pros and cons of the screening program. Judith said she would think about it and left.

The central controversy remains whether or not mammography is effective at preventing mortality from breast cancer. For those who believe the answer to this question to be yes, the controversies are over how a mammogram should be carried out, how screening programs should be established and what age groups should be targeted.

For those who believe that mammography is ineffective, questions remain about whether women should be actively encouraged and taught to engage in breast self-examination and whether or not clinical breast examination is an effective screening tool.

What is the evidence?

Until recently, and after heated controversy, there appeared to be general acceptance that the benefit of screening for breast cancer with mammography had been well documented.[9] Large randomised trials, covering a total of half a million women, had been carried out in New York, USA[10]; Edinburgh, Scotland[11]; Canada[12]; and Malmö[13], Kopparberg[14], Östergötland, Stockholm[15] and Göteborg[16] in Sweden.

These trials focused primarily on comparing mortality from breast cancer in those women invited to be screened with women who had had no intervention. The most quoted study supporting the efficacy of mammography is a meta-analysis published in *The Lancet* in 1993[17] of the Swedish trials. This review found the largest reduction of

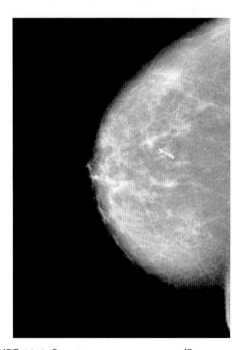

FIGURE 12.1 Breast cancer mammogram (From Silverberg[107])

breast cancer mortality (29%) in women aged 50–69 at randomisation. In women aged 40–49, a non-significant 13% reduction was demonstrated. Screening had only a marginal impact in women aged 70–74 years. Another review published in 1995 in the *Journal of the American Medical Association* was supportive of these figures, quoting a mortality benefit approaching 30% in women over 50 years of age 7–9 years from the start of the trials.[18]

The efficacy of regular mammography at reducing mortality from breast cancer is best estimated at about 15–20% in women aged between 50 and 70 years.

In 2000, another meta-analysis of the randomised controlled trials in mammography was published in *The Lancet*, this time by Gøtzsche & Olsen.[19] With the perilous title 'Is screening for breast cancer with mammography justifiable?', the authors reviewed the methodology of each of the eight trials in meticulous detail. They concluded that there were significant problems in the randomisation procedures of several of the trials and that only two of the eight trials were therefore valid. When the results of these two trials were then pooled, the outcome showed no significant difference in either total mortality or mortality secondary to breast cancer in those screened with mammography compared with controls. This work was subsequently included in the Cochrane database.[20] Nystrom et al updated their review of the Swedish RCTs and answered some of the criticisms levelled at these trials in the Cochrane review. Their results confirmed a 21% (RR = 0.79, 95% CI 0.70–0.89) reduction in breast cancer mortality overall, with the reduction being greatest in the 60–69 year age group (33%).[21] The most recent review[22] has determined that mammography brings about a reduction in breast cancer mortality of 20%; however, the effect is lower in the highest-quality trials and a more reasonable estimate is a 15% relative risk reduction. Based on the risk level of women in these trials, the absolute risk reduction was 0.05%.

Should a mammographic screening program carry the warning: 'screening can damage your health'?

Those who argue against mammography point out the fact that as a screening test it results in a significant amount of morbidity. There is an estimated 30% increase in overdiagnosis and overtreatment, or an absolute risk increase of 0.5%.[22] Overdiagnosis refers to the detection of abnormalities that will never cause symptoms or death during a patient's lifetime.

Overdiagnosis of cancer occurs when the cancer grows so slowly that the patient dies of other causes before it produces symptoms or when the cancer remains dormant (or regresses). Because doctors don't know which patients are overdiagnosed, we tend to treat them all. Overdiagnosis therefore results in unnecessary treatment.[23] For every 2000 women invited for screening throughout 10 years, only one will have her life prolonged. In addition, 10 healthy women who would not have been diagnosed if there had not been screening will be diagnosed as breast cancer patients and will be treated unnecessarily.[24]

Table 12.1 shows the morbidity generated by the UK National Health Service (NHS) screening program in 1 year (1997–98).[25] These data demonstrate that, while 5% of all women screened are recalled for further assessment, the number of cancers detected are 5.9/1000.

The high level of morbidity generated by mammography has been very well demonstrated by Elmore et al.[26] They performed a 10-year retrospective cohort study of breast cancer screening and diagnostic evaluations among 2400 women who were 40–69 years old. These women received a median of four mammograms and five clinical breast examinations per woman over the 10-year period. Of the women who were screened, 23.8% had at least one false-positive mammogram, 13.4% had at least one false-positive breast examination, and 31.7% had at least one false-positive result for either test.

TABLE 12.1 Screening activity generated by the UK NHS Breast Cancer Screening Program (1997–1998) (From NHS Breast Screening Programme Review[25])

Number of women invited	1,668,476
Acceptance rate (% of invited)	75.1%
Number of women screened (invited)	1,252,324
Number of women screened (self/GP referrals)	97,780
Total number of women screened	1,350,104
Number of women recalled for assessment	71,255
Per cent of women recalled for assessment	5.3%
Number of benign biopsies	2212
Number of cancers detected	7932
Number of cancers detected per 1000 women screened	5.9
Number of in situ cancers detected	1718
Number of invasive cancers less than 15 mm	3381

The estimated cumulative risk of a false-positive result was 49.1% (95% CI, 40.3–64.1%) after 10 mammograms and 22.3% (95% CI, 19.2%–27.5%) after 10 clinical breast examinations. The false-positive tests led to 870 outpatient appointments, 539 diagnostic mammograms, 186 ultrasound examinations, 188 biopsies and 1 hospitalisation. They estimated that among women who do not have breast cancer, 18.6% (95% CI, 9.8–41.2%) will undergo a biopsy after 10 mammograms, and 6.2% (95% CI, 3.7–11.2%) after 10 clinical breast examinations. For every $100 spent for screening, an additional $33 was spent to evaluate the false-positive results.

Studies have also documented the psychological distress caused by abnormal mammograms and being recalled for further tests. Women with high-suspicion mammograms had substantial mammography-related anxiety (47%) and worries about breast cancer (41%). Such worries affected the moods (26%) and daily functioning (17%) of these women, despite diagnostic evaluation that excluded malignancy.[27] In general, women have not been informed about the risk of false-positive results and the accompanying anxiety they generate,[28] nor have they been warned about the risk of receiving the diagnosis of carcinoma in situ.[29]

Many women undergoing mammographic screening will have a false-positive result, which will generate a significant amount of anxiety and morbidity as a result of unnecessary breast biopsies.

The other issue that should not be discounted when discussing mammography related morbidity is that many women find mammography very painful.[30]

Women generally exaggerate the benefits and are unaware of the harms of screening and invitations to women to participate in breast cancer screening reinforce this as they are information-poor and biased in favour of participation.[31] Box 12.2 lists the points that such invitations and related pamphlets and websites should emphasise to give a more accurate representation of the risks and benefits of mammography.[32]

What other issues need to be considered when evaluating whether mammography is worthwhile?

The other issues to consider, apart from the morbidity generated by the screening test, is the cost and whether or not the funds would be better directed elsewhere, such as to treatment or at least to research into better treatment. Some have suggested that this should be the case.[33]

BOX 12.2 Suggested contents of evidence-based leaflet on mammography (From Jorgensen and Gotzsche[32])

- It may be reasonable to attend for breast cancer screening with mammography, but it may also be reasonable *not* to attend because screening has both benefits and harms.
- If 2000 women are screened regularly for 10 years, one will benefit from the screening, as she will avoid dying from breast cancer.
- At the same time, 10 healthy women will, as a consequence, become cancer patients and will be treated unnecessarily. These women will have either a part of their breast or the whole breast removed, and they will often receive radiotherapy and sometimes chemotherapy.
- Furthermore, about 200 healthy women will experience a false alarm. The psychological strain until one knows whether it was cancer, and even afterwards, can be severe.

For those countries that have yet to develop and implement a screening program, it must be remembered that mammography is only the start of the process. There need to be in place proper facilities and treatment protocols to implement best practice in treatment if a country is going to go to the bother of screening in the first place. This requires trained personnel, equipment and ongoing quality assurance and evaluation programs to ensure that the program is delivering a quality service.

Are any other screening tests effective?

One that deserves attention is clinical breast examination—that is, examination carried out by specially trained doctors or nurses and carried out in the medical setting. When comparing mammography with clinical breast examination, it is worth considering the outcomes of mammography:

- 60% of cancers detected are >1 cm in size— clinical breast examination should detect these.
- 18% of cancers detected are in situ—it is uncertain whether these will progress to cancer.
- 22% of cancers are <1 cm in size.[34]

Clinical breast examination should be able to detect lesions >1 cm in size. It is likely that some cancers <1 cm in size will be detectable by clinical examination. This means that if mammography is to be more effective than clinical examination, it has to do so through those 22% of cancers <1 cm in size and the 18% in situ cancers. The question is whether these lesions are clinically significant in terms of causing morbidity or mortality.

The only study to address this issue has been the Canadian National Breast Screening Study.[35] It enrolled 40,000 women from 1980–1985 into either clinical breast examination and mammography or clinical breast examination alone. After 13 years of follow-up, there was no sign that mortality was lower in the mammography group.[35] The combined group had 107 and the examination-only group 105 deaths attributable to breast cancer, giving a cumulative rate ratio of 1.02 (95% CI, 0.78–1.33).

As far as pick-up rates of breast cancer is concerned:

- 622 invasive and 71 in situ breast carcinomas were detected in the mammography plus physical examination group
- 610 invasive and 16 in situ were ascertained in the physical examination-only group.

Although longer follow-up may reveal a benefit, currently there is no evidence to suggest that the detection of non-palpable cancers by mammography contributes to reducing mortality from breast cancer.[36] However, the study did highlight the morbidity brought about by mammography, with the rate of biopsy of benign lumps being three times higher in the combined examination/mammography group compared with that in the group undergoing clinical breast examination alone.[35]

In order to determine whether clinical breast examination can be implemented as a screening tool, however, more research needs to be carried out. This research must be a randomised, controlled trial comparing clinical breast examination on its own with no screening at all. Until this research is carried out, the US Preventive Services Task Force concludes that the evidence is insufficient to recommend for or against routine clinical breast examination (CBE) alone to screen for breast cancer.[37]

If the implementation of clinical breast examination is also controversial, then what about breast self-examination?

Women's health advocates have vigorously promoted this form of 'screening' as a way for women to take screening into their own hands. But is it effective?

Unfortunately, while breast self-examination (BSE) can detect symptomatic breast cancer at an earlier stage, it does not appear to have any influence on mortality. An American Cancer Society study compared 177,602 women who practised BSE during the preceding 13 years with 272,554 women who did not and found similar breast cancer death rates in the two groups.[38] The UK Trial of Early

Detection of Breast Cancer (TEDBC)[39] involved 300,000 women in eight health districts—two with mammographic screening centres, two where BSE was taught by trained nurses and four where neither form of intervention was available. At 16 years, the relative risk of death from breast cancer in women attending the two screening clinics was reduced by 27% (RR, 0.73; 95% CI, 0.63–0.84), but there was no risk reduction in the two BSE centres (RR, 0.99; 95% CI, 0.87–1.12).

Three randomised trials to evaluate the effect of BSE on breast cancer mortality have been undertaken in St Petersburg and Moscow[40] and in Shanghai.[41] The final results of the Shanghai study,[42] which included more than 250,000 women, found a similar incidence and an identical number of breast cancer deaths among BSE subjects and controls. BSE has however greatly increased biopsy rates, with the number of benign lesions detected in the BSE group being twice those of the controls. These findings indicate that women should be aware of their breasts as part of general body awareness and seek medical help when their breasts look or feel abnormal, but the promotion of regular BSE is not justified.[22]

A large randomised, controlled trial has shown no benefit from the regular practice of breast self-examination.

Conclusions

Since 1990 there *has* been a decrease in breast cancer mortality in the order of 30%.[43–45] The problem is that this decrease may either be due to screening and early diagnosis or it may be secondary to improved therapy, or both. When the original mammography trials were being undertaken, systemic therapy was not as widespread as it is today, when most women will receive some kind of adjuvant therapy.[46]

Screening programs now exist in 22 countries around the world. Millions of dollars are being spent on these programs. While the literature remains confused and conflicting, it is perhaps best to continue to encourage women to undergo mammography screening but to be aware that the benefits are more modest than originally believed. Patients need to understand the pros and cons and particularly that there maybe significant morbidity as a result of the screening process.

Hopefully, research in the areas of aetiology, optimising therapy and achieving better and longer survival will progress, so that breast cancer will no longer be the scourge that it is today.

Summary of key points

- Breast cancer is the most common malignancy in women.
- There is controversy as to whether screening mammography actually decreases mortality from breast cancer in women.
- Screening mammography results in significant morbidity for women resulting from false-positive scans.
- Further research is needed to determine whether clinical breast examination alone might be an effective screening tool.
- Breast self-examination does not result in decreased mortality from breast cancer.
- Over the last 10 years there has been a decrease in mortality from breast cancer in the order of 30%, but it is unclear if this is due to mammography or better treatment.

PREVENTING CERVICAL CANCER

How big a problem is cervical cancer?

Compared to breast cancer, cervical cancer is completely different: its aetiology, pathophysiology and development is much better understood and entirely different screening tests (compared with those for breast cancer) exist.

Since the advent and widespread use of the Papanicolaou (Pap) smear—a test that detects asymptomatic preinvasive lesions at the earliest stages—the incidence of cervical cancer has dramatically decreased. With the introduction of the National Cervical Screening Program in Australia, new cases of cervical cancer among women of all ages almost halved, from 13.2 new cancers per 100,000 women in 1991 to 6.9 in 2005. Mortality also halved, from 4 deaths per 100,000 women in 1991 to 2 in 2005.[13] However, in many parts of the developing world, cervical cancer continues to cause significant morbidity and mortality.

The greatest burden of disease occurs in developing countries, where unfortunately there are no organised cervical screening programs. In terms of absolute number, the Asian region has an incidence of 265,884 cases of cervical cancer per year.[47] In contrast, Australia had 734 new cases of cervical cancer and 221 deaths in 2005.[48]

Human papillomavirus (HPV) has now been causally related to cervical cancer,[49] with HPV DNA detected in at least 95% of cervical cancers (of which HPV types 16 and 18 are the most commonly isolated[50]). The association between persistent HPV DNA detection and cervical cancer is more than 10 times the association between smoking and lung cancer.[51]

CASE STUDY: 'I thought if you weren't having sex you didn't need to have a Pap smear.'

Maude was 72 years old; she was a very active lady who enjoyed her tennis and was involved in community groups. She had been widowed for the last 25 years and was surprised when asked by her new GP when the last time was that she had had a smear. 'Oh, I haven't bothered with them since my husband died. I thought if you weren't having sex, you didn't need to have them any more', she replied. The GP explained that guidelines recommended that women should continue to have regular smears until the age of 70 and that, as Maude hadn't had a smear in more than 25 years, she should have at least one. Two weeks later Maude returned for her smear and was pleasantly surprised at how easy it was. 'They used to hurt when I had them all that time ago,' she mused. Another 2 weeks passed and the GP found that she had to call Maude in to see her for the results. The smear had shown suspected cancer of the cervix. Maude had not had any symptoms and seemed genuinely surprised at the result. The GP explained that she would need to see a gynaecologist for confirmation of the smear result and organised an urgent appointment. One month later Maude came back to see her GP with a bunch of flowers. She had had surgery to remove the tumour and was requiring further treatment, but wanted to thank her GP for convincing her to have the smear and for 'saving her life'. Maude's case illustrates the importance of undertaking smears in 'underscreened' women—those who are past their reproductive years and women of non-English-speaking backgrounds.

For more information about the natural history of HPV infection see Box 12.3 and Figure 12.2 (p 204).

How can cervical cancer be prevented?

Until recently, the most effective mechanism for cervical cancer prevention was organised cervical cancer screening with a Pap smear. Pap screening detects cellular changes in the cervix caused by persistent HPV infection. If HPV infection is left untreated, it has been estimated that about 30% of women with high-grade lesions would develop cancer over a 30-year period.[58] Detection of high-grade lesions through Pap screening allows treatment prior to the development of cancer and as such is a secondary prevention strategy.

The recent introduction of HPV vaccination now offers a primary preventive approach. Two HPV vaccines, exist:

- the bivalent Cervarix (HPV types 16 and 18)
- the quadrivalent Gardasil (HPV types 16, 18, 6 and 11).

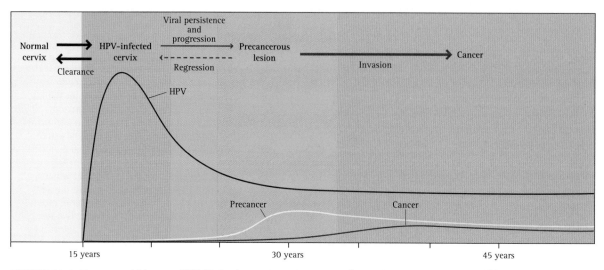

FIGURE 12.2 The natural history of HPV infection and cervical cancer (From Schiffman and Castle.[108] Copyright © 2005 Massachusetts Medical Society. All rights reserved.)

HPV types 16 and 18, worldwide, are responsible for about 70% of cervical cancer cases, 50% of high-grade precancerous lesions and 25% of low-grade lesions.[59] HPV 6 and 11 infections are associated with most genital warts and around 8–10% of low-grade cervical lesions.[60]

Who should receive the HPV vaccine?

Administering the vaccines to the pre-adolescent population maximises the chances of most of the population achieving immunity before HPV exposure (i.e. before sexual activity commences). As a more robust immune response to vaccination is achieved at this age, protection is likely to endure through the years of maximal exposure. However, extended follow-up of populations in clinical trials will help to determine whether a booster is required.[61]

Favourable estimates of the cost-effectiveness of a catch-up immunisation program for women up to the age of 26 years in economic models adapted to Australian data led to federal government funding of a universal immunisation program for girls aged 12 and 13 in Australia, with a 2-year catch-up program for older adolescent and young adult women.[57] This catch-up program, run through schools and general practitioners, ended in 2009. Australia was the first country in the world to roll out a national HPV vaccination program and has established a register of women who received the vaccine. This register will facilitate cross-referencing of vaccination data with information from cervical cytology (Pap smear) or cervical cancer registries for evaluation purposes in the future.

BOX 12.3 HPV infection: natural history

- Up to 75% of women will become infected with human papillomavirus (HPV) at some stage in their lives,[52] usually in the first few years after becoming sexually active. (One study showed a cumulative incidence of HPV of about 40% in women after sexual debut or after a new sexual partner, over a 24-month follow-up.[53])
- Most infections are subclinical[52] and transient,[54] with the immune system clearing detectable virus over time.
- Median duration of detectable HPV infection has ranged from 8 to 17 months in studies.[54]
- High-risk HPV (such as HPV16 & 18) persist longer on average than low risk HPV (such as HPV 6 and 11).[54]
- Most infections, including those with high-risk types, do not lead to dysplasia and will clear spontaneously within 2 years, leaving no residual detectable HPV DNA.[55]
- Women who do develop cytologically or histologically detectable cervical lesions in response to HPV infection will eventually mount an effective cell-mediated immune response, which causes lesion regression.[56]
- In a small proportion of women, persistent infection continues; this is linked to the development of high-grade cervical lesions and cervical cancer.[57]

Both Cervarix and Gardasil are registered in Australia for women up to the age of 45. Many question the utility of vaccinating women who are already been sexually active and therefore have already been exposed to HPV. However, the following questions remain to be conclusively addressed[61]:

- whether an older woman newly infected with HPV has a risk of cervical cancer similar to that of a younger woman
- whether the vaccine provides protection against new infection at this age
- whether new infections occur in older age
- whether the vaccine has a role in preventing reactivation of latent infection.

And until these issues are resolved, vaccination in women up until the age of 45 can be considered to be like taking out 'insurance'. Advice for 'older' women related to HPV vaccination is given in Box 12.4.

Should women be tested for HPV prior to vaccination?

No. While women who receive the vaccination who are already sexually active are likely to have been exposed to one or more strains of HPV, it is unlikely they have been exposed to both HPV 16 and 18 and therefore the vaccine will still provide them with some protection. Currently there are no validated, approved and readily available HPV type-specific polymerase chain reaction or serological assays.[61] Were they available and used, the process would add considerable expense to an already expensive intervention.[61]

What is the role of HPV vaccination in women who have already had dysplasia?

The HPV vaccine is a prophylactic, not therapeutic, vaccine. It will therefore have no effect on current HPV infection or current or previous dysplasia. Its aim is to prevent the acquisition of new HPV (primarily types 16 and 18, although there is some evidence of cross-protection with other strains).[62]

CERVICAL CANCER SCREENING

Which women should be screened for cervical cancer?

One of the most basic questions to ask when implementing a screening test is who should have it done? To answer this question one needs to have an understanding of the risk factors and

> **BOX 12.4 Advice about HPV vaccination for women up to the age of 45 years (From Skinner et al[61])**
>
> **Are human papillomavirus (HPV) vaccines appropriate for sexually experienced women?**
> Even with increasing age and numbers of sexual partners, most women do not have evidence of past exposure to HPV types 16 or 18. Older women have robust immune responses to the bivalent HPV vaccine, and so should derive benefit from the vaccine if exposed to HPV 16 or 18 in the future.
>
> **Is it too late to vaccinate a woman if she has a history of HPV disease shown by clinical evidence such as an abnormal Pap test or genital warts?**
> Evidence to date indicates that vaccination will have no effect on current or prevalent disease due to any HPV type. However, vaccination would ensure protection from future infection with oncogenic HPV types covered by the vaccine.
>
> **Can a woman's ongoing risk of acquiring HPV be determined?**
> Future risk of exposure is difficult to determine accurately on the basis of past and current sexual history. This is because of patterns and changes in sexual behaviour through life, the potential for transmission through successive monogamous relationships, and inaccuracies in predictions about concurrency of sexual partners.
>
> **Should there be an age cut-off for vaccination?**
> As a woman ages, natural immunity to HPV wanes, but also the incidence of new HPV infection decreases and the time to develop cancerous lesions from HPV must be balanced against the likelihood of other age-related diseases. Both the bivalent and quadrivalent vaccines are licensed for use in women up to 45 years.

pathophysiology of cervical cancer. Traditionally we have been told that all women who are having or have ever had sexual intercourse are at risk of cervical cancer, the reason being that they may have acquired HPV as a result of their sexual activity. This is slightly simplistic, however, especially when considering whether virgins, lesbians and women in monogamous relationships should be screened.

The recent introduction of polymerase chain reaction (PCR) testing has revealed that HPV infections are much more common among young, asymptomatic women than previously suspected. The site-specificity of genital HPV led to the assumption that HPVs were primarily transmitted by sexual contact. However, since HPVs have been detected in virgins, infants and children, and after juvenile laryngeal papillomatosis was shown to be caused by these viruses, there has been acknowledgment of the fact that HPV may be transmitted by other non-sexual routes as well.[63] Despite this, women who have never engaged in sexual intercourse with a man have a minimal risk of developing squamous cell cancer of the cervix.

At what age should cervical cancer screening commence?

The question of when to start screening is slightly more complex, requiring an understanding of the natural history of HPV infection. In Australia the recommendation is to commence screening at 18–20 years of age or 2 years after first intercourse, whichever is later. In America screening guidelines advocate annual smears from the age of 18 until consecutive smears are normal, after which time screening can revert to 2-yearly.

As seen in Figure 12.3, between 20% and 25% of women have acquired HPV in their 20s. There is a steep decline in HPV prevalence up to the age of 35, and after the age of 55 the prevalence is <5%.

In most women, there is resolution of the infection after a year or two.[64] This is explained in Figure 12.4. The incubation period is in the order of 1–8 months, after which time the first lesion/s may appear; over the next 6–12 months there is initially growth of the virus, followed by host containment after the immune response is mobilised. Most women then clear the virus, with a small group having persistent or recurrent disease.

The highest risk of testing positive for HPV is in the first few years after initiation of intercourse. Thereafter, HPV positivity declines, reflecting the transient nature of most HPV infections due to immune suppression.

If the ramifications of this for cervical cancer screening are then considered, many abnormalities are likely to be found in young women who have recently acquired HPV. Often we are detecting and treating areas infected with HPV before the immune system has had the chance to respond.

What this also means is that older women who have cleared any HPV they may have had while younger and who have a history of normal smears are probably at very low risk of cervical cancer.

It is for these reasons that the UK NHS Cervical Screening Programme[65] invites women to commence screening only from the age of 25 and offers screening at different intervals, depending on age (Table 12.2). This means that women are provided with a more targeted and effective screening program.

At what age can screening for cervical cancer stop?

In Australia the recommendation is that screening may cease at the age of 70 if the last two smears have been normal. In the UK, the corresponding age is 64.

Recent publications have suggested, however, that women can be withdrawn from the screening program at an earlier age to that currently recommended,[66] saving them from unnecessary screening and anxiety and saving the government money. The age proposed for withdrawal is 50.[67] Although over half of all cases of invasive cervical cancer occur among women aged over 50,[68] few have been found in women with histories of regular smear tests with normal results. While there is

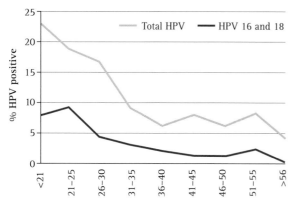

FIGURE 12.3 HPV prevalence by age (From ARHP[64])

TABLE 12.2 Screening intervals of the UK NHS screening program (From National Cervical Screening Program[79])

Age group (years)	Frequency of screening
25	First invitation
25–49	3-yearly
50–64	5-yearly
65+	Only screen those who have not been screened since age 50 or who have had recent abnormal tests.

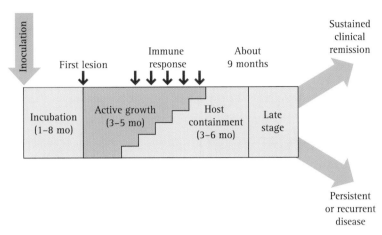

FIGURE 12.4 The natural history of HPV infection (From ARHP[64])

evidence that women with certain types of HPV infection are at high risk of developing high-grade precancerous lesions,[50,69,70] the risk of acquiring new HPV infection is believed to decrease as women get older, so postmenopausal women without previous HPV infection may have little risk of developing invasive cancer.[71] Therefore, by taking account of recent smear test results or the results of HPV tests, a sizeable population of older women at low risk of cervical disease might be identified, and their early removal from the screening program would have little impact on the incidence of invasive cancer.

What should the interval for cervical cancer screening be set at?

Many of us are faced with patients who are extremely anxious and request smears on a yearly basis or even 6-monthly. It is important to explain to them that a yearly screening policy would only reduce the cumulative incidence of cervical cancer by 1%, while at the same time doubling the cost to the government.

Annual smears have the potential to prevent only another 1% of cancers in addition to those prevented by 2-yearly smears.[72]

The extra effort needed to conduct a yearly screening program would be better spent in trying to encourage underscreened women to enter the program and have regular smears than by reducing the screening interval. In the future, given the advent of large cohorts of women being vaccinated against HPV and the likelihood of using HPV as the triage tool rather than the smear result, it is likely that screening intervals will be extended to 3–5 years, but until official guidelines are altered women should continue to have regular smears every 2 years.

Which cervical sampling tools should GPs use to optimise the quality of Pap smears?

Figure 12.5 (p 208) illustrates the wide variety of cervical sampling tools available for use in general practice. Which tools ensure the best-quality smear? Previously, wooden spatulas and cotton swabs have been used to collect cervical cells. A meta-analysis published in *The Lancet*[73] looked at this issue and came up with the following results. Wooden spatulas are not recommended now that plastic ones are available, as the former trap cells, reducing the amount transferred to the slide. The same reasoning is behind the abandonment of use of cotton swabs. When trying to choose between spatulas, the ones with an extended tip are superior for collecting endocervical cells, with an odds ratio of 2.25 (CI 2.06–2.44). A spatula alone is inferior to a spatula used in conjunction with an endocervical sampling device. The best combination by far is a spatula and cytobrush.

How can the number of false-negative smears be reduced?

One of the major issues in Pap smear screening is the incidence of false-negative smears. A number of measures can be put in place to reduce these. First, Pap smears must be performed correctly, using good technique. This entails visualising the

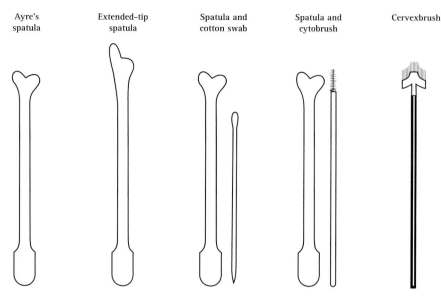

FIGURE 12.5 Cervical sampling tools

cervix and removing any mucus or blood covering it before taking the smear. Good technique also requires sampling the transformation zone, from which most squamous cervical cancer arises, and therefore the use of correct instruments. Figure 12.6 gives examples of appearances of the cervix.

The next step involves having good quality assurance measures in place at the laboratory level. This involves setting workload limitations on cytopathologists so that they screen no more than 100 slides a day and ensuring that at least 10% of those smears read as 'normal' are manually rescreened.

False-negative smears can be reduced mainly by improving Pap smear technique and by improving quality assurance in laboratories.

Another suggestion to improve the quality of Pap smear results is to use automated rescreening. This involves passing the slides through a computer that identifies areas of potential abnormality for examination by a cytopathologist.

What is automated rescreening?

The goals of automated rescreening are to improve Pap smear interpretation, increase laboratory productivity and increase the detection of cancerous precursors. While automation and computerisation have the potential to extend human resources and decrease fatigue in a very labour-intensive profession, it does add considerably to the cost of screening and actually involves manual rescreening anyway. Evaluation of this technology has found that, while automated rescreening does result in detection of 7% more abnormalities compared with manual screening, most of these are low-grade lesions of questionable significance.[74] The technology can also be used as the primary screen before a cytopathologist sees the slide. In this scenario, it may be possible for computers to separate those cases that require manual screening from those that do not and thus significantly reduce the manual screening load in a laboratory.

What is liquid-based cytology?

Liquid-based cytology (LBC) involves placement of the Pap smear instruments in solution so that the cells fall off into the fluid. The fluid is then spun down to remove mucus and blood and other debris and the cells are placed as a monolayer on the slide, providing an easier specimen for the cytologist to read.

Fluid-based technology makes excellent smears and can eliminate smears that are unsatisfactory or less than optimal because of blood or inflammation. The collection of cervical cytology samples into an LBC medium also provides the opportunity for reflex-testing of a range of pathogens, including HPV, *Chlamydia trachomatis* and *Neisseria gonorrhoeae*.

The studies that have compared monolayer slides to conventional smears have shown monolayers to be more sensitive and better at predicting the presence of dysplasia.[75] However, many problems exist with its use

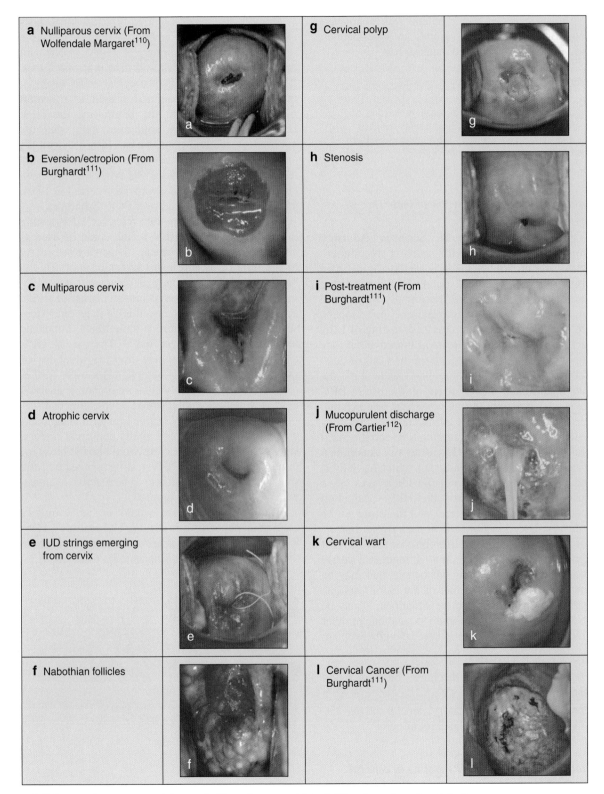

FIGURE 12.6 Appearances of the cervix (From Papscreen Victoria[109], unless otherwise stated)

as a primary screening tool. Problems with monolayers relate to the detection of glandular abnormalities, scanty smears and increased material costs.

Liquid-based cytology and automated rescreening may decrease the rate of false-negative smears reported, but the clinical significance of the abnormalities these methods pick up is questionable.

Should GPs recommend the use of these two technologies to women?

In Australia, the Medical Services Advisory Committee (responsible for making recommendations about which medical technologies gain public funding) reviewed the evidence regarding these technologies in 2009. Essentially they found that, in comparison to conventional pap smears, LBC and automated (computerised) testing of LBC specimens are safe and at least as effective but they are not currently recommended on the basis of cost-effectiveness. Their decision was made with the understanding that the evidence on the use of LBC was available mainly through overseas research and its use in the UK, Europe, Canada and the USA; they felt that assessment of international research needed to take into account the effectiveness of Australia's cervical cancer screening program, which has halved rates of cervical cancer, and the likely preventive impact of the recently introduced HPV vaccination program.[76] These technologies will therefore not be publically funded in Australia at the current time.

It is essential, therefore, to emphasise that the most important aspect of screening is regular 2-yearly smears and that any additional benefit that may be gained from carrying out one of the extra tests is a small increment only. In some situations, it may be reasonable to encourage women to have one or other of these tests. Such situations[77] are when the woman:

- is extremely anxious
- has excessive mucus, discharge or even blood present
- has recurrent 'inflammatory' smears or unsatisfactory results due to a paucity of cells.

What roles are there for HPV testing in cervical cancer screening?

One of the most exciting areas in cervical cancer screening currently in development is the use of HPV testing as either a screening, triage or management tool.

One of the most commonly used HPV tests is the hybrid capture technique (Digene). It is a second-generation commercial HPV DNA kit that detects five low-risk and nine high-risk types. It is fairly simple, with a cervical swab taken of the transformation zone and placed in transport medium (Fig 12.7). In the laboratory, the HPV DNA is 'captured' by antibodies and, after the addition of alkaline phosphatase, light is given off and measured. The hybrid capture 2 test is the only test for cervical high-risk HPV types that has been clinically validated and approved by the US FDA, and is therefore preferred over PCR techniques.

There are several possible roles for HPV testing in cervical screening. HPV testing could be used as either an adjunct to Pap smears (to increase sensitivity of the test) or as a primary screening tool. This is being looked at increasingly for older women, as HPV infection in young women is more a marker of sexual activity, whereas persistence of HPV in an older (less sexually active population) is more likely to indicate increased cervical cancer risk.[78] The use of HPV testing alongside smears may offer the possibility of extending the screening interval. However, further research is necessary, as well as an economic analysis to show whether or not it would be cost-effective.

Another role for HPV testing is in the management or triage of borderline and mildly abnormal smears. HPV positivity in these cases would be the basis for rapid referral. Where HPV testing is negative, the smear results are more likely to be reactive changes, which can probably be ignored.

Another possible use would be as a quality assurance mechanism in cytology laboratories. Here it could be used as a marker of potential high-grade disease, requiring those smears to be rescreened.

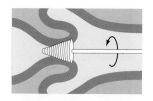
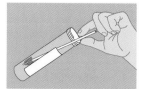
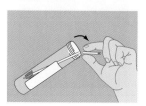
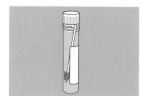

FIGURE 12.7 Taking a sample for the hybrid capture HPV test (From Papscreen Victoria and Victorian Cytology Service[109])

A fourth role is in post-treatment surveillance of women who have had high-grade dysplasias diagnosed and treated, to determine more quickly whether or not there has been complete excision of the lesion and to reduce the surveillance if there has. While almost all these lesions are HPV-positive initially, HPV-negativity after treatment is a very good indication that the disease has been completely excised. If they remain HPV-positive, there's probably residual disease that needs attention.

HPV testing as a test of cure has been adopted in current Australian Cervical Screening Guidelines (see below), but its use as a triage tool or as a primary screen is still awaiting further evaluation.

HPV testing in cervical cancer screening may have many roles, the most established of which is triage of borderline and mildly abnormal smears.

What impact has our understanding of HPV and its role in cervical cancer had on current cervical screening programs?

In 2005, in response to our increasing understanding of the role of HPV in cervical cancer, Australia's cervical screening guidelines were changed. The major changes are listed in Box 12.5 and the current screening pathway is represented by an algorithm in Figure 12.8 (p 212).

Will the cervical screening program as we know it change as a result of the introduction of HPV vaccination?

Despite HPV vaccination being in place, cervical screening in one form or another will remain necessary, and it is in fact very important to stress to women that they should continue to have regular Pap smears even if they have been vaccinated. This is because:

- the vaccine does not protect against all strains of HPV. While 50% of high-grade lesions are due to HPV types 16 and 18 (the strains found in the vaccine), 50% are not.[80]
- The sexually active women who received the vaccine may already have been infected with HPV and therefore a proportion of these may develop dysplasia and are at risk of cancer.

In the future, it is likely that HPV vaccination and testing may allow the onset of cervical screening to be delayed, lengthen the intervals between screens and shorten the total duration of screening.

BOX 12.5 Six key areas of change in Australian cervical screening guidelines (From National Cervical Screening Program[79])

1. A new terminology system is now used for Pap smear cytology.
2. Repeat a Pap smear for most women with low-grade squamous change.
3. Do not treat women with biopsy proven CIN1.
4. Refer all women with atypical glandular cell reports for colposcopy.
5. Use HPV testing as test of cure following treatment for high-grade abnormalities.
6. Do not report normal endometrial cells in postmenopausal women.

As mentioned above, our method of screening may change too. Meanwhile GPs should follow national guidelines and watch this space for future developments.

Why do cervical cancer and Pap smears attract so much media attention?

Despite the clear success of Pap smear screening programs on a macro scale, on a micro scale a lot of attention is given to those unfortunate women who develop cervical cancer despite being screened. These women often have aggressive tumours that seem to develop in the interval between their screening tests. In some cases, the 'failure' to detect the cancer has been due to a laboratory error. However, these cases are very rare.[81]

Up to 85% of women who develop cervical cancer have either not had a smear or have a history of inadequate screening in the past 10 years.

Conclusions

In conclusion, with the advent of HPV vaccination primary prevention of cervical cancer is now available, as well as secondary prevention through organised cervical screening programs. Like all screening programs, cervical screening relies on high levels of recruitment, an effective screening tool with high sensitivity and specificity, and effective follow-up mechanisms. When considering the use of measures to optimise the screening tool itself, it is probably more important to take smears

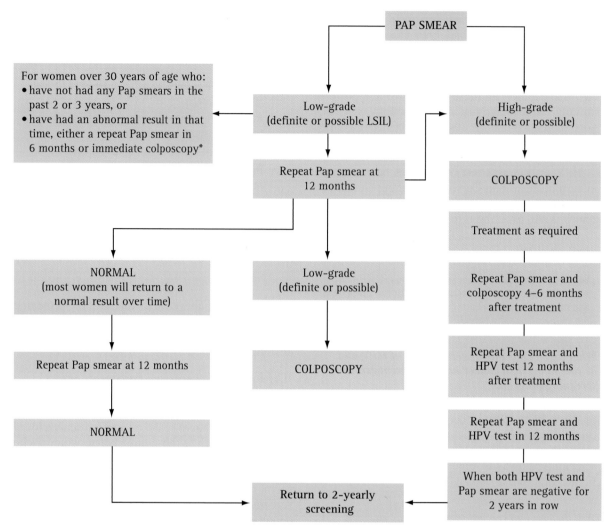

FIGURE 12.8 Pathway for the management of abnormal smear results (From National Cervical Screening Program[114])

regularly every 2–5 years across whole population than to use the newer devices. HPV testing is going to play an increasingly important role in cervical screening in the future and, while at present it is recommended only as a test of cure, other uses are still being evaluated. From a GP's perspective, we need to ensure that we use good technique and that we are using a laboratory with good quality control. Finally, very stringent measures for follow-up and management of abnormalities need to be put in place so that when and if abnormalities are detected they are followed up and managed appropriately.

Summary of key points
- HPV vaccination allows for the primary prevention of cervical cancer.

- Current Australian cervical screening guidelines recommend that Pap screening commences at approximately 18–20 years of age and continues every 2 or more years on a regular basis.
- The majority of cervical cancers occur in women with poor screening histories.
- HPV testing may emerge as either an adjunct to or a replacement for Pap smears in the future.

Tips on taking pap smears
What should be used to lubricate a speculum when taking a Pap smear?

The speculum should be lubricated with warm water. The use of any other material may result in contamination of the smear. This may make it difficult for the cytopathologist to read the slide.

What strategies can be used to better visualise the cervix?

Sometimes when undertaking a Pap smear, it can be difficult to visualise the cervix (Fig 12.9). If this occurs, the following advice should be followed:

- It is best to remember that the cervix is located in the distal sixth of the anterior wall of the vagina, not at the vaginal apex (Fig 12.10).
- When using a duckbill speculum, the handle of the speculum is best directed downward in order to visualise the cervix (Fig 12.10). In patients with an anteverted uterus, attempting to insert the speculum with the handle directed upwards

makes cervical exposure difficult, as the long blade pushes the cervix out of view while the short blade fails to control bulging of the cul de sac and upper rectal wall.

- Tilting the pelvis upwards by placing a small cushion under the patient's buttocks will assist the practitioner to see the cervix.
- A broad-billed speculum may assist with women who have a cystocoele or rectocoele.
- It may be helpful to wipe away any mucus from the cervix with a cotton bud, so as to better visualise the cervix and in order to collect cervical cells and not just mucus for the smear.

Why is it important to sample from the transformation zone when taking a Pap smear?

The transformation zone is the area on the cervix where columnar cells lining the endocervical canal undergo metaplasia to become squamous cells (Fig 12.11). Squamous cell carcinoma almost always arises in the transformation zone and it is therefore vital that cells are taken from this area when taking a Pap smear (Fig 12.12, p 214).

How and when should fixative be applied?

Air-drying can occur within 30 seconds (especially in summer); therefore, it is important to fix the smear immediately after the cells have been transferred

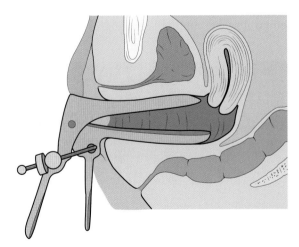

FIGURE 12.9 Visualisation of a normal cervix and vagina prior to taking a smear

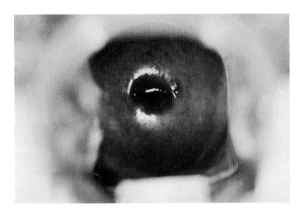

FIGURE 12.10 Location of the cervix in the distal sixth of the anterior wall of the vagina, not at the apex of the vagina

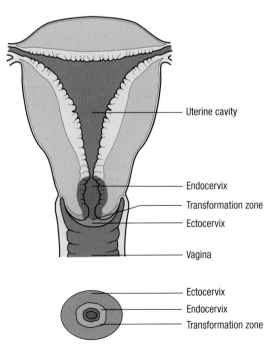

Uterine cavity

Endocervix

Transformation zone

Ectocervix

Vagina

Ectocervix

Endocervix

Transformation zone

FIGURE 12.11 The transformation zone

onto the slide (thus, before removing the speculum from the patient and clearing away the instruments). Most clinicians use an aerosol or pump-action alcohol spray. Ideally two brisk sprays should be given from a distance of 10–15 cm. Spraying closer than this can cause freezing artifact.

Is an ectropion the same as an eversion and what is it exactly?

An 'ectropion' is the same as an 'eversion', which is the same as an 'erosion'. It is present when endocervical cells are present and visible on the surface of the cervix. They have a velvety, red appearance, in contrast to the pink plastic-looking cells of the ectocervix. The endocervical cells present within the boundaries of an ectropion are more friable than those found on the ectocervix and therefore tend to bleed more easily. Hormonal status impacts on whether or not an ectropion is present in an individual woman. For example, pregnant women and those who are using a combined oral contraceptive pill are more likely to have a cervical ectropion, while in menopause the squamocolumnar junction may recede into the endocervical canal.

Summary of key points

- When taking a smear, water is the only medium that should be used to lubricate a speculum.
- The cervix is located at the end of the anterior vaginal wall, not at the apex of the vagina.
- Squamous cell carcinoma almost always arises from the transformation zone, so it is vital to sample from this area when taking a Pap smear.
- Fixative should be applied immediately after a smear is taken.
- An ectropion is a normal variation occurring when endocervical cells appear on the surface of the cervix.

Pap smears in special situations

Do lesbians need Pap smears?

Previous studies of lesbians and bisexual women have suggested that negative experiences with healthcare practitioners, combined with misinformation about the health needs of this diverse population, have led to an underutilisation of medical services. This group of women may have risk factors for cervical cancer, including multiple past or current sexual partners (both male and female), early age at first coitus, history of sexually transmissible infections, and cigarette smoking. In one study, a quarter of respondents had not had a Pap test within the last 3 years, including 39 (7.6%) who had never had a Pap test. Women who reported that their healthcare providers were more knowledgeable and sensitive to lesbian issues were significantly more likely to have had a Pap test within the last year, even when controlling for age, education, income and insurance status.[82] Lesbians are at risk of cervical cancer and should receive routine cervical screening.[83] The quality of clinician–patient interactions strongly influences care-seeking within the population sampled. One Australian paper has recommended that Pap smears should be taken every 2 years in lesbian patients.[84]

Should Pap smears be taken in pregnant women?

Pap smears may be taken during pregnancy if indicated, but use of a cytobrush should be avoided because of the risk of rupturing the membranes and chorioamnionitis.

How should a GP undertake a smear in a woman with moderate to severe vaginal atrophy?

It is still important that these women are screened, but in order to achieve this the vaginal atrophy will need to be treated with a local oestrogen preparation. Either ovestin (cream or pessaries) or vagifem (pessaries) can be used each night for a week or two and ceased at least 2 days before the procedure is reattempted.

Do women who have had a hysterectomy still need a Pap smear?

Because of the low prevalence (about 0.13–0.15%) of vaginal dysplasia after a hysterectomy for benign disease, routine screening is not felt to be

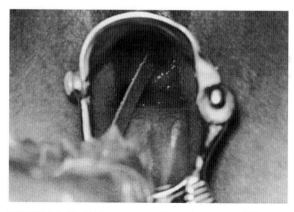

FIGURE 12.12 Taking a smear (From James et al[113])

necessary. If the cervix is still present, the usual guidelines apply. There is evidence, however, that women who have had a hysterectomy because of cancer of the cervix or carcinoma in situ do benefit from routine screening of the vaginal vault.[85] Papanicolaou testing does not help detect ovarian cancer.

Do women with a current or past history of genital warts require more frequent Pap smears?

HPV types 6 or 11 usually cause visible anogenital warts, and lesions may appear on the vulva, cervix, vagina, penis, scrotum, urethra and anus. Intra-anal warts are seen predominantly in patients who have had receptive anal intercourse. These warts are distinct from perianal warts, which can occur in men and women who have not had receptive anal sex. HPV types 6 and 11 have also been associated with conjunctival, nasal, oral and laryngeal warts. HPV types 6 and 11 have low oncogenic potential and are rarely associated with invasive squamous cell carcinoma in the genital tract.

Other anogenital HPV types (e.g. 16, 18, 31, 33 and 35) are strongly associated with vulval, penile, anal and cervical intraepithelial neoplasia (CIN) and squamous cell carcinoma. These oncogenic types are found occasionally in visible genital warts and have also been associated with vulvar intraepithelial neoplasia (VIN), penile intraepithelial neoplasia (PIN) and anal intraepithelial neoplasia (AIN).

Women with a current or past history of genital warts may go on to develop CIN, but it would be extremely rare for the visible wart type to be responsible for this development. If the woman did develop CIN, it would most likely be due to concurrent infection with a different subtype that does not cause visible warts. For this reason, women with a current or past history of genital warts do not need more frequent smears.

Summary of key points

- Lesbians require Pap smear screening.
- Pap smears may be taken during pregnancy, but a cytobrush should not be used.
- In a woman with atrophic vaginitis, oestrogen pessaries or cream should be used for at least a week and ceased a couple of days before a smear is attempted.
- Women with a current or past history of genital warts do not require more frequent smears.

Management of reported Pap smear abnormalities

What should a GP do if no endocervical cells are seen on a patient's Pap smear report?

An endocervical sampling rate of 75% is a reasonable expectation for GPs taking smears. However, collection of an endocervical component is not possible in all women, particularly in pregnant women, postmenopausal women and women who have had previous ablative or excisional treatment for a cervical lesion. In these cases, the rate may even be considerably lower.

It is recommended that negative smears be repeated at 2 years, irrespective of the endocervical status. Six randomised, controlled trials[86–91] have failed to demonstrate that increasing the proportion of smears with an endocervical component is associated with increasing the detection of high-grade abnormalities. A longitudinal study of women whose index smear was not reported to include an endocervical component did not show a higher rate of abnormality at the next screening when an endocervical component was present.[92] Analysis of data from the Victorian Cytology Service[93] shows that while the proportion of smears with an endocervical component increased from around 50% during 1987–89 to around 75% during 1990–91, no parallel increase in the rate of reporting of high-grade epithelial lesions occurred.

What if inflammation is seen on the smear?

Inflammation seen by cytologists may be due to thrush or a sexually transmissible infection (STI). *Chlamydia* is the most common bacterial STI in women and is particularly prevalent in younger women who have recently had a change in sexual partner. Bacterial vaginosis, while not an inflammatory condition, is also associated with mucus production that may make the collection of a quality smear more difficult.

Removing excessive mucus means that the smear is more likely to contain cervical cells and ordering fluid cytology such as the ThinPrep test will also remove many of the inflammatory cells.

If definite or possible low-grade change is found on the smear (LSIL), what is the next step?

Low-grade cytology mostly represents HPV infection of squamous cells. As such, the guidelines recommend repeating the Pap smear at 12 months in order to give an opportunity for the HPV to clear. If the woman is 30+ years and has no negative cytology in previous 2–3 years, repeat the Pap smear in 6 months or order immediate colposcopy. Colposcopy is also recommended for women <30 years who have a second possible or definite LSIL 12 months after the first. Colposcopy, with directed biopsy where indicated, ensures accurate diagnosis, whereas Pap smear results are only a screen. The Victorian Cervical Cytology Registry has documented that 10% of women with a cervical smear report of HPV change (LSIL) have been found to have CIN 2 or 3 on biopsy. Of the women whose smear report was HPV and who had a biopsy, 0.4% (2/508) were found to have invasive cancer. Both of these women had abnormal bleeding at the time of the cytology report of HPV.[94]

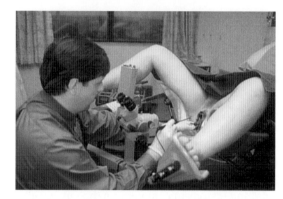

FIGURE 12.13 Colposcopy clinic (From James et al[113])

What advice should be given to women who are reported to have high-grade changes (possible or definite HSIL) on their smear?

Current recommendations are that all women with HSIL on a smear should be referred for colposcopy. With biopsy-confirmed CIN 2, the cited regression rate varies from 35% to 57%, with a mean of 45%. Some 16–49% of lesions have been shown to persist, with a mean of 32%, while 18–27% progress to CIN 3, with a mean of 23%.[95,96] Current recommendations are for women with HSIL to be referred for colposcopic assessment and directed biopsy where indicated, with definitive treatment once the lesion is confirmed.

What does a colposcopy involve?

Colposcopy is the examination of a woman's cervix with a special microscope called a colposcope (Fig 12.13). A colposcopy is performed to evaluate an abnormal Pap smear or persistent postcoital bleeding, or to examine for abnormal growths in the woman's genital tract inside or on the outside of the vagina. While the Pap smear is a good screening test, a colposcopy is a more accurate diagnostic test, which allows the location of cell changes and assessment of the extent of changes picked up on a Pap smear.

A colposcopy is similar to having a Pap smear. A speculum is inserted into the vagina. A weak acetic acid solution is then applied to the cervix to highlight any abnormal areas, which will appear white (Fig 12.14). The colposcope is placed at the entrance to the vagina and the cervix is viewed through the colposcope. If the cervical tissues stain white, then biopsies are taken. The biopsies generally are not painful, but some local anaesthetic may be sprayed onto the cervix to help. The tissue collected is then sent to a laboratory for histological examination in order to confirm the diagnosis and determine if treatment is necessary.

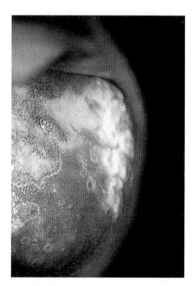

FIGURE 12.14 Florid mosaicism, an acetowhite change seen on the cervix as a result of HPV disease (From James et al[113])

Do Pap smears also pick up adenocarcinoma?

Adenocarcinoma of the cervix comprises about 15% of all cases of cervical cancer and the incidence is possibly increasing. Screening is less effective in preventing adenocarcinoma, as there is a lower detection rate for this kind of cancer. This is because:

- the malignancy arises in an anatomically inaccessible location (for example, high in the endocervical canal or below the mucosal surface, in an endocervical gland)
- the lesion fails to shed cells
- the cytologist, colposcopist or histopathologist may fail to recognise the precursor lesions of adenocarcinoma.

Summary of key points

- Negative smears should be repeated at 2 years, irrespective of the presence of endocervical cells.
- Inflammatory changes seen on a smear may be due to thrush or an STI such as *Chlamydia*.
- If low-grade changes (possible or definite LSIL) persist at 12 months, colposcopy is indicated.
- For women over 30 years of age who either have not had any Pap smears in the last 2–3 years or who have had an abnormal result in that time, either a repeat Pap smear in 6 months or immediate colposcopy is recommended.
- All women with possible or definite HSIL on a smear should be referred for colposcopy.
- Adenocarcinoma makes up 15% of all cervical cancer and is not picked up by Pap smear screening as well as the more common squamous cell carcinoma.

OVARIAN CANCER SCREENING

Ovarian cancer, while rare, is the leading cause of death from gynaecological malignancy. The incidence in Australia is 10 per 100,000.[97] The problem with ovarian cancer is that, although 5-year survival rates are >90% in women diagnosed with early disease,[98] most ovarian cancer is diagnosed at an advanced stage because symptoms and signs occur late in the disease and can be non-specific. Many believe that if breast cancer and cervical cancer screening exist, so too should ovarian cancer screening. However, in order to improve the mortality rate for ovarian cancer, detection in the early stages of the disease is required.

CASE STUDY: An email urging women to demand ovarian screening

Monique, 39 years of age, is a lawyer. She presents to her GP demanding ovarian cancer screening. A woman in her office has recently been diagnosed with ovarian cancer and it has prompted a round of emails urging women to seek screening for the disease. Monique shows you a copy of the email. It implies that there is a conspiracy of silence by doctors concerning the availability of a simple blood test (CA 125) to detect ovarian cancer and that because it is a disease that can have only vague symptoms women should have the blood test done on a regular basis.

Many patients attend requesting screening for ovarian cancer. How should a GP respond?

This is a very difficult consultation, in which GPs often have to overcome fear in their patient and a lot of misinformation that is circulating in the public arena. Basically, there is no current evidence to support the use of any test or combination of tests for ovarian cancer screening in asymptomatic women.[99]

The utility of CA 125, a serum biomarker for ovarian cancer is limited by its poor sensitivity in early stage disease. CA 125 levels are elevated in only 50% of patients with stage 1 disease, whereas levels are elevated in over 90% of patients with advanced disease. The specificity of CA 125 is also limited, due in part to elevation of the marker in other conditions, including other cancers, benign diseases and physiological conditions (Box 12.6).[100]

Transvaginal ultrasound (TVUS) utilises morphology and ovarian volume to detect changes that may signify developing malignancy; however, it has limitations in distinguishing between benign and malignant masses owing to the complexity of ovarian morphology.[99] The specificity of the test is low and the high rate of false-positive results can lead to unnecessary surgery.

Results of trials incorporating combinations of CA 125 and TVUS tests and repeat CA 125 measurements over time are awaited.[98]

OvPlex™ is a commercially available blood test developed by HealthLinx Limited (Australia) that is marketed as a test for the early detection of ovarian cancer. The test measures CA 125 and four additional protein biomarkers. Results remain unpublished and no data have been reported from prospective controlled clinical trials.[99]

As the National Breast and Ovarian Cancer Centre points out, should the woman decide to proceed with ovarian cancer screening despite current evidence, she should be aware that she may need to repeat the test, or to undertake further tests, which may include surgery to investigate the abnormal result.[99] The discovery and investigation of abnormal findings can

---

BOX 12.6 Causes of CA125 elevation other than ovarian cancer (From Nossov et al[100])

- Ovulation
- Menstruation
- Endometriosis
- Benign ovarian cysts
- Liver or kidney disease
- Other cancers such as breast or lung cancer

result in unnecessary anxiety and the investigations can carry significant risks.

Summary of key points
There is currently no evidence to support the use of any test, including pelvic examination, CA 125 or other biomarkers, ultrasound (including transvaginal ultrasound) or a combination of tests to screen for ovarian cancer at a population level in asymptomatic women.

STI SCREENING

What questions need to be asked in taking her sexual history?

- Does she have male partners, female partners or both?
- Age of first sexual activity
- How many current or recent (over the last 6 months) sexual partners?
- Does she use condoms? Every time?
- Ascertain other risk factors for blood-borne viruses in both herself and her partner:
  – intravenous drug use
  – tattoos
  – transfusions
  – body piercing
  – overseas travel
  – bisexual contacts.
- Does she have any symptoms?
  – discharge
  – ulcers
  – itches
  – lumps
  – abnormal bleeding
  – abdominal pain
  – dysuria
  – dyspareunia.

CASE STUDY: 'How do I get checked for STIs?'

Julie is 21 years old and presents for a Pap smear. She has recently started a new relationship and is using a 30 mg monophasic pill as contraception. She states she wants to be checked out for STIs and asks what this involves. Sexual history reveals that she has been sexually active for 4 years and has had approximately six partners during this time. She does not know how many partners her boyfriend has previously had. Neither Julie nor her boyfriend has ever used intravenous drugs and she is currently asymptomatic.

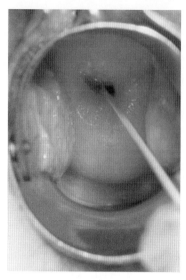

FIGURE 12.15 Taking an endocervical swab (From James et al[113])

Should Julie have STI screening?
Julie should be offered an examination and screening for genital STIs at the same time as her smear. Ideally, the following investigations should be undertaken:

- A vaginal swab taken from the posterior fornix. A smear should be prepared and air-dried, and the swab and slide sent for microscopy and culture. This will test for trichomoniasis but will also pick up any *Candida* or bacterial vaginosis that is present.
- An endocervical swab for PCR testing for *Chlamydia* and gonorrhoea (Fig 12.15). Alternatively, a first-pass urine sample can also be tested for *Chlamydia* and gonorrhoea using PCR.

Viral swabs for genital herpes should be taken if any blisters, ulcers or fissures are visible. Julie should also be offered counselling regarding her risks for the blood-borne viruses and tested for syphilis, hepatitis B and C, and HIV. If she has not been already immunised, Julie should be offered vaccination against hepatitis B.

Should genital swabs be taken before or after the Pap smear?
This is a controversial issue. The most important points are to:

- visualise the cervix well
- wipe away any mucus that is present before taking any specimens

obtain a good specimen for *Chlamydia* testing by rotating the swab 360 degrees in the endocervix. *Chlamydia* is an intracellular organism and so cells need to be picked up on the swab for the testing to be accurate.

Julie asks if her boyfriend needs testing too?

Yes, even if he is totally asymptomatic and has no findings on examination, he still requires screening. He should provide a first-pass urine specimen for PCR *Chlamydia* and gonorrhoea testing and tests for syphilis, hepatitis B and C, and HIV. Again vaccination against hepatitis B is warranted.

Can Julie just have a urine test?

A cervical swab is the preferred specimen when a woman is symptomatic of an STI, is due a pap smear or has been in contact with someone infected with chlamydia. Urine testing is acceptable when a woman refuses a pelvic examination, if she is menstruating or when she is not due a pap smear.

What guidelines exist regarding **Chlamydia** *screening for sexually active young people?*

Australian guidelines[101] recommend screening for *Chlamydia* as follows:

in any two of the following circumstances

- age less than 25 years
- recent change of sexual partner
- no contraceptive, non-barrier method or unplanned pregnancy
- cervical ectopy
- patient's request

in any one of the following circumstances

- any current STI
- a partner with urethritis or another STI
- cervical cervicitis or inflammatory change on smear.

While this refers to women, some 50% of men with *Chlamydia* are asymptomatic, providing a strong case for screening all men who report a change of sexual partner and who are not consistently using condoms.

GPs should undertake *Chlamydia* screening in young women with a recent change of sexual partner.

Summary of key points
- STI screening involves taking a sexual history, as well as performing examination and investigations for STIs such as *Chlamydia*, gonorrhoea and *Trichomonas* and blood-borne diseases such as syphilis, hepatitis B and HIV.

- Vaccination against hepatitis B is indicated in all sexually active young people.
- Risk factors for *Chlamydia* infection in women include:
  – age <25 years
  – recent change of sexual partner
  – no contraceptive, barrier method or where there is an unplanned pregnancy
  – cervical ectropion
  – any current STI
  – a partner with urethritis or an STI.

IS ROUTINE PELVIC EXAMINATION ESSENTIAL?

Pelvic examinations for most women are a source of great anxiety and uneasiness. Not only are women fearful that the examination will cause discomfort or actually be painful, but they also feel (quite understandably) uncomfortable about exposing their genitals to a stranger and having him/her feel inside their vagina. There is fear and uncertainty about whether their genitals are 'normal' and about the way they look and the way they smell.

Many women may never in fact have felt inside their vagina and do not really know much about the structure of their reproductive tract or the nature of their cervix. It is also often quite unclear why a doctor is doing a pelvic examination in the first place, especially when the woman is asymptomatic. What is the doctor looking for?

As women become increasingly more vocal consumers in the healthcare system, much emphasis has been given in recent years to training doctors to perform a sensitive pelvic examination. We have been taught to focus on consent and privacy, to be aware of the woman's modesty and to enable the woman to understand what we are doing by talking to her as we perform the examination.

Like many things in medicine, however, the routine pelvic examination has not been adequately critiqued in terms of its viability as a diagnostic tool and its cost-effectiveness in psychological terms for the patient. Few of us know what evidence exists in favour of or against routinely performing a pelvic examination at the time of a Pap smear.

How should pelvic examinations be conducted?

The essentials involve making the woman feel comfortable by explaining the procedure and obtaining her consent before proceeding. If it is her first examination, show her a speculum and any other equipment you will use if a smear or swabs are taken.

Give her the opportunity to empty her bladder before the examination takes place. Then ask her to disrobe and to lie on the couch, covering herself with a sheet. Pull a curtain around the couch so that she feels secure. A good light source is used to visualise the genitalia. The correct speculum is chosen to ensure that the best visualisation with the least discomfort is achieved and the speculum is warmed with warm tap water.

After the cervix and vagina are visualised and the necessary specimens obtained, the speculum is removed and lubricant applied to the gloved fingers. While holding the labia minora apart two fingers are gently inserted into the vagina and the cervix felt. It is important to reiterate to the woman at this point that she will feel some pushing and that you will now try to assess the size of the uterus. With one hand pushing down gently above the symphysis pubis, the uterus is ballotted between the fingertips of both hands. At this point the woman can be told the size of the uterus and its axis. She can also be asked if she can feel her uterus between the GPs fingers, as often this is the only time that she will have a sensation of the size of this organ.

The uterine size is then assessed. Next, you should make a mental note of whether there is any tenderness when rocking the cervix, before proceeding to palpate the fornices bimanually, feeling for lumps or cysts and watching for tenderness. At the end of the examination, the woman should be offered some tissues to wipe away any lubricant before she dresses again.

Should a pelvic examination be part of a regular gynaecological check-up?

The American Cancer Society and National Cancer Institute recommend a pelvic examination as part of a regular gynaecological check-up in association with a Pap smear and breast examination.[102] But is there any justification in performing a bimanual pelvic examination routinely at the time of a Pap smear in normal healthy women?

It has in the past been thought that a pelvic examination could act as a screen for pelvic pathology. However, the routine introduction of a pelvic examination as a screening test is questionable. At this point it must be reiterated that we are discussing pelvic examinations as opposed to Pap smears, and that the one does not necessarily involve the other.

What pathology can be accurately detected at the time of a pelvic examination in otherwise asymptomatic women?

Theoretically, the diseases could involve the vagina, the cervix, the uterus, the fallopian tubes or the ovaries. Given that the Pap smear is an effective

screening tool for squamous cell carcinoma of the cervix, the other cancers that could be said to be prevalent in women are ovarian or endometrial cancer. Neither of these cancers is all that common, however, and they are usually found in older women. Nor is pelvic examination necessarily sensitive in detecting these cancers.

Grover and Quinn[103] looked at these very issues. In their study, more than 2500 women aged between 25 and 92 years had pelvic examinations and blood taken for serum CA 125 antigen estimation (elevation being associated with ovarian cancer). This was followed up with an ultrasound if women had abnormal adnexal findings or an elevated serum CA 125. On examination, only 1.5% of the women were found to have abnormal adnexal findings, and the positive predictive value for a subsequent diagnosis of benign adnexal abnormalities was 22%. Approximately 13% of the women were found to have a 'bulky or fibroid' uterus on examination, but the detection of this abnormality is of no clear benefit, as progression to malignancy is rare. Grover and Quinn concluded that 'bimanual pelvic examination is of questionable value as a screening strategy in view of the low incidence of ovarian cancer in healthy women and the relatively high prevalence (1.5%) of relatively unimportant adnexal abnormalities'.

Another disease that may be considered as important to look for on routine pelvic examination is endometriosis. This is particularly so because of the possible long-term effects on fertility. Again, however, endometriosis does not fit into the criteria for screening. There is a lack of understanding about the pathogenesis of this disease and poor evidence about treatment efficacy. Pelvic examination is therefore only useful in eliciting signs of endometriosis in women who are symptomatic.[104]

Routine pelvic examination is not a good screening tool for pelvic pathology and so should be conducted only when the patient is symptomatic.

Should a rectal examination be a routine component of a pelvic assessment along with a vaginal examination?

The diagnostic utility of a digital rectal examination as part of a routine pelvic examination has been assessed. After performing a rectal examination in over 270 women under the age of 40, the diagnostic yield of this procedure was zero, suggesting there was no reason to perform this test in asymptomatic young women as part of a pelvic examination.[105]

So in what context is pelvic examination recommended?

Obviously it is certainly needed when women are symptomatic. This is particularly so when there is a suspicion of infection, ectopic pregnancy or ovarian disease. The examination should be followed by appropriate investigation such as microbiological tests and an ultrasound. Routine examinations, however, are questionable, especially in the younger patient population. So think hard before you do your next pelvic examination!

Successful speculum examinations

For all of us there are occasions when the cervix is difficult to visualise or take a smear from. The problem usually arises from a lack of understanding of where the cervix actually lies, poor equipment or a poor light source. If you are having difficulty with a speculum examination, one of the following tips might be helpful.

- Position the woman correctly. Place a small cushion under her buttocks to tilt the pelvis forward. Some GPs have made a habit of asking a woman to clench her fists and to place them underneath her bottom. Not only is this very uncomfortable but it takes away control from the woman, making her feel more vulnerable and unable to reach out and stop you if the examination is painful.
- Some people recommend that if you cannot 'find' the cervix (as if it is lost somewhere) you should do a digital examination to locate it. This is usually not necessary if the woman is relaxed and you are relaxed. If you do need to do this, use water as a lubricant rather than gel, as water will not affect the collection of specimens.
- Have a range of speculums available for use. If you use plastic ones, make sure your surgery also has a wide-blade speculum available for use with women who have degrees of vaginal prolapse. If the woman suffers from significant vaginal prolapse, cut off the thumb of a large glove so that it resembles a tube and place it like a sheath over the speculum so that once inserted the rubber holds back the lateral vaginal walls.
- If you are using a duckbill speculum, insert it with the handle pointing towards the couch. You may need to use a cushion (as described above) to avoid the handle hitting the couch. Speculums are designed so that the blade closest to the handle is the longest and sits in the posterior fornix. The shorter, top blade will therefore allow the cervix

to be visualised as the cervix actually sits at the end of the anterior vaginal wall. When the handle points towards the woman's abdomen, the longer, bottom blade can obscure the cervix.

- Postmenopausal women with a significantly atrophic vagina should use oestrogen cream or pessaries two or three times a week for a couple of weeks before a smear is attempted.
- Remember that the vagina points downwards and backwards, so if you have inserted the speculum too horizontally you may need to reposition the speculum. Often the two blades are made to sit in the posterior fornix or anterior fornix and only vaginal wall is visualised. Pull the speculum towards you a little bit and point it towards the woman's coccyx so that the top blade is in front of the cervix and the bottom one is behind the cervix.
- If the woman is very tense and pushing the speculum out by contracting her vaginal muscles, ask her to bear down as if she is trying to defecate. This action results in relaxation of the vaginal muscles and an easier speculum examination for both patient and doctor.
- Purchase a set of sponge forceps and a tenaculum in case you need to use them.
- Have some thick cotton swabs available. These are useful for wiping away any mucus that is emerging from the cervix and for soaking up any vaginal discharge that may be present. This allows for better inspection of the cervix, better smears (containing cells and not mucus) and correct sampling from the endocervix for *Chlamydia* testing.

TIPS FOR PRACTITIONERS

- A woman's cervix can vary in appearance, depending on the age of the woman, her parity, the presence of infection, pregnancy and previous surgery.
- Pap smears must be performed correctly, using good technique. This entails visualising the cervix and removing any mucus or blood covering the cervix prior to taking the smear.
- Only use water when lubricating a speculum, as other agents may decrease the quality of the smear taken.
- Be suspicious of *Chlamydia* infection when a smear is reported as having 'inflammatory changes'.
- If a woman still has a cervix after a hysterectomy, the usual Pap smear screening guidelines apply.
- Lesbians need Pap smears, too.

- When counselling women about ovarian cancer screening, point out that only 1 in 77 women will be diagnosed with ovarian cancer in her lifetime and that the risk of ovarian cancer increases with age, with approximately 80% of all new cases of ovarian cancer diagnosed in women 50 years or older and a median age of first diagnosis of 64 years.[99]

REFERENCES

1. Wald NJ. Guidance on terminology. J Med Screen 2001; 8:56.
2. Wallace RB. Screening for early and asymptomatic conditions. In: Wallace RB (ed). Public health and preventive medicine. 14th edn. Norwalk: Appleton & Lange; 1998: 907–908.
3. McPherson K, Steel CM, Dixon JM. Breast Cancer—epidemiology, risk factor and genetics. BMJ 2000; 321:624–628.
4. Feuer EJ, Wun LM, Boring CC, et al. The lifetime risk of developing breast cancer. J Natl Cancer Inst 1993; 85: 892–897.
5. American Cancer Society. Cancer facts and figures, 2001–2002. Atlanta, Georgia: American Cancer Society; 2002. Online. Available: http://www.cancer.org [accessed 18.02.2002].
6. Brinkley B, Haybittle JL. The curability of cancer. Lancet 1975; 2:951.
7. Kerr GR, Kunkler IH, Langlands AO, et al. (In)curability of breast cancer: a 30 year report of a series of 3933 cases. Breast 1998; 7:90–94.
8. US Preventive Services Task Force. Screening for breast cancer: US Preventive Services Task Force recommendation statement. Ann Intern Med 2009; 151(10):716–726, W-236.
9. Dickersin K. Breast screening in women aged 40–49 years: what next? Lancet 1999; 353:1896–1897.
10. Chu KC, Smart CR, Tarone RE. Analysis of breast cancer mortality and stage distribution by age for the Health Insurance Plan clinical trial. J Natl Cancer Inst 1988; 80:1125–1132.
11. Alexander FE, Anderson TJ, Brown HK, et al. 14 years of follow-up from the Edinburgh randomised trial of breast-cancer screening. Lancet 1999; 353:1903–1908.
12. Miller AB, Baines CJ, To T, et al. Canadian National Breast Screening Study: 1 Breast cancer detection and death rates among women aged 40–49 years. Can Med Assoc J 1992; 147:1459–1476, 1477–1488.
13. Andersson I, Aspegren K, Janzon L, et al. Mammographic screening and mortality from breast cancer: the Malmo mammographic screening trial. BMJ 1988; 297:943–948.
14. Tabar L, Fagerberg G, Chen HH, et al. Efficacy of breast cancer screening by age: new results from the Swedish Two-county Trial. Cancer 1995; 75:2507–2517.
15. Frisell J, Lidbrink E, Hellstrom L, et al. Follow-up after 11 years: update of mortality results in the Stockholm mammographic screening trial. Breast Cancer Res Treat 1997; 45:263–270.
16. Bjurstam N, Bjorneld L, Duffy SW, et al. The Gothenburg breast screening trial: first results on mortality, incidence, and mode of detection for women ages 39–49 years at randomization. Cancer 1997; 80:2091–2099.
17. Nystrom L, Rutqvist LE, Wall S, et al. Breast cancer screening with mammography: overview of Swedish randomised trials. Lancet 1993; 341:973–978.
18. Kerlikowske K, Grady D, Rubin SM, et al. Efficacy of screening mammography. A meta-analysis. JAMA 1995; 273:149–154.
19. Gøtzsche PC, Olsen O. Is screening for breast cancer with mammography justifiable? Lancet 2000; 355:129–134.
20. Olsen O, Gøtzsche PC. Screening for breast cancer with mammography (Cochrane Review). In: The Cochrane Library, Issue 1, 2002. Oxford: Update Software; 2002.
21. Nystrom L, Andersson I, Bjurstam N, et al. Long-term effects of mammography screening: updated overview of the Swedish randomised trials. Lancet 2002; 359:909–919.
22. Kösters, JP, Gøtzsche PC. Regular self-examination or clinical examination for early detection of breast cancer. Cochrane Database Syst Rev 2003; 2:CD003373.
23. Welch HG. Overdiagnosis and mammography screening. BMJ 2009; 339(jul09_1):b1425.
24. Gøtzsche PC, Nielsen M. Screening for breast cancer with mammography. Cochrane Database Syst Rev 2009; 4: CD001877.pub3.
25. NHS Breast Screening Programme Review. , Sheffield: National Co-ordinating Centre:1999. Online. Available: http://www.cancerscreening.nhs.uk/breastscreen/publications/nhsbsreview.pdf [accessed 7.02.2003].
26. Elmore JG, Barton MB, Moceri VM, et al. Ten-year risk of false positive screening mammograms and clinical breast examinations. N Engl J Med 1998; 338:1089–1096.
27. Lerman C, Trock B, Rimer BK, et al. Psychological and behavioral implications of abnormal mammograms. Ann Intern Med 1991; 114:657–661.
28. Slaytor EK, Ward JE. How risks of breast cancer and benefits of screening are communicated to women: analysis of 58 pamphlets. BMJ 1998; 317:263–264.
29. Thornton H. The voice of the breast cancer patient—a lonely cry in the wilderness. Eur J Cancer 1997; 33:825–828.
30. Miller D, Martin I, Herbison P, et al. Interventions for relieving the pain of screening mammography (protocol for a Cochrane Review). In: The Cochrane Library, Issue 2. Oxford: Update Software; 2001.
31. Jorgensen KJ, Gøtzsche PC. Content of invitations for publicly funded screening mammography. [See comment.] BMJ 2006; 332(7540):538–541.
32. Jorgensen KJ, Gotzsche PC. Overdiagnosis in publicly organised mammography screening programmes: systematic review of incidence trends. BMJ 2009; 339(jul09_1):b2587.
33. Baum M, Tobias JS. Investment in treatment would be more effective (letter). BMJ 2000; 321:1528.
34. Patnick J. Review NHS breast screening programme. Sheffield: NHS Breast Screening Programme; 1998.
35. Miller AB, To T, Baines CJ, et al. Canadian National Breast Screening Study 2: 13 year results of a randomised trial in women aged 50–59 years. J Natl Cancer Inst 2000; 92: 1490–1498.
36. Mittra I, Baum M, Thornton H, et al. Is clinical breast examination an acceptable alternative to mammographic screening? BMJ 2000; 321:1071–1073.
37. US Preventive Services Task Force. Screening for breast cancer. Recommendations and rationale. Rockville, MD: Agency for Healthcare Research and Quality; 2002. Online. Available: http://www.ahrq.gov/clinic/3rduspstf/breastcancer/brcanrr.htm [accessed 7 Mar 2002].
38. Holmberg L, Ekbom A, Calle E, et al. Breast cancer mortality in relation to self reported use of breast self examination. A cohort study of 450,000 women. Breast Cancer Res Treat 1997; 43:137–140.
39. UK Trial of Early Detection of Breast Cancer Group. Sixteen-year mortality from breast cancer in the UKTEDBC. Lancet 1999; 353:1909–1914.
40. Semiglazov VF, Sagaidak VN, Moiseyenko VM, et al. Study of the role of the breast self examination in the reduction of mortality from breast cancer. The Russian Federation/World Health Organization study. Eur J Cancer 1993; 29A:2039–2046.

41. Thomas DBV, Gao DL, Self SG, et al. Randomised trial of breast self-examination in Shanghai. Methodology and preliminary results. J Natl Cancer Inst 1997; 89:355–365.

42. Thomas DBV, Gao DL, Ray RM, et al. Randomized trial of breast self-examination in Shanghai: final results. J Natl Cancer Inst 2002; 94:1445–1457.

43. Brown D. UK death rates from breast cancer fall by a third. BMJ 2000; 321:849.

44. Chu KC, Tarone RE, Kessler LG, et al. Recent trends in US breast cancer incidence, survival and mortality rates. J Natl Cancer Inst 1996; 88:1571–1579.

45. Peto R, Boreham J, Clarke M, et al. UK and USA breast cancer deaths down 25% in year 2000 at ages 20–69 years. Lancet 2000; 355:1822.

46. Gelmon KA, Olivotto I. The mammography screening debate: time to move on. Lancet 2002; 359:904–905.

47. International Agency for Research on Cancer. Globocan 2002 [database]. Lyon: International Agency for Research on Cancer; 2005. Online. Available: http://www-dep.iarc.fr [accessed 31.08.2009].

48. Australian Institute of Health and Welfare (AIHW). Cancer Australia and Australasian Association of Cancer Registries: cancer survival and prevalence in Australia—cancers diagnosed from 1982 to 2004. Canberra: AIHW; 2008.

49. Bosch FX, Lorincz A, Muñoz N, et al. The causal relation between human papillomavirus and cervical cancer. J Clin Pathol 2002; 55(4):244–265.

50. Bosch FX, Manos MM, Muñoz N, et al. Prevalence of human papillomavirus in cervical cancer: a worldwide perspective. J Natl Cancer Inst 1995; 87:796–802.

51. Bosch FX, Muñoz N. HPV infection and cervical disease. Meeting report. European HPV Clinical Summit Meeting, 1998.

52. Koutsky L. Epidemiology of genital human papillomavirus infection. Am J Med 1997; 102(5A):3–8.

53. Winer RL, Lee SK, Hughes JP, et al. Genital human papillomavirus infection: incidence and risk factors in a cohort of female university students. Am J Epidemiol 2003; 157(3):218–226.

54. Franco EL, Villa LL, Sobrinho JP, et al. Epidemiology of acquisition and clearance of cervical human papillomavirus infection in women from a high-risk area for cervical cancer. J Infect Dis 1999; 180(5):1415–1423.

55. Trottier H, Franco EL. The epidemiology of genital human papillomavirus infection. Vaccine 2006; 24(Suppl 1):S1–S15.

56. Stanley M. Immune responses to human papillomavirus. Vaccine 2006; 24(Suppl 1):S16–S22.

57. Schiffman M, Herrero R, Desalle R, et al. The carcinogenicity of human papillomavirus types reflects viral evolution. Virology 2005; 337(1):76–84.

58. McCredie MR, Sharples KJ, Paul C, et al. Natural history of cervical neoplasia and risk of invasive cancer in women with cervical intraepithelial neoplasia 3: a retrospective cohort study. Lancet Oncol 2008; 9(5):425–434.

59. Clifford G, Franceschi S, Diaz M, et al. Chapter 3: HPV-type distribution in women with and without cervical neoplastic diseases. Vaccine 2006; 24(Suppl 3):S3/26–S3/34.

60. Clifford GM, Rana RK, Franceschi S, et al. Human papillomavirus genotype distribution in low-grade cervical lesions: comparison by geographic region and with cervical cancer. Cancer Epidemiol Biomarkers Prev 2005; 14(5):1157–1164.

61. Skinner SR, Garland SM, Stanley MA, et al. Human papillomavirus vaccination for the prevention of cervical neoplasia: is it appropriate to vaccinate women older than 26? Med J Aust 2008; 188(4):238–242.

62. Brown DR, Kjaer SK, Sigurdsson K, et al. The impact of quadrivalent human papillomavirus (HPV; types 6, 11, 16, and 18) L1 virus-like particle vaccine on infection and disease due to oncogenic nonvaccine HPV types in generally HPV-naive women aged 16–26 years. J Infect Dis 2009; 199(7):926–935.

63. Czegledy J. Sexual and non-sexual transmission of human papillomavirus (a short review). Acta Microbiol Immunol Hung 2001; 48:511–517.

64. ARHP (Association of Reproductive Health Professionals). Human papillomavirus (HPV) and cervical cancer. Clinical proceedings, electronic edn. 2001. Online. Available: http://www. arhp.org/healthcareproviders/onlinepublications/clinicalproceedings/cphpv/ [accessed 07.03.2002].

65. National Health Service (UK). NHS Cervical Screening Programme. 2009. Online. Available: http://www.cancerscreening.nhs.uk/cervical/index.html [accessed 06.09.2009].

66. Van Wijngaarden WJ, Duncan ID. Rationale for stopping screening in women over 50. BMJ 1993; 306: 967–971.

67. Sherlaw-Johnson C, Gallivan S, Jenkins D. Withdrawing low risk women from cervical screening programmes: mathematical modelling study. BMJ 1999; 318: 356–361.

68. Office for National Statistics (UK). Estimates of newly diagnosed cases of cancer: England and Wales 1993–1997. London: DoH; 1998(Monitor MB1 98/2).

69. Jenkins D, Sherlaw-Johnson C, Gallivan S. Assessing the role of HPV testing in cervical cancer screening. Papillomavirus Reports 1998; 9:89–101.

70. Koutsky LA, Holmes KK, Critchlow CW, et al. A cohort study of the risk of cervical intraepithelial neoplasia grade 2 or 3 in relation to papillomavirus infection. N Engl J Med 1992; 327:1272–1278.

71. Schiffman MH, Sherman ME. HPV testing to improve cervical cancer screening. In: Srivastava S, Lippman SM, Hong WK, et al (eds). Early detection of cancer: molecular markers. Armonk, New York: Futura Publishing; 1994: 265–277.

72. Hakama M, Miller AB, Day NE. Screening for cancer of the uterine cervix. Lyon: International Agency for Research on Cancer; 1986:207.

73. Martin-Hirsch P, Lilford R, Jarvis G, et al. Efficacy of cervical-smear collection devices: a systematic review and meta-analysis. Lancet 1999; 354:1763–1770.

74. Farnsworth A, Chambers FM, Golschmidt CS. Evaluation of the PAPNET system in a general pathology service. Med J Aust 1996; 165:429–431.

75. Sheets EE, Constantine NM, Dinisco S, et al. Colposcopically directed biopsies provide a basis for comparing the accuracy of ThinPrep and Papanicolaou smears. Obstetrical & Gynecological Survey 1995; 50(9):659–661.

76. Medical Services Advisory Committee. Medical Services Advisory Committee public summary document, application no. 1122—liquid based cytology (LBC). 2009. Online. Available: http://www.health.gov.au/internet/msac/publishing.nsf/Content/2AD0E9BD12315EB9CA257 5C5002872A9/$File/1122_MSAC_PSD.pdf [accessed 05.01.2010].

77. Heley S. Is a Pap smear enough? Aust Fam Physician 2001; 30:535–538.

78. Herrington CS, Evans MF, Charnock FM, et al. HPV testing in patients with low grade cervical cytological abnormalities: a follow-up study. J Clin Pathol 1996; 49:493–496.

79. National Cervical Screening Program, Dr Stella Heley FAChSHM, Senior Liaison Physician, Victorian Cytology Service. Presentation on the revised guidelines. 2006. Online. Available: http://www.health.gov.au/internet/screening/publishing.nsf/Content/cv-presentation/$File/presentation-june06.pdf [accessed 06.09.2009].

80. Harper DM, Franco EL, Wheeler CM, et al. Sustained efficacy up to 4.5 years of a bivalent L1 virus-like particle vaccine against human papillomavirus types 16 and 18: follow-up from a randomised control trial. Lancet 2006; 367(9518):1247–1255.

81. Mitchell H, Medley G. An audit of women who died from cancer of the cervix in Victoria, Australia. Aust NZ J Obstet Gynaecol 1996; 36:73–76.

82. Rankow EJ, Tessaro I. Cervical cancer risk and Papanicolaou screening in a sample of lesbian and bisexual women. J Fam Pract 1998; 47:139–143.

83. Marrazzo JM, Koutsky LA, Kiviat NB, et al. Papanicolaou test screening and prevalence of genital human papillomavirus among women who have sex with women. Am J Public Health 2001; 91:947–952.

84. Wray L. Lesbians and cervical cancer: do lesbians need Pap smears? Venereology 1992; 5:121–122.

85. Pearce KF, Haefner HK, Sarwar SF, et al. Cytopathological findings on vaginal Papanicolaou smears after hysterectomy for benign gynaecologic disease. N Engl J Med 1996; 335:1559–1162.

86. Buxton J, Luesley D, Woodman C, et al. Endocervical sampling with a cytobrush does not improve cervical cytology. J Exp Clin Cancer Res 1990; 9(Suppl):FC/78.

87. Goorney BP, Lacey CJN, Sutton J. Ayre v Aylesbury cervical spatulas. Genitourin Med 1989; 65:161–162.

88. Pretorius RG, Sadeghi M, Fotheringham N, et al. A randomised trial of three methods of obtaining Papanicolaou smears. Obstet Gynaecol 1991; 78:831–836.

89. Selvaggi SM, Malviya V. Sampling accuracy of the modified Ayre spatula/Zelsmyr Cytobrush versus the modified Ayre spatula/bulb aspirator in the collection of cells from the uterine cervix. Diagn Cytopathol 1991; 7:318–322.

90. Szarewski A, Cuzick J, Nayagam M, et al. A comparison of four cytological sampling techniques in a genitourinary medicine clinic. Genitourin Med 1990; 66:439–443.

91. Wolfendale MR, Howe-Guest R, Usherwood MM, et al. Controlled trial of a new cervical spatula. BMJ (Clin Res Ed) 1987; 294:33–35.

92. Mitchell H, Medley G. Longitudinal study of women with negative cervical smears according to endocervical status. Lancet 1991; 337:265–267.

93. Mitchell H, Medley G. Cytological reporting of cervical abnormalities according to endocervical status. British J Cancer 1993; 67:585–588.

94. Mitchell H. Management of women with HPV change on Pap smears. Med J Aust 1992; 156 69.

95. Chanen W. The CIN saga-the biological and clinical significance of cervical intraepithelial neoplasia. Aust NZ J Obstet Gynaecol 1990; 30:18–23.

96. Nasiell K, Roger V, Nasiell M. Behaviour of mild cervical dysplasia during long-term follow-up. Obstet Gynaecol 1986; 67:665–669.

97. Australian Institute of Health and Welfare and Australasian Association of Cancer Registries. Cancer in Australia: an overview, 2008. AIHW Cancer Series no. 46. Canberra: AIHW; 2008.

98. Jacobs IJ, Menon U. Progress and challenges in screening for early detection of ovarian cancer. Mol Cell Proteomics 2004; 3(4):355–366.

99. National Breast and Ovarian Cancer Centre. Population screening and early detection of ovarian cancer in asymptomatic women—NBOCC Position statement 2009. Online. Available: http://nbocc.org.au/our-organisation/position-statements/population-screening-and-early-detection [accessed 05.01.2010].

100. Nossov V, Amneus M, Su F, et al. The early detection of ovarian cancer: from traditional methods to proteomics. Can we really do better than serum CA-125? Am J Obstet Gynecol 2008; 199(3):215–223.

101. National Health & Medical Research Council. Working Party Report: Pelvic inflammatory disease. Woden: ACT: NHMRC; 1988:10–11.

102. American Cancer Society. Cancer risk report 1995. Atlanta, Georgia: American Cancer Society; 1995.

103. Grover SR, Quinn MA. Is there any value in bimanual pelvic examination as a screening test? Med J Aust 1995; 162: 408–410.

104. Evers JL, Dunselman GA, Van der Linden PJ. Markers for endometriosis. Baillière's Clin Obstet Gynaecol 1993; 7: 715–739.

105. Campbell KA, Shaughnessy AF. Diagnostic utility of the digital rectal examination as part of the routine pelvic examination. J Fam Pract 1998; 46:165–167.

106. Hart CR. Theory and its application. In: Hart CR, Burke P (eds). Screening and surveillance in general practice. Edinburgh: Churchill Livingstone; 1992.

107. Silverberg SG. Atlas of breast pathology. New York: Saunders; 2002.

108. Schiffman M, Castle PE. The promise of global cervical-cancer prevention. New England J Medicine 2005; 353(20): 2101–2104.

109. Papscreen Victoria and Victorian Cytology Service. Cervix Sampling Card. 2009. Online. Available http://www.papscreen.org.au/downloads/resources/other/Cervical_sampling_card.pdf [accessed 01.09.09].

110. Wolfendale M. Taking cervical smears. British Society for Clinical Cytology; 1995:12.

111. Burghardt E. Colposcopy cervical pathology textbook and atlas. Germany: Georg Thiem Verlag; 1984:162, 174.

112. Cartier R. Practical colposcopy. Switzerland: Laboratoire Cartier; 1984:168.

113. James D, Pilai M, Rymer J, et al. Obstetrics, gynaecology, neonatology: interactive colour guides. CD-ROM. Edinburgh: Churchill Livingstone; 2002.

114. National Cervical Screening Program. Management summary. 2006. Online. Available from: http://www.health.gov.au/internet/screening/publishing.nsf/Content/cv-management-kit/$File/mgmt-summary.pdf.

Genital tract disorders

CHAPTER CONTENTS

OBJECTIVES

- To be able to recognise, diagnose and treat the various causes of vaginitis
- To be able to diagnose and manage genital herpes and warts
- To differentiate between conditions causing vulvovaginal infection and those causing cervical infection
- To understand the rationale for *Chlamydia* screening
- To be aware of the common vulval dermatoses

VULVOVAGINAL CONDITIONS

Vaginitis: thrush

What do the normal flora of the vagina consist of?

The vagina is lined by squamous epithelium. It is highly sensitive to oestrogen, which induces the production of glycogen. Local enzymes and bacteria break down glycogen. Lactobacilli predominate in this environment. They lower the vaginal pH by producing lactic acid and hydrogen peroxide, inhibiting the growth of many organisms.

The vagina is colonised by a wide variety of both aerobic and anaerobic bacteria. The most common are lactobacilli, diphtheroids, streptococci and staphylococci. It is important to note that *Candida albicans* can be present in the vaginal flora of up to 20% of normal asymptomatic women.

What is thrush?

Thrush (vulvovaginal candidiasis) is an infection caused by *Candida* species. *Candida albicans* accounts for 90% of infections and *C. glabrata* 5%. Less than 5% of cases are caused by *C. tropicalis, C. parapsilosis, C. krusei, C. kefyr, C. guilliermondii* or *Saccharomyces cerevisiae*.[1] These organisms are all yeasts, that is they are microscopic single-celled fungi that reproduce by budding.

When is it most likely to occur?

Vaginal infections occur when there are changes to the 'ecological' environment that favour one or more types of organism over the status quo.

Despite the fact that thrush is probably one of the most common conditions affecting women, its aetiology and epidemiology remain poorly understood. The development of thrush has been linked to several factors including the recent use of antibiotics and oral contraceptives, the presence of diabetes mellitus, dietary practices, gastrointestinal colonisation by the organism, clothing and sanitary protection practices, sexual communicability of

the organism and specific immunological defects. However, the data supporting each of these factors are conflicting, and to date none is predictive of infection. The evidence related to each of these risk factors is summarised in Table 13.1.

TABLE 13.1 Epidemiological associations with vulvovaginal candidiasis (VVC)

Risk factor	Summary of the evidence
Antibiotics	• Antibiotics are a short-term risk factor. • Associated with increasing duration of use of antibiotic.[113]
Sexual factors	• Asymptomatic male partners do not need to be treated.[114] • VVC is not a sexually transmitted disease, as it can occur in celibate women and because *Candida* is considered part of normal vaginal flora.[6] • *Candida* organisms, however, may be transmitted by vaginal sexual intercourse and other forms of sexual activity.[115,116] • The relationship between frequency of coitus and VVC is controversial.[117] • Receptive oral sex is related to incidence of VVC.[118]
Oral contraceptive use	• Associated with a higher risk of VVC.[119] • Risk is higher, the higher the dose of oestrogen in the COCP.[120]
Other methods of contraception	There is a higher risk with: • recent use of a diaphragm and spermicide[121] • vaginal contraceptive sponge[120] • intrauterine contraceptive device.[120]
Sanitary pads and tampons	Studies have failed to establish a link between thrush and either douching, tampons or sanitary pads.[122,123]
Tight-fitting clothing	Is anecdotal and unproven.[6]
Dietary factors	Are anecdotal and unproven; one RCT is too small to draw any conclusions.[124]

CASE STUDY: Recurrent vaginal itch

Helen is 32 years old and presents to you complaining of vulval itchiness. It has been present on and off for the last 3 months and tends to be worse before her period. She is currently using condoms for contraception. She has had thrush before on several occasions and usually buys 'thrush cream' over the counter and after using it feels better. This time it has kept recurring and she can't seem to clear herself of it.

CASE STUDY: Diabetes as a cause of thrush

Patricia is 62 and presents to you complaining of vulval irritation and dyspareunia. She has never previously had thrush. Her menopause occurred at the age of 50 and was uneventful. She does not use any HRT and is on no other medications. On examination, the vulva and vagina is very inflamed. You suspect candidiasis and take a random blood sugar measurement. It turns out to be 12 mmol/L. Patricia has non-insulin-dependent diabetes mellitus (NIDDM), presenting as thrush.

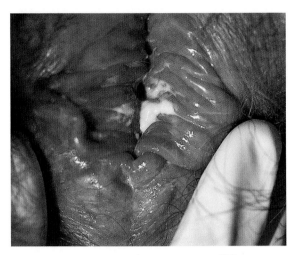

FIGURE 13.1 Candidiasis (From Morse et al[125])

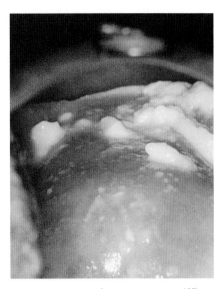

FIGURE 13.2 Candidiasis (From Morse et al[125])

What are the classic symptoms and signs?

Classically, when women have thrush they complain of vulvovaginal itchiness. There may also be associated vaginal discharge that is white and resembling 'curd' or 'cottage cheese'. As opposed to other forms of vaginitis, thrush is odourless. No symptoms, either individually or collectively, are diagnostic of thrush, as other diseases can cause a very similar pattern of symptoms. On examination, GPs may note vulval erythema with fissuring and the characteristic discharge. For examples of vulvovaginal candidiasis (VVC), see Figures 13.1 and 13.2.

Is it necessary to obtain microbiological confirmation of candidiasis every time a woman presents with symptoms of thrush?

There are several ways to confirm a diagnosis of vulvovaginal candidiasis. Vaginal cultures of swabs taken from the anterior fornix or the lateral vaginal wall will identify the organism. They are not routinely required, however, but should be considered in all symptomatic cases where microscopy and pH tests are inconclusive and in repeated treatment failures, recurrence or suspicion of non-albicans species.[2]

An easier option is to have some litmus paper available in the surgery. In cases of thrush, vaginal pH is normal (i.e. slightly acidic pH 4.0–4.5). If the pH is 5.0 or above, another diagnosis such as bacterial vaginosis or trichomoniasis should be considered.

If a microscope is handy, microscopy with saline solution may show yeast budding or pseudohyphae in up to half of infections (Fig 13.3) but will still not pick up all cases. Non-albicans strains are more difficult to recognise.

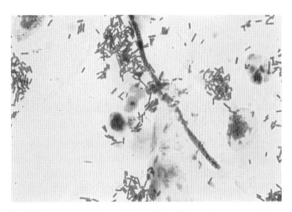

FIGURE 13.3 Hyphae of Candida albicans in gram stain of vaginal smear (From Morse et al[125])

What is the differential diagnosis of thrush?

When looking at the differential diagnosis of thrush, GPs should consider other conditions that give rise to the two classic symptoms (pruritus and discharge). Herpes simplex, contact dermatitis, psoriasis, lichen sclerosus or allergies can give rise to acute pruritus vulvae, while trichomoniasis, bacterial vaginosis and, less commonly, the cervical infections Chlamydia or gonorrhoea (the discharge from these two organisms is actually cervical but may emerge from the introitus and appear to be vaginal in origin) can produce vaginal discharge. Table 13.2 (p 228) compares and contrasts three different forms of vaginitis. It is worth remembering that of the three bacterial vaginosis is the most common, followed by candidiasis and trichomoniasis.[3]

TABLE 13.2 A comparison of the most common vaginal infections (not all the symptoms described occur in each case)

	Bacterial vaginosis (BV)	Thrush (vaginal candidiasis)	Trichomoniasis (*Trichomonas vaginalis*)
Cause	An alteration in the pH of the vagina associated with change in levels of different bacteria	An overgrowth of *Candida* organisms in the vagina	A sexually transmissible infection
Vaginal odour	'Fishy' or musty; unpleasant	None	'Fishy'; unpleasant
Vaginal itching/ irritation	No itch; mild irritation only	Usually present	Usually present and pronounced
Additional symptoms		Superficial dyspareunia and dysuria	Dysuria and lower abdominal pain
Vaginal discharge	Thin; milky white or grey	Thick, cottage cheese–like; white	Frothy; yellow-green
Signs	Discharge coating vagina and vestibule; no vulval inflammation	Normal findings or vulval erythema, oedema, fissuring satellite lesions	Vulvitis and vaginitis; so-called strawberry cervix (uncommon, 2%)
Treatment	Metronidazole, tinidazole or clindamycin cream; available only on prescription	Creams or pessaries such as miconazole or nystatin; available over the counter from pharmacies	Oral metronidazole; available only on prescription

There are many different products available to manage acute thrush: which are the best to use?

Women and their doctors are often confused by the wide variety of products and formulations available for the treatment of candidiasis. Importantly, none of the available drugs are fungicidal. While they can reduce *Candida* to below detectable levels, they are not necessarily able to eradicate the organism completely. Azoles such as clotrimazole, econazole or miconazole (topical and oral) give an 80–95% clinical and mycological cure rate in acute thrush in non-pregnant women. By comparison, nystatin, an older product, gives a 70–90% cure rate under these circumstances.[4]

Differences in formulation are not thought to affect treatment outcome, and are more a function of patient preference.[5]

Women have the option of either topical or oral therapy. Creams are effective and give quicker initial relief than oral agents. Oral azoles, such as fluconazole or itraconazole as a 1-day course, are equally as effective as topicals (but a more expensive option), but they may have a delay in onset of action of 12–24 hours. They may also result in systemic side effects in 10% of users. These effects include gastrointestinal intolerance, headache and rashes, but are usually mild and transient.[6] Oral ketoconazole is

indicated only in cases not responsive to other agents. It should not be used for superficial fungal infections because of the potential risk of liver toxicity.

In the treatment of vulvovaginal candidiasis, creams are effective and give quicker initial relief than oral agents, which are more expensive and have more side effects.

It is important to be aware of the fact that antifungal vaginal agents can produce local side effects characterised by burning, itching, soreness, erythema and oedema, especially with repeated application. For this reason, if the vulva is very inflamed oral treatment may be preferred. Another reason for using oral therapy is if the woman doesn't feel comfortable using pessaries or products requiring the use of intravaginal applicators.

Routine use of corticosteroids is not recommended. In severe infections, low-potency topical corticosteroids may rapidly reduce local inflammation and burning, but the application of higher-dose corticosteroids often exacerbates the burning sensation.[6]

What duration of therapy is recommended?

Topical and oral azoles are effective in short courses. The term 'short course' can mean single dose, 3-day or sometimes even 5–7 day courses. As treatment courses have become shorter, the doses used have become higher, with the assumption that the total dose is more important than the duration of treatment, especially in uncomplicated infection.[6]

Are there any other steps that should be recommended to a patient commencing therapy?

Patients should continue taking their combined oral contraceptive pills but avoid sexual activity until their symptoms clear, if only for comfort's sake. Patients who rely on condoms or diaphragms for contraception should be made aware that the antifungal agents can damage these products and make them unsafe for use as contraception.

They should also avoid the application of anything to the vulva that may increase irritation. They should therefore wear cotton underwear rather than nylon, wash with warm water rather than soap, not use vaginal douches or perfumes, and avoid perfumed sanitary pads and panty liners.

Current evidence does not support concurrent treatment of male partners.[7]

Many antifungal agents are available over the counter. Should women use these therapies rather than see a GP?

While over-the-counter topical azoles are convenient for women and more cost-effective to the health system, their availability is of some concern. First, women may misdiagnose themselves, particularly if they have not had the condition before. Second, recurrent or prolonged applications of azoles to the vulva may in fact irritate the skin, causing secondary dermatitis. For these reasons it is wise to advise women to see a GP if their symptoms do not resolve with treatment so that an accurate diagnosis can be made.

What about natural therapies like yoghurt?

There are currently no conclusive data on the effectiveness of *Lactobacillus*-containing yoghurt, administered either orally or vaginally, for the treatment or prevention of thrush.[8,9] In addition, the use of oral or vaginal forms of *Lactobacillus* to prevent post-antibiotic vulvovaginitis[10] has not been shown to be effective in a randomized, controlled trial.

BOX 13.1 Reasons for failure of treatment of an isolated episode of thrush

- Has the patient been compliant with the medication prescribed?
- Is the thrush caused by a non-*albicans* species such as *Candida glabrata*, which tends to be more resistant to treatment with azoles? Confirm the diagnosis with vaginal swabs sent for culture. Nystatin may be effective in cases where azoles have failed.
- 10% of women with thrush have mixed infections and bacteria may be present. In this scenario, both infections should be treated.
- Underlying factors such as long-term antibiotic use, diabetes mellitus, immunodeficiency or corticosteroid use may be present.

Women may use probiotics (live yoghurts) in the management of vulvovaginal candidiasis or bacterial vaginosis, but evidence of effectiveness is poor.[7]

What if treatment of an isolated episode fails?

As in any case of treatment failure, a GP should first ascertain that the patient has been compliant with the medication. If the answer is yes, the checklist given in Box 13.1 should be followed. If none of these factors are relevant, a longer course of treatment can be tried (e.g. 7 days if a 1- or 3-day treatment was initially used, or 14 days if a 7-day treatment was initially used). Another option is to combine oral with topical treatment.

What approach should be taken if the woman gets recurrent thrush (>4 episodes per year)?

In these women, it is essential to be sure that what you are really dealing with is thrush. For this reason, with each individual episode vaginal swabs should be taken for microscopy and culture, and topical contact dermatitis, hypersensitivity or allergic reactions excluded. The patient should also be screened for diabetes, immunodeficiency, corticosteroid use and frequent antibiotic use.[4]

Recurrent thrush can be a very problematic condition that can prove frustrating to treat, not only for the woman but also for the doctor. The suggested approach is to use a two-phase line of attack. An induction period reduces the *Candida* and alleviates symptoms. A maintenance period then follows, aimed at preventing recurrence.[1]

Although the optimal induction period is not currently known, recurrent infections tend to respond less well to short courses of anti-mycotics (e.g. single-dose fluconazole or 7 days of a topical). Therefore, 'induction' therapy is recommended with at least 1 week of oral products or 1–2 weeks of topical products.[1,6]

The maintenance period usually lasts for 6 months. A wide variety of different regimens have been recommended. Commonly cited ones include oral fluconazole 100 mg weekly for 6 months, or topical clotrimazole (in the form of a pessary) 500 mg weekly for 6 months.[1,4,6]

Unfortunately cessation of therapy results in relapse in at least 50% of women[4] and a small percentage of women may require maintenance azoles for years.[6]

If the woman is using a combined oral contraceptive pill, some advocate switching the pill to a less oestrogenic one (see Chapter 3). In women who are not on the pill who experience recurrent thrush in the week prior to the onset of menstruation, oral fluconazole can be used on a monthly basis at this time.

Another more novel way of treating recurrent or persistent candidiasis is through the use of Depo-Provera®.[11] Its mechanism of action is thought to be through its action of lowering oestradiol levels in the blood.

Is there any difference to management if the woman is pregnant or breastfeeding?

While thrush in pregnancy does not pose a risk to the fetus, it can cause considerable distress to the mother, because of persistence and recurrence. Asymptomatic colonisation with *Candida* species is higher in pregnancy (30–40%) and symptomatic candidosis is more prevalent throughout pregnancy.[4]

Topical azoles can safely be used in pregnancy. Clotrimazole is safe and effective. Miconazole and econazole can also be used and systemic absorption is negligible.[12] Topical imidazole appears to be more effective than nystatin for treating symptomatic vaginal candidiasis in pregnancy. Treatments for 7 days may be necessary in pregnancy rather than the shorter courses more commonly used in non-pregnant women.[13]

Oral therapy should not be given. Although the small amount of data available for fluconazole has not found any significant teratogenic effect, the amount of data is too small to draw firm conclusions.

Summary of key points
- Pruritus vulvae and vaginal discharge are the cardinal symptoms of thrush.
- *Candida albicans* accounts for about 90% of infections and *C. glabrata* for 5%.
- *C. glabrata* infections are often resistant to azoles.
- Recurrent episodes require clinical examination, culture of swabs and consideration of underlying disease.
- Male partners who do not have symptoms need not be examined, have swabs taken for culture or be treated.
- Reduction of intestinal colonisation is of no value in preventing recurrence.

Vaginitis: bacterial vaginosis

What exactly is bacterial vaginosis?

Bacterial vaginosis (BV) is regarded as a fairly innocuous condition but it is the most common cause of vaginal discharge in women of childbearing age.[14] The condition comes about when the normal hydrogen peroxide-producing *Lactobacillus* spp in the vagina is replaced by high concentrations of polymicrobial anaerobic bacteria. Women with bacterial vaginosis have complex and diverse vaginal infections, with many newly recognised species, including three bacteria in the Clostridiales order that are highly specific for bacterial vaginosis.[15]

BV 'infection' is a superficial one and is characterised by a lack of an inflammatory reaction and an absence of white cells in the discharge. This is why it is called a 'vaginosis' rather than a 'vaginitis'. Previously the condition was known as *Gardnerella* vaginosis, because the organism *Gardnerella vaginalis* was commonly found in increased numbers in women with BV. However, it is not always present and has been reported in 16–42% of women with no signs or symptoms of vaginitis.[16]

CASE STUDY: 'Unpleasant discharge'

A 30-year-old woman presents with what she calls 'unpleasant discharge'. She describes it as smelly and slightly irritating but not itchy. She had a similar episode 6 months ago which she thought was thrush and which resolved spontaneously. She wants to know if it's anything serious and how she can get rid of it.

What causes BV?

The literature has yet to show a real understanding of why BV occurs or how its recurrence can be stopped. The prevalence of BV varies with ethnicity (with rates of >33% in studies of Indigenous Australian women,[17] and >50% in sub-Saharan African and African American women[18]), low socioeconomic status, a history of STDs, large numbers of sexual partners and a recent change in sexual partner. A high concordance of BV between women in lesbian relationships has also been reported.[19]

What is the significance of BV?

BV puts women at greater risk of developing other STIs, especially HIV.[20] It can also lead to infective complications after surgery and premature birth (see p 233).

What are the symptoms of BV?

Characteristically, women notice a thin, watery, homogenous discharge and an associated malodorous, 'fishy' smell (Figs 13.4 and 13.5). Often women can be completely asymptomatic. Characterised by an overgrowth of anaerobic bacteria, it can occur and remit spontaneously.[21]

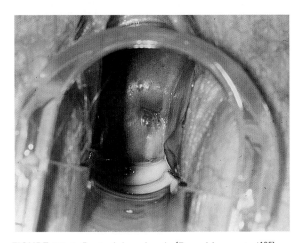

FIGURE 13.4 Bacterial vaginosis (From Morse et al[125])

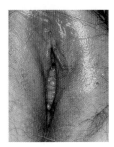

FIGURE 13.5 Bacterial vaginosis (From Habif [130])

How is the diagnosis of BV made?

Examination of a woman with a complaint of a vaginal discharge or odour should include an evaluation for the clinical criteria (Amsel criteria)[23] of BV (Box 13.2). At least three of these criteria must be present for a diagnosis of BV to be made.

The odour of the vaginal secretions can be tested by smelling the withdrawn speculum (the 'whiff test'); normal vaginal secretions do not have an unpleasant odour. If this test is negative, a more sensitive procedure for detecting the amines produced is performed by adding a few drops of 10% potassium hydroxide (KOH) to a few drops of vaginal secretions. The mixture should be smelt ('whiffed') immediately for the transient 'dead fish' odour characteristic of BV. KOH increases the pH to the point at which the volatilisation of polyamines, such as putrescine, cadaverine and trimethylamine, occurs. (Many women first notice vaginal malodour immediately following intercourse, because semen, which has a pH of 8.0, alkalinises vaginal fluid, thus releasing the volatile amines.)

The pH of vaginal secretions can be determined by using a strip of narrow-range pH paper (about pH 4.0–5.5), which may be applied to the withdrawn speculum or directly pressed against the vaginal wall with a swab.

Lastly, a wet mount of vaginal secretions should be tested to look for 'clue' cells. These are epithelial cells covered with *G. vaginalis* (Fig 13.6, p 232). They have a ground glass appearance and are the clues to the diagnosis of BV. By comparison, vaginal epithelial cells from women without BV have clear borders.

The Gram stain is the single, best laboratory test for diagnosis of BV. This method is preferable to culture because it has greater specificity. To prepare a vaginal smear for a Gram stain, a swab should be used to obtain vaginal fluid and cells

---

BOX 13.2 Diagnostic criteria for bacterial vaginosis

- Homogenous vaginal discharge (colour and amount may vary)
- Presence of clue cells (greater than 20% of the epithelial cells on the wet prep should be clue cells)
- Amine ('fishy') odour when potassium hydroxide solution is added to vaginal secretions (commonly called the 'whiff test')
- Vaginal pH greater than 4.5
- Absence of normal lactobacilli

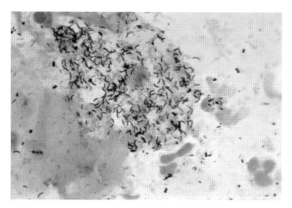

FIGURE 13.6 Clue cells (From Morse et al[125])

from the vaginal wall (not the cervix). This swab should then be rolled across a slide and the material allowed to air-dry. There is no need to fix the smear prior to shipment to the laboratory: air-dried vaginal smears are stable at room temperature for months.

Is BV a sexually transmissible infection?

This is a very controversial issue. A recent systematic review and meta-analysis has found that there are associations between BV and increasing number of partners and a decrease in the incidence of condom use.[24] However, there is opposition to this view because:

- urethral colonisation rates of *Gardnerella* and *Mobiluncus* species among male partners of women with BV are no higher than those for partners of normal women.[25]
- Co-treating the male partner has not been shown to reduce the recurrence risk in females.[26,27,28]
- BV has been diagnosed in women who have not been sexually active.[29]

How is BV treated?

There are two options, either oral or topical treatment. First-line treatment of BV is either oral metronidazole (Flagyl) or tinidazole (Fasigyn) or the use of the vaginal cream clindamycin. These treatments are outlined in Box 13.3. Oral and topical therapy have the same efficacy, with cure rates of 70–90%.[30] There is no evidence of teratogenicity of metronidazole in women during the first trimester of pregnancy.[31–33] Regardless of which therapy is used, BV will recur in over half of the women in which treatment seemed effective.[34] In this group it may be helpful to suggest condom use because of the associated decreased incidence of BV among

---

> **BOX 13.3 Treatment of bacterial vaginosis in non-pregnant women**
>
> **Oral treatment**
> - Metronidazole (Flagyl) 400 mg b.d. for 7 days or 2 g stat
> - Tinidazole (Fasigyn) 2 g stat
>
> **Topical treatment**
> - Clindamycin 2% vaginal cream (Dalacin). Use one applicator-full intravaginally at bedtime for 7 consecutive days.

female partners[35] (perhaps because the pH of semen does not affect the vaginal ecosystem when condoms are used).

Recent meta-analyses have established the safety of metronidazole use by pregnant women in the first trimester of pregnancy.

If a woman has no symptoms (many women have possible BV reported as an incidental finding on smear), should it be formally diagnosed and treated?

Recent research has shown that BV is associated with post-abortion pelvic inflammatory disease[36] and post-hysterectomy vaginal cuff cellulitis.[37] In pregnancy BV is associated with:

- amniotic fluid infection[38]
- clinical chorioamnionitis[39]
- spontaneous abortion, postpartum endometritis and post-caesarean wound infections[40]
- premature rupture of membranes (7.3 times more likely in the presence of BV)[41]
- preterm delivery[42,43]
- low birth weight.[44]

Because of its association with these adverse events women who are seen prior to having an abortion or hysterectomy or when pregnant should therefore be tested for BV and treated if it is present.

What is the association between BV and premature birth?

There are many and varied reasons why premature birth occurs. In up to 40% of cases, the cause is infection,[45] with one of the strongest correlations with premature delivery being the existence of chorioamnionitis. This condition is also associated with failure of the tocolytic drug therapy that is used to delay or reverse the onset of labour. Examination of the amniotic fluid or chorioamniotic membranes of women who experience premature labour and premature rupture of membranes commonly finds evidence of infection manifested by the presence of organisms and inflammatory cytokines. Most of these microorganisms are thought to come from the vagina, particularly from women with BV.[46]

In typical obstetric populations, BV is prevalent in 10–30% of women.[47] In a study of high-risk pregnant women, the prevalence was 50%.[48] Studies looking at the association between BV in pregnancy and premature delivery have found relative risks ranging from 0 to 6.9. A recently published meta-analysis reviewed 19 studies looking at the association and found a 60% increased risk of premature delivery given the presence of BV, or an odds ratio of 1.6.[49]

This association has enormous clinical significance, but the association between BV and premature delivery is not clear-cut. It is thought that BV is only a marker for something else—presumably subclinical infection of the upper genital tract that then leads to premature delivery. Interestingly, spontaneous regression of BV during pregnancy as assessed by vaginal Gram stain does not appear to improve perinatal outcomes.[50]

Does treatment of BV decrease the risk of premature birth?

A Cochrane review[51] has found that antibiotic therapy was highly effective in eradicating infection during pregnancy. They also found that, while treating BV during pregnancy resulted in a trend towards fewer births before 37 weeks' gestation, it only significantly prevented births before 37 weeks' gestation in the subgroup of women with a previous premature birth (odds ratio 0.37, 95% CI 0.23–0.60).

This means that the current evidence does not support screening and treating all pregnant women for BV to prevent premature birth and its consequences. However, a proportion of those women with a history of premature birth may benefit from detection and treatment, preventing a further premature birth.

What guidelines for the management of this problem currently exist?

The American College of Obstetrics and Gynecology (ACOG) recommends that women be screened for BV during pregnancy only if they have a history of premature delivery or if they weigh less than 50 kg before the commencement of the pregnancy.[52] On the basis of current evidence, ACOG maintains that screening for other women is not warranted.

Summary of key points
- BV is the most common cause of vaginal discharge in women of reproductive age.
- The characteristic symptoms are a 'fishy' smell and a thin, watery, homogeneous discharge.
- BV is not a sexually transmissible infection.
- BV has been found to be associated with post-abortion pelvic inflammatory disease, post-hysterectomy vaginal cuff cellulitis and premature rupture of membranes.
- Women should be screened for BV in pregnancy if they have a history of premature birth.

Vaginitis: trichomoniasis

What is trichomoniasis?

Trichomoniasis is caused by a flagellated protozoan that is sexually transmitted. In men the infection occurs in the urethra, but in women infection can occur in the vagina, urethra and paraurethral glands. In fact, urethral infection occurs in 90% of cases but is the only site of infection in less than 5% of cases.

How does it present?

Symptoms in women can range from being asymptomatic to intense pruritus, dyspareunia and dysuria. Patients may notice some discharge and odour.

How can a diagnosis be made?

Classically vaginal discharge is frothy, yellowy-green in colour and malodorous (Figs 13.7 and 13.8, p 234). The vulva and vagina appear inflamed (in contrast to BV) and a 'strawberry cervix' (this appearance is due to punctuate haemorrhages) is visible to the naked eye in 2% of patients.

CASE STUDY: Vaginal irritation and odour

Amanda was a 35-year-old woman with chronic schizophrenia who was not very compliant with her medications. This resulted in frequent readmissions to the local psychiatric hospital. She tended to have many sexual partners (especially when in hospital) and after the last admission presented with vaginal irritation and odour. The diagnosis was suggested on examination when frothy malodourous discharge was seen pooling in the posterior fornix of the vagina. This was later confirmed on microscopy. Amanda had contracted trichomoniasis. In this instance it was going to be difficult to carry out contact tracing.

The clinical features are not sufficiently sensitive to diagnose *Trichomonas vaginalis* infection.[53] Diagnosis should therefore occur either through microscopy or culture of the organism. A swab is taken from the pool of discharge in the posterior fornix of the vagina. If a microscope is to hand, the *Trichomonas* can be seen as a unicellular flagellated protozoan in a saline wet mount. Culture requires a special medium. Sometimes *Trichomonas* infection is detected on a Pap smear as an incidental finding. Cervical cytology has a sensitivity of only 60–80% for *Trichomonas,* however, and a false positive rate of 30%, so its use as a diagnostic test is not recommended.[54]

What treatment is there?

Trichomonas is effectively treated with metronidazole. It can be taken either as a stat dose of 2 g or a twice-daily dose of 400 mg for 7 days. While compliance and expense favour the stat dose, the failure rate (5%) may be higher with single-dose therapy, possibly because of failure to treat partners concurrently. Side effects of metronidazole include nausea, a metallic taste and the need to abstain from using alcohol during use and for 48 hours afterwards.

Contrasting with BV, vaginal preparations such as metronidazole gel are not effective at treating *Trichomonas* (50%). Topically applied antimicrobials are unlikely to achieve therapeutic levels in the urethra or perivaginal glands and are therefore not recommended for use.

Some strains of *T. vaginalis* have diminished susceptibility to metronidazole. Thankfully, most of these will respond to higher doses of metronidazole. If treatment fails with either regimen, the patient should be re-treated with metronidazole 500 mg twice a day for 7 days. If treatment fails again, the patient should be treated with a single, 2 g dose of metronidazole once a day for 3–5 days.[55]

As with all STIs, sexual partners need to be treated simultaneously, contacts traced and screening for concurrent STIs undertaken.

Patients should be instructed to avoid sex until they and their sex partners are cured, i.e. when therapy has been completed and patient and partner(s) are asymptomatic (in the absence of a microbiologic test of cure).

What if the patient is pregnant?

Like BV, vaginal trichomoniasis has been associated with enhanced HIV transmission and increased adverse pregnancy outcomes, such as premature rupture of the membranes, preterm delivery, and low

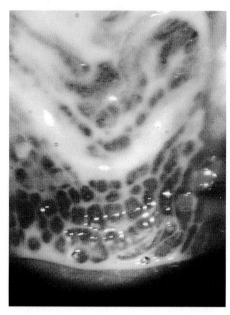

FIGURE 13.7 Trichomoniasis (From Morse et al[125])

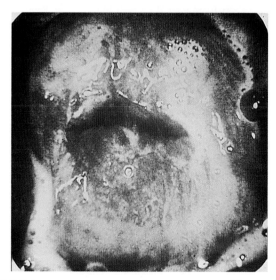

FIGURE 13.8 Trichomoniasis (From Morse et al[125])

birth weight.[56] Unfortunately a study examining the consequences of treatment of pregnant women with metronidazole resulted in increased morbidity.[57]

Summary of key points
- *Trichomonas vaginalis* is a protozoan.
- Patients with *T. vaginalis* infection can range from being asymptomatic to having intense pruritus and inflammation.
- Infection of the vagina occurs but also of the urethra.

- Neurotropism
- Skin manifestations
- Latency (site being the trigeminal or sacral ganglia)
- Recurrence

- Metronidazole orally is the treatment of choice, in either a single dose or as a 7-day course.
- Treatment failure may be due to not treating partners concurrently or because the dose is too low.

Herpes

What causes herpes?

The herpes simplex virus (HSV) belongs to the Herpetoviridae family, the properties of which are described in Box 13.4. It gains access to sensory neurones through abraded skin, causes latency and persists for the life of the host. There are two types of HSV, type 1 and 2. Both types can cause oral and/or genital herpes, although type 1 favours oral sites and type 2 genital infections.

How common is it?

The prevalence and epidemiology of the two types of HSV are quite different. HSV1, traditionally associated with oral infection, is prevalent in about 20% of children <5 years of age and the prevalence rises in a linear fashion thereafter.[58] Eventually about 80% of people acquire HSV1.[59] Interestingly only a third report ever having a 'cold sore'.[60] HSV1 genital herpes may be increasing in incidence, especially in younger people. In a Melbourne study, the proportion of first-episode genital herpes due to HSV1 increased from 15.8 to 34.9% of cases between 1980 and 2003.[61] The rising incidence of HSV1 genital herpes could be the result of decreasing HSV1 seroprevalence and consequently a larger susceptible population and/or an increase in the popularity of oral sex.[62]

In contrast HSV2 is extremely rare in young people, with most disease being acquired between the ages of 15 and 40, as would be expected of an STD. Approximately 20–25% of sexually active people contract HSV2 during this time.[63] Prior infection with HSV1 modifies the clinical manifestations of first infection by HSV2.[64]

What is the natural history of herpes?

One of the key features of herpes infection that has become more evident in recent years is the fact that the majority of herpes remains undiagnosed, probably because most outbreaks are not recognised and are only mildly symptomatic.[65] Less than 25% of HSV2 seropositive people report a clinical diagnosis of genital herpes.[60] However, 50–60% of 'asymptomatic' HSV2 seropositive people can identify clinical outbreaks if taught how to do so.[66] Reasons for failure to diagnose genital herpes infection are given in Box 13.5.

A patient who contracts herpes for the first time may or may not have the classical primary presentation of the disease. They may instead have any one or more of the clinical manifestations of genital herpes that are listed in Box 13.6. How primary herpes manifests depends on preexisting immunity. The severity of symptoms is much greater for people with primary genital HSV infection (HSV2 acquisition by a person without preexisting HSV1 immunity or HSV1 acquisition by a seronegative person) than with initial non-primary HSV2 infection (HSV2 acquisition by a person with preexisting HSV1 immunity).[67] Following initial infection, the virus becomes latent, during which time asymptomatic shedding and clinical recurrences can occur.

What are the characteristics of primary herpes?

The characteristic features of primary herpes include severe pain and systemic symptoms such as headache, fever and inguinal lymphadenopathy.

- Anatomically hidden
- Microscopic ulceration
- No clinical abnormality
- Atypical symptoms not correctly diagnosed
- Failure of presentation to the doctor
- Insensitivity of current diagnostic tests

- Painless ulcers
- Dysuria
- Urethral and vaginal discharge
- Vulvar irritation
- Perianal and vulvar fissures
- Classical vesicopustular lesions

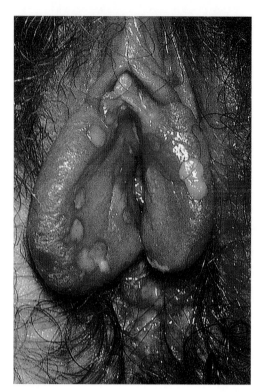

FIGURE 13.9 Primary vulval herpes infection (From James et al[126])

CASE STUDY: Primary herpes

Miranda, 18 years old, presented 2 weeks after attending her end-of-school party. She complained of dysuria and in the consultation room seemed very uncomfortable. On examination she had the unmistakable signs of primary herpes with small ulcers and a couple of small vesicles scattered over the vulva associated with inguinal lymphadenopathy. On further questioning, she started crying, saying that her first sexual encounter had occurred after the party with a boy from her class. She had been a little intoxicated and they had not used a condom.

BOX 13.7 Management of primary genital herpes

Management of primary genital herpes involves:
- symptomatic treatment
- salt baths
- changing pads frequently
- betadine
- xylocaine jelly
- antiviral therapy
- provision of written information about herpes infection.

Patients may notice some tingling and irritation followed by the development of genital sores that are extremely painful. In women, the vulva is very swollen with clusters of clear fluid-filled vesicles, which burst, develop into open ulcers and then crust over and dry out (Fig 13.9). The ulcers are very tender. Sometimes the pain is so severe that acute urinary retention and constipation ensue. Primary herpes occurs between 2 and 20 days after exposure and is much more severe than recurrent attacks.

What is the management of primary herpes?

Patients should be advised to cleanse the vulva with warm water, to allow air-drying and then to use Betadine and some local anaesthetic jelly. The woman can also use analgesics and should keep the sores clean and dry. She can commence with an antiviral medication such as Acyclovir 200 mg five times daily for 5 days or until resolution of infection, after taking a swab for culture or PCR. Valacyclovir (500 mg twice daily) can also be prescribed. The patient should be recalled for a STI screen when she can tolerate a speculum examination, as if she has contracted herpes she

will also be at risk of having contracted other STIs. For a summary of the management of primary genital herpes, see Box 13.7.

In genital herpes:
- 20% are truly asymptomatic
- 20% have been diagnosed because of symptoms
- 60% have symptomatic but undiagnosed infection.

What is the nature of a recurrent attack?

Compared with primary herpes, secondary or recurrent episodes of genital herpes are more likely to present with less severe pain and ulceration (Fig 13.10) and can often just manifest with atypical symptoms such as fissures and rashes. Recurrences are often triggered by factors such as those listed in Box 13.8 and over time decrease in frequency and severity. Recurrent episodes of genital HSV1 are much less frequent than those experienced by

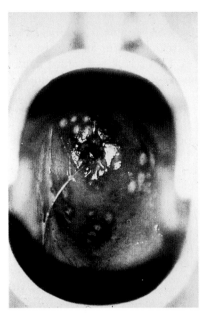

FIGURE 13.10 Genital herpes: cervical lesions identified by speculum examination (From Black and Mackay[22])

BOX 13.8 Triggers to recurrence of genital herpes

- Immunosuppression
- Menstruation
- Trauma
- UV radiation

---

patients infected with HSV2 which accounts for 95% of recurrence cases.[68]

When treating recurrences, the dose of Famciclovir is 125 mg twice daily and the dose of Valacyclovir is 500 mg twice daily.

About 70–90% of people with symptomatic HSV2, and 20–50% with symptomatic genital HSV1 will have a recurrence within the first year.[68]

What occurs during the latent phase of infection?

Patients are said to be in the 'latent phase' of the infection if they are symptom-free, although asymptomatic viral shedding can still occur in this phase. It is hard to tell when asymptomatic shedding is occurring. Known predictive factors for asymptomatic viral shedding are listed in Box 13.9,

---

BOX 13.9 Factors involved in asymptomatic viral shedding

- How recently the herpes was acquired
- Type of HSV (HSV2 sheds more commonly than HSV1)
- Use of antiviral therapy
- Immunosuppression

---

and include time since acquisition of the infection (shedding being more frequent in the first year), type of virus (shedding is more common with type 2) and annual number of symptomatic recurrences.[69,70] It is not related to contraception or menstruation. Asymptomatic viral shedding of HSV2 has been found to occur on up to 20% of days when HSV2 is tested for with polymerase chain reaction (PCR) technology.[66,71] This has important implications when counselling patients regarding their risks of transmitting HSV, as they may not know when they are infectious.

How is herpes transmitted?

Given that an estimated 80% of people with the disease remain undiagnosed, about 70% of cases of first-episode herpes are contracted from asymptomatic individuals.[72] Transmission from asymptomatic individuals in monogamous relationships can occur after several years, causing severe psychological distress. Because intercourse involves greater trauma to female genitalia, male to female transmission is much higher than female to male.

Previous HSV1 infection does not reduce the rate of HSV2 infection, but it does increase the likelihood of asymptomatic seroconversion, as compared with symptomatic seroconversion.[64]

In discordant couples what are the chances of catching herpes?

Couples are serodiscordant when one partner is seropositive for herpes and the other is seronegative. In a study of HSV serodiscordant couples advised to abstain from sexual contact during HSV recurrences, transmission occurred in 3.8% and 16.9% of susceptible male and female partners respectively over 12 months.[73] Condoms offer significant protection against male to female transmission of HSV, but not vice-versa.[74] This is because the herpes virus affects all the genital skin area, not just the penis. Condom use should still be recommended, however, as protection against other STIs.

When counselling discordant couples, a good rule of thumb is that the non-infected partner has a 10% chance of becoming infected after a year of unprotected intercourse.

What is the best method of diagnosing herpes?

Several methods can be used to diagnose herpes virus infection. The direct detection tests include HSV culture, immunofluorescence or DNA detection. These tests are type- and site-specific and are therefore useful only for those patients presenting with clinical lesions.

Conventional viral culture followed by viral typing has been until recently the diagnostic method of choice.[75] In order to culture HSV, the best results are obtained when a swab is taken of vesicular fluid from a blister that has had the top removed. Vesicular fluid is filled with live virus, whereas open sores and mucus will more generally contain bacteria and pus cells. The sensitivity of viral culture is notoriously low, however, leading to false negative results, often because patients present with dry sores that give very little live viral material to culture.

The Western blot assay is the gold standard for type-specific HSV serology. More recently ELISA tests have become commercially available, although they are limited by the window period of 12 weeks for the patient to develop IgG antibodies.

PCR testing has emerged as an alternative method for herpes diagnosis because it is up to four times more sensitive, less dependent on collection and transport conditions, and potentially faster than viral culture.[76]

Is it necessary to undertake viral typing?

In the absence of lesions, or with negative virus detection tests, serological testing can identify HSV infection. Type-specific IgG testing directed against glycoprotein G of HSV1 or that of HSV2 can distinguish HSV1 infection from HSV2 infection. There is little utility in screening for HSV; however, viral typing of the herpes virus into HSV1 or HSV2 is important:

- when counselling discordant couples regarding their risks of transmission
- when counselling the patient about long-term outcomes
- to demonstrate maternal seronegativity or discordant serology between partners in pregnancy.

Viral typing is also useful for advising patients about long-term outcomes, particularly because HSV2 is associated with an increased number of recurrences. HSV2 is also regarded more seriously when women develop herpes at the time of delivery (whether as a primary or secondary infection), because of the higher degree of risk it poses to the infant.

Type-specific serology and direct virus-testing can help to establish whether the episode is new acquisition of HSV infection or reactivation (Table 13.3). Type-specific HSV antibodies can take from 2 weeks to 3 months to develop. Thus, in a person with newly acquired herpes, the initial absence of IgG antibodies specific for glycoprotein G and subsequent development of such antibodies after 12 weeks confirms new HSV infection.[77]

What advice should be given to a woman who contracts or has herpes while pregnant?

HSV poses a significant threat to the fetus/neonate at the time of delivery. The worst-case scenario is for a woman to develop a primary infection in the last trimester of pregnancy. The neonate may then become infected from the mother's genital tract before she has produced type-specific neutralising antibodies, which seem at least partially protective. This is why recurrent infections (where the antibodies already exist) pose less risk to the neonate.[78]

When a baby is delivered through a genital tract infected with primary herpes, neonatal infection occurs in 50% of cases. The neonatal mortality rate of those infected is in the order of 50–65%, and serious neurological sequelae occur in 75% of survivors of neonatal infection.

If couples are discordant, pregnant women should be advised to use condoms throughout the pregnancy during sexual activity. Should acute infection occur, delivery via caesarean section is currently preferred, despite the lack of evidence to support this intervention.[79]

How do antivirals work in the treatment of herpes?

Acyclovir decreases the duration and severity of the illness and viral shedding. It works by inhibiting viral replication, inhibiting the formation of new lesions and reducing viral shedding. It will not affect the chances of having a recurrent attack of herpes, however, as it does not eliminate the virus from the dorsal root ganglia.

The major differences between the antivirals currently available are their different bioavailabilities and therefore dosing frequency. Acyclovir is equally as effective as famciclovir and valacyclovir, but it

TABLE 13.3 Virological and serological approach to HSV2 diagnosis in the presence and absence of genital lesions

	HSV2 positive by culture, antigen detection or PCR	Type-specific HSV1 IgG antibody	Type-specific HSV2 IgG antibody	Interpretation
First assessment of genital lesions	Positive	Positive or negative	Negative	Acute HSV2 infection can check convalescent HSV2 antibody
	Positive	Positive or negative	Positive	Recurrent HSV2 infection, with HSV2 infection acquired at least 6 weeks ago
No lesions	N/A	Negative	Negative	At risk of orolabial or genital HSV1 infection and HSV2 infection; if healed genital lesions or new sexual exposure, check convalescent HSV1 and HSV2 serology
	N/A	Positive	Negative	At risk of acquiring HSV2 infection; if healed genital lesions or new sexual exposure, check convalescent HSV2 serology
	N/A	Positive	Positive	HSV1 and HSV2 infection
Recurrent genital lesions	Positive	Positive or negative	Positive	Recurrent HSV2 infection
	Negative	Negative	Positive	Recurrent HSV2 infection; need to consider other potential causes of genital ulcerative disease

has reduced bioavailability and therefore requires a five-times daily dosage for initial episodes and a t.d.s. or b.d. dosage for suppressive therapy. It is much less expensive than either of these drugs, however. Topical acyclovir can reduce the duration of viral shedding and the length of time before all lesions become crusted, but it is much less effective than oral therapy.

Antiviral therapy can be taken episodically for individual outbreaks or as daily suppressive therapy in those patients whose recurrences are too frequent to be tolerable or where a decrease in asymptomatic viral shedding is required. The dosage of the various antivirals available is given in Table 13.4.

Is the vaccine against herpes viable?

The herpes vaccine is still being evaluated and has yet to be commercially released.

Summary of key points

- Following primary infection, HSV becomes latent in local sensory ganglia, periodically reactivating to cause symptomatic lesions or asymptomatic, but infectious, viral shedding.
- More than 80% of people with HSV2 are asymptomatic, yet shed virus from the genital tract.
- Many people who acquire infection subclinically subsequently develop clinical recurrences.

TABLE 13.4 Antivirals used in the treatment of genital HSV (From Gupta et al[77])

Name	Primary herpes	Recurrent herpes	Suppressive therapy
Acyclovir	200 mg 5 times daily for 5–10 days	200 mg 5 times daily for 5 days	200 mg t.d.s. or 400 mg b.d.
Valacyclovir	500 mg b.d. for 5–10 days	500 mg b.d. for 5 days	500 mg daily; increase to b.d. if <10 episodes per year
Famciclovir	Not indicated	125 mg b.d. for 5 days	250 mg b.d.

- Recurrence rates decline over time in most individuals.
- Transmission can occur in long-standing monogamous couples.

Genital warts

What causes genital warts?

Human papilloma virus (HPV) can appear anywhere in the genital region, from the vulva to the perianal area. Most anogenital warts are benign and caused by types 6 and 11. Genital warts and those present on the hands and feet are generally of different types and therefore not thought to be transmissible from one site to the other.

How is HPV transmitted?

The highest rates of genital HPV infections are found in adults 18–28 years of age. Although risk factors for infection are difficult to assess because of the high frequency of subclinical infection, the statistical likelihood of acquiring genital HPV increases according to the number of different sexual partners a person has. Direct skin-to-skin contact spreads HPV infection most efficiently. The virus is not transmitted via blood or body fluid, e.g. semen. Genital forms of the virus target the mucous membranes and adjacent genital skin.

How soon after exposure do they come about?

The incubation period of HPV, while usually in the order of 3–6 months, may vary.[80]

How common is HPV?

HPV infection is widespread, with approximately 75% of women being exposed to at least one HPV infection in their lifetime.[81] The highest prevalence is in young women (20–25% around age 20) falling to 10% at age 30 and falling slightly thereafter.[81] A small increase in women over 65 years may reflect reactivation of previously undetectable infection acquired earlier in life, new infections or a cohort effect.[82] Visible warts are only present in 1% of adults aged 15–49 years. Most genital HPV infections are subclinical, with 4% of women having the wart virus on colposcopy and 10% of the community having subclinical infection.[83] This is graphically represented in Figure 13.11. Indeed many women are surprised to hear that changes attributable to HPV have been found on their

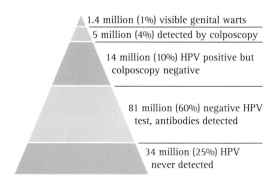

FIGURE 13.11 The prevalence of HPV (From Koutsky[83])

smear test, as they have never noticed any obvious warts. This situation necessitates explaining to them the concept of subclinical infection, a good analogy for which is that obvious genital warts represent only the 'tip of the iceberg' where HPV is concerned.

What do genital warts look like?

Genital warts occur in the anogenital area. They are usually visible on clinical examination and may be discrete or coalesce into confluent plaques[84] (Figs 13.12 and 13.13). Genital warts can be either multifocal, where one or more lesions occur at one anatomic site (e.g. vulva), or multicentric, where lesions occur at different sites (e.g. perineum and cervix). Smooth papular warts tend to occur on fully keratinised skin, while condylomata accuminata occur most commonly on moist surfaces and flat-topped papular external genital warts can occur on either surface.[85] A characteristic lesion of HPV found on the vulva is the so-called 'kissing lesion', where warts are present on adjacent sides of the labia in women. Wart virus does not form cysts, ulcers or vesicles.

What is the differential diagnosis of genital warts?

The differential diagnosis of genital warts includes lesions that cause papules and flat erythematous lesions. This includes vestibular papillae, sebaceous glands, molluscum contagiosum, skin tags, melanocytic nevi and condylomata lata (found in secondary syphilis).

What is the natural history of HPV?

The natural history of HPV is outlined under 'Cervical cancer screening' in Chapter 12.

What management of genital warts can a GP use?

If left untreated, only 20% of warts would resolve spontaneously.[86] The others would either remain unchanged or increase in size and/or number. Most patients will therefore choose to treat. There are

---

CASE STUDY: 'He didn't have any diseases.'

Pam was very distressed. She was a 19-year-old girl who presented saying that she had felt something growing down below. After an examination, the GP told her that she had genital warts. The GP explained that having warts wasn't so bad and that most people picked up the wart virus if they were sexually active, but that some never knew they had it. On further history, Pam said that she had been sexually active with her current boyfriend for about 4 months and that he had told her that he didn't have any diseases. She was now concerned how she was going to tell him that she had warts and that she thought she had got them from him!

The image content (Figure 13.11):

1.4 million (1%) visible genital warts
5 million (4%) detected by colposcopy
14 million (10%) HPV positive but colposcopy negative
81 million (60%) negative HPV test, antibodies detected
34 million (25%) HPV never detected

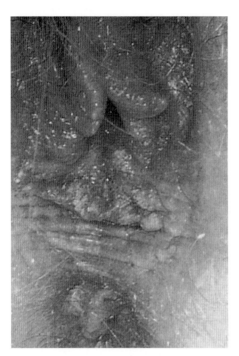

FIGURE 13.12 Vulval warts (From James et al[126])

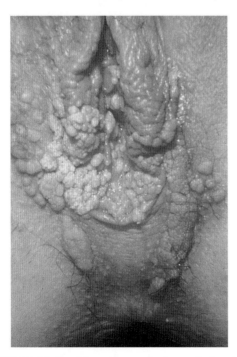

FIGURE 13.13 Condylomata acuminata – vulval and perineal (From Morse et al[125])

numerous treatment options (Box 13.10). Key principles when considering treatment for genital warts are listed in Box 13.11.

Podophyllotoxin is dispensed in 0.5% concentrations and causes tissue necrosis. Patients should be instructed to apply the solution to the warts while protecting surrounding skin through the application of Vaseline. It should be used twice a day for 2 or 3 days then the area should be rested for 4 days. This cycle can then be repeated several times.

If, however, the wart does not resolve, an alternative method should be used. Podophyllotoxin should not be used for large areas of warts or during pregnancy.

Imiquimod (Aldara cream) is a relatively new topically active immune enhancer that stimulates production of interferon and other cytokines. A thin layer of cream should be applied prior to sleep and rubbed in until no longer visible, three times a week for 16 weeks. The treated area should not be bandaged or wrapped occlusively. Sexual contact (genital, anal and oral) should be avoided while the cream is on the skin. About 6–10 hours following application of the cream, the treated area should be washed with mild soap and water. It is common for patients to experience skin reactions such as redness, flaking or oedema at the treatment site, and these reactions are usually mild or moderate in intensity. This treatment may worsen preexisting inflammatory skin conditions.

The cream is available only on prescription and the patient purchases a set of twelve sachets, which is equivalent to approximately 1 month of therapy. Imiquimod is not recommended for use for the treatment of urethral, intravaginal, intra-anal, cervical or rectal HPV infections, nor is it recommended for use during pregnancy. It may be that future trials of imiquimod will show benefit for the treatment of other viral conditions such as molluscum contagiosum; the results of these trials are eagerly awaited.

Of the physician-applied therapies, GPs would most commonly use cryotherapy. This destroys the wart tissue by freeze/thawing. Liquid nitrogen can either be applied using a 'cryogun', which delivers a very focused spray, or through application with loosely wound cotton on a wooden applicator. The full thickness of the wart should be frozen with whitening of the skin around the wart to 2 mm. Cryotherapy is the treatment of choice during pregnancy. The patient should be warned that the procedure is painful and that blistering sometimes occurs. Often patients will need to return for further applications to the same area.

How can large bulky warts be treated?

Most forms of treatment are eventually successful for patients with small numbers of warts. Where the warty area is large and bulky, ablative therapy to 'debulk' the warts is probably necessary.

Is there any indication to biopsy a lesion or lesions?

Biopsy and pathological examination should be considered when:

- lesions are surrounded by either thickened skin or colour changes
- lesions are slightly raised, red or pigmented
- presumed genital warts do not respond to several office treatments
- 'chronic dermatoses' do not respond to medical therapy
- when any suspicion of neoplasia exists.

Do genital warts recur?

After successful treatment, genital warts may recur. This usually happens in about 1 in 3 people. After the warts have resolved, some experts believe that the ability to transmit HPV decreases with time, but at present we do not know whether the immune system completely clears the virus from the body or whether the virus remains at undetectable levels.

If a woman finds out that she has HPV, what should she advise her sexual partner/s?

As far as the partner's risk of contracting HPV is concerned, condoms provide a barrier to the penis but do not prevent all genital skin-to-skin contact. Genital HPV infection is regional and not confined to the warts themselves; therefore condom use does not prevent the transmission of HPV.[87,88] While it is believed that transmission is more likely in the presence of visible warts, it is also possible when there is subclinical infection. Infection with one strain of genital wart virus does not confer immunity from infection from another strain. Once one HPV infection has resolved, a person is immune to infection by the same HPV type, but may be susceptible to future infection by other HPV types. It is therefore likely that if one member of a stable partnership has genital HPV infection, the other will be either infected or immune to that infection.

What patient characteristics are associated with resistance to therapy?

Patients who are pregnant, those who are immunosuppressed or smokers often have difficulty clearing HPV lesions.

What happens to genital warts during pregnancy?

Genital warts can proliferate and become friable during pregnancy because of altered immunity as well as increased blood supply. Rarely, laryngeal papillomatosis occurs in infants of mothers with genital warts, but how this happens is not clear. Imiquimod, podophyllin and podophyllotoxin should not be used during pregnancy, but warts can be treated using cryotherapy, trichloro-acetic acid (TCA), or surgical removal and laser ablation.[85]

Patients who are pregnant, immunosuppressed or smokers often have difficulty clearing HPV lesions.

What are the dangers of HPV infection?

Human papilloma virus has now been causally related to cervical cancer,[89] with HPV DNA detected in at least 95% of cervical cancers (of which HPV16 and HPV18 are the most commonly isolated types[90]).

The recent introduction of HPV vaccination now offers a primary preventive approach. Two HPV vaccines, exist:

- the bivalent Cervarix (HPV16 and 18)
- and the quadrivalent Gardasil (HPV16, 18, 6 and 11).

Worldwide, HPV types 16 and 18 are responsible for about 70% of cervical cancer cases, 50% of high-grade precancerous lesions and 25% of low-grade lesions.[91] HPV types 6 and 11 infections are associated with most genital warts and around 8–10% of low-grade cervical lesions.[92]

More information concerning the natural history of HPV and the HPV vaccine can be found in Chapter 12, under 'Cervical cancer screening'.

Summary of key points
- HPV types causing cancer are different from those which cause warts.
- HPV is common in people who have recently become sexually active.
- Most genital HPV is subclinical.
- Partners of those infected with HPV will either be infected themselves or have immunity to that infection.
- Biopsy is indicated only when the diagnosis is in doubt, where lesions are large and confluent or when the warts do not respond to treatment.
- No one treatment is ideal for all patients.

Non-infective causes of vaginal irritation

What kind of conditions can occur in the vulvovaginal region?

When trying to diagnose the cause of a genital rash or irritation, most GPs will start by thinking of an infective cause, as after all 'common things occur commonly'. However, one of the pitfalls is in isolating the genital area and treating it as removed from the array of dermatological conditions that can manifest elsewhere on the skin. Indeed, it is sometimes only when treatment for an infectious condition has failed that non-infectious causes are considered. In some cases the diagnosis may need

---

CASE STUDY: 'Things aren't quite right.'

Sandra, 60 years old, came in complaining of chronic vaginal irritation. On closer questioning she revealed she had had this for many years. Before going through the menopause around the age of 50, she remembered having endless treatments for thrush, with only minor improvements in symptoms. Since the menopause, she had seen a couple of different gynaecologists about her condition, which was put down to atrophic vaginitis. Since then she had used oestrogen pessaries religiously but she still felt that things weren't quite right. On examination, the vulva appeared pale and atrophic-looking despite Sandra's use of local oestrogen. There were excoriations and fissuring present. A small punch biopsy was taken and lichen sclerosus diagnosed. Sandra was prescribed topical steroids and returned for follow-up a couple of months later saying she felt a vast improvement.

---

to be confirmed with the use of a small punch biopsy under local anaesthetic and perhaps the placement of a small stitch.

Chronic dermatological vulvovaginal conditions are often misdiagnosed as having an infectious aetiology.

The range of conditions causing papulosquamous lesions in the genital area and their characteristic features are outlined in Table 13.5 (p 244).

For most GPs, the common conditions such as psoriasis (Fig 13.14, p 244), seborrhoeic dermatitis, tinea cruris and chronic dermatitis are easily diagnosable. The others, lichen simplex chronicus, planus and sclerosus are less common and therefore less familiar. In vulval dermatology clinics, lichen sclerosus is the most commonly diagnosed vulvar dermatosis; approximately one-third of the women have this disorder. Vulvar dermatitis is observed in 20–25% of new patients, and lichen planus is rare.[93]

What is lichen planus?

Lichen planus is a condition that can be described using the four 'Ps'—purple, polygonal, pruritic papules.

What is the aetiology and epidemiology of this condition?

Lichen planus is an uncommon skin complaint whose cause is unknown. It is thought to be due to an abnormal immune reaction, possibly started by a

TABLE 13.5 The differential diagnosis of common papulosquamous disorders of the genitals

Condition	Erythema	Skin changes (thickening)	Pruritus	Associated lesions
Psoriasis	++	+++	±	Red plaques with silvery scales on knees, elbows, scalp; nail pitting; little or no scaling in genital psoriasis
Seborrhoeic-dermatitis	++	+	+	Scaling/erythema on eyebrows, nasolabial folds, hairline and occasionally on axillae, inguinal folds or genitals
Tinea cruris	++	Raised border	++	Annular plaque with central clearing and peripheral scale
Candidiasis	++	Oedema	+++	Acute erythema, oedema, peeling, satellite lesions
Lichen simplex	++	+++	+++	May be limited to vulva, but other common sites include ankle, nape of neck and arm
Chronic dermatitis (contact or irritant)	+++	++	++	Often eczematous and oozing; may generalise
Lichen planus	Violaceous	++	++	Purple, polygonal, papules and plaques, especially on wrists and legs. Lacy, white pattern on buccal mucosa
Lichen sclerosus	+	−	±	Usually limited to the vulva and anus in 'keyhole' distribution; white and non-scaly, dermis thick and epidermis atrophic

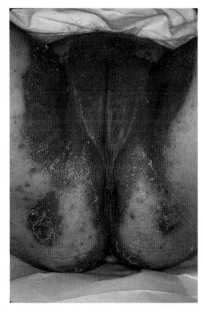

FIGURE 13.14 Psoriasis of the vulva (From Black and Mackay[22])

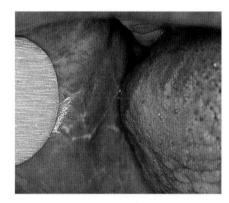

FIGURE 13.15 Wickham's striae (From Black and Mackay[22])

viral infection. Inflammatory cells seem to mistake the skin cells as foreign and attack them.

Where can this condition occur?

1. The genital areas of both men and women
2. The gums and lining of the mouth (oral lichen planus)
3. The skin of the arms (usually wrists and forearms), legs, and trunk of the body.

Oral lichen planus showing Wickham's striae, the fine white lines across the papules, is a characteristic feature of lichen planus (Fig 13.15). It is characterised by itchy, purple bumps on the shins, the inner wrist and the hands. In some cases, it can also affect the mouth (the inner cheeks, gums and tongue) and the genital and perianal (Fig 13.16) areas. About a third of those who have oral lichen planus will also have it on the skin. It often involves the vagina as well as the vulva, where it may resemble other vulvar skin conditions (Fig 13.17). In most cases, lichen planus goes away within 2 years, but it may leave a little brown discoloration that fades with time.

The exact cause of lichen planus is unknown but it is not an infectious disease. It is therefore not possible to 'catch' the disease or to 'give' it to someone else. The lesions consist of inflamed skin, but what causes the inflammation is unknown. The thin mucous

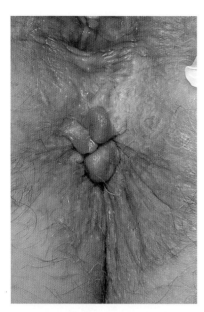

FIGURE 13.16 Lichen planus: typical white striae can occur on perianal skin as well. (From Habif[130])

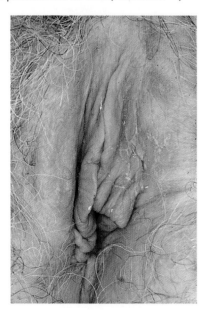

FIGURE 13.17 Lichen planus of the vulva (From Black and Mackay[22])

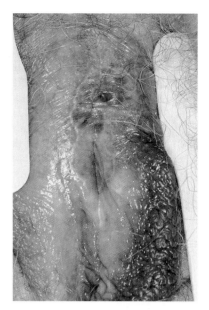

FIGURE 13.18 Lichen planus: lacy, reticulated pattern with periclitoral scarring (From Fisher and Margesson[131])

- increased vaginal discharge
- redness, soreness, burning associated with raw areas of the vulva and vagina
- bleeding and/or pain with intercourse.

Often the onset of lichen planus is slow, taking months to reach its peak. It usually clears within 18 months, but in a few people it persists for many years. People aged 30–60 years make up two-thirds of cases of lichen planus, with a preponderance of cases being in females.

Oral lichen planus is associated with diabetes, and more recently an association between hepatitis C and lichen planus has been revealed.[94]

Can complications arise from lichen planus?

If lichen planus becomes erosive, the lesions in the mouth become painful. If erosions occur in the vagina, they can become secondarily infected and lead to scarring and narrowing of the vagina, making intercourse difficult.

How is it diagnosed?

Lichen planus is diagnosed by biopsy. This is a minor procedure, often done in the GP's office under local anaesthesia. A small area of skin is removed and sent for analysis.

What treatment is appropriate?

Treatment is usually with various steroid creams and ointments that act to decrease the inflammation.

membranes inside the mouth and vagina lose their top layer when they become involved with lichen planus, so red erosions rather than bumps develop in these areas. Erosive lichen planus (Fig 13.18) may be painful in the mouth and vagina, and secondary infection may occur. If the areas touch one another, scarring may occur, resulting in a narrowing of the vagina.

Lichen planus can vary from mild to severe, but when erosions are present the following symptoms may occur:

If vaginal discharge occurs, it may indicate an erosion or secondary infection. Medication is most often used on a regular basis to maintain optimal tissue status, rather than only with flare-ups of the disease. There may be a small association with the development of vulvar carcinoma.

Treatment is not always necessary. Topical steroids can be used by applying a thin smear that is rubbed in accurately once a day and stopped when the lesions have flattened with the normal skin. This may take between 4 to 6 weeks. Brown marks are often left at the sites, which take several months to fade.

In extensive cases systemic steroids such as prednisolone may be prescribed for a few weeks or longer. This will lessen the itch and often clear up the lichen planus completely. However, it may recur later.

What is lichen sclerosus?

Lichen sclerosus has been described as the 'classic, pruritic, chronic dermatosis of the postmenopausal vulva'.[129] It is an inflammatory condition, its unknown aetiology perhaps linked to autoimmune disorders.[95] Women with vulval lichen sclerosus (Figs 13.19 and 13.20) complain of itch and irritation, soreness, dyspareunia and urinary symptoms. It can however be asymptomatic. On examination, the vulval skin is pale and atrophic-looking (Figure 13.21), with erosions and fissuring either in a localised or 'figure-of-eight' distribution in the perianal area (Fig. 13.22).

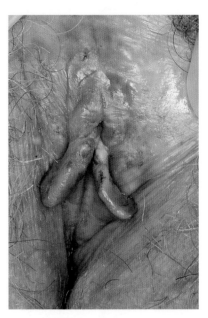

FIGURE 13.20 Lichen sclerosus et atrophicus of the vulva (kraurosis vulvae). The crease areas are atrophic and wrinkled, the labia is hyperpigmented, and the introitus is contracted and ulcerated. (From Habif[130])

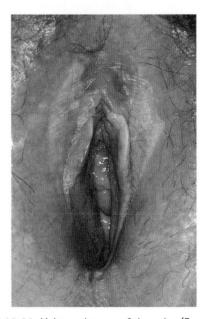

FIGURE 13.21 Lichen sclerosus of the vulva (From Black and Mackay[22])

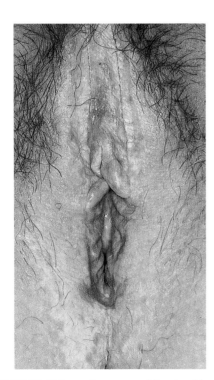

FIGURE 13.19 Lichen sclerosus: a white atrophic plaque encircles the vagina and the anus (inverted keyhole pattern). (From Habif[130])

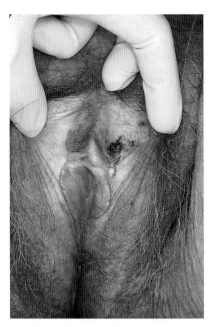

FIGURE 13.22 Lichen sclerosus of the vulva is often extremely pruritic. The thin epidermis is easily traumatised by scratching and petechiae and purpura are very characteristic findings in this disorder. (From Black and Mackay[22])

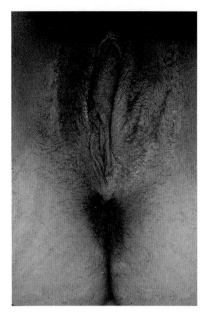

FIGURE 13.23 Lichen simplex chronicus (From Black and Mackay[22])

A complication of lichen sclerosus is loss of architecture in the vulval region, with loss of the labia or midline fusion as well as the development of squamous cell cancer. Diagnosis is by biopsy, and treatment consists of topical steroids, preferably in an ointment format twice a day for 3–4 months. Once the skin texture normalizes, the frequency of application can be decreased.

What is vulvar lichen simplex chronicus?

It is a chronic pruritic inflammatory dermatosis characterised by a plaque of cutaneous thickening usually affecting only one of the labia majora but sometimes both[96] (Fig 13.23). Patients complain of severe pruritus with nocturnal exacerbations. Treatment is with topical steroids.

CERVICAL CONDITIONS

Chlamydia

How common is Chlamydia?

Chlamydia is the most common bacterial sexually transmissible infection.[97] Notification rates have risen dramatically, from 47.4 per 100,000 population in 1997 to 273.8 per 100,000 in 2008.[98] It is unclear whether this is atributable to more testing, better testing methods or a true increase in prevalence. The answer is probably all three.

Studies have found that 16% of women attending STI clinics and 8% of women attending clinics for a termination of pregnancy have *Chlamydia*, and in family planning clinics the prevalence of *Chlamydia* among women patients is 5%.[99] Rates of infection

---

CASE STUDY: *Chlamydia* **in a woman under 25**

Marie, 21 years old, attended for a repeat prescription of her oral contraceptive pill. In passing, she mentioned that she had a new partner and had restarted the pill after stopping several months ago when she had broken up with her last boyfriend. The GP asked her if she had started back on the pill well before recommencing sexual activity, and Marie reassured her that she had been very responsible about it, as last year she had had an abortion because of exactly that reason and she had not wanted to repeat her mistake. The GP asked if Marie was also using condoms since she was with a new partner. Marie shook her head. 'Well how about having an STI screen then, to make sure you haven't picked up anything?' the GP asked. Marie agreed. One of the tests undertaken was a first-catch urine specimen to be tested by PCR for *Chlamydia*. The results came back several days later. Marie was positive for *Chlamydia*. She had had no symptoms and, when she asked her boyfriend about it, neither had he. They came in together for a prescription of azithromycin and Marie's boyfriend also underwent an STI screen.

are highest among young women aged 16–19.[100] In general practice, the prevalence of *Chlamydia* infection has been reported to be between 2% and 12%.[101]

How do you know if you have it?

The problem with *Chlamydia* is that it is generally an asymptomatic infection. Estimates are that over 80% of infections in men and women are asymptomatic, making screening the only way to detect cases and reduce the duration of infection and the risk of complications.[102,103] If there *are* symptoms, they are likely to be cervical discharge (perceived by women to be mucopurulent vaginal discharge), urinary symptoms, intermenstrual or postcoital bleeding or bleeding with pelvic pain, or dyspareunia due to the development of pelvic inflammatory disease (PID) (Fig 13.24).

What are the risk factors for Chlamydia?

Several studies have looked at the risk factors for *Chlamydia* in an effort to help determine who should be screened for infection. These studies have shown that *Chlamydia* is more likely to be found in women who[104]:

- are aged 25 years or under
- have a new or multiple partners
- are single
- are of ethnic background
- left school at an early age
- have genital symptoms
- have another STI.

Adolescent girls may indeed be at increased risk of acquiring *Chlamydia* compared with older women, because the adolescent cervix has a greater area of ectopy and because adolescents tend to engage in serial monogamy or have concurrent sexual partners.

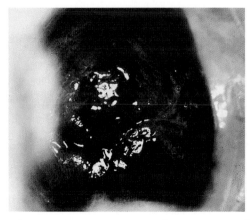

FIGURE 13.24 Chalmydial cervicitis (From Morse et al[125])

What are the consequences of Chlamydia infection?

Despite being a generally asymptomatic infection, *Chlamydia* can have devastating outcomes. The possible consequences of *Chlamydia* infection are listed in Box 13.12. Of note is the fact that 15–40% of women with untreated *Chlamydia* infection will develop pelvic inflammatory disease (PID).[105] Repeated PID episodes increase a woman's risk of infertility, with 11% infertile after one episode of PID and 23% infertile after two.[106]

Despite being the most prevalent bacterial STI, *Chlamydia* often goes undiagnosed, causing morbidity later in life.

What investigations should be undertaken if Chlamydia is suspected?

PCR and ligase chaine reaction (LCR) testing (nucleic acid amplification tests [NAATs]) have surpassed culture for the diagnosis of *Chlamydia*. The specimen can either be an endocervical or urethral swab or, more conveniently for the patient, a first-catch urine sample. The advantages of urine testing is that it is an ideal specimen for screening purposes, has high patient acceptability because it is not invasive and the specimen can be produced by the patient, and the urine can be used for testing of other infectious agents such as gonorrhoea.

Should GPs be screening for Chlamydia?

Given the high morbidity associated with *Chlamydia* infection, especially in terms of future infertility, screening for *Chlamydia* was introduced in Sweden, Denmark and the USA in the 1990s. While there were some initial reductions in the prevalence of *Chlamydia* following the introduction of these programs, prevalence has begun to increase again. The reasons for this are unclear but may involve changes in sexual behaviour, with a trend

---

BOX 13.12 The possible consequences of *Chlamydia* infection

- Urethritis
- Cervicitis
- Pelvic inflammatory disease (PID)
- Chronic pelvic pain
- Tubal infertility
- Ectopic pregnancy
- Reiter's syndrome (urethritis, arthritis and conjunctivitis)
- Fitz-Hugh–Curtis syndrome (perihepatitis with associated 'violin string' adhesions under the diaphragm)

to increasing numbers of sexual partners in young people.[107]

Australia is working towards the introduction of a national *Chlamydia* screening program. Various methods of *Chlamydia* screening are being considered, such as the possibility of a central *Chlamydia* screening registry that sends out invitations for screening or screening packs, screening through sports clubs and schools, and screening through general practice.[107]

What is the treatment for Chlamydia?

Previously, *Chlamydia* was treated with doxycycline 100 mg b.d. for 7 days. If the woman was pregnant or unable to take doxycycline, the alternative treatment was erythromycin 500 mg q.i.d. for 7 days. Having to take the medication for 1 week in multiple doses did not aid compliance. Azithromycin given as a 1 g stat dose is now the treatment of choice . It has helped address the compliance issues, has very few side effects and is very effective at eradicating *Chlamydia*.

Test of cure is not routinely recommended if standard treatment has been given, there is confirmation that the patient has adhered to therapy and there is no risk of reinfection. However, if these criteria cannot be met or if the patient is pregnant, a test of cure is advised. This should be taken using the same technique as used for the initial testing. Ideally, a minimum of 3–5 weeks post-treatment is required as nucleic acid amplification tests will demonstrate residual DNA/RNA even after successful treatment of the organism.[108]

What other issues should a GP be aware of with regard to Chlamydia?

Many women who have been diagnosed with *Chlamydia* and treated are often found to have what appears to be persistent infection or reinfection. The most likely reasons for this are probably reinfection from an untreated partner, inappropriate antibiotic treatment or non-compliance.

Contact tracing has been encouraged as a means of treating asymptomatic partners of infected patients. However, it is fraught with difficulties, as patients may not want to disclose that they have an STI to previous partners or indeed to current ones. Indeed, the mere fact that they have contracted an STI may suggest that one partner has been unfaithful, leading to all sorts of problems in their relationship. Male partners may also be very reticent to present to a doctor for a check-up, fearing intrusive examinations and painful investigations. For these reasons, many advocate the use of patient-delivered partner medication (PDPM). This is where the patient is given the antibiotic along with instructions to convey to their partner. The problem is that there is no way of ensuring compliance or testing the partner for other STIs.

The other issue to be aware of is the need to test the woman for other STIs. The fact that she has picked up *Chlamydia* puts her at high risk for having other concurrent STIs of which she is not aware.

Women diagnosed with *Chlamydia* require STI screening for other concurrent infections.

Gonorrhoea

Should GPs be concerned about gonorrhoea in their female patients?

Gonorrhoea is more common in the developing world than in the Western world, where it tends to be more prevalent in homosexual men and in men (and subsequently their female partners) who have engaged in sexual activity in developing countries.

Gonorrhoea is a Gram-negative diplococcus found in columnar epithelium (Fig 13.25). In women it can infect the urethra, cervix, rectum and the pharynx and tonsils. While in men the classic symptom is mucopurulent urethral discharge, in women the infection, like *Chlamydia*, can often be asymptomatic. The incubation period is 4–7 days. Like *Chlamydia*, this organism can cause PID and also bartholinitis.

Management consists of treatment with one of the following:

- ciprofloxacin 500 mg orally as a single dose
- ofloxacin 400 mg orally as a single dose

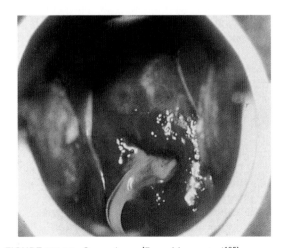

FIGURE 13.25 Gonorrhoea (From Morse et al[125])

ampicillin 2 g or 3 g plus probenecid 1 g orally as a single dose, where regional prevalence of penicillin-resistant *Neisseria gonorrhoeae* <5%.

Summary of key points
- Chlamydia is the most common bacterial STI.
- It is usually asymptomatic but responsible for a great deal of morbidity later in life.
- GPs should undertake routine screening for women <25 or for those >25 who have had a new or multiple partners in the past year.
- A first-catch urine specimen can be used for screening, using nucleic acid amplification tests such as LCR or PCR.
- The treatment of choice is azithromycin 1 g stat.
- Contact tracing is essential in order to decrease the prevalence of *Chlamydia*.
- Women who screen positive for *Chlamydia* should be tested for other STIs.

TIPS FOR PRACTITIONERS

- General advice to women for maintaining vaginal health:
  - avoid douching, as this may alter the pH of the vagina and its ecology
  - avoid perfumed soaps and feminine hygiene sprays, which can irritate the vagina
  - avoid tight, hot clothing that can trap moisture and create a good growth environment for infections
  - change pads and tampons frequently
  - when bathing wash the genital area with warm water only
  - during sex, use water-based lubricants such as KY jelly if the vagina feels too dry.
- A woman of reproductive age presenting with vaginal discharge who is low risk for STIs and without symptoms indicative of upper reproductive tract infection may be given empirical treatment, based on symptoms, without taking swabs at first presentation.[7]
- A woman of reproductive age complaining of vaginal discharge should be investigated if[7]:
  - she requests investigation
  - she is deemed to be at higher risk of STIs
  - there are symptoms indicative of upper reproductive tract infection
  - previous treatment has failed
  - it occurs postnatally
  - it occurs after miscarriage or abortion
  - she is within 3 weeks of intrauterine contraceptive insertion.

- Risk factors for STIs to be sought are[7]:
  - age <25 years
  - change in sexual partner in the last year
  - more than one partner in the last year.
- Group B streptococcus is often reported on vaginal swabs, but is not usually thought to cause discharge and needs treatment only in pregnancy.[109]
- Treatment of recurrent thrush involves a two-phase approach:
  - 'induction', with at least 1 week of oral products or 1–2 weeks of topical products
  - a maintenance period of 6 months using either oral fluconazole 100 mg weekly or topical clotrimazole (in the form of a pessary) 500 mg weekly.
- Isolation of *Gardnerella vaginalis* cannot be used to diagnose BV because it can be cultured from the vagina of more than 50% of normal women.
- Alcohol should be avoided when taking metronidazole because of the possibility of a disulfiram-like action. Clindamycin cream can weaken condoms, which should not be used during such treatment. Pseudomembranous colitis has been reported with both oral clindamycin and clindamycin cream.[110]
- HSV is one of the three most prevalent STIs (together with *Chlamydia* and human papilloma virus)[111] and, apart from HIV, is of greatest concern to sexually active people.[112]
- Acyclovir inhibits viral replication and new lesion formation and reduces viral shedding, infectivity and risk of autoinfection in first episodes. There is no effect on chance of recurrence, however.
- Acyclovir 3% ointment is not effective for the treatment of genital herpes.
- Specific counselling messages concerning genital herpes should include the following:
  - Education should be given about the natural history of the disease, with emphasis on the potential for recurrent episodes, asymptomatic viral shedding and attendant risks of sexual transmission.
  - Suppressive and episodic antiviral therapy is available and is effective in preventing or shortening the duration of recurrent episodes.
  - The patient should be encouraged to inform current sex partner(s) that they have genital herpes and to inform future partners before initiating a sexual relationship.
  - Sexual transmission of HSV can occur during asymptomatic periods.

- Abstain from sexual activity with uninfected partners when lesions or prodromal symptoms are present.
- Latex condoms, when used consistently and correctly, can reduce the risk of contracting genital herpes when the infected areas are covered or protected by the condom.
- Sex partners of infected persons should be advised that they might be infected even if they have no symptoms.
- Pregnant women who are not infected with HSV2 should be advised to avoid intercourse during the third trimester with men who have genital herpes. Similarly, pregnant women who are not infected with HSV1 should be counselled to avoid genital exposure to HSV1 during the third trimester (e.g. cunnilingus with a partner with oral herpes and vaginal intercourse with a partner with genital HSV1 infection).
- When counselling patients about genital warts, the following points should be covered:
  - Genital warts are caused by a viral infection that is very common among sexually active adults.
  - Infection is almost always sexually transmitted.
  - Sexual partners are almost always infected by the time of the patient's diagnosis, although they may have no symptoms or signs of infection.
  - The types of HPV that usually cause external genital warts are not associated with cancer.
  - Recurrence of genital warts within the first several months after treatment is common and usually indicates recurrence rather than reinfection.
  - Use of condoms has been associated with a lower rate of cervical cancer, an HPV-associated disease.
  - Because genital HPV is common among people who have been sexually active and because the duration of infectivity is unknown, the value of disclosing a past diagnosis of genital HPV infection to future partners is unclear.
- When treating warts, it is helpful to record lesions on genital maps, thereby providing a visual record of approximate number, distribution and response to treatment.
- Perianal warts can occur in women who have not had receptive anal intercourse. They are distinct from intra-anal warts and are seen predominantly where this practice has occurred.

- When taking a swab for *Chlamydia* testing, it is important to remove any discharge from the cervix and then to swab the endocervix vigorously by rotating the swab for about 10 seconds. Swabbing discharge is inappropriate, as *Chlamydia* is an intracellular organism and therefore cellular material is required to aid the diagnosis.
- The urine specimen for *Chlamydia* testing is 'first-catch' as opposed to the 'mid-stream' specimen required for urine microscopy culture.

REFERENCES

1. Bingham JS. What to do with the patient with recurrent vulvovaginal candidiasis. Sex Transm Infect 1999; 75: 225–227.
2. Sobel JD. Vaginitis. N Engl J Med 1997; 337:1896–1903.
3. O'Dowd TC, Parker S, Kelly A. Women's experiences of general practitioner management of their vaginal symptoms. Br J Gen Pract 1996; 46:415–418.
4. CEG (Clinical Effectiveness Group), Association for Genitourinary Medicine and the Medical Society for the Study of Venereal Diseases. National guidelines for the management of vulvovaginal candidiasis. 2001. Online. Available: http://www.agum.org.uk/ceg2002/candida0601.htm or http://www.mssvd.org.uk/PDF/CEG2001/candida% 2006%2001.PDF [accessed 13.02.2003].
5. Nurbhai M, Grimshaw J, Watson M, et al. Oral versus intra-vaginal imidazole and triazole anti-fungal treatment of uncomplicated vulvovaginal candidiasis (thrush). Cochrane Database Syst Rev 2007(4):CD002845.
6. Sobel JD, Faro S, Force RW, et al. Vulvovaginal candidiasis: epidemiological, diagnostic and therapeutic considerations. Am J Obstet Gynaecol 1998; 178:203–211.
7. Faculty of Family Planning and Reproductive Health Care Clinical Effectiveness Unit. The management of women of reproductive age attending non-genitourinary medicine settings complaining of vaginal discharge. J Fam Plann Reprod Health Care 2006; 32(1):33–42; quiz 42.
8. Elmer GW, Surawicz CM, McFarland LV. Biotherapeutic agents: a neglected modality for the treatment and prevention of selected intestinal and vaginal infections. JAMA 1996; 275:870–876.
9. Shalev E, Battino S, Weiner E, et al. Ingestion of yoghurt containing *Lactobacillus acidophilus* compared with pasteurised yoghurt as prophylaxis for recurrent candidal vaginitis and bacterial vaginosis. Arch Fam Med 1996; 5:593–596.
10. Pirotta M, Gunn J, Chondros P, et al. Effect of lactobacillus in preventing post-antibiotic vulvovaginal candidiasis: a randomised controlled trial. BMJ 2004; 329(7465):548.
11. Dennerstein G. Pathogenesis and treatment of genital candidiasis. Aust Fam Physician 1998; 27:363–369.
12. Reef SE, Levine WC, McNeil MM, et al. Treatment options for vulvovaginal candidiasis, 1993. Clin Infect Dis 1995; 20(Suppl 1):S80–S90.
13. Young GL, Jewell D. Topical treatment for vaginal candidiasis (thrush) in pregnancy (Cochrane Review). In: The Cochrane Library, Issue 3. Oxford: Update Software; 2002.
14. Eschenbach DA, Hillier S, Critchlow C, et al. Diagnosis and clinical manifestations of bacterial vaginosis. Am J Obstet Gynecol 1988; 158:819–828.

15. Fredricks DN, Fiedler TL, Marrazzo JM. Molecular identification of bacteria associated with bacterial vaginosis. N Engl J Med 2005; 353(18):1899–1911.
16. Hill GB. The microbiology of bacterial vaginosis. Am J Obstet Gynecol 1993; 169:450–454.
17. Smith KS, Tabrizi SN, Fethers KA, et al. Comparison of conventional testing to polymerase chain reaction in detection of Trichomonas vaginalis in indigenous women living in remote areas. Int J STD AIDS 2005; 16(12):811–815.
18. Koumans EH, Sternberg M, Bruce C, et al. The prevalence of bacterial vaginosis in the United States, 2001–2004; associations with symptoms, sexual behaviors, and reproductive health. Sex Transm Dis 2007; 34(11): 864–869.
19. Marrazzo JM, Koutsky LA, Eschenbach DA, et al. Characterization of vaginal flora and bacterial vaginosis in women who have sex with women. J Infect Dis 2002; 185(9):1307–1313.
20. Taha TE, Hoover DR, Dallabetta GA, et al. Bacterial vaginosis and disturbances of vaginal flora: association with increased acquisition of HIV. AIDS 1998; 12(13):1699–1706.
21. Wilson J. Managing recurrent bacterial vaginosis. Sex Transm Infect 2004; 80(1):8–11.
22. Black M, Mackay M, eds. Obstetric and gynaecologic dermatology. 2nd edn. London: Mosby; 2002:84.
23. Amsel R, Totten PA, Spiegel CA, et al. Nonspecific vaginitis. Diagnostic criteria and microbial and epidemiologic associations. Am J Med 1983; 74:14–22.
24. Fethers KA, Fairley CK, Hocking JS, et al. Sexual risk factors and bacterial vaginosis: a systematic review and meta-analysis. Clin Infect Dis 2008; 47(11):1426–1435.
25. Holmes KK. Lower genital tract infections in women: cystitis/urethritis, vulvovaginitis, and cervicitis. In: Sexually transmitted diseases. 2nd edn. New York: McGraw Hill; 1990:527–545.
26. Centers for Disease Control and Prevention. Sexually transmitted diseases treatment guidelines. Washington, DC: US Department of Health and Human Services; 1993.
27. Colli E, Landoni M, Parazzini F. Treatment of male partners and recurrence of bacterial vaginosis: a randomised trial. Genitourin Med 1997; 73:267–270.
28. Moi H, Erkkola R, Jerve F, et al. Should male consorts of women with bacterial vaginosis be treated? Genitourin Med 1989; 65:263–268.
29. Bump RC, Buesching WJ 3rd. Bacterial vaginosis in virginal and sexually active adolescent females: evidence against exclusive sexual transmission. Am J Obstet Gynecol 1988; 158:935–939.
30. Koumans EH, Markowitz LE, Hogan V. Indications for therapy and treatment recommendations for bacterial vaginosis in nonpregnant and pregnant women: a synthesis of data. Clin Infect Dis 2002; 35(Suppl 2):S152–S172.
31. Burtin P, Taddio A, Ariburnu O, et al. Safety of metronidazole in pregnancy: a meta-analysis. Am J Obstet Gynecol 1995; 172:525–529.
32. Caro-Paton T, Carvajal A, Martin de Diego I, et al. Is metronidazole teratogenic? A meta-analysis. Br J Clin Pharmacol 1997; 44:179–182.
33. Czeizel A, Rockenbauer M. A population based case-control teratologic study of oral metronidazole treatment during pregnancy. Br J Obstet Gynaecol 1998; 105:322–327.
34. MacDermott R. Bacterial vaginosis. Br J Obstet Gynaecol 1995; 102:92–94.
35. Pheifer TA, Forsyth PS, Durfee MA, et al. Nonspecific vaginitis: role of *Haemophilus vaginalis* and treatment with metronidazole. N Engl J Med 1978; 298:1429–1434.
36. Eschenbach DA. Bacterial vaginosis and anaerobes in obstetric—gynecologic infection. Clin Infect Dis 1993; 16(Suppl 4):S282–S287.
37. Larsson PG, Platz-Christensen JJ, Forsum U, et al. Clue cells in predicting infection after abdominal hysterectomy. Obstet Gynecol 1991; 77:450–452.
38. Newton ER, Piper J, Peairs W. Bacterial vaginosis and intra-amniotic infection. Am J Obstet Gynecol 1997; 176:672–677.
39. Gibbs RS. Chorioamnionitis and bacterial vaginosis. Am J Obstet Gynecol 1993; 169:460–462.
40. McGregor JA, French JI. Bacterial vaginosis in pregnancy. Obstet Gynecol Surv 2000; 55:S1–S19.
41. McGregor JA, French JI, Seo K. Premature rupture of membranes and bacterial vaginosis. Am J Obstet Gynecol 1993; 169:463–466.
42. Meis PJ, Goldenberg RL, Mercer B, et al. The preterm prediction study: significance of vaginal infections. National Institute of Child Health and Human Development Maternal-Fetal Medicine Units Network. Am J Obstet Gynecol 1995; 173:1231–1235.
43. Hay PE, Lamont RF, Taylor-Robinson D, et al. Abnormal bacterial colonization of the genital tract and subsequent preterm delivery and late miscarriage. BMJ 1994; 308:295–298.
44. Hillier SL, Nugent RP, Eschenbach DA, et al. Association between bacterial vaginosis and preterm delivery of a low-birth-weight infant. N Engl J Med 1995; 333:1737–1742.
45. Lettieri L, Vintzileos AM, Rodis JF, et al. Does idiopathic preterm labour resulting in premature birth exist? Am J Obstet Gynecol 1993; 168:1480–1485.
46. Hillier SL, Martius J, Krohn M, et al. A case-controlled study of chorioamniotic infection and histologic chorioamnionitis in prematurity. N Engl J Med 1988; 319:972–978.
47. Lamont RF, Fisk NM. The role of infection in the pathogenesis of preterm labour. In: Studd JW, ed. Progress in obstetrics and gynaecology. London: Churchill Livingstone; 1993:135–158.
48. Fiscella K. Racial disparities in preterm births: the role of urogenital infections. Public Health Rep 1996; 111:104–113.
49. Flynn CA, Helwig AL, Meurer LN. Bacterial vaginosis in pregnancy and the risk of prematurity: a meta-analysis. J Fam Pract 1999; 48:885–892.
50. Gratacos E, Figueras F, Barranco M, et al. Spontaneous recovery of bacterial vaginosis during pregnancy is not associated with an improved perinatal outcome. Acta Obstet Gynecol Scand 1998; 77:37–40.
51. Brocklehurst P, Hannah M, McDonald H. Interventions for treating bacterial vaginosis in pregnancy. Cochrane Database Syst Rev 2000; (2):CD000262.
52. Committee on Obstetric Practice. Bacterial vaginosis screening for prevention of preterm delivery. ACOG committee opinion. Washington DC: American College of Obstetricians and Gynecologists; 1998.
53. Wolner-Hanssen P, Kreiger JN, Stevens CE, et al. Clinical manifestations of vaginal trichomoniasis. JAMA 1989; 264:571–576.
54. Wiese W, Patel SR, Patel SC, et al. A meta-analysis of the Papanicolaou smear and wet mount for the diagnosis of vaginal trichomoniasis. Am J Med 2000; 108:301–308.
55. Workowski KA, Levine CW. Sexually transmitted diseases treatment guidelines 2002. MMWR Morb Mortal Wkly Rep 2002; 51:1.
56. Cotch MF, Pastorek JG 2nd, Nugent RP, et al. Trichomonas vaginalis associated with low birth weight and preterm delivery. The Vaginal Infections and Prematurity Study Group. Sex Transm Dis 1997; 24(6):353–360.
57. Klebanoff MA, Carey JC, Hauth JC, et al. Failure of metronidazole to prevent preterm delivery among pregnant women with asymptomatic Trichomonas vaginalis infection. N Engl J Med 2001; 345(7):487–493.
58. Johnson RE, Nahmias AJ, Magder LS, et al. A seroepidemiologic survey of the prevalence of herpes simplex virus type 2 infection in the United States. N Engl J Med 1989; 321:7–12.

59. Mindel A, Taylor J, Tideman RL, et al. Neonatal herpes prevention: a minor public health problem in some communities. Sex Transm Infect 2000; 76:287–291.

60. Tideman RL, Taylor J, Marks C, et al. Sexual and demographic risk factors for herpes simplex type 1 and 2 in women attending an antenatal clinic. Sex Transm Infect 2001; 77(6):413–415.

61. Tran T, Druce JD, Catton MC, et al. Changing epidemiology of genital herpes simplex virus infection in Melbourne, Australia, between 1980 and 2003. Sex Transm Infect 2004; 80(4):277–279.

62. Sheary B, Dayan L. Herpes simplex virus serology in an asymptomatic patient. Aust Fam Physician 2005; 34(12):1043–1046.

63. Fleming DT, McQuillan GM, Johnson RE, et al. Herpes simplex virus type 2 in the United States, 1976 to 1994. N Engl J Med 1997; 337:1105–1111.

64. Langenberg AG, Corey L, Ashley RL, et al. A prospective study of new infections with herpes simplex virus type 1 and type 2. Chiron HSV Vaccine Study Group. N Engl J Med 1999; 341:1432–1438.

65. Corey L, Simmons A. The medical importance of genital herpes simplex virus infection. International Herpes Management Forum. 1997. Online. Available: http://www.ihmf.org/library/ monograph/M_Ob.pdf [accessed 16.09.2003].

66. Wald A, Zeh J, Selke S, et al. Reactivation of genital herpes simplex virus type 2 infection in asymptomatic seropositive persons. N Engl J Med 2000; 342:844–850.

67. Corey L, Adams HG, Brown ZA, et al. Genital herpes simplex virus infections: clinical manifestations, course, and complications. Ann Intern Med 1983; 98(6):958–972.

68. Benedetti J, Corey L, Ashley R. Recurrence rates in genital herpes after symptomatic first-episode infection. Ann Intern Med 1994; 121:847–854.

69. Wald A, Zeh J, Selke S, et al. Virologic characteristics of subclinical and symptomatic genital herpes infections. N Engl J Med 1995; 333:770–775.

70. Koelle DM, Benedetti J, Langenberg A, et al. Asymptomatic reactivation of herpes simplex virus in women after the first episode of genital herpes. Ann Intern Med 1992; 116: 433–437.

71. Wald A, Corey L, Cone R, et al. Frequent genital herpes simplex virus 2 shedding in immunocompetent women. Effect of acyclovir treatment. J Clin Invest 1997; 99: 1092–1097.

72. Mertz GJ, Schmidt O, Jourden JL, et al. Frequency of acquisition of first-episode genital infection with herpes simplex virus from symptomatic and asymptomatic source contacts. Sex Transm Dis 1985; 12:33–39.

73. Mertz GJ, Benedetti J, Ashley R, et al. Risk factors for the sexual transmission of genital herpes. Ann Intern Med 1992; 116(3):197–202.

74. Wald A, Langenberg AG, Link K, et al. Effect of condoms on reducing the transmission of herpes simplex virus type 2 from men to women. JAMA 2001; 285(24): 3100–3106.

75. Tetrault I, Boivin G. Recent advances in management of genital herpes. Can Fam Physician 2000; 46:1622–1629.

76. Ramaswamy M, McDonald C, Smith M, et al. Diagnosis of genital herpes by real time PCR in routine clinical practice. Sex Transm Infect 2004; 80(5):406–410.

77. Gupta R, Warren T, Wald A. Genital herpes. Lancet 2007; 370(9605):2127–2137.

78. Prober CG, Sullender WM, Yasukawa LL, et al. Low risk of herpes simplex virus infections in neonates exposed to the virus at the time of vaginal delivery to mothers with recurrent genital herpes simplex virus infections. N Engl J Med 1987; 316:240–244.

79. Marrazzo JM, John GC, Krohn MA, et al. Cesarean delivery in women with genital herpes in Washington State 1989–1991. Infect Dis Obstet Gynecol 1997; 5:29–35.

80. Beutner KR, Tyring S. Human papillomavirus and human disease. Am J Med 1997; 102:9–15.

81. Burchell AN, Winer RL, de Sanjosé S, et al. Chapter 6: Epidemiology and transmission dynamics of genital HPV infection. Vaccine 2006; 24(Suppl 3):S3/52–S3/61.

82. Trottier H, Franco EL. The epidemiology of genital human papillomavirus infection. Vaccine 2006; 24(Suppl 1):S1–S15.

83. Koutsky LA. Epidemiology of genital papillomavirus infection. Am J Med 1997; 102:3–8.

84. Trofatter KF. Diagnosis of human papillomavirus genital tract infection. Am J Med 1997; 102:21–27.

85. Australia and New Zealand HPV Project. Guidelines for the medical management of genital HPV and or genital warts in Australia and New Zealand. 3rd edn. 2002. Online. Available: http://www.hpv.org.nz/pdf/hpvguidelines2002.pdf [accessed 13.02.2003].

86. Ho GY, Bierman R, Beardsley L, et al. Natural history of cervicovaginal papillomavirus infection in young women. N Engl J Med 1998; 338:423–428.

87. Ferenczy A, Mitao M, Nagai N, et al. Latent papillomavirus and recurring genital warts. N Engl J Med 1985; 313:784–788.

88. Rymark P, Forslund O, Hansson BG, et al. Genital HPV infection not a local but a regional infection: experience from a female teenage group. Genitourin Med 1993; 69:18–22.

89. Bosch FX, Lorincz A, Muñoz N, et al. The causal relation between human papillomavirus and cervical cancer. J Clin Pathol 2002; 55(4):244–265.

90. Bosch FX, Manos MM, Muñoz N, et al., Prevalence of human papillomavirus in cervical cancer: a worldwide perspective. International biological study on cervical cancer (IBSCC) Study Group. J Natl Cancer Inst 1995; 87(11):796–802.

91. Clifford G, Franceschi S, Diaz M, et al. Chapter 3: HPV type distribution in women with and without cervical neoplastic diseases. Vaccine 2006; 24(Suppl 3):S3/26–S3/34.

92. Clifford GM, Rana RK, Franceschi S, et al. Human papillomavirus genotype distribution in low-grade cervical lesions: comparison by geographic region and with cervical cancer. Cancer Epidemiol Biomarkers Prev 2005; 14(5):1157–1164.

93. Ball SB, Wojnarowska F. Vulvar dermatoses: lichen sclerosus, lichen planus, and vulval dermatitis/lichen simplex chronicus. Semin Cutan Med Surg 1998; 17:182–188.

94. Marshman G. Lichen planus. Aust J Dermatol 1998; 39:1–13.

95. Meyrick Thomas RH, Ridley CM, McGibbon DH, et al. Lichen sclerosus et atrophicus and autoimmunity—a study of 350 women. Br J Dermatol 1988; 118:41–46.

96 Virgili A, Bacilieri S, Corazza M. Managing vulvar lichen simplex chronicus. J Reprod Med 2001; 46:343–346.

97. National Notifiable Diseases Surveillance System. Annual report, 1998. Australia's notifiable disease status. Commun Dis Intell 1999; 23:277–305.

98. Australian Government Department of Health and Ageing. National Notifiable Diseases Surveillance System. Number of notifications of chlamydial infection, Australia, 2008, by age group and sex. 2009. Online. Available: http://www9.health.gov.au/cda/Source/Rpt_5.cfm [accessed 07.09.2009].

99. Pimenta J, Catchpole M, Gray M, et al. Evidence based health policy report. Screening for genital chlamydial infection. BMJ 2000; 321:629–631.

100. Lamagni TL, Hughes G, Rogers PA, et al. New cases seen at genitourinary medicine clinics: England 1998. Commun Dis Rep CDR Suppl 1999; 9:S1–S12.

101. Stokes T. Screening for Chlamydia in general practice: a literature review and summary of the evidence. J Public Health Med 1997; 19:222–232.

102. Peipert JF. Clinical practice. Genital chlamydial infections. N Engl J Med 2003; 349(25):2424–2430.

103. Sutton TL, Martinko T, Hale S, et al. Prevalence and high rate of asymptomatic infection of Chlamydia trachomatis in male college Reserve Officer Training Corps cadets. Sex Transm Dis 2003; 30(12):901–904.

104. Chief Medical Officer's expert advisory group. Main report of the CMOs expert advisory group on *Chlamydia trachomatis*. London: Department of Health; 1998.

105. McCormack WM, Alpert S, McComb DE, et al. Fifteen-month follow-up study of women infected with *Chlamydia trachomatis*. N Engl J Med 1979; 300:123–125.

106. Westrom L. Incidence, prevalence, and trends of acute pelvic inflammatory disease and its consequences in industrialized countries. Am J Obstet Gynecol 1980; 138:880–892.

107. Hocking JS, Walker J, Regan D, et al. Chlamydia screening—Australia should strive to achieve what others have not. Med J Aust 2008; 188(2):106–108.

108. Clinical Effectiveness Group. British Association for Sexual Health and HIV. Sexually Transmitted Infections: UK National Screening and Testing Guidelines. 2006. Online. Available: http://www.bashh.org/documents/59/59.pdf [accessed 07.09.2009].

109. Shaw C, Mason M, Scoular A. Group B streptococcus carriage and vulvovaginal symptoms: causal or casual? A case-control study in a GUM clinic population. Sex Transm Infect 2003; 79(3):246–248.

110. Trexler MF, Fraser TG, Jones MP. Fulminant pseudomembranous colitis caused by clindamycin phosphate vaginal cream. Am J Gastroenterol 1997; 92:2112–2113.

111. Corey L, Handsfield HH. Genital herpes and public health: addressing a global problem. JAMA 2000; 283:791–794.

112. Catotti DN, Clarke P, Catoe KE. Herpes revisited. Still a cause of concern. Sex Transm Dis 1993; 20:77–80.

113. Spinillo A, Capuzzo E, Acciano S, et al. Effect of antibiotic use on the prevalence of symptomatic vulvovaginal candidiasis. Am J Obstet Gynecol 1999; 180:14–17.

114. Bisschop MP, Merkus JM, Scheygrond H, et al. Co-treatment of the male partner in vaginal candidosis: a double blind randomised control study. Br J Obstet Gynecol 1986; 93:79–81.

115. Horowitz BJ, Edelstein SW, Lippman L. Sexual transmission of *Candida*. Obstet Gynecol 1987; 69:883–886.

116. Spinillo A, Carratta L, Pizzoli G, et al. Recurrent vaginal candidiasis. Results of a cohort study of sexual transmission and intestinal reservoir. J Reprod Med 1992; 37:343–347.

117. Foxman B. The epidemiology of vulvovaginal candidiasis: risk factors. Am J Public Health 1990; 80:329–331.

118. Hellberg D, Zdolsek B, Nilsson S, et al. Sexual behavior of women with repeated episodes of vulvovaginal candidiasis. Eur J Epidemiol 1995; 11:575–579.

119. Spinillo A, Capuzzo F, Nicola S, et al. The impact of oral contraception on vulvovaginal candidiasis. Contraception 1995; 51:293–297.

120. Barbone F, Austin H, Louv WC, et al. A follow-up study of methods of contraception, sexual activity, and rates of trichomoniasis, candidiasis, and bacterial vaginosis. Am J Obstet Gynecol 1990; 163:510–514.

121. Hooten TM, Roberts PL, Stamm WE. Effect of recent sexual activity and use of diaphragm on vaginal flora. Clin Infect Dis 1994; 19:274–278.

122. Geiger AM, Foxman B. Risk factors in vulvovaginal candidiasis: a case-control study among college students. Epidemiology 1996; 7:182–187.

123. Reed BD. Risk factors for *Candida* vulvovaginitis. Obstet Gynecol Surv 1992; 47:551–560.

124. Hilton E, Isenberg HD, Alperstein P, et al. Ingestion of yogurt containing Lactobacillus acidophilus as prophylaxis for candidal vaginitis. Ann Intern Med 1992; 116:353–357.

125. Morse SA, Holmes KK, Ballard RC. Atlas of sexually transmitted diseases and AIDS. 3rd edn. St Louis: Mosby; 2002.

126. James D, Rymes J, Hyer W, et al. Obstetrics, gynaecology, neonatology interactive colour guides. CD-ROM. Edinburgh: Churchill Livingstone; 2000.

127. Australia and New Zealand HPV Project. Guidelines for the management of genital HPV in Australia and New Zealand. 5th edn. 2007. Online. Available from: http://www.hpv.org.nz/health/guidelines.htm [accessed 07.09.09].

128. Edwards L. Lichen planus. In: Black M et al, eds. Obstetric and gynecologic dermatology. 3rd edn. London: Mosby, Elsevier; 2008:147–156.

129. Edwards L. Lichen sclerosus. In Black M et al, eds. Obstetric and gynecologic dermatology. 3rd edn. London: Mosby Elsevier; 2008:133–147.

130. Habif T. Clinical Dermatology, 5th edn. St Louis: Mosby; 2010.

131. Fisher BK, Margesson LJ. Genital Disorders: Diagnosis and Treatment. St Louis: Mosby; 1998.

14

Menopause and osteoporosis

CHAPTER CONTENTS

OBJECTIVES

- To understand the aetiology and natural history of the menopause
- To understand the indications, limitations, risks and benefits of hormone therapy (HT)
- To be able to prescribe HT appropriately and manage common side effects
- To be aware of the evidence base for alternatives to HT for the treatment of menopausal symptoms
- To understand the World Health Organization (WHO) criteria for osteoporosis
- To be able to advise women about the risks of osteoporosis and prevention strategies
- To be able to detect and manage osteoporosis appropriately

FEATURES OF THE MENOPAUSE

What exactly is the menopause?

Menopause by definition is the time of cessation of menstruation. Women are said to be postmenopausal after 1 year of amenorrhoea. This occurs on average at 51.4 years[1]; in smokers, those with a hysterectomy and chronic disease, however, it occurs earlier.[2] The perimenopause refers to those years leading up to and including the menopause. Premature menopause (that which occurs before the age of 40) occurs in up to 2.5% of women.[3] It is usually iatrogenic, coming about as a result of bilateral oophorectomy, radiation or chemotherapy.

Menopause occurs on average at 51.4 years but is earlier in smokers, those with a hysterectomy and chronic disease.

The current nomenclature used to describe stages of reproductive aging[4] is described in Box 14.1 and shown in Figure 14.1.

From just after menarche (stage –5) cycles can be irregular for several years, but should then occur every 21 to 35 days for a number of years (stages –4 and –3). In the early menopausal transition (stage 2), the menstrual cycle remains regular but the length changes by 7 days or more (regular cycles are now every 24 instead of 31 days). The late menopausal transition (stage +1) is characterised by two or more skipped menstrual cycles and at least one intermenstrual interval of 60 days or more.[4]

Follicle-stimulating hormone (FSH) levels gradually increase throughout the menopausal transition, but the variability is high and an FSH level of 40 IU/L or more is not necessarily as predictive of the late menopausal transition as amenorrhoea of 60 days or more.[5]

Why does the menopause come about?

The menopause commences when there are only a few thousand primordial follicles remaining in the ovary, an insufficient number to stimulate cyclical activity. Oestrogen levels fall in the course of about 5 years and this has a positive feedback on the pituitary, increasing the production of FSH and luteinising hormone (LH). Eventually the ovary produces only androstenedione (also produced by the adrenal glands), which is converted by peripheral fat into the weak oestrogen, oestrone.

BOX 14.1 Staging reproductive ageing (short version of STRAW[4] definitions)

- Late reproductive: no change in menstrual cycle
- Early menopausal transition: change in menstrual frequency by ≥7 days
- Late menopausal transition: >2 skipped cycles, ≥60 days of amenorrhoea
- Postmenopause: 12 months or more of amenorrhea.

How can women tell if the menopause is imminent?

The dominant feature of the early menopausal transition is cycle length variability of 7 days or more, with cycle irregularity marking for most women the approach of their final menstrual period. The time when a woman is most likely to experience menopausal symptoms is during the late menopausal transition when there is amenorrhoea of 60 days or more. An indicator of the approach of menopause (less than 20 cycles remaining) is a rise in cycle length to 42 days or greater.[6] Bleeding patterns are most indicative sign of menopausal stage, not necessarily hot flushes.[5]

Bleeding patterns rather than hot flushes are most indicative of menopausal stage.

Are there any investigations that can be used to determine whether menopause has occurred?

In women still experiencing menstrual bleeding, FSH levels measured on day 2 or day 3 after the onset of bleeding are considered increased when they exceed 10–12 IU/L, which is an indication of diminished ovarian response.[7] FSH levels over 40 IU/L are indicative of the late menopausal transition.[5] However, studies show that a single FSH determination alone poorly predicts menopausal status and cannot be used to predict final menstrual period.[8] It has been common practice to consider ovarian failure highly likely when two measurements of FSH >30 IU/L are obtained at least 1 or 2 months apart. FSH should be measured when the woman is not taking either HT or hormonal contraception.

A single FSH determination alone poorly predicts menopausal status.

Final menstrual period
(FMP)

Stages	−5	−4	−3	−2	−1	0	+1	+2
Terminology	Reproductive			Menopausal transition			Postmenopause	
	Early	Peak	Late	Early	Late*		Early*	Late
				Perimenopause				
Duration of stage	Variable			Variable			ⓐ 1 yr / ⓑ 4 yrs	Until demise
Menstrual cycles	Variable to regular	Regular		Variable cycle length (>7 days different from normal)	≥2 skipped cycles and an interval of amenorrhoea (≥60 days)	Amenorrhoea: 12 months	None	
Endocrine	Normal FSH		↑ FSH	↑ FSH			↑ FSH	

*Stages most likely to be characterised by vasomotor symptoms   ↑ = elevated

FIGURE 14.1 Nomenclature used to describe stages of reproductive aging (From Soules et al[4])

What are the true signs and symptoms of the menopause?

Despite the fact that all women pass through the menopause if they live long enough, the symptoms directly attributable to the menopausal transition are difficult to quantify because of confounding factors such as age, social class and education. One study[9] found that vasomotor symptoms (hot flushes and night sweats), difficulty falling asleep, decreased sexual interest and vaginal dryness are all associated with menopause after controlling for the effects of age. Sexual satisfaction, however, was not related to menopausal status and symptoms often associated with menopause, such as cognitive difficulties, depression and irritability, were more strongly associated with social class and employment. Dennerstein et al[10] found that from early to late perimenopause increasing numbers of women reported five or more symptoms (+14%), hot flushes (+27%), night sweats (+17%) and vaginal dryness (+17%). Breast soreness/tenderness decreased with the meno-

pausal transition (−21%). Figure 14.2 (p 258) illustrates the association between hormone status and symptoms in the women they studied. A list of the common signs and symptoms associated with menopause is given in Box 14.2 (p 259).

Only 10% of women going through menopause seek help from healthcare providers.

Another important point to note about menopausal symptoms is that, while a large proportion of women may experience menopausal symptoms, the proportion of women who experience the symptom as a problem is much less. For example, a British study[11] found that 57% of women experienced hot flushes but only 22% said they were a problem, 66% reported sleep problems but only 33% said this was a problem. Interestingly, only 10% of women seek help from healthcare providers.[12]

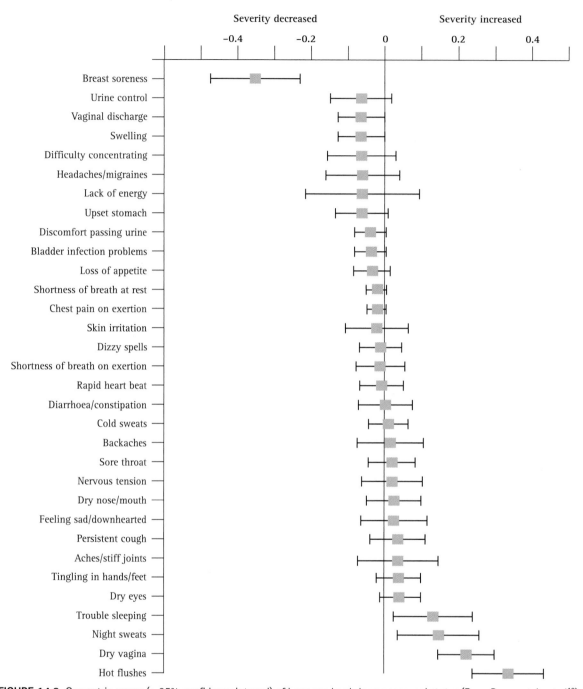

FIGURE 14.2 Geometric means (± 95% confidence interval) of hormone levels by menopausal status (From Dennerstein et al[10])

How long do menopausal symptoms usually last?

For most women, symptoms are transient, with 30–50% of women improving within several months. Hot flushes usually last for 4–5 years and in some women may take longer to resolve. A recent meta-analysis has shown peak vasomotor symptom prevalence at 1 year after the final menstrual period, with 50% of women reporting symptoms after 4 years and 10% reporting symptoms as long as 12 years later[13] (Fig 14.3).

What are the long-term health implications of the menopause?

Osteoporosis, urogenital atrophy, cardiovascular disease and stroke all increase in incidence in women after menopause. While twice as many women as men suffer from Alzheimer's disease (the most common cause of dementia among the elderly), this may in part be due to longer life expectancy.[14] Interestingly, limited clinical trial evidence suggests that HT does not improve symptoms or slow disease progression in Alzheimer's disease and that it may actually increase dementia risk when initiated after age 64 years.[15,16,17] Observational studies suggest that HT used by younger women around the time of menopause is associated with lower risk of Alzheimer's disease. However, further research is needed to determine whether there might exist an early window during which HT effects on Alzheimer's disease risk are beneficial rather than harmful.

BOX 14.2 Signs and symptoms commonly attributed to the menopause

- Changes to the menstrual pattern
- Vasomotor symptoms—hot flushes and night sweats
- Sleep disturbance
- Urogenital symptoms such as vaginal irritation, dyspareunia, urinary tract infection and urinary incontinence
- Mood changes
- Loss of libido
- Thinning of the skin, brittle nails and hair loss
- Generalised aches and pains

What can a GP do for women with atrophic vaginitis?

First, it is important always to examine these patients, as their symptoms may in fact be due to a condition other than atrophic vaginitis. Treatment of atrophic vaginitis involves oestrogen replacement, either systemically or locally. An alternative if symptoms are not severe is the use of lubricant to assist sexual activity.

Oestrogen can be delivered transvaginally either through the use of creams, pessaries or a hormone-releasing ring. Initially, creams and pessaries should be used daily for about 2 weeks, but once symptoms improve the dosage can be reduced to once or twice a week. The advantages of creams and pessaries are that they are effective in treating symptoms and have fewer systemic effects, thereby lessening the risk of endometrial carcinoma. However, they involve vaginal manipulation and the twice-weekly dosage may lead to decrease of patient compliance. The transvaginal ring offers an alternative, as the ring can remain in the vagina and deliver a constant low dose of hormones. It can be easily removed and reinserted and can still be worn during sex.

Summary of key points

- Menopause occurs on average at 51.4 years.
- Premature menopause is that which occurs before the age of 40.
- An FSH of 40 IU/L is considered to be in the postmenopausal range, but must be tested for when the woman is not using HT or hormonal

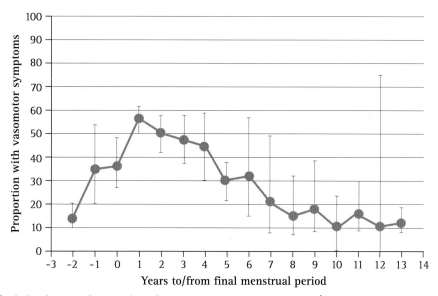

FIGURE 14.3 Pooled estimates of proportion of vasomotor symptoms by years to/from final menstrual period (From Politi et al[13])

contraception and confirmed with a repeat test 4–8 weeks later.

- The classic menopausal symptoms are the vasomotor ones of hot flushes and night sweats.
- Long-term consequences of menopause include osteoporosis, urogenital atrophy and cardiovascular disease.

HORMONE THERAPY (HT)

What has been the uptake and usage of HT by women in recent times?

The use of HT by menopausal and postmenopausal women has been controversial since first suggested. The medical profession has been subject to intense pressure

---

CASE STUDY: 'Should I take hormones if I have a family history of breast cancer?'

Marion was a 60-year-old woman who had been taking HT oestrogen (0.625 mg/day) for the last 20 years since having a bilateral oophorectomy and hysterectomy at the age of 40 for refractory endometriosis. She had been very happy taking the oestrogen replacement therapy (ET) all this time and had only once tried to come off it 10 years ago by tapering the dose slowly. At that time, however, she had had a severe recurrence of vasomotor symptoms with hot flushes occurring sometimes hourly and terrible night sweats. She had therefore recommenced her ET and not thought much more about it till she heard some press reports about the relationship between HT and breast cancer. Marion's family history was of some concern. While there was no cardiovascular disease in the family, her sister had developed breast cancer in her late 30s. Marion had no risk factors for osteoporosis.

Today, she presented wanting to discontinue her ET. After taking a history, an examination was undertaken, which was normal. Marion's case highlights some of the complexities of giving advice about ET or HT use. Given her family history, she is right to be cautious, but the oestrogen-only arm of the Women's Health Initiative (WHI) study found no increased risk of breast cancer after 7 years of use compared to the oestrogen/progestogen arm of the study.[18] The only two reasons to be on HT/ET are for the treatment of menopausal symptoms and the prevention of osteoporosis. While Marion is not at increased risk of the latter, some women continue to have hot flushes for many years after the menopause. In about 1 in 10 women who discontinue hormone therapy, the recurrence of menopausal symptoms is severe and persistent.[19] Marion could try again to come off the ET; if this were not tolerated, other treatments for vasomotor symptoms could be offered such as a selective serotonin reuptake inhibitor (SSRI) (e.g. venlafaxine or paroxetine) or clonidine.

---

by pharmaceutical companies to prescribe HT as both a therapeutic and preventive agent, as the potential market for HT is enormous (all women over 45).

Despite this, it is interesting to note that less than 20% of population samples of postmenopausal women in the USA have ever had HT prescribed. In addition, less than 40% of women who commence HT are still using it 1 year later,[20] and after 3 years that percentage drops further to 25%.[21] The reasons for this poor compliance may be related to the side effects that women experience when they use HT, such as bloating, breast tenderness and withdrawal bleeds, or to the perceived risks, especially breast cancer.

Up until 2002, when the Women's Health Initiative (WHI) study results were publicised,[22] use of HT in postmenopausal women varied from <10% in the UK, to 30–40% in the US. Australia was slightly less than the US with 28% of postmenopausal women taking HT and 12–22% throughout Europe.[23] In Australia, prescriptions for oestrogen/medroxyprogesterone acetate fixed-dose preparations dropped by 55.4% in the following 12 months; uptake of HT preparations decreased by about 30% in the same period and continued to fall at a lower rate following publication of the oestrogen-only (9%) and memory arms of the WHI (4%).[24]

What advice should general practitioners give patients seeking information about the pros and cons of HT?

In recent years, controversy has raged over the indications for HT and the risks and benefits of using HT in peri- and postmenopausal women. Much of this controversy stems from the undue fears and confusion that have resulted from the misinterpretation of clinical studies and the overrepresentation of risks arising from these studies,[25] in particular:

- inappropriate extrapolation of findings from one population of women to another
- reliance on a single clinical trial over and above a large amount of basic science and clinical research
- generalisation of results from one oestrogen and progestin, one dose and one route of administration to all forms of HT
- a lack of understanding of the concept of risk amongst both health professionals and their patients.

In counselling women about HT, it is essential that GPs are skilled in representing risk accurately (Box 14.3). Common non-cancer risks and benefits are outlined in Table 14.1.

A statistical association between an exposure and an outcome does not necessarily mean that the exposure caused the outcome.

Relative risk (RR)

- RR is a ratio—the rate of disease in the exposed group divided by the rate of the disease in the unexposed group.
- RR describes the number of events per number of individuals per time interval (e.g. 23 per 10,000 per year).
- If the annual rate of deep vein thrombosis (DVT) in postmenopausal women using oral ET is 22 per 10,000 and the annual rate is 11 per 10,000 in non-users of ET, the RR associated with ET use is 2.0.
- An RR of 1.2 means there is a 20% increase in risk in the exposed group.
- A RR of 0.3 means that there is a 70% lower risk in the exposed group.

Absolute risk (AR)

- The impact of RR on a population and individual depends on the incidence (the number of new cases).
- AR is the difference between the incidence rates in the exposed and unexposed groups.
- AR quantifies the effect of an exposure on a population basis, providing a measure of public health impact.
- AR is clinically more useful in explaining risk to patients than RR.
- With regard to risk of DVT in women using oral ET, the AR is from 22 per 10,000 per year to 11 per 10,000 per year.

Practice tips
Consider the following when explaining and presenting risk to patients[18]:

- For percentages, say 2 out of 10 may experience a side effect rather than 20%.
- Use the same denominator throughout the discussion, such as 1000 or 10,000 (e.g. 20 per 1000 developed headache on treatment whereas 12 per 1000 did not).
- Explain that an individual may develop the disease in question even without the proposed intervention.
- Don't overstate risk, particularly if studies of the population in question indicate a very low rate.

TABLE 14.1 The benefits and harms of using HT for 1 year in 10,000 women aged 65–74 years (From Nelson et al[82])

	Consequences	Number of cases
Benefits (events prevented)	Hip fractures	9
	Wrist fractures	37.5
	Vertebral fractures	57
Harms (events caused)	Strokes	3
	Thromboembolic events	1.5
	Cholecystitis with short-term use (<5 years)	25
	Cholecystitis with long-term use (>5 years)	53.5

- Be aware that words such as high, moderate, low, very low and minimal risk have different meanings for different patients.
- Individuals bring their own values, education, needs and preferences to the consultation, all of which will affect their perception of risk.
- Some individuals may fear certain outcomes more than others (e.g. stroke versus breast cancer).
- Media reports impact the perception of research reports among individuals, even though the media may not provide complete information.

Guideline recommendations

The following is a summary of the NAMS position statement on HT[18] and represents current guidelines on HT use.

HT should be used only after an individual assessment of the benefits and risks for that individual woman and confirmation of her treatment goals. This assessment will necessarily change with her age and the severity of her symptoms, but should always take into account her:

- baseline disease risks
- age
- age at menopause
- cause of menopause
- time since menopause
- prior use of hormones, and the types, dosages and routes of administration used
- emerging medical conditions during treatment.

Vasomotor symptoms

HT is the most effective treatment for hot flushes and night sweats. These symptoms remain the primary indication for HT.

Vaginal symptoms

The cause of symptoms related to vaginal atrophy is oestrogen deficiency, and the most appropriate treatment is local oestrogen therapy (ET) through low-dose intermittent application.

Sexual function

Dyspareunia (painful intercourse) that is caused by vaginal atrophy can be overcome by systemic ET/oestrogen & progestogen therapy (EPT) or local ET. However, these products are not recommended as the sole treatment for other problems of sexual functioning such as diminished libido.

Urinary health

In the presence of vaginal atrophy, local ET may benefit urge incontinence where there are symptoms of frequency and urgency in the absence of painful urination. If the latter is present, suspect a urinary tract infection and treat accordingly. Local ET may also reduce recurrent urinary tract infection.

There is no evidence to support systemic ET or EPT for the alleviation of true stress urinary incontinence.

Change in body weight/mass

Peak body mass index (BMI) occurs between the ages of 50 and 59, but there is no significant difference in mean weight gain or BMI between those women using HT and those that don't.

Quality of life (QOL)

There is good evidence to suggest an improvement in health-related quality of life in symptomatic women treated with hormones. Whether HT improves health-related QOL in asymptomatic women is unknown.

Osteoporosis

HT reduces postmenopausal osteoporotic fractures, including hip fractures, even in women without osteoporosis. Extended use of HT is an option in women who have established reduction in bone mass regardless of menopausal symptoms, for prevention of further bone loss and/or reduction in osteoporotic fracture when alternate therapies are not appropriate or cause side effects, or when the benefit–risk ratio of the extended use of alternate therapies is unknown.

Cardiovascular effects

Coronary heart disease (CHD)

The variation noted between observational studies and randomised controlled trials examining the effects of HT on cardiovascular outcome is now understood to be due to the timing of initiation of HT in relation to age and proximity to menopause.

Women who reach menopause at the typical age and who start HT within no more than 5 years of menopause are likely to gain some CHD protection, but, starting HT 10 or more years beyond menopause may increase risk. The absolute risks are rare, but nevertheless exist.

Fortunately, virtually all symptomatic women are in close proximity to menopause, so timing is not a real point of debate. The only reason for beginning systemic HT a long time after menopause would be for protection against osteoporosis, and in that context topics for discussion include risk, benefit and alternative bone-sparing therapies.

Another issue to consider, however, is the duration of therapy. For women in close proximity to menopause, the longer they remain on HT, the greater the protection. On the other hand, remaining on EPT for a long time adversely affects breast cancer risk.

Stroke

While the incidence of haemorrhagic stroke is not an issue in relation to HT, the WHI EPT and ET trials demonstrated an increased risk of ischaemic stroke of 8 additional strokes per 10,000 women per year of EPT use and 11 additional strokes per 10,000 women per year of ET use when data from all the age groups in the entire cohort were analysed. Younger women in the WHI (aged 50–59 years at study entry) had no significant increase in risk of stroke. Even though the risk of stroke in older women is rare, this is a serious event, and women with risk factors for cardiovascular disease should usually not be considered for HT. Nor can HT be considered for younger women for stroke prevention.

Venous thromboembolism (VTE)

The risk of VTE for all women starting HT is rare, but present. Growing evidence suggests that women with a prior history of VTE or women who possess factor V Leiden are at increased risk of VTE with HT use. Observational studies suggest that non-oral oestrogen (transdermal) use may be safer, as may lower doses of oral ET; however, there is no evidence as yet from randomised trials to support this.

Diabetes mellitus (DM, or type 2 diabetes)

DM is not a contraindication for HT. Limited evidence suggests that HT may actually reduce the incidence of DM in the order of 15 per 10,000 women per year of therapy, but this is not a reason in itself to prescribe. When prescribing oestrogen for a woman with DM, non-oral preparations may be preferred because of their reduced impact on raising triglycerides.

Endometrial cancer

Unopposed oestrogen significantly increases the incidence of endometrial cancer in women with an intact uterus. This risk increases with duration of use and persists for some years after discontinuation. Women must always receive progestogen when being prescribed oestrogen with an intact uterus.

Breast cancer

EPT use beyond 5 years is associated with increased breast cancer risk in the order of 4–6 additional invasive cancers per 10,000 women per year. It is unclear whether the risk differs between continuous and sequential use of progestogen. This absolute risk falls into the rare category. This risk needs careful explanation to women, and the decision to assume the risk is a personal one.

Interestingly, ET use did not demonstrate an increase in breast cancer risk after an average of 7.1 years use.

Evidence also suggests that EPT increases breast-cell proliferation, breast pain and mammographic density, negatively affecting the diagnostic interpretation of mammograms, which could lead to further, costly diagnostic tests, including biopsy.

Table 14.2 describes cancer risks and benefits associated with HT and may be helpful when counselling patients. Box 14.4 (p 264) contains the current recommendations of the National Breast and Ovarian Cancer Centre (NBOCC) regarding breast cancer risks and hormone therapy.[28]

Mood and depression

While ET may enhance the sense of wellbeing, for postmenopausal women without clinical depression evidence is mixed concerning the effects of HT on mood. Progestogens may actually induce symptoms similar to premenstrual syndrome. There is no evidence to justify use of HT as an antidepressant.

Cognitive ageing/decline and dementia

HT cannot be recommended at any age for the sole purpose of preventing cognitive ageing or dementia. The WHIMS study[16] showed an increase in dementia when HT was initiated in women over 65. Available data do not currently address whether HT used soon after the onset of menopause increases or decreases later dementia risk.[29]

Premature menopause and premature ovarian failure

Women <40 years of age experiencing premature menopause have a lower risk of breast cancer but an earlier risk of onset of osteoporosis and cardiovascular disease. There is inadequate data concerning this patient group in relation to HT. Existing data concerning women who reach menopause at the average age of 51 years should not be extrapolated to this younger patient group. However, the risk attributable to HT use by the younger women with premature menopause is likely to be smaller and the benefits potentially greater. Limited evidence favours these women being prescribed HT at least up to the typical age of menopause (51 years). Thereafter, the decision becomes the same as for all other women.

Total mortality

HT may reduce total mortality when initiated soon after menopause.

Summary of key points

- When counseling women risks should be conveyed in absolute numbers rather than percentages to avoid misinterpretation and alarm.

TABLE 14.2 Cancer risks associated with HT (Data derived from WHI[22], Stephanick et al[26] and Beral et al[27])

Type of cancer	Baseline risk for non-users of HT	Additional risk compared to non-users	
		With estrogen-only therapy	With combination estrogen and progestogen therapy
Breast	30 per 10,000 women years	No additional risk with up to 7 years of use	4–6 *extra* cases per 10,000 women years
Colorectal	10 per 10,000 women years		6 *fewer* cases per 10,000 women years
Endometrial	5 per 1000 women over 5 years	4 *extra* cases per 1000 women treated for 5 years 10 *extra* cases per 1000 women treated for 10 years	No changes in women treated for 5–10 years
Ovarian	2.2 per 1000 women over 5 years		2.6 per 1000 users over 5 years = 1 *extra* case per 2500 women treated for 5 years

BOX 14.4 Recommendations regarding HRT and breast cancer risk

Women with no personal or family history of breast cancer

- Women who are considering using combined HRT should be advised that the use of combined HRT (oestrogen and progestogen) is associated with an increased risk of breast cancer, which increases with duration of use. Although this risk appears to be associated with more than 3 years usage, it is not possible to determine a safe interval for use of combined HRT. For this reason, combined HRT should be considered only as a short-term option for the control of severe menopausal symptoms.
- Women who are already using combined HRT should be aware that there are both benefits and risks associated with the use of HRT. Women should review their needs every 6–12 months in consultation with their general practitioner, as their menopausal symptoms and underlying risk of breast cancer will have changed over time.
- Women using combined HRT should be advised that the risk of breast cancer decreases with increasing time since ceasing HRT usage, returning to the level of 'never-users' within 5 years of ceasing use.
- Women with a prior hysterectomy should be advised that the use of oestrogen-alone HRT for up to 8 years appears to have little or no effect on risk of breast cancer.

- Women should be advised that there is limited evidence indicating that combined oestrogen and testosterone HRT is associated with an increased risk of breast cancer that increases with each year of use.
- Women should be advised that there is limited evidence indicating that tibolone is associated with an increased risk of breast cancer.

Women with a personal or family history of breast cancer

- Women with a personal history of breast cancer should be advised that there is limited evidence indicating that the use of HRT is associated with an increased risk of breast cancer recurrence.
- Women with a family history of breast cancer should be advised that family history has no additive impact on risk of breast cancer with HRT usage.
- Women with a family history of breast cancer with a prior hysterectomy should be advised that short-term, oestrogen-only HRT would appear preferable to combined HRT.

'Natural' therapies

- Women should be advised that the risks of 'natural' HRT in relation to breast cancer are unknown.

- In women with premature menopause, HT improves quality of life and should be used for primary prevention of cardiovascular disease and skeletal risk.
- Young and healthy postmenopausal women can be started on HT when clinically warranted without fear of increased risk of cardiovascular disease.
- Use of oestrogens, even at ultra-low doses, should be opposed with adequate doses of progestogen to minimise the risk of endometrial carcinoma.
- HT is effective in relieving vasomotor symptoms.
- HT prevents the development of osteoporosis but its protective effect lasts only as long as the HT is taken.
- A window of opportunity for some degree of cardiovascular protection exists in women who reach menopause at the typical age and who start HT within no more than five years of menopause. However starting HT 10 or more years beyond menopause is likely to increase risk.
- There is no good evidence to support a role for HT in the primary prevention of Alzheimer's disease.

- HT use is associated with increased risk of breast cancer, endometrial cancer, cholecystitis, stroke and venous thromboembolus.

Practical therapeutic issues

Class versus specific product effect

Oestrogens and progestogens share some common features and effects, as well as potentially different properties. Without randomised controlled trial (RCT) evidence, results obtained in clinical trials from one agent are likely to be generalised to others, even though there are likely to be differences within each family, based on factors such as relative potency of the compound, androgenicity, glucocorticoid effects, bioavailability and administration route.

Progestogen indication

Progestogen is indicated to safeguard the endometrium. Given the evidence suggesting that progestogen added to oestrogen increases breast cancer risk, cardiovascular risk and adverse symptoms, it would obviously be best to reduce exposure to the least amount necessary in order to protect the endometrium.

Dosages

As with all medications, HT should be commenced using the lowest effective dose of oestrogen and corresponding low dose of progestogen to counter the adverse effects of systemic oestrogen on the uterus. Lower doses are better tolerated and may have a better benefit-risk profile than standard doses but have not been tested in long-term trials.

Routes of administration

Observational evidence suggests that transdermal ET may be associated with a lower risk of DVT, but there is no evidence from RCTs. Local ET is preferred when treating solely vaginal symptoms. Systemic progestogen is required for endometrial protection from unopposed ET. Topical progestogen is not recommended. With the exceptions referred to above, the route of administration and selection of pill, patch, cream, gel, spray, vaginal tablet or ring is really a personal preference.

Regimens

Research findings are inadequate to favour one regimen of dosing over another. There is insufficient evidence regarding endometrial safety to recommend as an alternative to standard EPT regimens the off-label use of: long-cycle regimens (14 days of progestogen every 2–6 months), vaginal administration of progestogen, the Mirena or low-dose oestrogen without progestogen. If any of these regimens are used, close surveillance is warranted. For a definition of the different EPT regimens, see Table 14.3.

Duration of use

When started in close proximity to menopause, the only long-term risk (beyond 5 years) might be an increased risk of breast cancer. Women who have reasons to remain on HT must have regular and appropriate follow-up, including mammography. As stated by the North American Menopause Spciety (NAMS),[18] provided that a woman is on the lowest effective dose, is well aware of the potential benefits and risks and has clinical supervision, extending HT use for individual treatment goals is acceptable under some circumstances for:

- the woman for whom, in her own opinion, the benefits of menopause symptom relief outweigh risks, notably after failing an attempt to stop HT
- further prevention of osteoporotic fracture and/or preservation of bone loss (regardless

TABLE 14.3 Terminology defining some types of EPT regimens (From North American Menopause Society[18])

Regimen	Oestrogen	Progestogen
Cyclic	Day 1–25	Last 10–14 days of ET cycle
Cyclic combined	Day 1–25	Day 1–25
Continuous–sequential	Daily	10–14 days every month
Long cycle	Daily	14 days every 2–6 months
Continuous–combined	Daily	Daily
Continuous–pulsed	Daily	Repeated cycles of 3 days on and 3 days off

of symptoms) in the woman with established reduction in bone mass when alternative therapies are not appropriate or cause unacceptable side effects, or when the benefit–risk ratio of the extended use of alternative therapies is unknown.

Discontinuance

There is no evidence to show that stopping HT cold turkey provides any difference in symptom recurrence than tapering.

One area of debate is whether there is residual increased risk for breast cancer after discontinuance. Recent data presented by the WHI suggest this may be so. On the other hand, the National Cancer Institute's Surveillance, Epidemiology and End Results (SEER) data showed a distinct drop in incidence of breast cancer in 2002 to 2003 after large numbers of women stopped HT. You cannot have it both ways, and the truth is probably in the middle, which is no effect.

Individualisation of therapy

Individualisation is what the art of menopause management is all about. Know the data, help a woman understand the risk, and weigh the level of potential risk and benefit for her personal circumstances. The informed woman will make the best decision for herself.

What should a GP do before starting a woman on HT?

GPs should give women the opportunity to discuss their understanding and fears about menopause. The pros and cons of HT should be discussed and written information given to the patient. It is also important to talk about alternatives and to take the opportunity to discuss lifestyle issues.

While taking the history the GP should assess:

1. the woman's menopausal state by inquiring about the last menstrual period, recent patterns of bleeding and whether or not she is experiencing any acute menopausal symptoms.
2. current contraceptive practice, as women who are currently taking the combined oral contraceptive pill (COCP) will not be experiencing any acute menopausal symptoms; as HT does not provide contraceptive cover, the patient's requirements for contraception will need to be considered if she is not on the COCP.
3. contraindications to HT (Box 14.5).
4. the family history of cardiovascular disease, osteoporosis, venous thromboembolism and breast, bowel and ovarian cancer.
5. Risk factors for cardiovascular disease (Box 14.6).
6. Risk factors for osteoporosis.

The woman's body mass index (BMI) and blood pressure should be recorded, and a breast examination and Pap smear should be carried out. Women should be encouraged to participate in the national breast-screening program.

No routine investigations are recommended before starting HT. FSH levels fluctuate during the perimenopause and if the woman is symptomatic and has no contraindications, a therapeutic trial of HT is warranted. In particular there is no place for endometrial assessment or mammography unless the woman is in a high-risk group. If there is a family history of venous thromboembolism, then thrombophilia screening can be carried out. This involves the tests listed in Box 14.7.[30]

For how long should women take HT?

Following on from the results of the HERS[31] and WHI[22] trials, women should be taking HT only for the management of menopausal symptoms and/or, if there are no alternatives, for the prevention of osteoporosis. This is because the incidence of some risks increases with increasing duration of use of HT, for example, breast cancer risk. Since hot flushes resolve in most women within a few years, it is now good practice to stop HT 2–3 years after starting, unless there is an indication to continue for the prevention of osteoporosis.

Which hormones, what dose and what regimen should be used?

Most of the complexity in managing women with the menopause lies in the vast array of products available and trying to ascertain what works best for individual women. The first question facing GPs when prescribing HT is which hormone or hormones to use:

- **Oestrogen** usually comes in the form of oestradiol or conjugated oestrogen. It should be given alone only to women without a uterus. Table 14.4 sets out the terminologies for dosing different oestrogens in hormone replacement preparations.
- **Progestogen** is necessary for the prevention of endometrial hyperplasia and cancer. The

---

BOX 14.5 Contraindications to HT

- Hormone-dependent malignancy, e.g. breast, endometrium
- Venous thromboembolic disease or pulmonary embolus
- Current pregnancy
- Severe active liver disease
- Undiagnosed breast mass
- Uninvestigated abnormal vaginal bleeding

BOX 14.6 Cardiovascular risk factors

- Cigarette smoking
- Hypertension
- Sedentary lifestyle
- Family history of premature myocardial infarction or stroke
- Diabetes mellitus
- Obesity (in particular central android obesity)

BOX 14.7 Screening women with a family history of venous thromboembolism

- Prothrombin time
- Protein C&S levels
- Antithrombin III level
- Lupus anticoagulant
- Antiphospholipid antibodies
- Full blood count, including platelets
- Urea and electrolytes
- Liver function tests
- Urinalysis
- Factor V Leiden DNA studies

Table 14.4 Terminologies for dosing of different oestrogens in hormone replacement preparations. Available doses may vary in different countries. Bioequivalence not tested (Adapted from Birkhäuser et al[32])

	High	Standard	Low	Ultra-low
Conjugated equine oestrogens (mg)	1.25	0.625	0.3	
Micronised 17β-oestradiol (mg)	4.0	2.0	1.0	0.5
Oestradiol valerate (mg)		2.0	1.0	
Transdermal 17β-oestradiol (μg)	100	50	25	14

progestogens most commonly used in HT are almost all synthetic and include:

– dydrogesterone and medroxyprogesterone
– norethisterone and levonorgestrel
– drospirenone.

Medroxyprogesterone and dydrogesterone are sometimes better tolerated than norethisterone or levonorgestrel because they are less androgenic. Drospirenone is also less androgenic and has aldosterone antagonistic activities, making it is useful for women who complain of fluid retention during the progestogen phase.

- **Tibolone** is a synthetic oral steroid with mixed oestrogenic/progestogenic and androgenic properties. Taken continuously it is used to treat acute menopausal symptoms as well as to prevent osteoporosis.
- **Androgen** testosterone is used by some in the treatment of low libido (see later).

The next question is whether to use a continuous or cyclical regimen (Table 14.5) or to use local treatment only.

- **Cyclical regimens** are best used in perimenopausal women with a uterus. They involve the use of oestrogen on a daily basis and progestogen given for a 14-day spell, preferably combined with the oestrogen in order to aid compliance. Cyclical regimens produce predictable withdrawal bleeding. Because of this many postmenopausal women will be adverse to their use, being unwilling to continue with the inconvenience of regular bleeds.
- **Continuous regimens** are more suitable for postmenopausal women and those who have had their uterus removed. Although there may be some spotting for the first few months, by 6 months, this kind of regimen should have resulted in endometrial atrophy and therefore amenorrhoea.
- **Local treatment** is appropriate for women who have urogenital atrophy but no systemic menopausal symptoms and who do not require preventive treatment for osteoporosis.

TABLE 14.5 Accepted doses of progestogen for endometrial protection (Data from BNF[78])

Progestogen type and route	Accepted endometrial protection dosage
Cyclical preparations	
Norethisterone oral	1 mg for last 12–14 days of 28-day cycle
Norethisterone patch	170–250 μg for last 14 days of a 28-day cycle
Levonorgestrel oral	75–250 μg for last 12 days of 28-day cycle
Levonorgestrel patch	10 μg for last 14 days of 28-day cycle
Norgestrel oral	150–500 μg for last 12 days of 28-day cycle
Medroxyprogesterone acetate oral	10 mg for last 14 days of 28-day cycle 20 mg for last 14 days of 3-month cycle
Dydrogesterone oral	10–20 mg for last 14 days of 28-day cycle
Continuous regimens	
Norethisterone oral	0.5–1 mg
Norethisterone patch	170 μg
Levonorgestrel patch	7 μg
Medroxyprogesterone acetate oral	2.5–5 mg
Dydrogesterone	5 mg

Cyclical regimens are best used in perimenopausal women with a uterus and *continuous* regimens are more suitable for postmenopausal women and those who have had their uterus removed.

The question of what dosage to prescribe can be confusing, given the different products available on the market. The golden rule of 'always prescribe the lowest dose necessary to achieve symptom control' is relevant here: if a woman is going to use HT, she should at least take a dose of oestrogen that has a bone-sparing effect. Low and ultra-low doses of HT have been shown to prevent postmenopausal bone loss only slightly less than that seen with standard doses, although there may be more non-responders. There are no data on fracture prevention using these low doses of HT.[32] The bone protective dosage of tibolone is 2.5 mg daily. The dose of progestogen a woman takes (presuming she is on combined HT) should also assure her of endometrial protection. Table 14.5 sets out these dosages.

What delivery method for HT is best?

The final decision to be made when prescribing HT is what delivery method to use. Currently there are tablets, transdermal methods (patches or gels), implants, intrauterine systems and vaginal products (Fig 14.4).

Oral tablets are usually the cheapest delivery mode but are easier to forget to take. The issue with putting the oestrogen in oral form is that the oestrogen is absorbed through the gut and undergoes first-pass metabolism in the liver before reaching the rest of the body, giving variable levels of hormone in the blood. The oral route should also be avoided in women using hepatic enzyme-inducing drugs.

Patches and gels come as oestrogen alone or combined with progestogen. Here, the oestrogen is absorbed directly through the skin into the systemic circulation, bypassing the liver. Hormone levels delivered by patch are higher and more constant than if given by mouth. The patches are usually placed on the buttocks. The problem with patches is that some women complain of skin reactions and lack of adhesiveness.

Another alternative is implants, particularly for women without a uterus. These are inserted subcutaneously and release oestradiol over several months. They may cause tachyphylaxis,[33] however, and flushing symptoms and cannot easily be removed. It is wise, therefore, to check that oestradiol levels have returned to normal (<1000 pmol/L) before inserting the next implant.

One method of progestogen delivery that may attract some women is to have in place a levonorgestrel intrauterine releasing system (Mirena). This provides continuous progestogen to the endometrium with little systemic side effect. After several months, a woman with the device in situ will become amenorrhoeic, so this may be the preferred method of endometrial protection in perimenopausal women, who do not want to continue a cyclical regimen that results in regular bleeding. It

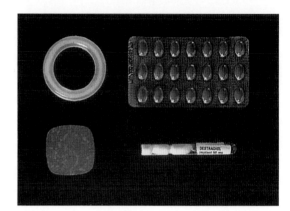

FIGURE 14.4 Different forms of HT: implant, patch, oral tablets and vaginal ring (From James et al[80])

is important to note that when Mirena is used for endometrial protection rather than contraception it is recommended to be changed after 4 years (instead of the usual 5 years).

Vaginal oestrogens are often used in the management of urogenital atrophy and come in the form of pessaries, tablets, creams and a silicone ring.

Proven effective starting doses at which symptom relief can be expected in the majority of women are[32]:

- 0.5–1 mg 17β-oestradiol (per orally)
- 0.3–0.45 mg conjugated equine oestrogens (per orally)
- 25–37.5 μg transdermal (patch) oestradiol
- 0.5–1.0 mg oestradiol gel

Symptoms should be reassessed after a couple of months and a decision made as to whether the dose should be altered. Approximately 20% of women will require a higher dose.[32] Table 14.6 sets out equivalent doses of HT—a handy reference when tailoring dosage to women's individual needs.

What are the side effects of HT?

Common side effects and their management are given below.[34]

Complaints of weight gain

Reassure the woman that weight gain is very common around the time of the menopause and that hormone therapy does not cause significant further weight gain.

Oestrogen–related adverse effects

These include fluid retention, bloating, breast tenderness or enlargement, nausea, headaches, leg cramps and dyspepsia and may occur continuously or randomly throughout the cycle.

TABLE 14.6 Equivalent doses of different types of oestrogen and progestogen combination HT (From Australian Menopause Society[79])

Cyclical oestrogen and progestogen combinations (use these at perimenopause or if less than 12 months amenorrhoea)		
Medium-dose		
Product	Presentation	Composition
Trisequens	Tablet	1,2 mg oestradiol/1 mg norethisterone
Estalis sequi 50/140	Transdermal patch	50 μg oestradiol/140 μg norethisterone acetate
Estalis sequi 50/250 (same oestrogen, more progestogen than Estalis sequi 50/140), Estracombi	Transdermal patch	50 μg oestradiol/250 μg norethisterone acetate
Continuous oestrogen and progestogen combinations (should be used if 12 months since LMP or after 12 months cyclical HRT)		
Low dose		
Product	Presentation	Composition
Angeliq1/2	Tablet	1 mg oestradiol/2 mg drospirenone
Kliovance	Tablet	1 mg oestradiol/0.5 mg norethisterone
Livial (generally suitable for older women or at least 2 years postmenopause)	Tablet	2.5 mg tibolone
Medium dose		
Product	Presentation	Composition
Femoston	Tablet	2 mg oestradiol/10 mg dydrogesterone
Kliogest	Tablet	2 mg oestradiol/1 mg norethisterone
Nuvelle	Tablet	2 mg oestradiol/0.075 mg levonorgestrel
Premia 2.5 Continuous	Tablet	0.625 mg conjugated equine oestrogens/2.5 mg medroxyprogesterone acetate
Premia 5 Continuous (same oestrogen, more progestogen than Premia 2.5 Continuous)	Tablet	0.625 mg conjugated equine oestrogens/5 mg medroxyprogesterone acetate
Estalis continuous 50/140	Transdermal patch	50 μg oestradiol/140 μg norethisterone acetate
Estalis continuous 50/250 (same oestrogen, more progestogen than Estalis continuous 50/140)	Transdermal patch	50 μg oestradiol/250 μg norethisterone acetate

- *Leg cramps* can improve with lifestyle changes, including exercise and regular stretching of the calf muscles.
- *Nausea/gastric upset* may be helped by adjusting the timing of the oestrogen dosage or taking with food.
- *Breast tenderness* may be alleviated by a low-fat, high-carbohydrate diet. Gamolenic acid (evening primrose oil) has no proven efficacy.
- *Migraine* triggered by fluctuating oestrogen levels may respond to transdermal therapy, as this produces more stable oestrogen levels.

Progestogen-related adverse effects

Many women are surprised when they find that they experience 'premenstrual'-type symptoms when taking HT. For some, these symptoms along with a recurrence of bleeding are enough to make them discontinue. The following strategies may assist in alleviating such symptoms:

- *Changing the type of progestogen in the HT,* for example, from more androgenic ones, such as norethisterone and norgestrel, to less androgenic ones, such as medroxyprogesterone or dydrogesterone.

- *Changing the route of progestogen,* for example, from oral to transdermal, vaginal or intrauterine progestogen. This may be most beneficial when the woman is nauseous while receiving oral HT. If the oestrogen is to be delivered by a different route from the progestogen, the woman can easily miss out the progestogen as desired if it is causing unpleasant adverse effects. However, the woman must fully understand that the progestogen is being given to provide endometrial protection.
- *Reducing the duration of progestogen adminis-tration*—progestogens can be taken for 12–14 days of each monthly sequential regimen, so swapping from a 14-day to a 12-day product may provide benefit.
- *Changing to a product with a lower dose of progestogen* (dosages are preparation-dependent).
- *Reducing the frequency* of progestogen dosing. This can be achieved by switching to a long-cycle regimen, administering progestogen for 14 days every 3 months (but this strategy is suitable only for women without natural regular periods).
- *Changing to continuous combined therapy* or tibolone often reduces progestogenic adverse effects with established use (as these products contain lower dosages of progestogen), but this is suitable only for postmenopausal women.

When confronted with these side effects a GP can suggest:

- that the woman persist for 3 months, as adverse effects generally resolve with time
- lowering the dose (being aware of the minimum bone-sparing and endometrial protection dosages)
- changing the oestrogen or progestogen type— some women who get side effects using conjugated oestrogens will be less affected by oestradiol; similarly if the side effects are more progestogenic in nature, it may be beneficial to swap from the more androgenic types (norethisterone and norgestrel) to the less androgenic (medroxyprogesterone acetate and dydrogesterone)
- changing the route of delivery (mostly from tablets to patches).

What is the role of tibolone in the management of menopausal symptoms?

Tibolone is a compound that can be selectively metabolised by individual tissues to its oestrogenic, progestogenic or androgenic metabolites, exhibiting tissue-specific hormonal effects. Tibolone appears to be at least as efficacious as other forms of HT for climacteric symptoms and alleviates symptomatic atrophic vaginitis. It has also been demonstrated to reduce lumbar fractures in an elderly population (mean age 68).[32] It may cause irregular bleeding, however, unless used with at least 1 year of amenorrhoea and is therefore not indicated in perimenopause.[35]

Tibolone also has positive effects on mood and aspects of memory and is associated with improvements in sexual function that seem to be greater than those achieved with standard hormone therapy. It therefore provides another option for menopausal women who are experiencing loss of libido as part of their symptomatology or who have persistent low libido despite adequate oestrogen/ progestogen therapy.[36]

Tibolone is associated with a small increased risk of stroke when used in women over 60 but has no increased risk of VTE. While it has a minimal effect on breast tenderness and mammographic density, data on tibolone and outcomes such as breast cancer and cardiovascular disease are awaited from randomised trials.[32] The recent results of the LIBERATE (Livial Intervention Following Breast Cancer: Efficacy, Recurrence, and Tolerability Endpoints) trial[37] unfortunately found that tibolone significantly increases the risk of recurrence in breast cancer patients and so it should not be prescribed to any woman with current, past or suspected breast cancer.

What if the woman develops irregular bleeding while taking HT?

It is important to rule out any pathology before altering the hormone therapy, so conduct an examination, visualise the cervix, check that smears are up to date and refer for transvaginal ultrasound to exclude pelvic abnormalities. Also be sure to check compliance and whether there are any ongoing drug interactions (e.g. anticonvulsants) or have been gastrointestinal problems.

In women encountering problems on monthly cyclical regimens, altering the progestogen part of the regimen may improve bleeding problems[34]:

- Heavy or prolonged bleeding: increase the duration or dosage of the progestogen, or change the type of progestogen. Idiopathic menorrhagia may be helped by using the levonorgestrel-releasing intrauterine system, combined with an oestrogen delivered orally or transdermally.
- Bleeding early in the progestogen phase: increase dosage or change the type of progestogen.
- Irregular bleeding: change regimen or increase the dosage of progestogen.

- No bleeding while taking a cyclical regimen reflects an atrophic endometrium and occurs in 5% of women.

Pregnancy needs to be excluded in perimenopausal women. Check compliance if the progestogen component is taken separately.

In women taking continuous combined or long-cycle HT regimens, irregular breakthrough bleeding or spotting is common in the first 3–6 months. However, bleeding beyond 6 months or after a spell of amenorrhoea requires further investigation or referral.

What follow-up should women taking HT receive?

There is no set rule for how often a woman on HT should be monitored. If the woman has just started on HT or changes regimen it is probably wise to follow up in 3 months, looking for any adverse effects. In the longer term, GPs should keep an eye on the total duration of the HT and review the necessity of staying on HT for longer than 5 years in view of the increased risk of breast cancer. Women should also be encouraged to adhere to national guidelines on breast cancer and cervical cancer screening by undertaking clinical examination, mammography and Pap smears when indicated.

Is HT suitable as contraception?

The short answer is no: HT is not contraceptive as the case below illustrates.

When do women stop needing contraception?

As a general rule, non-hormonal contraception should be continued for 1 year after the last menstrual period for women over 50 years old, or for 2 years after the last menstrual period for women under the age of 50 years.[38] This gives the woman some margin of safety in the unlikely event that an ovulatory cycle ensues after some months of amenorrhoea.

Non-hormonal contraception should be continued for 1 year after the last menstrual period for women over 50 years old, or for 2 years after the last menstrual period for women under the age of 50 years.

Is it OK to recommend combined oral contraception during perimenopause?

The answer is yes. Previously, when we had only relatively high-dose oestrogen-containing COCPs to use, the recommendation was to stop using the pill after the age of 35, mainly because of the increasing risk of cardiovascular disease. Now the recommendation is that women (provided there are no contraindications) can continue on COCP (low-dose oestrogen) until the age of 50. At that time, women should be counselled about the benefits and risks of combined contraception and about suitable alternative methods such as barrier methods or the progestogen-only pill (POP). After stopping combined contraception, barrier methods can be used until the menopause is confirmed (1 year of amenorrhoea or 2 years if aged <50 years). Alternatively, a POP may be a suitable option for women who wish to continue with an oral regimen.[39]

COCP has several benefits in the perimenopausal period. Not only will it prevent pregnancy efficiently when taken correctly, but it will also make bleeding regular, lighter and relatively painless. The COCP will also provide oestrogen to the woman, thereby ensuring bone protection and prevention of the development of osteoporosis.[40]

As they approach menopause, many women pay increasing attention to their risks of cancer. They can be assured by the fact that incidence of both ovarian[41] and endometrial cancer[42] is lowered with COCP use. The relationship between breast cancer and the pill is another matter, however, having been the subject of numerous studies. Collectively they suggest the following[43]:

- Past users (>10 years since use) are at no increased risk for breast cancer.
- Current and recent users (<10 years since stopping) have a small increase in risk of breast cancer, which is not related to duration of use.
- The small, excess risk seems largely confined to tumours localised in the breast. Such tumours have a better prognosis than those that have spread beyond the breast.

Perimenopausal women should therefore be told of this small increase in breast cancer risk and consider it in the light of their own personal risk factors and family history.

How should a GP change a woman over from the COCP to HT?

Menstrual bleeding patterns are unhelpful when a woman is using exogenous hormones. Amenorrhoea may be due to contraceptive hormones: POPs, injectables, implants or the levonorgestrel-releasing intrauterine system (LNG-IUS, or Mirena). Regular bleeding may be due to contraceptive hormones (COCP). Assessments of FSH levels are unreliable when women are using combined contraception, even

CASE STUDY: 'Is my HT contraceptive?'

Claudia was 43 years old. She presented on a Monday afternoon seeking advice about the results of some blood tests done (by another GP) 3 months beforehand. At that time she had complained to the GP about hot flushes and feeling 'terrible'. She had wondered whether or not she may have been menopausal, as her mother and aunt both went through the menopause at around 40 years of age. At the time she had been on a triphasic combined oral contraceptive pill and had been taking this since the birth of her first and only child 7 years previously. As a result of the tests she had done, her GP had discontinued the pill and placed her on cyclical combined HT. She now wanted to know if the HT was contraceptive, as she and her partner had had unprotected sex on Saturday night. She handed over copies of the results of the blood tests.

Test results

- HCG: <5 U/L negative
- TSH 1.18 mIU/L (0.40–4.70)
- Serum oestradiol 108 pmol/L

Reference ranges:

Follicular phase 70–670

Luteal phase 200–600

Pre-ovulatory 550–2000

Postmenopausal <120

Prepubertal <40

- Follicle stimulating hormone (FSH): 0.9 IU/L
- Luteinising hormone (LH): <1.0 IU/L

Reference ranges for FSH and LH:

	FSH	LH
Follicular phase	3.5–16.0	<15.0
Midcycle peak	8.0–30.0	15.0–75.0
Luteal phase	1.8–12.0	<15.0
Postmenopausal	>5.0	5.0–50.0

It seemed Claudia's results had been poorly interpreted by her GP. The key finding in postmenopausal women is that the FSH level usually sits at 40–50 IU/L. While Claudia's serum oestradiol level is in the postmenopausal range, it is also in the range of women in the follicular phase of their cycle. In Claudia's case, the serum oestradiol level reflects the fact that she is taking HT. The exogenous oestrogen acts to suppress FSH and LH in order to prevent ovulation, hence the low levels of these hormones. Claudia had originally wanted to know if she was menopausal. In order to make an accurate diagnosis of menopause in this woman, she would need to cease all forms of hormone ingestion for a minimum of 6 weeks. At the end of this time, a FSH level could be taken and then repeated 1–2 months later. If it was above 30 on both occasions, she could be presumed to be menopausal. At this consultation, Claudia requires emergency contraception, as HT is not contraceptive and there is no evidence as yet that she is truly postmenopausal. Although women approaching menopause are not as fertile as they were in their 20s, they are still at risk of unplanned pregnancy. Ovulation continues sporadically during the several years approaching menopause. Among women of perimenopausal age with irregular menses, as many women return to regular menses as enter menopause.[45] Although some mid-life couples welcome pregnancies, most are unplanned.

The second question in this case is whether Claudia should go back to using hormonal contraception at her age. The health benefits of hormonal contraceptive use for older women are both contraceptive (i.e. related to the health benefits of avoiding unintended pregnancy) and non-contraceptive. While a barrier method of contraception for a woman in her 40s might be suitable, hormonal contraception will regulate her periods and provide her with symptom control as she approaches menopause. However, it is important to check her blood pressure and make sure she is not smoking and has no other contraindications should she choose to use hormonal contraception. Claudia would be best on a low-dose oral contraceptive (with either 20 or 30 mg of ethinyl oestradiol). The choice of progestogen in the pill is less important. Another valuable option to consider is the use of the progestogen-releasing IUS (Mirena).

if measured in the pill-free interval.[39] However, FSH levels can be measured while using progestogen-only contraception (POPs, injectables, implants and the LNG-IUS).[44] FSH may be assessed 6 or more weeks after discontinuing combined hormones. A level of >30 IU/L on two or more occasions, at least 1 or 2 months apart, with accompanying amenorrhoea is highly suggestive of ovarian failure.

For an algorithm of when to stop contraception, see Figure 14.5.

Assessments of FSH levels are unreliable when women are using combined contraception, even if measured in the pill-free interval.

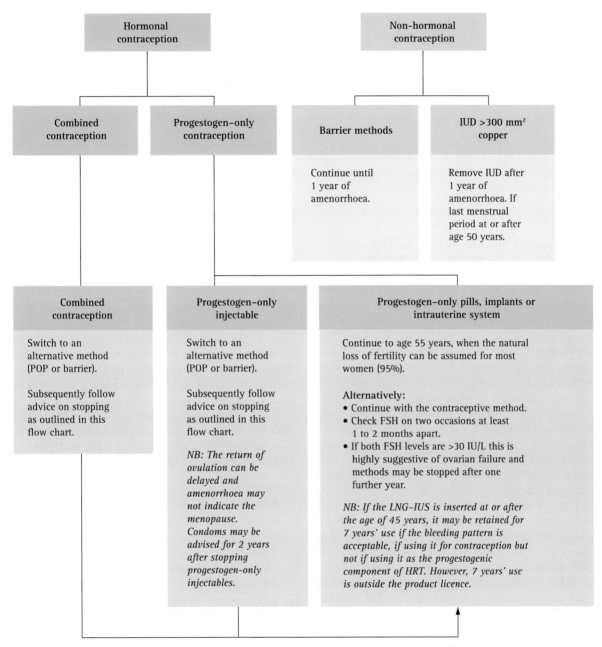

FIGURE 14.5 Advice for women at age 50 years on stopping contraception (From FFPRHC[39]). FSH, follicle-stimulating hormone; IUD, intrauterine device; LNG-IUS, levonorgestrel-releasing hormone; POP, progestogen-only pill.

What is the role of androgens in the treatment of menopausal symptoms?

Although it is generally believed that testosterone plays a vital role in female sexual functioning, there is no good study that demonstrates a clear correlation between circulating testosterone levels and sexual functioning. There is, however, some limited evidence from randomised trials that exogenous testosterone can have a positive effect on sexual function—primarily desire, arousal and orgasmic response—in women after spontaneous or surgically induced menopause.[18]

Androgen therapy should be considered only in women who have a physiological reason for reduced androgen concentrations. As sexual dysfunction and additional symptoms associated with androgen insufficiency are characteristic of many other medical, psychological and psychosocial problems, alternative causes of the presenting symptoms must be identified and treated before considering androgen therapy.

As sexual dysfunction and additional symptoms associated with androgen insufficiency are characteristic of many other problems, alternative causes of the presenting symptoms must be identified and treated before considering androgen therapy.

HT remains first-line therapy for lack of desire and symptoms of tiredness and lethargy in the postmenopausal woman, mainly because of its relative safety compared with the use of androgens. The synthetic steroid tibolone is also an option because it has some androgenic-like actions. While not as effective as conventional HT in controlling hot flushes, it has a low incidence of adverse side effects, and many women do report an improvement in libido and well-being after 4–5 months of use.[46]

Postmenopausal women who are significantly distressed by decreased sexual desire and have no other identifiable cause may be candidates for testosterone therapy, but it should be used only concomitantly with oestrogen therapy. Table 14.7 lists possible treatment regimens for women having androgen therapy.

The potential risks of androgen therapy, particularly when administered at supraphysiologic doses, include hirsutism, acne, liver dysfunction, lowering of the voice, adverse lipid changes and virilisation of the female fetus. Women who elect for a trial of therapy should be informed of these potential risks and made aware that it is not known whether testosterone therapy increases the risk of breast cancer, cardiovascular disease or thromboembolic events. Monitoring of liver function tests and a serum lipid profile may be indicated in long-term users.

It is important to note that clinically available laboratory assays do not accurately detect testosterone concentrations at the values typically found in women, and that laboratory testing of testosterone levels should be used only to monitor for supraphysiologic levels before and during therapy, not to diagnose testosterone insufficiency.[47]

Transdermal patches and topical gels or creams are preferred over oral products because of first-pass hepatic effects documented with oral formulations.

TABLE 14.7 Treatment regimens for women having androgen therapy

Product	Dosage
Androderm (testosterone patch)	1/8 of a patch daily
Sustenon injection (multiple testosterone compounds)	50–100 mg by deep intra-muscular injection monthly
Testosterone implants	50–100 mg every 6–12 months, with serum testosterone assay indicated before insertion of the next implant
Andro-feme cream (1% testosterone)	10 mg of cream applied to a 2 cm² area of skin on the forearm daily, with dose adjusted according to response

Custom-compounded products should be used with caution because the dosing may be more inconsistent than it is with government-approved products. Testosterone products formulated specifically for men have a risk of excessive dosing. Testosterone therapy is contraindicated in women with breast or uterine cancer or in those with cardiovascular or liver disease. It should be administered at the lowest dose for the shortest time that meets treatment goals. Counselling about the potential risks and benefits should be provided before initiating therapy.[47]

Summary of key points
- Women should take HT only for the management of menopausal symptoms and for the prevention of osteoporosis.
- Duration of HT use should probably be limited to <5 years unless there is a strong indication to continue.
- Tibolone is a useful agent in the management of decreased libido.
- HT is not contraceptive.

ALTERNATIVES TO HT

What are phytoestrogens?

Phytoestrogens are compounds derived from plants that are converted into oestrogenic substances in the gastrointestinal tract. They are increasingly being promoted as 'natural' alternatives to oestrogen replacement therapy. There are three main groups of phenolic plant oestrogens: isoflavones, lignans and coumestans.[48] These compounds or their metabolites can bind to oestrogen receptors and act as oestrogen agonists when endogenous oestradiol levels are low, such as in the menopause.[49] In premenopausal women, however, they may actually compete with oestradiol at the receptor site and act as oestrogen antagonists.[49]

The best known and most researched phytooestrogens are those derived from the soy bean; however, other herbs that are said to have oestrogenic properties include red clover (*Trifolium pratense*), black cohosh (*Cimicifuga racemosa*), licorice (*Glycyrrhiza glabra*), alfalfa (*Medicago sativum*), dong quai (*Angelica sinensis*) and hops (*Humulus lupulus*). The classification and food sources of phytoestrogens are given in Box 14.8.

What is the scientific basis for the claim that phytoestrogens may assist postmenopausal women?

The interest in phytoestrogens stems from the fact that women of Asian origin, particularly Japanese women, have a lower prevalence of hot flushes when compared with women from Western countries. This finding has been attributed to the fact that the Asian diet is rich in phytoestrogens.[50] Cardiovascular disease, osteoporosis and breast cancer—diseases that are known to be related to oestrogen status—are also lower in populations where the diet is high in phytoestrogens.[51,52]

BOX 14.8 Classification and food sources of phytoestrogens

Isoflavones
Legumes
Soybeans, lentils, beans (haricot, broad, kidney, lima/butter)
Chickpeas
Soy meal, soy grits, soy flour, tofu, soy milk

Lignans
Wholegrain cereals
Wheat, wheatgerm, barley, hops, rye, rice, brans, oats
Fruit, vegetables, seeds
Cherries, apples, pears, stone fruits, linseed
Sunflower seeds, carrots, fennel, onion, garlic
Vegetable oils including olive oil
Alcoholic sources: beer from hops, bourbon from corn

Coumestans
Bean sprouts
Alfalfa, soybean sprouts
Fodder crops
Clover

What evidence is there that phytoestrogens have a positive effect on menopausal symptoms?

A recent Cochrane review assessed the efficacy, safety and acceptability of foods and supplements based on high levels of phytoestrogens in reducing hot flushes and night sweats in postmenopausal women.[53] They found no evidence of effectiveness in the alleviation of menopausal symptoms with the use of phytoestrogen treatments. There was a strong placebo effect in most trials, with a reduction in frequency ranging from 1% to 59% with a placebo. There was no indication that the discrepant results were due to the amount of isoflavone in the active treatment arm, the severity of vasomotor symptoms or trial quality factors. There was also no evidence that the treatments caused oestrogenic stimulation of the endometrium (an adverse effect) when used for up to 2 years.

Do phytoestrogens have an effect on cardiovascular disease or breast cancer?

The large variance in the prevalence of breast cancer between Western and Asian countries points to a link between the presence of phytoestrogens in the diet and the prevention of breast cancer. Indeed, studies have shown a significantly reduced incidence of breast cancer among past phytoestrogen users and beneficial effects on surrogate parameters such as bone mineral density, vasodilation, platelet aggregation, insulin resistance and serum concentrations of triglycerides, high-density lipoprotein and low-density lipoprotein. No RCTs have documented a protective effect of phytoestrogens for the clinical end points of breast cancer, bone fracture or cardiovascular events.[54]

Based on the available evidence, phytoestrogens should be used only in selected women, that is, those presenting with mild to moderate vasomotor symptoms in early natural postmenopause. None of the compounds investigated so far have been proved to protect against breast cancer, bone fracture or cardiovascular disease.

Do phytoestrogens have any detrimental effects?

As with any other active agent, it would be naïve to assume that exposure to these compounds is always good. Toxic effects have not been rigorously sought out. Also, because phytoestrogens are often marketed in health-food shops and presented as 'natural' and therefore beneficial as supplements, the commercial preparations that are currently available may not have been subject to the controlled trials and standardisations of dose to which pharmaceutical products are subjected in order to obtain licensure for sale in countries such as Australia. It is important also to be aware that middle-aged women are the highest users of alternative therapies,[55] and many will have turned to non-prescription alternatives following media reports of the WHI study. In 2007, Australian authorities issued a warning of a very rare association between the use of black cohosh and liver damage, and advised health professionals to be on the lookout for signs of liver toxicity associated with the use of black cohosh medicines.[56]

What should I tell my patients when they ask about the usefulness of phytoestrogens?

While in theory phytooestrogens should work, there is no current evidence supporting their effectiveness. The placebo effect is likely to be high. No long-term data are available about safety. If women choose to use black cohosh, they should be aware of the rare side effect of liver toxicity.

What other non-hormonal options are there?

Several non-hormonal options have been recommended as an alternative to oestrogen for the management of vasomotor symptoms, particularly in breast cancer survivors. SSRIs (paroxetine) or SNRIs (venlafaxine), clonidine and gabapentin trials provide evidence of efficacy. However, effects are less than for oestrogen, and adverse effects and cost may restrict use for many women. These therapies may be most useful for highly symptomatic women who cannot take oestrogen but are not optimal choices for most women.[57]

The reported decrease in the number of hot flushes with SSRI use is only 1 per day.[57]

What is the role of selective oestrogen receptor modulators (SERMs)?

SERMs are synthetic compounds that bind oestrogen receptors and produce agonistic activity in some tissues while acting as oestrogen antagonists in other tissues.[58] The most common SERMs available include clomiphene, tamoxifen and raloxifene.

While clomiphene is widely used by gynaecologists in the treatment of infertility, tamoxifen has made a name for itself in the treatment of breast cancer and in the prevention of breast cancer in women at high risk. It is however associated with increased risk of thromboembolism and endometrial cancer. Raloxifene is effective in the prevention and treatment of women with osteoporosis (see later),

but it also is associated with increased risk of venous thromboembolism.

Some of my patients want to try 'bioidentical hormones'? What are they and should I recommend them?

Women are encouraged to believe that symptoms they experience are due to a 'hormone imbalance' and that, given all the bad publicity about HT, they should approach menopause using 'bioidentical hormones', which they believe are natural products. Bioidentical hormones are made up usually by compounding pharmacies into lozenges or troches or creams that are sucked in the cheek and absorbed through the lining of the cheek or through the skin. Oestrogen mixes are sometimes combined with progesterone, testosterone or dehydroepiandrosterone (DHEA), or they can each be prescribed alone. Of note, DHEA is not approved for use in Australia by the TGA. Progesterone is not used in conventional pharmaceutical HT, as it is filtered by the liver; therefore, altered progestin compounds are used.[59]

The term 'bioidentical hormone' has been deemed to be 'a marketing term that carries no scientific or medical merit'.[60] While the term implies that these products are non-synthetic, they are in fact derived from yam or soy and then manufactured synthetically using a similar process to that used for most hormones, including the pill, but once synthesised they are in forms that are produced in the body.

Bioidentical hormones are not supported by well-controlled studies examining the route of administration and pharmacokinetics. They are also not subject to the same government regulations imposed on pharmaceutical companies that require extensive safety and efficacy data. Of particular concern is the fact that there are no adequate data to show what dose of progestin (progesterone) is necessary to protect the lining of the uterus (endometrium). No evidence is available from any published study to show that progesterone absorbed through the cheek will protect the lining of the uterus from conditions such as uterine cancer.[59] Bioidentical hormones are also expensive, because they are individually prepared.

In addition, bioidentical hormone prescriptions are customised according to saliva tests and blood sera levels, in direct contradiction of evidence-based guidelines that support tailoring HT individually according to symptoms.[61]

To conclude, until these products are supported by rigorous evidence showing safety and efficacy, they cannot be supported.

Summary of key points

- Cardiovascular disease, osteoporosis and breast cancer are lower in populations where the diet is high in phytoestrogens.
- Randomised, controlled trials have not shown phytoestrogens to alleviate the vasomotor symptoms of menopause.
- There are no rigorous studies looking at adverse effects of phytoestrogens.
- It is currently premature to recommend the use of phytoestrogens to menopausal women.
- SSRIs, SNRIs, clomiphenes and gabapentin can be used in women for whom oestrogen is contraindicated for the management of hot flushes, although they are not as effective as oestrogen.
- SERMs are synthetic agents that bind to oestrogen receptors. Clomiphene is used in the treatment of infertility, tamoxifen in breast cancer and raloxifene in osteoporosis.
- Bioidentical hormones should not be recommended to women with menopausal symptoms.

MANAGING ESTABLISHED OSTEOPOROSIS

How common is osteoporosis?

A 50-year-old Caucasian woman has a 32% lifetime risk of spine fracture, 16% risk of hip fracture and 15% risk of fracture of the distal radius. These rates exceed her risk of developing endometrial or breast cancer.[62] Women have high rates of osteoporosis because they generally achieve a lower peak bone mass and have greater bone loss as a result of the hormonal changes associated with menopause.

How do I know if my patient has it?

The criteria for osteoporosis have been defined by the World Health Organization according to levels of bone mineral density (BMD), as low bone mass is the biggest risk factor for fragility fractures. The WHO criteria[63] (Table 14.8) use the 'T score', which compares the patient's BMD in standard deviations with the peak BMD in healthy young people. Therefore, a normal bone density is one within one standard deviation (SD) of the mean. Osteopenia is said to exist when the BMD is more than 1 SD but less than 2.5 SD below the mean. Osteoporosis is where the BMD is more than 2.5 SD below the mean.

Both peripheral (extremities) and central (spine and hip) bone sites can be used to measure BMD, but on whom BMD should be measured remains controversial. BMD screening is not recommended;

Table 14.8 WHO Criteria for osteoporosis (from WHO[83])

Osteoporosis	Osteopenia	Normal bone density
T < −2.5 SD	−2.5 SD < T <−1 SD	T > −1 SD

BOX 14.9 Risk factors for osteoporosis

- Prolonged oestrogen deficiency
- Age of woman
- Family history of osteoporosis
- Thin, underweight build
- Oriental or Caucasian origin
- Immobility/sedentary lifestyle
- Smoking
- Prolonged corticosteroid use
- Excessive alcohol intake
- Previous fragility fracture
- Low calcium or vitamin D intake or deficiency of vitamin D
- Malabsorption disorders
- Nulliparity
- Loss of height

rather an individualised approach should be adopted by assessing an individual woman's risk factors for osteoporosis (Box 14.9).

What imaging modality should be used to assess BMD?

The three major imaging modalities in use today are dual energy X-ray absorptiometry (DXA) scans, quantitative computerised tomography (QCT) and calcaneal ultrasound. Because these different techniques give different results, even at the same site, the T scores they produce cannot be used interchangeably.[64] DXA scans (Figs 14.6 and 14.7, p 278) are the most widely used modality and have a high level of precision.[65] They are the current 'gold standard' in the diagnosis of osteoporosis.[66] QCT allows for selective assessment of both cortical and trabecular bone, and since trabecular bone has a higher rate of turnover it may show metabolic changes earlier. However, QCT scans are more expensive and associated with a higher level of radiation.[64] Ultrasonography cannot be used for monitoring skeletal changes over time or for evaluating response to therapy.[65]

In general, calcaneal ultrasound can be used as a screening test when the osteoporotic risk is unknown or thought to be minimal. In women with multiple risk factors, the DXA scan or QCT is more appropriate.[67]

While some advocate universal screening of women for osteoporosis, one algorithm that can be used to select women for bone densitometry testing more effectively is the Osteoporosis Risk Assessment Instrument (ORAI). It is based on age, weight and current oestrogen. It selects the following women as candidates for DXA scanning[68]:

- all women >45 years and weighing <60 kg
- all women 55–64 years weighing <70 kg and not taking supplemental oestrogen
- all women >65 years, regardless of weight or current oestrogen usage.

When should treatment be initiated?

If a woman has a spinal fracture, if she has a non-spinal fracture and her BMD is in the osteoporotic range, or if she has major risk factors for osteoporosis, she should be treated.[66] An algorithm for the management of osteoporosis is given in Figure 14.8.

What non-drug measures can be instituted by a GP in the management of osteoporosis?

GPs should be sure to tackle lifestyle issues related to the development of osteoporosis when counselling patients about this condition. Bone loss is affected by diet, exercise, smoking and alcohol consumption. Women should have adequate levels of calcium in their diet and vitamin D and they should be advised to undertake weight-bearing exercise. The current recommended daily dose of calcium in postmenopausal women is 1200–1500 mg/day. Since the average intake of calcium for women is 500–700 mg/day, most women will require calcium supplementation to ensure adequate intake.

What medication can be used to treat osteoporosis?

The bisphosphonates alendronate and risedronate are the first-line agents in the treatment of postmenopausal osteoporosis, as is the SERM raloxifene. Bisphosphonates inhibit bone resorption: alendronate reduces the risk of vertebral, wrist and hip fractures by about 50%[68] and risedronate by about 40%.[70]

Bisphosphonates can cause oesophagitis, however, and patients with gastroesophageal reflux need to be monitored carefully. Patients should be advised that they must take the tablet with a large glass of water and that they should remain upright, either standing or sitting, for at least half an hour after swallowing it. Bisphosphonates should also be taken on an empty stomach (at least half an hour before eating) to aid absorption. Jaw osteonecrosis has been most commonly reported with the use

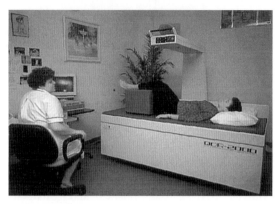

FIGURE 14.6 Bone density measurement (From James et al[80])

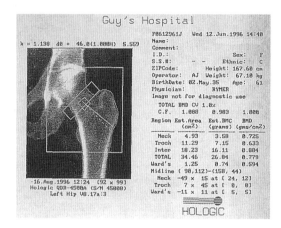

FIGURE 14.7 DEXA printout of bone density (From James et al[80])

of intravenous bisphosphonates (zoledronate and pamidronate) in cancer patients. Several cases have been reported in people taking oral bisphosphonates for osteoporosis, but these have mainly been the result of high IV doses (4–10 times higher than oral bisphosphonate doses).[71]

The SERM raloxifene is less effective than bisphosphonates. While it does bring about a 30% reduction in spinal fractures, non-vertebral fractures are not reduced with its use.[72] It does have the added benefit, however, of showing a 76% reduction in breast cancer, compared with a placebo, in women where raloxifene is used for 3 years.[73] On the downside is the risk of generating hot flushes.

Strontium ranelate is a newer agent for the prevention of fractures in postmenopausal women with osteoporosis, increasing bone formation markers and decreasing bone resorption markers. It reduces vertebral fractures by 50%, non-vertebral fractures by 16%, and hip fractures by 19%. It is a once-daily dose, taken as a powder mixed with water.

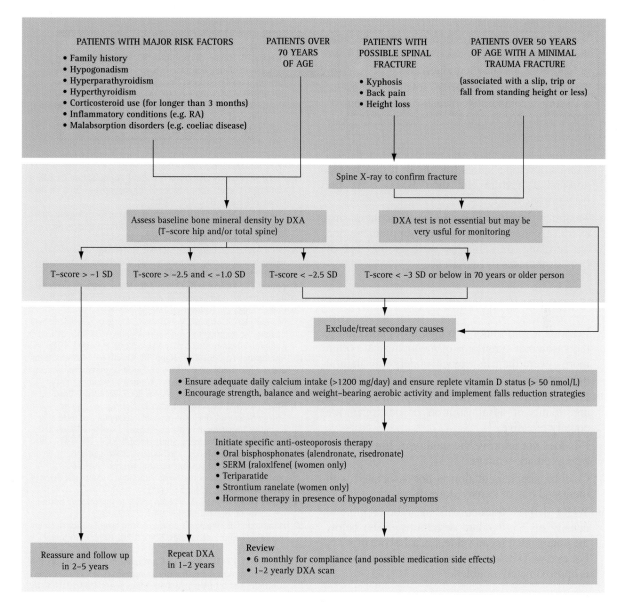

PATIENTS WITH MAJOR RISK FACTORS
- Family history
- Hypogonadism
- Hyperparathyroidism
- Hyperthyroidism
- Corticosteroid use (for longer than 3 months)
- Inflammatory conditions (e.g. RA)
- Malabsorption disorders (e.g. coeliac disease)

PATIENTS OVER 70 YEARS OF AGE

PATIENTS WITH POSSIBLE SPINAL FRACTURE
- Kyphosis
- Back pain
- Height loss

PATIENTS OVER 50 YEARS OF AGE WITH A MINIMAL TRAUMA FRACTURE
(associated with a slip, trip or fall from standing height or less)

Spine X-ray to confirm fracture

Assess baseline bone mineral density by DXA (T-score hip and/or total spine)

DXA test is not essential but may be very usful for monitoring

T-score > -1 SD

T-score > -2.5 and < -1.0 SD

T-score < -2.5 SD

T-score < -3 SD or below in 70 years or older person

Exclude/treat secondary causes

- Ensure adequate daily calcium intake (>1200 mg/day) and ensure replete vitamin D status (> 50 nmol/L)
- Encourage strength, balance and weight-bearing aerobic activity and implement falls reduction strategies

Initiate specific anti-osteoporosis therapy
- Oral bisphosphonates (alendronate, risedronate)
- SERM (raloxlfene((women only)
- Teriparatide
- Strontium ranelate (women only)
- Hormone therapy in presence of hypogonadal symptoms

Reassure and follow up in 2-5 years

Repeat DXA in 1-2 years

Review
- 6 monthly for compliance (and possible medication side effects)
- 1-2 yearly DXA scan

FIGURE 14.8 Algorithm for the management of osteoporosis (From Osteoporosis Australia[71]; developed by Dr Natalie Towers)

It is best taken at bedtime, at least 2 hours after food, calcium-containing products or antacids.[71]

The anabolic agent parathyroid hormone teriparatide (Forteo), which stimulates bone formation and hence bone density and strength, has been shown to reduce the incidence of spinal (65%) and non-spinal (55%) fractures in studies of postmenopausal women with prior spinal fractures. It is recommended for those with established osteoporosis who have had fractures, for whom other agents are considered unsuitable. It is given by daily subcutaneous injection, and maximum treatment duration is 2 years.[71]

In conclusion, where women have proven osteoporosis, either with a spinal fracture or T score in the osteoporotic range, treatment should commence to prevent further fractures. This treatment should include either alendronate, risedronate, raloxifene or strontium ranelate plus calcium and vitamin D. Patients should also begin exercising and fall prevention strategies should be implemented. In women who are in the osteopenic range, preventive therapy should be considered and can consist of either HT, or alendronate, risedronate or strontium ranelate in women > 0 years.

Summary of key points

- Women have higher rates of osteoporosis because they achieve a lower peak bone mass and have greater bone loss due to menopause.
- The definition of osteoporosis involves the use of a T score, a comparative measure of bone density.
- DXA scanning is the gold standard in bone density imaging.
- Treatment for osteoporosis should be initiated when women develop a spinal fracture or if they have a non-spinal fracture and their BMD is in the osteoporotic range.
- Treatment involves measures such as increasing exercise, calcium and vitamin D supplementation and ceasing smoking, as well as the use of bisphosphonates or raloxifene.

TIPS FOR PRACTITIONERS

- In women who undergo bilateral oophorectomy, the vasomotor symptoms of menopause are often more severe than in women undergoing natural menopause.[74]
- For treatment of menopausal symptoms, all types and routes of administration of oestrogen are equally effective.[75]
- HT does not improve the quality of life in older, asymptomatic women.[76]
- Calcium supplementation is not associated with increased risk of kidney stone disease.[77]
- WHO defines osteoporosis as a bone mineral density of 2.5 standard deviations (SDs) below the young adult mean value, i.e. a T score of <2.5. For every SD below the mean, the risk of fracture is approximately doubled.

REFERENCES

1. Gold EB, Bromberger J, Crawford S, et al. Factors associated with age at natural menopause in a multiethnic sample of midlife women. Am J Epidemiol 2001; 153:865–874.
2. Harlow BL, Signorello LB. Factors associated with early menopause. Maturitas 2000; 35(1):3–9.
3. Luborsky JL, Meyer P, Sowers MF, et al. Premature menopause in a multi-ethnic population study of the menopause transition. Hum Reprod 2003; 18(1):199–206.
4. Soules MR, Sherman S, Parrott E. Executive summary: Stages of Reproductive Aging Workshop (STRAW). Fertil Steril 2001; 76(5):874–878.
5. Randolph JF Jr, Crawford S, Dennerstein L, et al. The value of follicle-stimulating hormone concentration and clinical findings as markers of the late menopausal transition. J Clin Endocrinol Metab 2006; 91(8):3034–3040 [Epub 23.05.2006].
6. Taffe JR, Dennerstein L. Menstrual patterns leading to the final menstrual period. Menopause 2002; 9:32–40.
7. American Association of Clinical Endocrinologists. AACE medical guidelines for clinical practice for management of menopause. Endocr Pract 1999; 5:355–366.
8. Henrich JB, Hughes JP, Kaufman SC, et al. Limitations of follicle-stimulating hormone in assessing menopause status: findings from the National Health and Nutrition Examination Survey (NHANES 1999–2000)*. Menopause 2006; 13(2):171–177.
9. Hunter M, Battersby R, Whitehead M. Relationships between psychological symptoms, somatic complaints and menopausal status. Maturitas 1986; 8:217–228.
10. Dennerstein L, Dudley EC, Hopper JL, et al. A prospective population-based study of menopausal symptoms. Obstet Gynecol 2000; 96(3):351–358.
11. Porter M, Penney GC, Russell D, et al. A population based survey of women's experience of the menopause. Br J Obstet Gynaecol 1996; 103:1025–1028.
12. Woods NF, Mitchell ES. Symptoms during the perimenopause: prevalence, severity, trajectory, and significance in women's lives. Am J Med 2005; 118(Suppl 12B):14–24.
13. Politi MC, Schleinitz MD, Col NF. Revisiting the duration of vasomotor symptoms of menopause: a meta-analysis. J Gen Intern Med 2008; 23(9):1507–1513.
14. Launer LJ, Andersen K, Dewey ME. Rates and risk factors for dementia and Alzheimer's disease: results from EURODEM pooled analyses. Neurology 1999; 52:78–84.
15. Mulnard RA, Cotman CW, Kawas C. Oestrogen replacement therapy for treatment of mild to moderate Alzheimer disease: a randomized controlled trial. JAMA 2000; 283:1007–1015.
16. Shumaker SA, Legault C, Rapp SR. Oestrogen plus progestin and the incidence of dementia and mild cognitive impairment in postmenopausal women: the Women's Health Initiative Memory Study (WHIMS). JAMA 2003; 289:2651–2662.
17. Shumaker SA, Legault C, Kuller L. Conjugated equine estrogens and incidence of probable dementia and mild cognitive impairment in postmenopausal women: Women's Health Initiative Memory Study. JAMA 2004; 291:2947–2958.
18. North American Menopause Society. Oestrogen and progestogen use in postmenopausal women: July 2008 position statement of the North American Menopause Society. Menopause 2008; 15(4):584–602.
19. Grady D. A 60-year-old woman trying to discontinue hormone replacement therapy. JAMA 2002; 287:2130–2137.
20. Hammond CB. Women's concerns with hormone replacement therapy—compliance issues. Fertil Steril 1994; 62(6 Suppl 2): 157S–160S.
21. Ettinger B, Li DK, Klein R. Continuation of postmenopausal hormone replacement therapy; comparison of cyclic versus continuous combined schedule. Menopause 1996; 3:185–189.
22. WHI (Writing Group for the Women's Health Initiative Investigators). Risks and benefits of oestrogen plus progestin in healthy postmenopausal women. Principle results from the women's health initiative randomized controlled trial. JAMA 2002; 288:321–333.
23. Buick EL, Crook D, Horne R. Women's perceptions of hormone replacement therapy: risks and benefit (1980–2002): a literature review. Climactic 2005; 8:24–35.
24. Main P, Robinson M. Changes in utilisation of hormone replacement therapy in Australia following publication of the findings of the Women's Health Initiative. Pharmacoepidemiol Drug Saf 2008; 17(9):861–868.
25. Utian WH. NIH and WHI: time for a mea culpa and steps beyond. Menopause 2007; 14(6):1056–1059.
26. Stefanick ML, Anderson GL, Margolis KL, et al. Effects of conjugated equine estrogens on breast cancer and mammography screening in postmenopausal women with hysterectomy. JAMA 2006; 295(14):1647–1657.
27. Beral V, Bull D, Green J, et al. Ovarian cancer and hormone replacement therapy in the Million Women Study. Lancet 2007; 369(9574):1703–1710.

28. NBOCC (National Breast and Ovarian Cancer Centre). Hormone replacement therapy (HRT) and risk of breast cancer—NBOCC Position statement. 2009. Online. Available: http://www.nbocc.org.au/our-organisation/position-statements/hormone-replacement-therapy-hrt-and-risk-of-breast-cancer#rec [accessed 28.10.09].

29. Henderson VW. Alzheimer's disease and other neurological disorders. Climacteric 2007; 10(Suppl 2):92–96.

30. Royal College of Obstetricians and Gynaecologists. Guidelines 19: hormone replacement therapy and venous thromboembolism. 1999. Online. Available: http://www.rcog.org.uk/guidelines.asp?PageID 5 106&GuidelineID 5 11 [accessed 25.01.03].

31. Hulley S, Grady D, Bush T, et al. Randomized trial of estrogen plus progestin for secondary prevention of coronary heart disease in postmenopausal women. Heart and Estrogen/Progestin Replacement Study (HERS) Research Group. JAMA 1998; 280(7):605–613.

32. Birkhäuser MH, Panay N, Archer DF, et al. Updated practical recommendations for hormone replacement therapy in the peri- and postmenopause. Climacteric 2008; 11(2):108–123.

33. Garnett T, Studd JW, Henderson A, et al. Hormone implants and tachyphylaxis. Br J Obstet Gynaecol 1990; 97:917–921.

34. NHS Clinical Knowledge Summaries. Menopause (Sowerby Centre for Health Informatics at Newcastle). 2008. Online. Available: http://cks.library.nhs.uk/menopause/ [accessed 19.08.08].

35. Albertazzi P, Di Micco R, Zanardi E. Tibolone: a review. Maturitas 1998; 30:295–305.

36. Davis SR. The effects of tibolone on mood and libido. Menopause 2002; 9:162–170.

37. Kenemans P, Bundred NJ, Foidart JM, et al. Safety and efficacy of tibolone in breast-cancer patients with vasomotor symptoms: a double-blind, randomised, non-inferiority trial. Lancet Oncol 2009; 10(2):135–146.

38. Pitkin J. Contraception and the menopause. Maturitas 2000; 1:S29–S36.

39. FFPRHC (Faculty of Family Planning and Reproductive Health Care Clinical Effectiveness Unit). FFPRHC Guidance (January 2005) contraception for women aged over 40 years. J Fam Plann Reprod Health Care 2005; 31(1):51–63; quiz 63–4.

40. DeCherney A. Bone-sparing properties of oral contraceptives. Am J Obstet Gynecol 1996; 174(1 Pt 1):15–20.

41. Centers for Disease Control and the National Institute of Child Health and Human Development. The Cancer and Steroid Hormone Study. The reduction in risk of ovarian cancer associated with oral-contraceptive use. N Engl J Med 1987a; 316:650–655.

42. Centers for Disease Control and the National Institute of Child Health and Human Development. The Cancer and Steroid Hormone Study. Combination oral contraceptive use and the risk of endometrial cancer. JAMA 1987; 257:796–800.

43. IMAP statement on hormonal contraception. IPPF Medical Bulletin 2002; 36(5). Online. Available: http: //www.ippf.org/medical/ bulletin/pdf/oct_02_en.pdf [accessed 26.01.2003].

44. Beksinska ME, Smit JA, Kleinschmidt I, et al. Detection of raised FSH levels among older women using depot medroxyprogesterone acetate and norethisterone enanthate. Contraception 2003; 68:339–343.

45. Kaufert PA, Gilbert P, Tate R. Defining menopausal status: the impact of longitudinal data. Maturitas 1987; 9:217–226.

46. Egarter C, Topcuoglu A, Vogl S, et al. Hormone replacement therapy with tibolone: effects on sexual functioning in postmenopausal women. Acta Obstet Gynecol Scand 2002; 81:649–653.

47. North American Menopause Society. The role of testosterone therapy in postmenopausal women: position statement of the North American Menopause Society. Menopause 2005; 12(5):496–511.

48. Knight DC, Eden JA. A review of the clinical effects of phytoestrogens. Obstet Gynecol 1996; 87:897–904.

49. Davis SR, Murkies AL, Wilcox G. Phytoestrogens in clinical practice. Integr Med 1998; 1:27–34.

50. Boulet MJ, Oddens BJ, Lehert P, et al. Climacteric and menopause in seven South East Asian countries. Mauritas 1994; 19:157–176.

51. Hunter M. Psychological and somatic experiences of the menopause: a prospective study. Psychosom Med 1990; 52:357–367.

52. Messina MJ, Persky V, Setchell KD, et al. Soy intake and cancer risk: a review of in vivo and in vivo data. Nutr Cancer 1994; 21:113–131.

53. Lethaby AE, Brown J, Marjoribanks J, et al. Phytoestrogens for vasomotor menopausal symptoms. Cochrane Database Syst Rev 2007; (4):CD001395.

54. Tempfer CB, Bentz EK, Leodolter S, et al. Phytoestrogens in clinical practice: a review of the literature. Fertil Steril 2007; 87(6):1243–1249. [Epub 09.05.2007.]

55. Adams J, Sibbritt DW, Easthope G, et al. The profile of women who consult alternative health practitioners in Australia. Med J Aust 2003; 179(6):297–300.

56. Therapeutic Goods Administration. Department of Health and Ageing. Black cohosh (Cimicifuga racemosa): new labelling requirements and consumer information for medicines containing black cohosh. Online. Available: http://www.tga.gov.au/cm/0705blkcohosh.htm [accessed 20.08.08].

57. Nelson HD, Vesco KK, Haney E, et al. Nonhormonal therapies for menopausal hot flashes: systematic review and meta-analysis. JAMA 2006; 295(17):2057–2071.

58. American College of Obstetricians and Gynaecologists. Selective oestrogen receptor modulators. ACOG practice bulletin no. 39. Obstet Gynaecol 2002; 100:835–844.

59. Jean Hailes Foundation Fact Sheet. Bioidentical hormones. Online. Available. http://www.managingmenopause.org.au/content/view/103/130/ [accessed 21.08.08].

60. US Food and Drug Administration. Compounded menopausal hormone therapy questions and answers. 2008. Online. Available: http://www.fda.gov/Drugs/GuidanceComplianceRegulatoryInformation/PharmacyCompounding/ucm183088.htm#MenopausalHormoneTherapy [accessed 21.06.09].

61. Cirigliano M. Bioidentical hormone therapy: a review of the evidence. J Women's Health (Larchmt) 2007; 16(5):600–631.

62. Cummings SR, Black DM, Rubin SM. Lifetime risks of hip, Colles', or vertebral fracture and coronary heart disease among white postmenopausal women. Arch Intern Med 1989; 149:2445–2448.

63. Kanis JA. Assessment of fracture risk and its application to screening for postmenopausal osteoporosis: synopsis of a WHO report. WHO Study Group. Osteoporos Int 1994; 4:368–381.

64. Kanis JA, Gluer CC. An update on the diagnosis and assessment of osteoporosis with densitometry. Committee of Scientific Advisors, International Osteoporosis Foundation. Osteoporos Int 2000; 11:192–202.

65. Miller PD, Zapalowski C, Kulak CA, et al. Bone densitometry: the best way to detect osteoporosis and to monitor therapy. J Clin Endocrinol Metab 1999; 84:1867–1871.

66. Sambrook PN, Seeman E, Phillips SR, et al. Preventing osteoporosis: outcomes of the Australian Fracture Prevention Summit. Med J Aust 2002; 176:S11–S16.

67. Brunader R, Shelton DK. Radiologic bone assessment in the evaluation of osteoporosis. Am Fam Physician 2002; 65:1357–1364.

68. Cadarette SM, Jaglal SB, Kreiger N, et al. Development and validation of the Osteoporosis Risk Assessment Instrument to facilitate selection of women for bone densitometry. CMAJ 2000; 162:1289–1294.

69. Black DM, Cummings SR, Karpf DB, et al. Randomised trial of effect of alendronate on risk of fracture in women with existing vertebral fractures. Fracture Intervention Trial Research Group. Lancet 1996; 348:1535–1541.
70. Harris ST, Watts NB, Genant HK, et al. Effects of risedronate treatment on vertebral and nonvertebral fractures in women with postmenopausal osteoporosis: a randomized controlled trial. Vertebral Efficacy with Risedronate Therapy (VERT) Study Group. JAMA 1999; 282:1344–1352.
71. Osteoporosis Australia. Prevent the next fracture—a guide for GPs. 2008. Online. Available. http://www.osteoporosis.org.au/files/internal/oa_fracture_gp.pdf [accessed 21.08.08].
72. Ettinger B, Black DM, Mitlak BH, et al. Reduction of vertebral fracture risk in postmenopausal women with osteoporosis treated with raloxifene: results from a 3-year randomized clinical trial. Multiple Outcomes of Raloxifene Evaluation (MORE) Investigators. JAMA 1999; 282:637–645.
73. Cummings SR, Eckert S, Krueger KA, et al. The effect of raloxifene on risk of breast cancer in postmenopausal women: results from the MORE randomized trial. Multiple Outcomes of Raloxifene Evaluation. JAMA 1999; 281:2189–2197.
74. Berg G, Gottwall T, Hammar M, et al. Climacteric symptoms among women aged 60–62 in Linkoping, Sweden, in 1986. Maturitas 1988; 10:193–199.
75. MacLennan A, Lester S, Moore V. Oral oestrogen replacement therapy versus placebo for hot flushes. Cochrane Database Syst Rev 2001; (1):CD002978.
76. Hlatky MA, Boothroyd D, Vittinghoff E, et al. Quality-of-life and depressive symptoms in postmenopausal women after receiving hormone therapy: results from the Heart and Oestrogen/Progestin Replacement Study (HERS) trial. JAMA 2002; 287:591–597.
77. Delmas PD. Treatment of postmenopausal osteoporosis. Lancet 2002; 359:2018–2026.
78. BNF 60. British National Formulary. 66th edn. London: British Medical Association and Royal Pharmaceutical Society of Great Britain; 2010.
79. Australian Menopause Society. Equivalent doses of HRT. 2009. Online. Available: http://www.menopause.org.au/content/view/426/804/ [accessed 28.10.09].
80. James D, Pilai M, Rymer J, et al. Obstetrics, gynaecology, neonatology interactive colour guides CD-ROM. Edinburgh: Churchill Livingstone; 2002.
81. Murkies A. Phytoestrogens—what is the current knowledge? Aust Fam Physician 1998; 27(Suppl 1):S47–S51.
82. Nelson HD, Humphrey LL, Nygren P, et al. Postmenopausal hormone replacement therapy: scientific review. JAMA 2002; 288:872–881.
83. WHO. Assessment of fracture risk and its application to screening for postmenopausal osteoporosis. Report of a WHO Study Group. WHO Technical Report Series, no. 843. Geneva: World Health Organization; 1994.

15

Urinary problems

OBJECTIVES

- To be aware of the different causes of frequency and dysuria in women
- To be able to explain to women the factors that can predispose them to urinary tract infections (UTIs)
- To be able to diagnose, manage and prevent uncomplicated UTIs in women
- To understand the aetiology of urinary incontinence
- To be able to determine what form of incontinence a woman has
- To be able to implement pelvic floor muscle training
- To know when to refer women with incontinence for further management
- To explore the nature of painful bladder syndrome/interstitial cystitis

URINARY TRACT INFECTION (UTI)

How common are UTIs?

A total of 10–15% of healthy non-pregnant women will suffer from acute uncomplicated cystitis each year[1] with the highest incidence (17.5%) reported by women aged 18 to 24 years. By age 24, one-third of women will have at least one physician-diagnosed UTI that was treated with prescription medication.[1] Some 12% of women with an initial infection and 48% of those with recurrent infections will have a further episode in the same year.[2]

What are the classic symptoms and signs?

Classically, women present with urinary frequency, urgency and dysuria. Dysuria without vaginal discharge or irritation has a positive predictive value of 77% for a positive urine culture.[3] Affected patients may complain of pelvic discomfort pre- and post-voiding, passing small quantities of urine and sometimes of haematuria. Some may have suprapubic tenderness or pain.

In the majority of cases, infection is limited to the lower urinary tract (i.e. the bladder and urethra: cystitis) but infection can also affect the upper urinary tract causing pyelonephritis. In uncomplicated cystitis, it is rare for women to present with fever or constitutional symptoms. Pyelonephritis is more likely to be associated with back pain, fever, nausea and vomiting.

In uncomplicated cystitis, it is rare for women to present with fever or constitutional symptoms.

Is there anything else that it could be?

In about 50% of women who present with urinary symptoms, there is no bacteriuria. These women nevertheless present with dysuria, frequency and urgency.[4] Pyuria may be present or absent. They are said to have acute urethral syndrome, or interstitial cystitis or irritable bladder.

The aetiology of urethral syndrome is unclear, but it may be due to bacteria found in low concentrations or bacteria that are difficult to culture, or to nonspecific inflammation or muscular dysfunction. Other causes of dysuria and frequency include:

- the presence of fastidious organisms such as *Ureaplasma urealyticum*
- genital pathogens (such as *Chlamydia trachomatis*, *Neisseria gonorrhoeae*, herpes simplex virus)

- vaginal infections with *Trichomonas vaginalis* and *Candida albicans*
- infestation with pinworm/threadworm
- irritants (such as deodorants, bubble baths and detergents)
- atrophic urethritis (in postmenopausal women).

How can I explain in simple terms to women how UTIs come about?

Most UTIs occur via an ascending route. This means that bacteria that live around the urethral opening can enter the urethra and climb up, reaching the bladder and establishing an infection.

Are there any factors that predispose to UTIs?

When providing patient education about UTIs, there are a number of predisposing factors[1,5,6,7–9] that should be highlighted, the strongest of which, in young women, is recent sexual activity (the relative odds of acute cystitis increase by a factor of 60 during the 48 hours after sexual intercourse).[10] It is important to inform women of the risk factors, so that they can understand how their own behaviour is related to the onset of UTIs. These factors are listed in Box 15.1. GPs should also be aware of factors that may lead to a more complicated situation, such as abnormalities of urinary tract function (for example, indwelling catheter, neuropathic bladder, vesicoureteric reflux, outflow obstruction, other anatomical abnormalities), previous urinary tract surgery and states of immunocompromise,

- Previous UTIs
- Sexual intercourse
- The use of diaphragms and spermicides
- Young age at first UTI (below 15 years)
- Maternal history of UTI
- Use of condoms by male partner/s
- Intake of antibiotics within the last 2–4 weeks
- Genetic factors

BOX 15.2 Organisms responsible for urinary tract infections

- Common organisms causing UTI:
  - *Escherichia coli*
  - *Staphylococcus saprophyticus*
  - *Proteus mirabilis*
- Less common organisms causing UTI:
  - *Proteus vulgaris*, *Klebsiella* species, *Enterobacter* species, *Citrobacter* species, *Serratia marcescens*, *Acinetobacter* and *Pseudomonas* species and *Staphylococcus aureus*
  - *Candida albicans* infection is rarely found in the community but is common in hospital patients, with risk factors such as indwelling catheters, immunosuppression, diabetes mellitus and antimicrobial treatment

and neurological disorders. Pregnant women are also at increased risk of pyelonephritis associated with the relative ureteral obstruction during gestation. Risk factors for UTI in postmenopausal women include recurrent UTI, bladder prolapse or cystocele, and increased post-void residual urine.[11]

The relative odds of acute cystitis increase by a factor of 60 during the 48 hours after sexual intercourse.

In a general practice population, what are the common organisms responsible for UTIs?

Box 15.2 lists the common organisms responsible for UTIs in a general practice population. Approximately 80% are caused by *E. coli* and 13% by *Staphyococcus saprophyticus*.[12]

What should a GP do when a woman presents with symptoms of a UTI?

Besides taking a history and checking for fever and the possibility of upper urinary tract infection, GPs need to decide whether to investigate the urine or treat empirically.

A mid-stream specimen of urine can be tested either by a urine dipstick or by sending the sample to a laboratory for microscopy and culture. Urine microscopy and culture has long been the 'gold standard' for diagnosis of UTIs but it is expensive and slow to produce a result. Dipstick testing, on the other hand, can be performed on the spot by a GP or nurse. When it shows the presence of either leucocyte esterase or nitrites, it is highly predictive of a positive urine culture (whereas absence of either finding markedly reduces the likelihood of infection),[13] and it has been found to be a fairly reliable way to diagnose UTIs. It is important, however, to undertake urine culture if an accurate diagnosis is needed or in order to select

an effective antimicrobial (as in pregnancy, treatment failure or immunocompromise). Box 15.3 (p 286) outlines the tests commonly carried out by dipstick testing and Table 15.1 (p 286) advises how to use nitrite and leucocyte testing to guide management in symptomatic female general practice patients.

Management based on dipstick testing and empirical use of first-line antibiotics is still appropriate for GP patients with uncomplicated UTI.

Imaging of women with an uncomplicated UTI is not warranted, as there is a low yield of positive results.[14] Neither is a single episode of pyelonephritis associated with a clinically significant risk of anatomic abnormality.[15] However, in cases of recurrent pyelonephritis imaging with renal ultrasound, intravenous pyelogram or voiding cystourethrogram is indicated.

Imaging of women with uncomplicated urinary tract infection is not warranted.

Should all women presenting with a UTI have urine M&C carried out?

Uncomplicated UTI in non-pregnant women rarely causes severe illness or has significant long-term consequences, and in 50% of patients the condition

BOX 15.3 Pertinent findings on urine dipstick analysis in cases of UTI (From Fitzgerald[54])

- Leucocyte esterase (LE)
  - If positive, indicates presence of neutrophils >white blood cells/high power field.
  - As an indicator of UTI, this has a sensitivity of 75–90%.
- Nitrites
  - Are a surrogate marker for bacteriuria.
  - Presence indicates bacterial reduction of dietary nitrates to nitrites by selected Gram-negative uropathogens, including *E. coli* and *Proteus*.
  - A negative test does not therefore rule out UTI, because some pathogens do not produce nitrate reductase, and frequent urination (common in cystitis) reduces the time available for the enzyme to act.
  - Best done on well-concentrated urine (e.g. first morning void). For nitrites to be present, urine should be held in the bladder for >1 hour in order for nitrate-to-nitrite conversion to take place.
- Protein
  - Dipsticks are most sensitive for albumin, commonly present in febrile response or in presence of protein-containing substances such as blood cells, bacteria and mucus.
- pH
  - Normally urine is acidic. However, if the pH is found to be alkaline in the presence of UTI symptoms and positive LE, *Proteus* may be present, splitting urea into CO_2 and ammonia, causing a rise in pH.

TABLE 15.1 How to use dipstick testing in the management of women with symptoms of an uncomplicated UTI

Nitrites	Leucocytes	Likelihood of UTI	Use of antibiotic
Positive	Positive or negative	High	Justified
Negative	Negative	1 in 5	Not justified
Negative	Positive	Half will have a UTI, and half will not	Perform culture and await results

In 50% of non-pregnant women with an uncomplicated UTI, the condition improves without antimicrobials within 3 days.

What antibiotic choices are there?

Whether treatment is empiric or not, as with all antibiotic prescribing there are a few general rules to follow[19]:

- Because uncomplicated cystitis is so common, antibiotics that are seldom prescribed for other infections should be preferred.
- Individual doctors should vary their choice of antibiotic from time to time, because increased prescription of one antibiotic may result in higher levels of local resistance.
- Local antibiotic resistance levels should also be considered.

Box 15.4 outlines the preferred antibiotics for the management of uncomplicated cystitis in non-pregnant women.

What is the optimum duration of antibiotic use for women with an uncomplicated UTI?

GPs have a choice of prescribing single-dose, 3- or 5-day, or the more traditional 7- to 14-day therapies for treatment of UTIs. Three-day courses of antibiotics such as trimethoprim are recommended as first-line therapy for lower, uncomplicated UTIs in young women.[20,21] One-day treatments are less effective, and longer treatments are associated with increased risk of adverse effects without clinically meaningful improvement in effectiveness.[22]

In women over 65, short-course treatment (3–6 days) is probably sufficient for treating uncomplicated UTIs.[23]

improves without antimicrobials within 3 days.[16] Despite this, empiric treatment of uncomplicated UTIs has been advocated by some as the most cost-effective way to manage UTIs.[17,18] Those against empiric management argue on two grounds. First, they say that the urine should be examined to ascertain the diagnosis, limit unnecessary use of antibiotics and identify those patients who may require further investigation. Second, they argue that since uncomplicated UTIs account for a substantial proportion of all prescribed antibiotics, empiric management may lead to rising levels of antibiotic resistance in the community. With regard to this latter argument, however, levels of resistance found in the laboratory may overestimate levels of resistance in general practice.[19]

BOX 15.4 Antibiotic choices for the management of uncomplicated cystitis

Trimethoprim 300 mg orally daily (3 days for women, 14 days for men)

OR

Cephalexin 500 mg orally 12 hourly (5 days for women, 14 days for men)

OR

Amoxycillin/clavulanate 500 mg/125 mg orally 12 hourly (5 days for women, 14 days for men)

OR

Nitrofurantoin 50 mg orally, 6-hourly (5 days for women, 14 days for men)

If there is proven microbial resistance to other medications use:
Norfloxacin 400 mg orally 12-hourly (3 days for women, 14 days for men)

Is any follow-up required?

If therapy is clinically successful, the only patients requiring a follow-up examination of the urine for bacteria are pregnant women. The reason for this is that it is only in this group of women that treatment of asymptomatic bacteriuria is justified, because of the increased risk of pyelonephritis and preterm delivery.[24] Asymptomatic bacteriuria is not related to any increase in morbidity or mortality in other patient groups.

After antibiotic therapy, the only patients requiring a follow-up examination of the urine for bacteria are pregnant women.

What is the risk of recurrence?

Recurrence of dysuria and frequency can either mean failure to eradicate the initial infection or reinfection. Interestingly between 12% and 16% of women receiving empiric therapy for UTI required another course of antibiotics within 4 weeks of their initial symptoms, irrespective of the type or duration of initial antibiotic therapy.[25] In these women a longer course of antibiotic should be given rather than using a more sophisticated antibiotic.

What preventive measures or general advice can GPs give to women regarding UTIs?

Adjuvant treatment and preventive measures are frequently recommended in cases of UTI, but few have been rigorously evaluated.

While popular for treating urinary symptoms such as dysuria and frequency, urine-alkalinising agents such as potassium citrate, sodium citrate and sodium bicarbonate have yet to be proved in terms of their efficacy, over which there is some doubt.[26]

It is not helpful to pursue further diagnostic procedures in women complaining of recurrent uncomplicated cystitis.

What measures can be taken in women suffering from recurrent urinary tract infections?

Case control studies[6,10] have found no evidence that poor urinary hygiene predisposes women to recurrent infections, and there is no evidence to support giving women specific instructions regarding the frequency of urination, the timing of voiding (postcoital voiding), wiping patterns, douching, the use of hot tubs or the wearing of pantyhose in order to prevent the occurrence of UTIs.

In postmenopausal women with recurrent UTIs, topical vaginal oestrogen can be effective in reducing recurrence.[11]

In women who have three or more urinary tract infections a year, a GP has several options for management[27]:

1. The woman can self-initiate a short course of antibiotic therapy at the onset of symptoms suggesting cystitis.[28]
2. If the woman describes a relationship between sexual activity and the onset of symptoms, GPs can recommend that she take 100 mg of trimethoprim after sexual intercourse.[29]
3. Another option is for the woman to use either 50 mg of trimethoprim or 50 mg of nitrofurantoin daily for 6 months or more if necessary.[30]

If either of the last two options are put in place, prophylaxis should be started after active infection has been eradicated (confirmed by a negative urine culture at least one to two weeks after treatment is

If women have recurrent UTIs related to sexual activity, GPs can recommend 100 mg of trimethoprim to be taken after sexual intercourse, or the woman can take either 50 mg of trimethoprim or 50 mg of nitrofurantoin daily for 6 months or more.

stopped).[31] It is important to inform women starting prophylaxis that it works while it is taken but that upon discontinuation UTIs may recur.[31]

How effective is cranberry juice in the prevention and/or treatment of UTI?

A recent Cochrane review has found that cranberry products significantly reduced the incidence of UTIs at 12 months (RR 0.65, 95% CI 0.46 to 0.90) compared with a placebo/control. While they are more effective at reducing the incidence of UTIs in women with recurrent UTIs than in other groups, the optimum dosage or method of administration (e.g. juice, tablets or capsules) has yet to be established.[32]

Summary of key points
- 10–15% of non-pregnant women suffer from a UTI each year.
- 50% of women with urinary symptoms do not have bacteriuria and are said to have urethral syndrome.
- 80% of UTIs in women are caused by *E. coli*.
- Nitrite and leucocyte testing can guide management of women with suspected UTIs.
- The optimum duration of antibiotic therapy for an uncomplicated UTI in a young woman is 3 days.
- Postcoital or daily low-dose antibiotics can be used to treat women who suffer from recurrent UTIs.
- Cranberry products can prevent UTIs in women with recurrent UTIs, but dosage and method of administration is unclear.

URINARY INCONTINENCE

How common is urinary incontinence?

Urinary incontinence is a hidden condition, rarely brought up by women as a presenting complaint to their GP. It is surprisingly common, however. A community-based study in Norway[33] found that 25% of women over 20 years of age had some degree of urinary incontinence. Nearly 7% had significant incontinence, defined as moderate or severe incontinence that was experienced as bothersome. The prevalence of incontinence increased with increasing age. Half of the incontinence was of stress type, 11% had urge and 36% mixed incontinence.

What percentage of women discuss it with their GP?

Few women suffering from urinary incontinence discuss their problem openly, three-quarters are too embarrassed to discuss it with their spouse and one in three too embarrassed to talk about it with their GP.[34]

> **CASE STUDY: 'Having to wear a pad most days'**
>
> A GP received some new posters on urinary incontinence as a result of a government campaign. One was prominently placed behind the toilet door in the female toilet at the surgery. As a result of this simple move, the inquiries from women patients started to come in. One of these was from Ann, a 42-year-old woman who had had two children, the youngest some 15 years previously. Over the last few years she said that her incontinence had been increasing in severity. After her second child, the main problem had been a slight amount of leakage when she sneezed suddenly, but recently she had found herself having to wear a pad most days. She wondered if anything could be done to improve her symptoms.

While not a life-threatening condition, urinary incontinence interferes with many aspects of a woman's life. She may not be able to engage in exercise or sexual activity, and the constant wetness and odour may interfere with her occupation and other activities of daily living. Despite this degree of disturbance in day-to-day life sufferers of incontinence are reluctant to come forth, often because they believe that urinary incontinence is normal after childbirth or as one ages or that there is nothing that can be done to help.

> Women rarely present to GPs complaining of urinary incontinence; hence, it is a hidden condition despite its being very common.

How is urinary incontinence classified?

There are several major types of incontinence:
- stress
- urge (overactive bladder)
- functional
- overflow
- mixed
- true incontinence.

Stress incontinence is responsible for approximately 50% of the incontinence detected in general practice.[35] In stress incontinence, leakage of urine occurs when there is a rise in intra-abdominal pressure, such as with coughing, sneezing, laughing, bending or during exercise. It usually develops after childbirth, especially in multiparous women, but can

BOX 15.5 Risk factors for stress incontinence (From Weiss & Newman[52])

- **Age:** pelvic muscle relaxation accelerates after menopause.
- **Race:** incidence of stress incontinence is less in black women than in white, Hispanic and Asian women[46]
- **Childbirth and pregnancy:**
  - Incidence of incontinence 9 weeks postpartum is 21% following spontaneous birth and 36% following forceps.[47]
  - Prevalence of stress incontinence 5 years after first delivery is 30%. [48]
  - Episiotomy and instrumental delivery increase the risk of pelvic floor dysfunction.
- **Menopause:** oestrogen depletion leads to atrophy of urethral and vaginal mucosa.
- **Pelvic muscle weakness:** prolapse of the pelvic organs results in bladder, uterus and urethra lying below their normal positions, often below the pelvic floor.
- **Pelvic surgery:** among women 60 years or older who have had a hysterectomy, 60% will develop urinary incontinence.[49]
- **Smoking:** increases the risk of all forms of incontinence, but stress incontinence in particular, secondary to smoker's cough.
- **Obesity:** places increased pressure on the bladder.
- **Physical activities:** activities that cause increased pressure on the abdomen increase downward pressure on the bladder. It is estimated that 50% of women who exercise regularly have or will have some degree of stress incontinence[50]

also be a result of obesity, pelvic surgery or other trauma. A comprehensive list of risk factors for stress incontinence is given in Box 15.5.

Overactive bladder is characterised by involuntary bladder contractions, resulting in a sudden urge to urinate. This 'urge' incontinence is characterised by frequency, abdominal distension and suprapubic discomfort. It can seem psychological as women with this form of incontinence often describe leaking as a result of turning the key in the door when they return home. Urge incontinence makes up approximately 8% of incontinence suffered by women attending general practice.[35] Some cases of overactive bladder can be attributed to specific conditions, such as acute or chronic urinary tract infection, bladder cancer and bladder stones, but most cases result from an idiopathic inability to

suppress detrusor contractions. Conditions that increase this likelihood are stroke, dementia, diabetes mellitus and neurological conditions such as multiple sclerosis or Parkinson's disease.

The four major types of incontinence are stress incontinence, urge incontinence, mixed incontinence and overflow incontinence.

Functional incontinence occurs as a result of impaired cognitive function or mobility. In overflow incontinence the bladder continues to fill until it exceeds functional capacity and leakage or constant dribbling occurs. Overdistension is typically caused by an underactive bladder (detrusor) muscle and/ or outlet obstruction. The detrusor muscle may be underactive secondary to drug therapy (especially with psychotropic medications) or conditions such as diabetic neuropathy, low spinal cord injury, radical pelvic surgery and multiple sclerosis. Outlet obstruction in women is almost always a result of urethral occlusion from pelvic organ prolapse or previous anti-incontinence surgery.

Mixed incontinence or a combination of stress and urge incontinence characterises 40% of those suffering from incontinence.[35]

True incontinence is a continous loss of urine through the vagina: it is commonly associated with fistula formation, usually following surgery or radiotherapy in the developed world but more commonly associated with obstructed labour in the developing world.

What are the steps in the diagnostic evaluation of a woman with incontinence?

Diagnostic evaluation of women with urinary incontinence involves four steps:

1. seeking reversible causes for the incontinence
2. identification of problems that require special evaluation and that make it unlikely that the woman can be managed in the primary-care setting
3. determining what type of incontinence the woman has.

Box 15.6 (p 290) highlights the potentially reversible causes of urinary incontinence that should be identified through the history and examination.

Several conditions suggest the need for specialist referral for further investigation or management. These are listed in Box 15.7 (p 290).

BOX 15.6 Potentially reversible causes of urinary incontinence

- Delirium
- Urinary tract infection
- Atrophic vaginitis
- Drugs (see Table 15.3)
- Endocrine problems such as diabetes and hypercalcaemia
- Restricted mobility
- Faecal impaction

BOX 15.7 Conditions requiring specialist referral

- Haematuria without infection
- Gross pelvic prolapse
- Prior incontinence surgery
- Prior radical pelvic surgery
- Prior pelvic radiation
- Recent onset of overactive bladder or urge incontinence

TABLE 15.2 Questions that distinguish between stress and urge incontinence

Question	Type of incontinence
Do you leak urine when you cough, laugh, lift something or sneeze? How often?	Stress
Do you ever leak urine when you have a strong urge to go to the toilet, but don't make it in time?	Urge
How frequently do you empty your bladder during the day? (>8 times in 24 hours)	Urge
How many times do you get up to urinate after going to sleep? Is it the urge to urinate that wakes you?	Urge

Other factors that need to be addressed in the history include:

- the mobility of the patient
- her mental state
- the medical and surgical history, with a particular emphasis on any abdominal or pelvic surgery
- obstetric history
- fluid intake and diet
- drug history.

Table 15.3 lists the classes of drugs that may contribute to urinary incontinence in a particular patient.

The final step in the evaluation of a patient with incontinence is to distinguish what kind of incontinence the woman has. In reality this is usually an attempt to differentiate stress from urge incontinence. In order to do this, the questions listed in Table 15.2 are helpful.

Symptomatic categorisation of UI based on reports from the woman and history taking is sufficiently reliable to inform initial, non-invasive treatment decisions.[53]

What other features of the history are important?

It is important to also assess the severity of the incontinence by asking questions such as the following:

- Do you wear pads that protect you from leaking urine? How often do you have to change them?
- Have you ever found urine on your pads or clothes but were unaware of when the leakage occurred?

Dysuria should be noted, as it may point to an underlying urinary tract infection. The patient should also be asked, 'Do you ever feel that you are unable to completely empty your bladder?', searching for bladder outlet obstruction.

What aspects of the physical examination are important during the assessment?

While carrying out a general examination, GPs should look for factors that may be directly impacting on urinary function, such as abdominal masses and pulmonary or cardiovascular pathology that may be contributing to cough.

The most important part of the examination is probably the pelvic exam. It commences by looking for any signs of inflammation, infection and/or atrophy. The urethra and trigone are oestrogen-dependent tissues and oestrogen deficiency can contribute to urinary incontinence and urinary dysfunction. Signs of oestrogen deficiency include thinning and paleness of the vaginal epithelium, loss of rugae, disappearance of the labia minora and presence of a urethral caruncle.

The GP can test for stress incontinence by asking the patient to cough vigorously while watching for leakage of urine. Any genital prolapse should be noted, as well as how the prolapse is affected by

TABLE 15.3 Drug classes and other substances associated with urinary incontinence

Substance	Effect
Alcohol	Sedation, frequency, overactive bladder
Caffeine/coffee	Frequency, urgency, overactive bladder
Diuretics	Frequency, urgency, overactive bladder
Calcium channel blockers	Retention (overflow)
Narcotics	Retention, constipation, sedation (overactive bladder and overflow)
Beta-adrenergic agonists	Inhibited detrusor function, retention (overflow)
ACE inhibitors	Cough (stress incontinence)
Alpha-adrenergic blockers	Decreased urethral tone (stress incontinence)
Anticholinergics	Retention (overflow)
Antihistamines	Sedation, retention (overflow)
Antidepressants, antipsychotics, benzodiazepines/hypnotics/sedatives	Sedation, retention (overflow)

coughing. GPs should then assess the tone of the pelvic floor by inserting their second and third fingers into the patient's vagina and asking the woman to tighten her 'vaginal muscles' around the GP's fingers with as much force as possible and to hold the contraction for as long as possible. It is normal for a woman to be able to hold such a contraction for 5–10 seconds. Finally, a rectal examination should be undertaken to check for faecal impaction, the presence of occult blood or rectal lesions and anal sphincter tone.

Should any investigations for urinary incontinence be undertaken in the general practice setting?

All women who present with symptoms of UI should have a dipstick test, with a formal midstream specimen sent for culture in the presence of symptoms of UTI or where leucocytes and nitrates are detected.

Bladder diaries are a reliable method for quantifying the degree of urinary frequency and incontinence and should be used in the initial assessment of women with UI or overactive bladder

(OAB).[53] Women should be encouraged to complete a minimum of 3 days of the diary covering variations in their usual activities, such as both working and leisure days.

Bladder diaries are a reliable method for quantifying the degree of urinary frequency and incontinence and should be used in the initial assessment of women with UI or OAB.

The third step involves excluding an overflow bladder. This is done by measuring postvoid residual urine volume (PVR): the amount of urine left in the bladder after the patient urinates. In women this can be done either through urinary catheterisation or by ultrasound. The PVR is normally 50 mL. There is some controversy as to whether it is necessary to measure PVR routinely, particularly in younger women where the symptoms are typical of either stress or urge incontinence. Another approach is therefore to measure PVR when the diagnosis of an overflow bladder is suggested by the history or when the patient fails to respond to treatment for other causes of incontinence.

What treatment can a GP initiate in the management of urinary incontinence?

A wide range of treatments are used and recommended in the management of urinary incontinence. These vary from conservative interventions such as physical therapies, lifestyle interventions and behavioural training to pharmaceutical interventions and surgery.

Despite the paucity of good quality research into the effects of lifestyle interventions for UI,[53] weight loss,[36] smoking cessation and caffeine reduction are helpful in reducing symptoms.

Weight loss, smoking cessation and caffeine reduction are helpful in reducing symptoms.

Pelvic floor muscle training

Pelvic floor muscle training (PFMT) is the most commonly recommended physical therapy treatment for women with stress incontinence. First introduced in 1948 by Arnold Kegel, PFMT can also be used in the treatment of women with mixed incontinence, and less commonly for urge incontinence. Biofeedback (using either a perineometer, a pressure-sensitive device that measures the force of pelvic muscle contractions, or electromyography) or electrical stimulation are commonly used as an adjunct to pelvic floor muscle training.

Pelvic floor muscle training programs involve teaching the patient how to identify and isolate their pelvic floor muscles and then how to undertake a mixture of quick contractions with sustained (endurance) contractions of 5 seconds or longer. The nature of PFMT is highly variable, however, and can include:

- intensive versus standard approaches
- individual or group sessions
- adjunctive use of medication, weighted vaginal cones (Fig 15.1) and/or electrical stimulation.

Just how effective PFMT remains is controversial. A Cochrane review[37] tried to answer that question by trying to analyse research that suffers from small sample sizes, lack of control groups and differing outcome measures. The results of the Cochrane review are given in Box 15.8. In summary the review suggests that pelvic floor exercises appear to be an effective treatment for adult women with stress or mixed incontinence and should be offered as a first line therapy. Recommendations from recent guidelines in relation to PFMT are given in Box 15.9.

Pelvic floor exercises appear to be an effective treatment for adult women with stress or mixed incontinence and should be offered as a first-line therapy.

Most trials to date have studied the effect of treatment in younger, premenopausal women; the effectiveness of these exercises in older, postmenopausal women requires further study. Another question requiring further clarification is whether undertaking prenatal PFMT decreases the risk of postnatal incontinence.

Bladder training

Bladder training is used in the management of urge incontinence, but sometimes also for mixed or stress incontinence. It aims to increase the time interval between voiding, so that the patient gains control over her continence and overcomes the urges to urinate. In order to be successful, patients must be physically and cognitively able and motivated. It usually takes

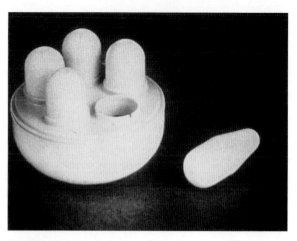

FIGURE 15.1 Vaginal cones (From James et al[51])

BOX 15.8 The effectiveness of pelvic floor muscle training (From NICE[53])

- Pelvic floor muscle training is better than no treatment or placebo treatment.
- There are few side effects of PFMT and these are minimal and reversible.
- PFMT should be offered as first-line conservative management to women with stress and/or mixed incontinence.
- 'Intensive' training where the woman has regular contact with a health professional with special skills in PFMT training is better than 'standard' training.
- Electrical stimulation does not appear to be better than PFMT alone.
- There is insufficient evidence to determine whether PFMT is better or worse than using vaginal cones (weights). Some women do not find cones acceptable or comfortable to use.

---

several months and involves patient education, scheduled voiding and positive reinforcement. Sometimes bladder training is used in conjunction with medication. A Cochrane review[38] suggests that while bladder training leads to some improvement in urge incontinence in the short term, its long-term efficacy has yet to be proven. Even so, the outcome of bladder training is not outstanding, with only 75% of patients using the technique reporting at least a 50% decrease in the number of incontinent episodes and 20% reporting complete dryness.[39] UK guidelines recommend that bladder training lasting for a minimum of 6 weeks should be offered as first-line treatment to women with urge or mixed UI and, if women do not achieve satisfactory benefit, that

- A trial of supervised pelvic floor muscle training of at least 3 months' duration should be offered as first-line treatment to women with stress or mixed UI.
- Pelvic floor muscle training programs should comprise at least eight contractions performed three times per day.
- If pelvic floor muscle training is beneficial, an exercise program should be maintained.
- Perineometry or pelvic floor electromyography as biofeedback should not be used as a routine part of pelvic floor muscle training.
- Electrical stimulation should not be used routinely in the treatment of women with OAB.
- Electrical stimulation should not be used routinely in combination with pelvic floor muscle training.
- Electrical stimulation and/or biofeedback should be considered in women who cannot actively contract pelvic floor muscles, in order to aid motivation and adherence to therapy.

the combination of an antimuscarinic agent with bladder training should be considered if frequency is a troublesome symptom.[53]

While bladder training leads to some improvement in urge incontinence in the short term, its long-term efficacy has yet to be proven.

Medications

Several classes of medications are used in the treatment of urinary incontinence:

1. Antimuscarinic drugs (oxybutynin) reduce the involuntary detrusor contractions that cause urgency. They also bring about an increased bladder capacity.
2. Duloxetine, a serotonin-noradrenaline reuptake inhibitor (SNRI), has been found to improve the quality of life of patients with stress urinary incontinence; however, adverse effects are common (nausea one in three) and about one in eight stop treatment as a consequence.[40] Propantheline and tricyclic antidepressants were used for urge incontinence but they are little used now because of their side effects. The use

of imipramine is limited by its potential to cause cardiac side effects. Alpha-adrenergic drugs such as pseudoephedrine are believed to improve the symptoms of stress incontinence by increasing resting urethral tone.

Until recently, oestrogen administered either intravaginally or systemically has been recommended for the treatment of urinary incontinence in postmenopausal women. While it is helpful in the treatment of vaginal atrophy, the effect of HT on urinary continence is controversial. A number of randomised, placebo-controlled trials have examined the effects of oestrogen, or oestrogen and progestogen together, in postmenopausal continence and concluded that oestrogens should not be used for the treatment of urge or stress incontinence.[41] There is evidence, however, to support the use of intravaginal oestrogens in the treatment of OAB symptoms in postmenopausal women with vaginal atrophy.[53]

Oestrogens should not be used for the treatment of urge or stress incontinence.

What management options are there at a specialist level?

Surgical procedures to remedy stress incontinence generally aim to lift and support the urethrovesical junction and can be undertaken when conservative management has failed. The precise mechanism by which continence is achieved is controversial. Choice of procedures is often influenced by coexistent problems, surgeon's preference and the physical features of the person affected. Numerous surgical methods have been described, but essentially they fall into seven categories:

- open abdominal retropubic suspension (e.g. colposuspension [Burch], Marshall-Marchetti-Krantz [MMK])
- laparoscopic retropubic suspension
- vaginal anterior repair (anterior colporrhaphy, e.g. Kelly, Pacey)
- suburethral slings
- needle suspensions (e.g. Pereyra, Stamey)
- peri-urethral injections
- artificial sphincters.

Retropubic midurethral tape procedures using a 'bottom-up' approach with macroporous polypropylene meshes are now the recommended treatment options for stress UI if conservative management has failed[53] and have a success rate of between 80% and 96%. With surgery, however, there is always the risk of complications and recurrence of the condition.

Summary of key points
- Women rarely present with incontinence so it is incumbent on the GP to ask about it.
- There are four major forms of incontinence: stress, urge, mixed and overflow incontinence.
- About 50% of the incontinence presenting to GPs is stress incontinence.
- GPs should look for potentially reversible causes of urinary incontinence.
- Pelvic floor muscle training should be promoted by GPs and is an effective form of treatment for stress incontinence.
- Oestrogens are not indicated for the treatment of urinary incontinence.

PAINFUL BLADDER SYNDROME/ INTERSTITIAL CYSTITIS (PBS/IC)

Interstitial cystitis is the existence of urinary symptoms of cystitis in the absence of urinary infection. It is more traditionally defined as chronic sterile inflammatory disease of the bladder. It overlaps with the condition 'painful bladder syndrome', which is described as suprapubic pain related to bladder filling, accompanied by other symptoms such as increased day and night-time frequency, in the absence of proven urinary infection or other obvious pathology. There is a lot of controversy about the definitions, diagnostic criteria and aetiologies of these conditions. For the general practitioner, they are best considered together.

How common is it?

Current estimates are that 1 in 500 adult women have PBS/IC,[42] and that the cases we recognise probably represent the more severe or advanced end of the spectrum of disease.[43] By the time women are given the diagnosis of interstitial cystitis, often many years have passed and they will have seen many doctors.[44]

What is the usual clinical course?

Typical symptoms include frequency, urgency, dysuria and lower abdominal, bladder, vaginal, urethral or perineal pain, in the absence of bacterial cystitis. Voiding often relieves the suprapubic discomfort, and drinking alcohol- and caffeine-containing drinks frequently exacerbates it.

What investigations are undertaken for diagnostic purposes?

While cystoscopy is undertaken in order to rule out major pathology, final diagnosis tends to be a diagnosis of exclusion.

What is the usual management?

The current trend for management of this frustrating condition is multimodal therapy.[45] This therapy consists of agents designed to restore epithelial function, prevent mast cell activation and inhibit neural activation and is usually initiated by urologists after cystoscopy.

TIPS FOR PRACTITIONERS

- Only freshly voided urine should be used for dipstick testing, as nitrite produced by contaminating bacteria can induce false-positive results in older specimens.
- There is no evidence basis for the recommendation to use a midstream or clean voided specimen for urine testing.
- Uropathogenic resistance to ampicillin and amoxycillin is between 25% and 30%, making their empiric use for cystitis questionable.
- Contamination of the urine specimen is suggested by the presence of one or more of the following:
  - bacteria, but no leucocytes (except in immuno-compromised people)
  - multiple organisms cultured
  - blood, if the woman is menstruating.
- The muscles involved in pelvic floor exercises can be identified by explaining that they are the same muscles used to stop the flow of urine or to stop defecation from occurring.
- Imaging is not of use in women suffering from urinary incontinence. Ultrasound is useful only to determine residual urine volume.

REFERENCES

1. Foxman B, Barlow R, D'Arcy H, et al. Urinary tract infection: self-reported incidence and associated costs. Ann Epidemiol 2000; 10:509–515.
2. Ikaheimo R, Siitonen A, Heiskanen T, et al. Recurrence of urinary tract infection in a primary care setting: analysis of a 1-year follow-up of 179 women. Clin Infect Dis 1996; 22: 91–99.
3. Bent S, Nallamothu BK, Simel DL, et al. Does this woman have an acute uncomplicated urinary tract infection? JAMA 2002; 287(20):2701–2710.
4. Brumfitt W. The urethral syndrome. In: Brumfitt W, Hamilton-Miller J, Bailey RR (eds). Urinary tract infections. London: Chapman and Hall Medical; 1998:147–154.

5. Hooton TM, Scholes D, Hughes JP, et al. A prospective study of risk factors for symptomatic urinary tract infection in young women. N Engl J Med 1996; 335:468–474.

6. Scholes D, Hooton TM, Roberts PL, et al. Risk factors for recurrent urinary tract infection in young women. J Infect Dis 2000; 182:1177–1182.

7. Handley MA, Reingold AL, Shiboski S, et al. Incidence of acute urinary tract infection in young women and use of male condoms with and without nonoxynol-9 spermicides. Epidemiology 2002; 13:431–436.

8. Omar HA, Aggarwal S, Perkins KC. Tampon use in young women. J Pediatr Adolesc Gynecol 1998; 11:143–146.

9. Smith HS, Hughes JP, Hooton TM, et al. Antecedent antimicrobial use increases the risk of uncomplicated cystitis in young women. Clin Infect Dis 1997; 25:63–68.

10. Strom BL, Collins M, West SL, et al. Sexual activity, contraceptive use, and other risk factors for symptomatic and asymptomatic bacteriuria. A case-control study. Ann Intern Med 1987; 107(6):816–823.

11. Perrotta C, Aznar M, Mejia R, et al. Oestrogens for preventing recurrent urinary tract infection in postmenopausal women. Cochrane Database Syst Rev 2008; (2):CD005131.

12. Jellheden B, Norrby RS, Sandberg T. Symptomatic urinary tract infection in women in primary health care. Bacteriological, clinical and diagnostic aspects in relation to host response to infection. Scand J Prim Health Care 1996; 14:122–128.

13. Hurlbut 3rd TA, Littenberg B. The diagnostic accuracy of rapid dipstick tests to predict urinary tract infection. Am J Clin Pathol 1991; 96(5):582–588.

14. Papanicolaou N, Pfister RC. Acute renal infections. Radiol Clin North Am 1996; 34(5):965–995.

15. Johnson JR, Vincent LM, Wang K, et al. Renal ultrasonographic correlates of acute pyelonephritis. Clin Infect Dis 1992; 14(1):15–22.

16. Christiaens TC, De Meyere M, Verschraegen G, et al. Randomised controlled trial of nitrofurantoin versus placebo in the treatment of uncomplicated urinary tract infection in adult women. Br J Gen Pract 2002; 52(482):729–734.

17. Barry HC, Ebell MH, Hickner J. Evaluation of suspected urinary tract infection in ambulatory women: a cost-utility analysis of office-based strategies. J Fam Pract 1997; 44:49–60.

18. Fenwick EA, Briggs AH, Hawke CI. Management of urinary tract infection in general practice: a cost-effectiveness analysis. Br J Gen Pract 2000; 50:635–639.

19. Baerheim A. Empirical treatment of uncomplicated cystitis. Br Med J 2001; 323:1197–1198.

20. Norrby SR. Short-term treatment of uncomplicated lower urinary tract infections in women. Rev Infect Dis 1990; 12:458–467.

21. Warren JW, Abrutyn E, Hebel JR, et al. Guidelines for antimicrobial treatment of uncomplicated acute bacterial cystitis and acute pyelonephritis in women. Infectious Diseases Society of America (IDSA). Clin Infect Dis 1999; 29:745–758.

22. French L, Phelps K, Pothula NR, et al. Urinary problems in women. Prim Care 2009; 36(1):53–71, viii.

23. Lutters M, Vogt-Ferrier NB. Antibiotic duration for treating uncomplicated, symptomatic lower urinary tract infections in elderly women. Cochrane Database Syst Rev 2008; (3):CD001535.

24. Smaill F. Antibiotics for asymptomatic bacteriuria in pregnancy. Cochrane Database Syst Rev 2001; (2):CD000490.

25. Lawrenson RA, Logie JW. Antibiotic failure in the treatment of urinary tract infections in young women. J Antimicrob Chemother 2001; 48:895–901.

26. Brumfitt W, Hamilton-Miller JM, Cooper J, et al. Relationship of urinary pH to symptoms of 'cystitis'. Postgrad Med J 1990; 66:727–729.

27. Car J, Sheikh A. Recurrent urinary tract infection in women. BMJ 2003; 327(7425):1204.

28. Gupta K, Hooton TM, Roberts PL, et al. Patient-initiated treatment of uncomplicated recurrent urinary tract infections in young women. Ann Intern Med 2001; 135(1):9–16.

29. Stapleton A, Latham RH, Johnson C, et al. Postcoital antimicrobial prophylaxis for recurrent urinary tract infection. A randomized, double-blind, placebo-controlled trial. JAMA 1990; 264:703–706.

30. Stamm WE, Counts GW, Wagner KF, et al. Antimicrobial prophylaxis of recurrent urinary tract infections: a double-blind, placebo-controlled trial. Ann Intern Med 1980; 92:770–775.

31. Car J. Urinary tract infections in women: diagnosis and management in primary care. BMJ 2006; 332(7533):94–97.

32. Jepson RG, Craig JC. Cranberries for preventing urinary tract infections. Cochrane Database Syst Rev 2008; (1):CD001321.

33. Hannestad YS, Rortveit G, Sandvik H, et al. A community-based epidemiological survey of female urinary incontinence: the Norwegian EPINCONT study. Epidemiology of Incontinence in the County of Nord-Trondelag. J Clin Epidemiol 2000; 53(11):1150–1157.

34. Seim A, Eriksen BC, Hunskaar S. A study of female urinary incontinence in general practice. Demography, medical history and clinical findings. Scand J Urol Nephrol 1996; 30:465–471.

35. Harrison GL, Memel DL. Urinary incontinence in women: its prevalence and its management in a health promotion clinic. Br J Gen Pract 1994; 44:149–152.

36. Subak LL, Whitcomb E, Shen H, et al. Weight loss: a novel and effective treatment for urinary incontinence. J Urol 2005; 174(1):190–195.

37. Hay-Smith EJC, Bø K, Berghmans LCM, et al. Pelvic floor muscle training for urinary incontinence in women (Cochrane review). In: The Cochrane Library, Issue 3. Oxford: Update Software; 2002.

38. Roe B, Williams K, Palmer M. Bladder training for urinary incontinence in adults (Cochrane Review). In: The Cochrane Library, Issue 3. Oxford: Update Software; 2002.

39. Fantl JA, Wyman JF, McClish DK, et al. Efficacy of bladder training in older women with urinary incontinence. JAMA 1991; 265:609–613.

40. Mariappan P, Alhasso Ammar A, Grant A, et al. Serotonin and noradrenaline reuptake inhibitors (SNRI) for stress urinary incontinence in adults. Cochrane Database of Systematic Reviews. Chichester, UK: John Wiley & Sons; 2005.

41. Quinn SD, Domoney C. The effects of hormones on urinary incontinence in postmenopausal women. Climacteric 2009; 12(2):106–113.

42. van de Merwe JP, Nordling J, Bouchelouche P, et al. Diagnostic criteria, classification, and nomenclature for painful bladder syndrome/interstitial cystitis: an ESSIC proposal. Eur Urol 2008; 53(1):60–67.

43. Clemens JQ, Meenan RT, Rosetti MC, et al. Prevalence and incidence of interstitial cystitis in a managed care population. J Urol 2005; 173(1):98–102; discussion.

44. Parsons JK, Kurth K, Sant GR. Epidemiologic issues in interstitial cystitis. Urology 2007; 69(4 Suppl):5–8.

45. Moldwin RM, Evans RJ, Stanford EJ, et al. Rational approaches to the treatment of patients with interstitial cystitis. Urology 2007; 69(4 Suppl):73–81.

46. Duong TH, Korn AP. A comparison of urinary incontinence among African American, Asian, Hispanic, and white women. Am J Obstet Gynecol 2001; 184:1083–1086.

47. Meyer S, Schreyer A, De Grandi P, et al. The effects of birth on urinary continence mechanisms and other pelvic-floor characteristics. Obstet Gynecol 1998; 92(4 Pt 1):613–618.

48. Viktrup L, Lose G. The risk of stress incontinence 5 years after first delivery. Am J Obstet Gynecol 2001; 185:82–87.

49. Brown JS, Sawaya G, Thom DH, et al. Hysterectomy and urinary incontinence: a systematic review. Lancet 2000; 356:535–539.

50. Nygaard IE, Thompson FL, Svengalis SL, et al. Urinary incontinence in elite nulliparous athletes. Obstet Gynecol 1994; 84:183–187.

51. James D, Pilai M, Rymer J, et al. Obstetrics, gynaecology, neonatology interactive colour guides CD-ROM. Edinburgh: Churchill Livingstone; 2002.

52. Weiss BD, Newman DK. New insight into urinary stress incontinence: advice for the primary care clinician. Clinical Update. Medscape Obs and Gyn Women's Health. 2002. Online. Available: http://www.medscape.com/viewprogram/1961 [accessed 06.11.02].

53. NICE (National Institute of Clinical Excellence). NICE Clinical Guideline 40. Urinary incontinence: the management of urinary incontinence in women. 2006. Online. Available: http://www.nice.org.uk/nicemedia/pdf/CG40fullguideline.pdf [accessed 15.06.09].

54. Fitzgerald MA. Urinary tract infection: providing the best care. Clinical Update. Medscape Obs and Gyn Women's Health. 2003. Online. Available: http://www.medscape.com/viewprogram/1920 [accessed 15.02.03].

16

Sexual problems

OBJECTIVES

- To describe the normal sexual response in women
- To understand the factors that contribute to female sexual dysfunction and the different ways it can manifest
- To assist women suffering from sexual dysfunction as a result of antidepressant use
- To understand the aetiology of dyspareunia and be able to manage it appropriately
- To understand the aetiology of vulvodynia and be able to manage it appropriately

NORMAL SEXUAL RESPONSE IN WOMEN

What are the characteristics of 'normal' sexual response in women?

Women's sexual response is characterised as highly variable and influenced by a wide range of determinants, including physiological, psychosocial and contextual factors. While aspects of sexual response such as vaginal lubrication and orgasmic contractions are seen to occur in most women who are adequately sexually stimulated, the subjective or emotional aspects of sexual responsiveness are highly individual and subject to learning and cultural factors.[1]

Subjective or emotional aspects of sexual responsiveness are highly individual.

In different places around the world, female sexuality is viewed very differently: in Western countries women are highly sexualised, especially through the media, whereas in some Asian and African countries the opposite is true. The most extreme example of this is the practice of female genital mutilation, which is used as a means of limiting or controlling sexual pleasure in women. Many cultures and some religions also mandate restrictions over sexual practice during menstruation, pregnancy and/or menopause. There is often no sense of equality in sexuality between men and women. Open communication and discussion of sexual matters is discouraged, and women in these cultures may find it hard to express their sexual needs to their partners or to initiate discussion about sexual difficulties.[1]

Our understanding of women's sexual response has changed over the years. Masters and Johnson spoke of four phases: excitement, plateau, orgasm and resolution, each of which has associated genital and extragenital responses. Kaplan's three-stage model (desire, excitement and orgasm) formed the basis of the *Diagnostic and Statistical Manual of Mental Disorders* (DSM) III and IV classification of sexual dysfunction:

- disorders of sexual desire (hypoactive sexual desire disorder)
- sexual excitement disorders (male erectile dysfunction, female sexual arousal disorder)
- orgasmic disorders (premature ejaculation, male and female anorgasmia).

Both of these models assumed linear progression from one phase to the next and did not adequately recognise individual variation or the importance to sexual satisfaction of the subjective experience, environment and stimuli that are conducive to sexual feelings.[2] In essence, they ignored the psychosocial components of women's sexual responsiveness.

A new and refreshingly different model of women's sexual response cycle has been proposed by Basson (Fig 16.1).[3] It is circular and includes multiple sexual and non-sexual reasons for engaging in sex, the psychological and biological influences on arousability, and subjective feelings of arousal and desire.[1] According to this model, women frequently enter into a sexual experience through a stance of neutrality with positive motivation for intimacy or relationship. While some may criticise the model as stereotyping women as sexually passive, Basson proposes that rather than initiate sexual activity out of sexual drive, as the traditional model would propose, a woman may instigate physical contact or be receptive to sexual initiation for various reasons, such as the desire for closeness, intimacy and commitment, and as an expression of caring.[1]

A new model to describe women's sexual response cycle includes multiple sexual and non-sexual reasons for engaging in sex, the psychological and biological influences on arousability, and subjective feelings of arousal and desire.

Other unique aspects of this model are also worth considering:

- Spontaneous desire, including sexual thoughts, feelings and fantasies, is not necessary for sexual excitement or orgasm to occur but may contribute to a woman's willingness to become receptive or to her psychological and biological processing of the sexual stimuli.[3]
- A lack of spontaneous sexual desire is considered normal rather than dysfunctional, in contrast to traditional models of sexual response.[4]
- Just because a woman is involved in sexual activity and stimulation, it does not mean she is necessarily aroused; her ability to be aroused may be influenced by biological and psychological factors, including issues such as previous abuse, low self-esteem and concerns about contraception and sexually transmissible infections.

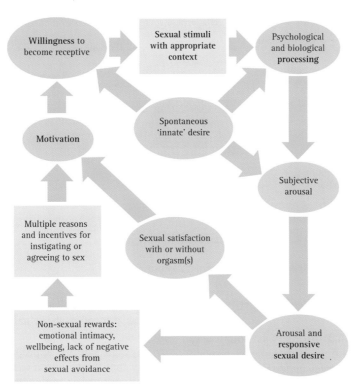

FIGURE 16.1 Sex response cycle, showing responsive desire experienced during the sexual experience, as well as variable initial (spontaneous) desire (Modified from Basson[4]; published with the permission of the American College of Obstetricians and Gynecologists)

- The type of stimulation and the time needed to become aroused as well as the context within which arousal occurs are all highly individual.
- Orgasm and resolution are not essential. Sexual satisfaction is viewed as occurring when a woman is able to focus on her sexual pleasure without negative outcome, such as pain, and may occur with or without orgasm.
- Arousal and desire are reciprocal processes whereby as a woman's sexual pleasure grows and intensifies she begins to feel desire for sex. Arousal may lead to sexual satisfaction and non-sexual rewards, such as emotional intimacy and wellbeing, both of which create continued motivational incentives for engaging in sexual activity.

SEXUAL DYSFUNCTION

How is female sexual dysfunction classified?

While an argument could be made that 'sexual dysfunction' is in reality a normal or logical response to difficult circumstances (e.g. a problem with the relationship, sexual context or cultural factors),[3] the *Diagnostic and statistical manual of mental disorders,* 4th edition (DSM-IV)[5] has utilised the term 'female sexual dysfunction' and subclassifed it into four categories: hypoactive sexual desire disorder, sexual arousal disorder (lubrication), orgasmic disorder and dyspareunia. Some have voiced concern that the classification of female sexual dysfunction has been engineered by the pharmaceutical industry in an effort to create the need for pharmacological intervention.[6] There are also other problems inherent in this classification. Loss of desire is not necessarily perceived as problematic for all women and there is little correlation between sexual thoughts and sexual satisfaction.[7,8] Additionally, while between 5% and 17%[8,9] of women say that they have problems with arousal, there are no objective measures to measure this.[10]

Loss of desire is not necessarily perceived as problematic for all women.

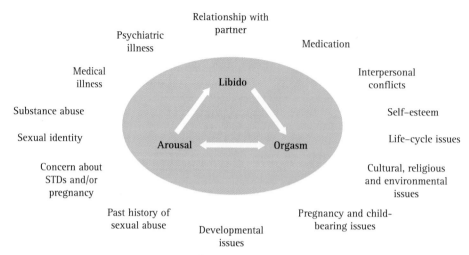

FIGURE 16.2 Potential causes of sexual dysfunction (From Zajecka[26])

How commonly do sexual problems present in general practice?

The prevalence of sexual disorders is notoriously difficult to assess, as different instruments provide different answers.[11] In a survey undertaken in London general practices,[12] 22% of men and 40% of women had some form of sexual dysfunction, but only 3–4% had an entry relating to sexual problems in their general practice notes. Among women with any sexual difficulty, on average, 64% experienced desire difficulty, 35% experienced orgasm difficulty, 31% experienced arousal difficulty, and 26% experienced sexual pain.[13] Of the sexual difficulties that occurred for 1 month or more in the previous year, 62–89% persisted for at least several months and 25–28% persisted for 6 months or more.[13] Only a proportion of women with sexual difficulty were distressed by it (21–67%).

What are the potential causes of sexual dysfunction in women?

Interpersonal issues and psychological and physiological factors can all contribute to sexual dysfunction (Fig 16.2).[3]

Interpersonal issues, psychological and physiological factors can all contribute to sexual dysfunction.

A national sample of American women found that their emotional relationship with the partner during sexual activity and general emotional wellbeing were the two strongest predictors of absence of distress about sex.[7] Contextual factors such as concerns about safety (risks of unwanted pregnancy and STDs, for example, or emotional or physical safety), appropriateness or privacy, or simply that the situation is insufficiently erotic, too hurried, or too late in the day may also contribute to dysfunction.[3]

Psychological factors associated with sexual dysfunction include low self-esteem, mood instability, tendency towards worry and anxiety[14] as well as memories of past negative sexual experiences (such as coercive or abusive ones), and expectations of negative outcomes to the sexual experience (e.g. dyspareunia or partner sexual dysfunction).[15]

Low self-esteem is strongly related to sexual dysfunction in women.

Myths and facts concerning the impact of hormonal factors and medications are outlined in Box 16.1.

How should GPs approach patients with sexual dysfunction?

In recognition of the multiple influences on sexual functioning, it has been suggested that doctors focus on the three factors that contribute to sexual dysfunction: past psychosexual development; current life context; and medical factors, including comorbid illness, drugs and previous surgery.[2] It is important to avoid 'pathologising' women by diagnosing a sexual disorder where symptoms are

> ### BOX 16.1 Myths and facts concerning the impact of hormonal factors and medications on sexual function
>
> - Oestrogen deficiency does not necessarily preclude adequate lubrication, provided that stimulation is sufficient.[16]
> - Up to 40% of postmenopausal women may have symptomatic vaginal atrophy that adversely affects sexual function.[17]
> - Testosterone and dopamine play a role in modulating sexual response, since testosterone supplementation or treatment with a dopaminergic agonist can augment response.[10]
> - Underproduction of androgen in women—as may occur with adrenal disease, after bilateral oophorectomy or during normal ageing—is sometimes associated with reduced desire and arousal.[10]
> - The proportion of women with low desire increases with age, while the proportion of women distressed about their low desire decreases with age.[18]
> - Large population studies have failed to find the expected positive correlations between sexual function and serum testosterone levels.[19,20]

> Physical examination infrequently identifies a cause of sexual dysfunction.

a normal response to an external factor.[3] Equally important is the identification of issues such as past sexual abuse or past or current intimate partner violence.

> It is important to avoid 'pathologising' women by diagnosing a sexual disorder where symptoms are a normal response to an external factor.

The history is the most important part of assessment and diagnosis in sexual dysfunction and should involve questions about the quality of the couple's relationship, the woman's mental and emotional health, the quality of past sexual experiences, specific concerns related to sexual activity (such as insufficient non-genital and non-penetrative genital stimulation), and the woman's thoughts and emotions during sexual activity.[10] The partner's perspective regarding the situation is also important to obtain. Physical examination infrequently identifies a cause of sexual dysfunction but may be helpful when there is associated dyspareunia.[10]

What are the recommended approaches to the management of sexual dysfunction in women?

The answer to this question really depends on the causative factors. GPs have a central role to play in educating women about the normal variation in women's sexual response and the factors that affect libido and arousal. This could be achieved by explaining the model given in Figure 16.1 to the woman. For many women, this explanation and reassurance that her symptoms are not due to 'hormone deficiency' may be all that is required. Other women may require other interventions.

Psychological interventions

Cognitive behavioural approaches and psychodynamic approaches are used during counselling. It is also helpful to work with the couple when there is loss of sexual desire, as this allows both partners' understanding of the problem to be examined and differences in sexuality and sexual needs to be explored. While many people expect their partner to have the same sexual needs as their own, counselling aims to encourage acceptance of difference, a concept sometimes described as 'benign variation'.[21] A brief outline of the kinds of psychological therapies that may assist are given in Box 16.2 (p 302).

Pharmacological interventions

With the advent of phosphodiesterase inhibitors such as Viagra for the treatment of male sexual dysfunction came the query as to whether such medication would assist women. Large randomised trials of sildenafil in women with arousal and desire disorders, however, showed no improvement in any measure of sexual desire, sensation, lubrication or satisfaction.[22]

Much focus has been given lately to the possibility that androgen therapy in the form of testosterone patches may improve symptoms in women with low libido. Current guidelines, however,

> recommend against making a diagnosis of androgen deficiency in women at present because of the lack of a well-defined clinical syndrome and normative data on total or free testosterone levels across the lifespan that can be used to define the disorder. Although there is evidence for short-term efficacy of testosterone in selected populations, such as surgically menopausal women, we recommend against the generalized use of testosterone by women because the indications are inadequate and evidence of safety in long-term studies is lacking.[23]

Of particular concern with long-term androgen use is a potential increase in insulin resistance, which could predispose a woman to the metabolic syndrome or exacerbate the syndrome if it is already present.[10]

The role of systemic oestrogen in increasing desire and subjective arousal remains unclear[10]; however it is logical that where vasomotor symptoms, insomnia or vaginal atrophy contributed to sexual dysfunction, use of oestrogen might assist. Tibolone (an agent with estrogenic, progestogenic and androgenic properties) has been shown in some small trials to bring about improved sexual function compared to a placebo or to women taking traditional HT.[24] However, there may be some concerns about the risk of breast cancer with long-term use of tibolone.

BOX 16.2 Psychological therapies for sexual dysfunction (From Basson and Basson[10])

Cognitive behavioural therapy
- Focuses on identifying and modifying factors that contribute to sexual dysfunction, such as maladaptive thoughts, unreasonable expectations, behaviours that reduce the partner's interest or trust (such as disrespectful behaviour or lack of honesty), insufficient erotic stimuli and insufficient non-genital physical stimulation.
- Strategies are suggested to improve the couple's emotional closeness and communication and to enhance erotic stimulation.
- Sessions vary in number and usually include both partners.

Sex therapy
Focuses on similar issues but also includes sensate focus techniques, consisting initially of non-sexual physical touch, with gradual progression towards sexual touch; partners are encouraged alternately to touch each other and to provide feedback about what touches are pleasurable. These techniques help change the undue focus on a performance goal (e.g. one partner's orgasm or mutual orgasms).

Short-term psychotherapy
Focuses on poor sexual self-image and on non-sexual experiences in childhood that are considered to relate to current sexual function (e.g. a chaotic upbringing that predisposed a woman to need to be in control could interfere with her 'letting go' sexually as an adult).

In conclusion pharmacological management options for women with sexual dysfunction are limited.

Sexual dysfunction related to antidepressant use

Is this scenario common?
Unfortunately, yes. Sexual dysfunction, that is decreased sexual interest and inhibited orgasm, are often the most troublesome side effects of selective serotonin-reuptake inhibitors (SSRIs). When the SSRIs were first released there was little information available regarding rates of sexual dysfunction associated with this new class of antidepressants. While sexual side effects were acknowledged on the patient information sheets and in information given to medical practitioners, the information was vague and rarely was the problem quantified. It was not until 5–6 years after the drugs were released that the right studies were carried out to find the extent of the problem. The prevalence of sexual disorders that are associated with the use of antidepressants in women is estimated at 22–58%, with higher rates reported for SSRIs and lower rates with some newer agents such as reboxetine and bupropion.[25] All classes of antidepressant medication are associated with sexual dysfunction.

CASE STUDY: 'My responsiveness has changed.'

Susie was a long-term patient of the practice in her late 30s. She had three children and was the local maternal and child-health nurse. Some 4 years ago, the birth of her last child had coincided with the death of her mother and soon after Susie began to show signs of depression. A partner in the practice had started her on paroxetine and she had made a quick recovery, but had continued on the medication all this time because of relapsing symptoms each time she had tried to stop.

Today Susie was in for a routine smear. Before carrying out the procedure the GP went through a routine list of questions. When was your last period? Are they regular? Are you having any bleeding between periods? Do you have any bleeding after intercourse? At this last question Susie laughed. 'Well, we don't have sex much any more, so there's no risk of that'. 'Why's that?' the GP asked. Susie hesitated and then said that since she had been on the antidepressants she felt her responsiveness had changed. She hadn't had an orgasm for 4 years and while she initially thought it was due to her depression, now that she felt really well she suspected it was due to the medication. Her husband felt so pressured to try to get her to achieve an orgasm that she was more likely to try not to have sex at all.

All classes of antidepressant medication are associated with sexual dysfunction.

What is the mechanism of interference with sexual functioning?

The mesolimbic system of the brain and more particularly dopamine as a neurotransmitter have been associated with maintenance of sexual interest. The potent and selective serotonin reuptake blockade associated with some antidepressants has been implicated in reducing dopamine activity in the mesolimbic system via the serotonin-2 ($5-HT_2$) receptor. While the central nervous system may have some impact, orgasm and ejaculation are primarily mediated at the peripheral spinal level. Sympathetic and parasympathetic tones are important and at least partially dependent upon norepinephrine and dopamine activity, which are again mediated by the $5-HT_2$ receptor. This may explain why agents that block the $5-HT_2$ receptor (e.g. nefazodone, mirtazapine) or have minimal or no effect on the serotonin reuptake system (e.g. bupropion) are not associated with decreased libido, arousal or anorgasmia.[26]

What solutions are there?

There are some general guidelines that GPs can follow when addressing antidepressant-induced sexual dysfunction with patients (Box 16.3).

A recent Cochrane review of strategies to ameliorate dysfunction associated with antidepressants did not recommend any particular drug, although the potential advantages of bupropion were noted[25] (in Australia bupropion is not indicated for treatment of depression). A drug holiday (e.g. halting the use of shorter-acting SSRIs over the weekend) seems to be a logical strategy but is not recommended, owing to withdrawal symptoms and compromise of compliance.

It is thought that, in some patients, over several months adaptation to the antidepressant medication will occur and sexual dysfunction will lessen. Antidepressant side effects are also dose-related, so that the higher the dose the more likely that sexual side effects will occur. As a general therapeutic principle, the lowest effective dose for the treatment of the depression should therefore be used.

Can a 'pharmacological antidote' be used?

Probably the least palatable strategy for reducing antidepressant-induced sexual dysfunction is the use of a 'pharmacological antidote'. While this therapeutic approach is widely used in other areas of medicine (e.g. the use of potassium in conjunction with diuretics), popping a pill before sex may

make the patient more aware of the problem, reduce spontaneity in sex and work against sexual functioning. Still, if the situation is that problematic, maybe patients will feel less apprehensive about their sexual functioning having taken the antidote.

When suggesting antidotes, most GPs will have to take into consideration several factors, including whether the antidepressant is efficacious in treating the underlying illness, the potential for drug interactions, potential new side effects, the cost of additional medication and potential additive effects of enhancing efficacy or managing other side effects. Table 16.1 (p 304) lists several pharmacological antidotes that have been reported to be effective in managing antidepressant sexual side effects and includes the typical doses needed, what antidepressant they are useful with and which phase of the sexual cycle they are helpful. Most of the antidotes, apart from sildenafil (Viagra) that can be used on an as-needs basis, require daily use.

Buspirone is one of the few 'antidotes' that has been shown to reverse SSRI-induced sexual dysfunction in a placebo-controlled study.[27] It is an anxiolytic that may be ideal for those patients on SSRIs or venlafaxine who could also benefit from further antidepressant augmentation.

Bupropion is devoid of serotonergic activity and is thought to have dopaminergic- and norepinephrine-enhancing properties; hence its ability to reduce sexual dysfunction in those on SSRIs and venlafaxine.[28] Its use, however, requires careful assessment because of possible interactions.

Sildenafil (Viagra) and *Gingko biloba* extract are thought to have a similar mode of action in reducing sexual dysfunction. Both are associated with increased peripheral blood flow to the genital organs. Yohimbine, on the other hand, probably works by increasing noradrenergic activity, but can also cause anxiety, agitation and panic attacks.

What approach should be taken for women suffering from female orgasmic disorder?

The role of orgasm for women is not well defined. For some it is extremely important and sought at every sexual encounter. However, for others it seems less important and sometimes of little relevance; many women can be quite content without it. An important issue is the male partner's understanding of the female orgasm. He often feels that, like him, his partner cannot fully enjoy sexual activity without orgasm, and this can put enormous pressure on the woman to achieve orgasm.

Anorgasmia is treated using a staged approach involving self-exploration, sensate focus, masturbation, use of adjuncts (vibrators), resolution of unconscious fears of orgasm, distraction, exercises to heighten sexual arousal, transfer to heterosexual situation and orgasm on sexual intercourse.

Dyspareunia

What is dyspareunia and how common is it?

Dyspareunia is the term used to describe genital pain experienced just before, during or after sexual intercourse.[29] The prevalence in women is about 7%.[30] A survey looking specifically at dyspareunia[31] found that 22 women out of 105

(21%) who had dyspareunia reported its occurrence as 'rare', 58 (55%) reported it as 'occasional' and 25 (24%) as 'frequent' or 'constant'. Although the actual frequency of intercourse was the same among all these groups, 49 (47%) of the women reported that they had less frequent intercourse because of dyspareunia, and 35 (33%) reported that their dyspareunia had an adverse effect on their relationship with a sexual partner.

The prevalence of dyspareunia in women is about 7%.

As noted above, the *Diagnostic and Statistical Manual of Mental Disorders* (DSM-IV),[32] the classification manual of psychiatry nominates dyspareunia as a sexual pain disorder, a subcategory of sexual dysfunction. The criteria used to define the condition are the following:

- Recurrent or persistent genital pain is associated with sexual intercourse in either a male or a female.
- The disturbance causes marked distress or interpersonal difficulty.

TABLE 16.1 Pharmacological antidotes for antidepressant-associated sexual dysfunction (From Zajecka[41])

Antidote	Dosage	Comments	Reported efficacy
Methylphenidate (Ritalin)	5–40 mg/d	For SSRIs or venlafaxine	Libido, arousal, orgasm
Dextroamphetamine	5–40 mg/d	Avoid night dosing for insomnia	Libido, arousal, orgasm
Gingko biloba extract	180–240 mg/d t.d.s.	Potential for increased clotting time and possible flatulence	Libido, arousal, orgasm
Amantadine (Symmetrel)	100 mg b.d.	Use with caution in patients predisposed to psychosis	Orgasm
Cyproheptadine (Periactin)	4–12 mg four times daily	MAOIs, TCAs, SSRIs, venlafaxine Watch for re-emergence of depressive symptoms. Is sedating.	Orgasm
Buspirone (Buspar)	30–60 mg/d b.d.		Libido, orgasm
Bupropion (Zyban)	75–150 mg/d either q.i.d. or b.d.	Useful for SSRIs or venlafaxine. Fluoxetine may raise bupropion levels; use usual precautionary measures for bupropion.	Libido, arousal, orgasm
Mirtazapine	15–45 mg/d	SSRIs or venlafaxine	Orgasm
Nefazodone	Start at 50 mg/d – up to 150 mg/d	SSRIs or venlafaxine	Orgasm
Sildenafil	50–100 mg/d	Contraindicated with nitrates	Libido, arousal, orgasm
Yohimbine	5.4 mg t.d.s.	Can be anxiogenic; safety uncertain with MAOIs	Libido, arousal, orgasm

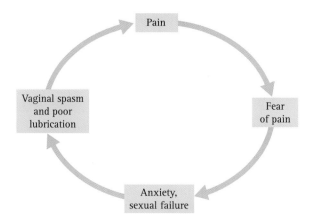

FIGURE 16.3 Cycle of pain in cases of dyspareunia

- The disturbance is not caused exclusively by vaginismus (pain resulting from attempted insertion of the penis into the vagina due to intense involuntary contraction of the perineal muscles surrounding the outer one-third of the vagina) or lack of lubrication.
- The disturbance is not better accounted for by another disorder (except another sexual dysfunction) from Axis I (clinical disorders, including major mental disorders, and learning disorders) and is not due exclusively to the direct physiological effects of a substance (e.g. a drug of abuse or a medication) or a general medical condition.

Is it a medical or psychiatric problem?

Finding it in the DSM-IV may make you think that dyspareunia is a psychiatric condition. It is probably more helpful, however, to consider dyspareunia as a 'pain syndrome', in which an initial instigating factor is then perpetuated by confounding factors.[33] This cycle is demonstrated in Figure 16.3.

Studies[34] have revealed that women with dyspareunia have more physical pathology on examination, report more psychological symptomatology, have more negative attitudes towards sexuality, and have higher levels of impairment in sexual function and lower levels of marital adjustment. They do not report more current or past physical or sexual abuse, however. Patients with dyspareunia are more likely than the general population to report pain with insertion of a tampon or digit, or during a gynaecological examination.[34]

Women who complain of dyspareunia have more pathology, more psychological symptomatology and more negative attitudes towards sexuality.

Rosa was a jovial 23-year-old woman who had recently married. She had been consulting her GP for various problems over the last 2 years. In the past year the GP had been badgering her about the need for a Pap smear and she had always blushed and said that she had her period but would make another time to do it. Finally, she attended for the smear. As the GP warmed the speculum with some warm water before approaching her, Rosa become very pale and stopped talking. She was asked to bend her knees, put her feet together and to then to let her knees go floppy. They parted about 30 centimetres. The GP asked her if she could go more floppy and try and get her knees down to the couch, as if in a yoga position. She made more of an effort, but her knees barely parted 45 degrees. Encouragingly, the GP remarked how the skin around the opening of the vagina all looked normal and told Rosa that she was now going to insert the speculum. The GP told her that she had made it slippery with some water and that Rosa should breathe out and relax her vaginal muscles while it was inserted. As the GP said this, she noticed Rosa's hands sliding down her abdomen getting ready to stop the procedure and her knees slowly coming together. The more the GP tried to insert the speculum, the more Rosa's back arched and her muscles clamped shut.

The GP put the speculum down and asked Rosa to think of the speculum as if it were a tampon. 'You know how you have to relax to get a tampon to slide in? Well, it's the same with this examination.' 'But I don't use tampons', Rosa replied. 'Well, another trick', the GP said, 'is for you to push out as if you want to do a poo while I'm inserting the speculum. That makes your muscles relax'. They tried again but ended up abandoning the procedure, as it was causing Rosa too much distress.

After Rosa had got dressed, the GP reassured her that she had encountered this kind of fear among many women when undertaking smears. Gently the GP asked Rosa if she had a similar problem when she had sex with her husband. Hearing this question Rosa burst into tears and disclosed that their sex life was non-existent because of her 'problem'. She told the GP that when they had first had sex it had been very painful, and that increasingly she was finding she was unable to allow intercourse to occur at all.

An approach to the classification of dyspareunia

The most helpful way to categorise dyspareunia is by determining the onset (primary versus secondary), frequency (complete versus situational) and location (superficial versus deep) of the pain.

When dyspareunia has been present the whole of the woman's sexual life, it is of primary onset and is probably related to psychosocial issues. The woman may have been brought up with negative attitudes towards sex and learned to associate sex with guilt and shame. She may be in an unwanted relationship or have had a painful first sexual experience. When the dyspareunia begins after a period of normal sexual functioning (secondary onset), a physical cause is more likely, although psychosocial issues may come into play and exacerbate the problem.

The location of the pain is very important when considering causation. When the pain is described as sharp, burning or pinching and occurring at the vaginal introitus at the time of penile insertion, it is likely that the pain is a learned response, perhaps to a negative experience. Deep pain experienced in the lower abdomen with deep thrusting of the penis is likely to be secondary to a pelvic problem such as endometriosis or a pelvic mass.

The classification of dyspareunia into primary or secondary, complete or situational, and superficial or deep helps the GP to understand the major causes of the problem and how to approach treatment.

When taking a history what features are important?

When dealing with patients with dyspareunia, GPs should ascertain:

- the nature of the pain
- duration of the pain
- intensity of the pain
- location of the pain
- exacerbating and ameliorating factors
- the partner's response to the woman's dyspareunia, and the impact of the problem on the individual and the relationship with her partner
- whether the woman has ever had a history of successful sexual experiences
- previous treatments and the degree of response to them.

Appropriate gynaecological questions include asking about the following[35]:

- symptoms of vaginitis
- a history of STDs, especially HSV or HPV
- a history of lacerations, episiotomies or other trauma at delivery
- abdominal or genitourinary surgical or radiation history
- endometriosis, fibroids or chronic pelvic pain
- current contraceptive method.

If the history points to primary dyspareunia or vaginismus, the woman's background should be explored with questions asked about the influence of her religion, culture and family in forming her attitudes towards sex. Exposure to either child or adult sexual abuse should also be explored.

How does a GP undertake an examination in a woman complaining of dyspareunia?

The GP needs to explain to the woman exactly what the examination will entail. Permission needs to be obtained to proceed and a woman should be given the option of delaying the examination until the next consultation should she so wish. A hand mirror can be offered to the woman so that she can watch the proceedings and understand the evaluation that is taking place.

The GP should note areas of erythema, atrophy, leukoplakia or discharge at the introitus, as well as any traumatic, surgical or episiotomy scars. Focal tenderness elicited by gently touching the vestibule with a cotton-tipped applicator is indicative of vestibulitis. This syndrome involves a constellation of findings consisting of vulvar erythema and severe pain or burning with touching of the vestibule or attempted vaginal entry.[36] The cause of vulvar vestibulitis is unknown.

Vulvar vestibulitis is a condition of unknown aetiology characterised by severe pain or burning when the vestibule is touched or on attempted vaginal entry.

Insertion of a small speculum, lubricated generously with water, can then be attempted. If pain is elicited, it is important to ask the woman if it is the same type of pain as the pain she experiences with intercourse. If speculum examination is tolerated, inspection of the vagina and cervix can occur. The inspection should note any lesions, signs of infection or atrophy, presence of congenital anomalies and evidence of trauma. If appropriate, swabs for microscopy and culture and for *Chlamydia* PCR testing, and a Pap smear can be taken.

Once the speculum is removed, vaginal examination using one digit can proceed. This examination allows the GP to assess the presence of vaginismus and to do a pelvic assessment, noting the presence of any adnexal masses, the size and position of the uterus and the presence of any localised tenderness.

At the conclusion of the examination, the GP should reassure the woman that all looks normal if this is in fact the case.

Are any investigations useful?

Investigations are of limited value in making a diagnosis in cases of dyspareunia. If vulvar disease is suspected, a colposcopy is recommended. A pelvic ultrasound may be of assistance if an ovarian mass or endometriosis is suspected. If a physical cause for the dyspareunia is thought to be likely, referral to a gynaecologist is indicated and for a laparoscopy to assess the pelvis.

What is the therapeutic approach to dyspareunia?

While treatment of dyspareunia should be directed at the underlying cause, all women should be offered simple reassurance and some will benefit from some sexual education. The importance of explaining the normal pattern of female sexual arousal cannot be overemphasised. Suggestions for modification of sexual technique may help to reduce pain with intercourse. Increasing the amount of foreplay and delaying penetration until maximal arousal has occurred will allow increased vaginal lubrication and thus decrease pain with penile entry. Lubricant can also be recommended.

The partner's actions, emotions and responses to the situation also need to be explored. The woman should therefore be asked whether she would like to include her partner in any further consultations so that they can both gain insight into a problem that they share.

When managing dyspareunia, the GP should encourage the woman to involve her partner in education and counselling sessions.

The most effective treatment approach for superficial dyspareunia/vaginismus is a combination of behaviour modification and emotional counselling.[37] The aim of the treatment is to achieve a situation where the woman feels that she owns her own vagina and can share it for sexual activity should she wish.[38] Several steps in the treatment of vaginismus have been suggested (Box 16.4).[38]

Vaginismus is caused by involuntary muscle spasm.

> **BOX 16.4 Steps in the treatment of vaginismus (From Butcher[21])**
>
> - Sexual education
> - Control of vaginal muscles
> - Self-exploration of sexual anatomy
> - Insertion of a trainer under controlled relaxation
> - Sharing of control with partner
> - Insertion of penis, with the woman in control
> - Transfer control of insertion of penis to partner
> - Exploration of phobia

The first step is to educate the woman regarding her reproductive anatomy and function and explain to her the pattern of female sexual responsiveness. The partner should be involved and agree to withhold from intercourse until such time as the woman is prepared to allow it to occur. The partner should be warned that this might take up to 6 months.

The behaviour modification component of the treatment involves learning how to control the vaginal musculature through relaxation and performing Kegel (pelvic floor) exercises. The woman can practise contracting and relaxing these muscles at home and should be encouraged to explore her own sexual anatomy at home using a mirror. When she feels comfortable, she can start practising the insertion of a small dilator (available from sexual counselling clinics) or something like a small syringe into the introitus. Initially lubricant should be used, and the woman should be encouraged to insert the dilator after she has contracted and relaxed the vaginal muscles three times. This should be practised three or four times a week. Gradually the size of the dilator is increased and then the partner allowed to insert it during sex play. Only after the woman feels comfortable inserting a penile-sized dilator into the vagina can intercourse be attempted. At all times the woman needs to feel in control and the partner must not thrust until the woman signals she feels ready.

The aim of treatment of superficial dyspareunia/vaginismus is to achieve a situation where the woman feels she 'owns' her vagina and can share it for sexual activity should she wish.

> **BOX 16.5 Therapy of vulvodynia—an algorithm (From Edwards[40])**
>
> - Nonspecific but important therapy
>   - patient education on vulvodynia
>   - counselling
>   - avoidance of irritants and unnecessary topical agents
>   - lidocaine jelly 2%/ointment 5%
> - Amitryptilline/Gabapentin/Venlaflaxine/Duloxetine/Pregalbin
> - Pelvic floor therapy
> - Surgery

Conclusions

Managing patients with dyspareunia involves a lot of time and patience. GPs need to feel entirely comfortable dealing with issues of this kind in order to be successful. It can be very rewarding, however, to assist patients with what are relatively simple measures.

Vulvodynia

What is vulvodynia?

Previously termed 'vulvodynia' and 'vestibulitis', vulvar pain syndromes have been reclassified by the International Society for the Study of Vulvovaginal Disease (ISSVD) under the common diagnosis of 'vulvodynia'. Vulvodynia is now classified as generalised or localised, depending on the distribution of the pain, and is further subtyped based on inciting factors—provoked pain, unprovoked pain, or mixed (both provoked and unprovoked).[39] It is characterised by chronic burning, stinging, irritation, soreness, rawness, stabbing or other painful sensations of the vulva in the absence of any clinical or laboratory abnormalities that could account for the symptoms. Itching is not a typical symptom.[40]

Vulvodynia is poorly recognised by primary-care doctors and some gynaecologists, and this may lead patients to seek a diagnosis repeatedly from a variety of clinicians over a long period of time, often thinking they are suffering from recurrent thrush.

Therapies for vulvodynia are wide-ranging and suboptimal in terms of efficacy and long-term outcomes. It is postulated that this is because of failure to address the CNS components of the condition, inadequate understanding of the contributory mechanisms and failure to appreciate the psychosocial context.[40] Chronic vulvar pain is probably best approached, therefore, as a systemic pain disorder.[40] An algorithm for therapy is given in Box 16.5

Summary of key points

- Traditional models of women's sexual response such as that proposed by Masters and Johnson ignored the psychosocial components of women's sexual responsiveness.
- Approximately one-quarter of women in the population at large suffer from low sexual desire.
- Sexual dysfunction is a side effect of many antidepressants.
- GPs should ask their patients about their sexual concerns.
- Dyspareunia is best considered as a 'pain syndrome', in which an initial instigating factor is perpetuated by confounding factors.
- Dyspareunia should be categorised as either primary or secondary, complete or situational, and superficial or deep.
- Superficial dyspareunia or vaginismus is probably more commonly seen in general practice.
- Vaginismus is caused by involuntary muscle spasm.
- Vulvodynia is often poorly recognised by health professionals, leading sufferers to believe they have recurrent thrush.

TIPS FOR PRACTITIONERS

- When asking a patient about sexual dysfunction GPs can normalise the question and put the patient at ease by asking something like: 'Everyone periodically has concerns and questions about sexual issues: what are yours at this time?'
- Dyspareunia should be considered as a pain syndrome, in which an initial instigating factor is prolonged and exacerbated by other personal, psychological and physical factors.

REFERENCES

1. Rosen RC, Barsky JL. Normal sexual response in women. Obstet Gynecol Clin North Am 2006; 33(4):515–526.
2. Basson R, Leiblum S, Brotto L, et al. Definitions of women's sexual dysfunction reconsidered: advocating expansion and revision. J Psychosom Obstet Gynaecol 2003; 24(4):221–229.
3. Basson R. Women's sexual dysfunction: revised and expanded definitions. CMAJ 2005; 172(10):1327–1333.
4. Basson R. Female sexual response: the role of drugs in the management of sexual dysfunction. Obstet Gynecol 2001; 98(2):350–353. [Erratum appears in Obstet Gynecol 2001; 98(3):522.]
5. American Psychiatric Association. Diagnostic and statistical manual of mental disorders. 4th edn revised: DSM-IV-R. Washington, DC: American Psychiatric Association; 2003.
6. Moynihan R. The making of a disease: female sexual dysfunction. BMJ 2003; 326(7379):45–47.

7. Bancroft J, Loftus J, Long JS. Distress about sex: a national survey of women in heterosexual relationships. Arch Sex Behav 2003; 32(3):193–208.

8. Avis NE, Zhao X, Johannes CB, et al. Correlates of sexual function among multi-ethnic middle-aged women: results from the Study of Women's Health Across the Nation (SWAN). Menopause 2005; 12(4):385–398.

9. Dunn KM, Croft PR, Hackett GI. Sexual problems: a study of the prevalence and need for health care in the general population. Fam Pract 1998; 15(6):519–524.

10. Basson R, Basson R. Clinical practice. Sexual desire and arousal disorders in women. N Engl J Med 2006; 354(14):1497–1506.

11. Hayes RD, Dennerstein L, Bennett CM, et al. What is the 'true' prevalence of female sexual dysfunctions and does the way we assess these conditions have an impact? J Sex Med 2008; 5(4):777–787.

12. Nazareth I, Boynton P, King M. Problems with sexual function in people attending London general practitioners: cross sectional study. BMJ 2003; 327(7412):423.

13. Hayes RD, Bennett CM, Fairley CK, et al. What can prevalence studies tell us about female sexual difficulty and dysfunction? J Sex Med 2006; 3(4):589–595.

14. Hartmann U, Heiser K, Ruffer-Hesse C, et al. Female sexual desire disorders: subtypes, classification, personality factors and new directions for treatment. World J Urol 2002; 20(2):79–88.

15. Graham CA, Sanders SA, Milhausen RR, et al. Turning on and turning off: a focus group study of the factors that affect women's sexual arousal. Arch Sex Behav 2004; 33(6):527–538.

16. van Lunsen RH, Laan E. Genital vascular responsiveness and sexual feelings in midlife women: psychophysiologic, brain, and genital imaging studies. Menopause 2004; 11(6 Pt 2):741–748.

17. Stenberg A, Heimer G, Ulmsten U, et al. Prevalence of genitourinary and other climacteric symptoms in 61-year-old women. Maturitas 1996; 24(1–2):31–36.

18. Hayes RD, Dennerstein L, Bennett CM, et al. Relationship between hypoactive sexual desire disorder and aging. Fertil Steril 2007; 87(1):107–112.

19. Santoro N, Torrens J, Crawford S, et al. Correlates of circulating androgens in mid-life women: the Study of Women's Health Across the Nation. J Clin Endocrinol Metab 2005; 90(8):4836–4845.

20. Davis SR, Davison SL, Donath S, et al. Circulating androgen levels and self-reported sexual function in women. JAMA. 2005; 294(1):91–96.

21. Butcher J. Female sexual problems II: sexual pain and sexual fears. Br Med J 1999; 318:110–112.

22. Basson R, McInnes R, Smith MD, et al. Efficacy and safety of sildenafil citrate in women with sexual dysfunction associated with female sexual arousal disorder. J Women's Health Gend Based Med 2002; 11(4):367–377.

23. Wierman ME, Basson R, Davis SR, et al. Androgen therapy in women: an endocrine society clinical practice guideline. J Clin Endocrinol Metab 2006; 91(10):3697–3710.

24. NathorstBoos J, Hammar M. Effect on sexual life—a comparison between tibolone and a continous estradiol–norethisterone acetate regimen. Maturitas 1997; 26(1):15–20.

25. Taylor MJ, Rudkin L, Hawton K. Strategies for managing antidepressant-induced sexual dysfunction: systematic review of randomised controlled trials. J Affect Disord 2005; 88(3):241–254.

26. Zajecka J. Strategies for the treatment of antidepressant-related sexual dysfunction. J Clin Psychiatry 2001; 62(Suppl 3):35–43.

27. Landen M, Eriksson E, Agren H, et al. Effect of buspirone on sexual dysfunction in depressed patients treated with selective serotonin reuptake inhibitors. J Clin Psychopharmacol 1999; 19:268–271.

28. Labbate LA, Grimes JB, Hines A, et al. Bupropion treatment of serotonin reuptake antidepressant-associated sexual dysfunction. Ann Clin Psychiatry 1997; 9:241–245.

29. American College of Obstetricians and Gynecologists. Sexual dysfunction. Technical Bulletin no. 211. Washington, DC: ACOG; 1995.

30. Laumann E, Paik A, Rosen RC. Sexual dysfunction in the United States: prevalence and predictors. JAMA 1999; 281:537–544 (published erratum appears in JAMA 281: 1174).

31. Glatt AE, Zinner SH, McCormack WM. The prevalence of dyspareunia. Obstet Gynecol 1990; 75:433–436.

32. American Psychiatric Association. Diagnostic and statistical manual of mental disorders. 4th edn. Washington, DC: American Psychiatric Association: 1994:511–518.

33. Meana M, Binik YM, Khalife S, et al. Dyspareunia: sexual dysfunction or pain syndrome? J Nerv Ment Disord 1997; 185:561–569.

34. Meana M, Binik YM, Khalife S, et al. Biopsychosocial profile of women with dyspareunia. Obstet Gynecol 1997; 90:583–589.

35. Phillips N. The clinical evaluation of dyspareunia. Int J Impot Res 1998; 10(Suppl 2):S117–S120.

36. Marinoff SC, Turner ML. Vulvar vestibulitis syndrome: an overview. Am J Obstet Gynecol 1991; 165:1228–1233.

37. Canavan TP, Heckman CD. Dyspareunia in women. Breaking the silence is the first step toward treatment. Postgrad Med 2000; 108:149–152, 157–160, 164–166.

38. Butcher J. ABC of sexual health: female sexual problems I: loss of desire—what about the fun? BMJ 1999; 318(7175):41–43.

39. Gunter J. Vulvodynia: new thoughts on a devastating condition. Obstet Gynecol Surv 2007; 62(12):812–819.

40. Edwards L. Vulvodynia. In: Black M, Ambros-Rudolph CM, Edwards L, et al, eds. Obstetric and gynecologic dermatology. 3rd edn. Mosby; 2008.

41. Zajecka JM. Clinical issues in long term treatment with antidepressants. J Clin Psychiatry 2000; 61(Suppl 2):20–25.

17

Violence against women

OBJECTIVES

- To understand the role of the general practitioner in managing a woman presenting after a sexual assault
- To be aware of the medical and psychological consequences of sexual assault
- To understand the epidemiology, causes and consequences of intimate partner violence
- To be able to screen for intimate partner violence in the general practice setting
- To effectively counsel women who have experienced intimate partner violence
- To develop an approach towards dealing with perpetrators who are also patients

RAPE

What is the difference between rape and sexual assault?

To most people, adult sexual assault equals rape. Rape is a legal term, however, not medical. Two elements are involved in its definition: sexual intercourse and commission of the act forcibly and without consent.[1] Adult sexual assault is a broader term, defined as occurrences of a sexual nature that happen without a person's consent. This definition includes events such as attempted rape, unwanted sexual advances from someone in authority, sexual advances from relatives, narrowly missing being sexually assaulted, and situations where there is violence or the threat of violence and at the same time fear of being sexually assaulted. All of these forms of sexual assault or threatened sexual assault are likely to have an effect on the victim.

When dealing with a topic such as rape, it is important that, as a GP, you recognise how you conceptualise sexual assault. In the past the attitude has been one of blaming the victim, that men cannot possibly control their sexual urges and that if women dressed and acted more modestly, rape would not occur. This mentality is characterised by the notion that 'No' doesn't necessarily mean 'No' and that if a woman asks a man into her home it is an invitation and permit for him to have sex with her. With the rise of feminism, our understanding of rape has come a long way. Sexual assault is typically an issue not of sexual motivation but of power and control. Assailants display anger, violence, hostility and aggression.[2] Their power over the victim is more satisfying than the actual sexual act.[3]

Sexual assault is an act of violence, not of sexual gratification. Sex is the weapon; it is a means, not the end.

Victim or survivor?

Many women feel offended at being labelled a 'victim', because it stereotypes them as helpless. The term survivor has therefore come into use, as it has better connotations than 'victim'. It suggests positive qualities of strength and courage and expresses the fact that these women have gone through a terrible trauma and survived. In this chapter, the words victim and survivor will be used interchangeably.

CASE STUDY: 'I think I was raped last night.'

Melissa walked into the consulting room. She was a fairly typical 19-year-old young woman who the GP had previously seen on several occasions with her mother. On this occasion she was alone and had obviously been crying. Her eyes were puffy and she sniffed as she sat down. 'You look very upset Melissa, what's the matter?' the GP asked. 'I think I was raped last night', she said and broke down in sobs.

Melissa had been to a party the night before. She had been persuaded to go to the home of a young man she knew only slightly. They were sitting drinking coffee when two friends of his arrived at the house. The three proceeded to rape her in turn. She only managed to escape, half clothed, later that night and had been driven home by a concerned stranger who had stopped to see if she was all right.

The GP explained to her that if she wanted to she could report the incident to the police, and that either a forensic doctor or the GP could examine her to see if she had any injuries or needed any treatment. Melissa decided she needed time to think about whether or not she would report the incident. She didn't feel that she had any injuries and didn't want to be examined. She did accept emergency contraception, however, as she was fearful of becoming pregnant. She agreed to return in a couple of days to talk over the incident some more and perhaps to allow an examination at that time.

How common is sexual assault?

The true prevalence of adult sexual assault is difficult to ascertain because it is often not reported to police. Indeed, one study[4] reported that only 12% of rape victims and 7% of those sexually assaulted had reported these crimes to the police, indicating that official rates greatly underestimate their true prevalence. In the USA, it has been estimated that one in six women will be raped during her lifetime.[5]

Studies of community samples show that the lifetime prevalence of sexual assault ranges from 13.5%[6] up to 59.9%, if all sexually stressful events (i.e. non-contact sexual assault) are considered.[7]

In studies of family practice patients,[8] approximately 40% recalled some form of sexual aggression since the age of 18; 7.5% had been raped and 17% had experienced attempted rape. In another study that surveyed women attending general practitioners, 13% of women over the age of 18 answered that they had experienced rape or attempted rape at some time during their adult life.[9]

A sample of student patients found a higher prevalence of rape or attempted rape of 28.7%,[8] consistent with the phenomenon of 'date rape',

CASE STUDY: Genital warts after being raped

Sally was 23. The GP had never met her before. She presented for the treatment of genital warts, which she said she had noticed for the first time over the past 2 weeks. When the GP took a sexual history from Sally, she appeared uncomfortable. She told the GP that she was not currently sexually active and had not been since she was raped 2 months previously. A man had entered her apartment, where she lived alone, at night through a window. He had been a burglar, but when she disturbed him he had assaulted and raped her before escaping.

Soon after, Sally had attended a rape crisis centre to receive counseling, but she described how she continued to feel extremely fearful and anxious. She had felt distracted and had not made much progress in her university studies. She had been unable to continue her sexual relationship with her boyfriend and often burst into tears for no particular reason. She felt like a complete mess and now realised that she had contracted the warts from the man who raped her. She felt dirty and 'marked' for life.

Sally needed treatment of her warts and reassurance that in time and with treatment the warts would disappear. After establishing the fact that she had already made a police report, the GP offered her ongoing support and counselling.

which would be more prevalent in a student population. In this same study, almost half of the victimised individuals felt they would have great difficulty discussing their experience with a medical professional or would not be able to discuss it at all. This suggests that the same factors that discourage the reporting of sexual assault to official authorities also discourage communication with doctors.

What role should a GP have?

In general, the role of the doctor is threefold. First, there are medical concerns. The woman may have experienced significant injuries that require diagnosis and treatment. Consideration should also be given to her risk of pregnancy and sexually transmissible infections. The second concern is for the emotional state of the woman. Doctors should provide emotional support not only at the time of the disclosure and any subsequent examinations or consultations, but also over the long term during the process of recovery or during any legal proceedings. Third, a doctor has a legal role: to collect and interpret evidence, should the victim undertake legal action. Sometimes these three roles are in conflict. For example, in some scenarios management of medical conditions may preclude the collection of specimens for legal purposes.

Women who have been sexually assaulted may have suffered physical injuries, are at risk of pregnancy and may have contracted sexually transmissible infections.

When responding to a disclosure of sexual assault, it is important to[10]:

- ensure privacy, safety and adequate time for the victim
- acknowledge her courage in speaking out
- accept the victim's story in a non-judgmental way—it is the role of police to investigate its veracity
- explain that reactions to rape—such as shock, arousal, anxiety and fear—are normal, emphasising that the victim is not to blame
- understand that the aim of management is to return control to the victim by enabling her to make choices about reporting, counselling and medical therapy.

GPs should accept the woman's story in a non-judgmental way and emphasise that she is not to blame for what occurred.

Further action is defined by whether the victim decides to make a formal complaint. A useful flowchart for the management of sexual assault is given below:

Should only forensic doctors see rape victims?

Many GPs feel reluctant to take on the care of rape victims and try to pass on the job to forensic services. This is appropriate when the woman has decided to make a formal report to the police and where there is the likelihood of legal ramifications. Forensic services are often difficult to access, however, and many women do not want to be examined by a stranger, or indeed by a male doctor, in these circumstances. Other women prefer their own GPs to conduct the necessary examinations, and still others are unsure at the time of presentation whether they will actually proceed to make a report. It is therefore important that all GPs have the skills to undertake the care of victims of sexual assault in their own practice and feel confident to do so.

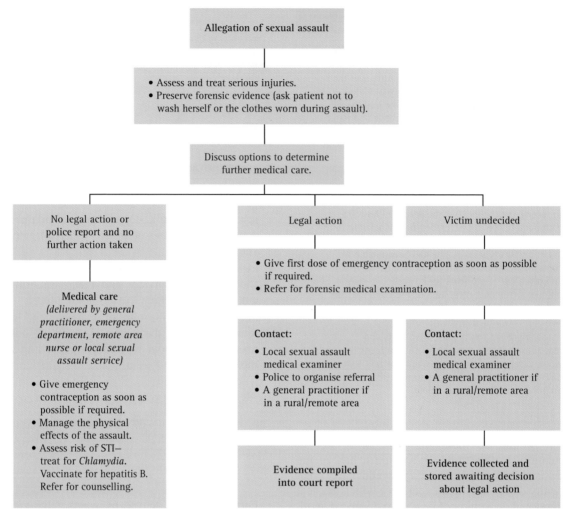

FIGURE 17.1 Flowchart for the management of sexual assault (From Mein et al[10])

What special consideration should be taken?

Taking a history, conducting an examination and undertaking the management of a patient who has undergone a sexual assault differs in many ways from a routine consultation. For a start, the emotional needs of the woman are paramount. The attending GP must ensure that the interview and subsequent examination takes place in a quiet, safe and private environment. Patient consent must be sought at every step of the consultation: history taking, physical examination, evidence collecting and photographing. This will help establish trust and confidence between the GP and the patient, and help the patient to regain some control over her circumstances. Box 17.1 summarises the needs of a sexual assault survivor.

Obtaining the history and performing the physical examination is time-consuming. Adequate time

should be scheduled, as at least 60 minutes will be required.

Lastly, when recording the history the GP should use terms such as 'alleged sexual assault', or 'sexual assault by history', not 'she was raped', as rape is not a medical term but rather a legal term and so should not enter the lexicon of a medical report.

How soon after the assault do women present?

The time when the patient is first seen in relation to the assault is highly variable. Sometimes women will present straight after they have been assaulted, but often there is a delay of days to weeks after the incident. This may be because of fear of retaliation, feeling too vulnerable to undergo 'questioning', or not wanting to be examined or 'labelled' as a rape victim. Often a woman will not present until friends or family members manage to convince her to report to authorities several days after the assault.

The timing of the history and examination in relation to the assault will have a great impact on the ability of a GP to collect evidence and to take action to prevent pregnancy and/or disease. Evidence collected more than 48–72 hours after an assault may be difficult to recover or may be invalid. It is important to explain this to the patient and to encourage her to proceed with examination and evidence collection at first presentation, so that even if she doesn't want to proceed with a police report at that time she has the option to do so later.

What key features of the history are important to document?

When taking a history from a woman who has been a victim/survivor of sexual assault, it is important to maintain a respectful and empathic attitude and to ask open-ended questions. Sometimes the patient may not be able to give a history or may have a friend or relative who tells part of the history if the woman is too upset. In these situations, it is important to record why the woman is unable to tell her story—for example she is too upset or crying uncontrollably. If others provide information, it is important to document this clearly. The issues listed in Box 17.2 should be covered and recorded in an objective fashion, as far as possible using the woman's own words.

Some features of the general medical history are also critical to record, as they may also impact on the long-term outcomes for the patient. These include:

- pre-existing medical conditions
- prescribed medications
- illicit drug use
- previous history of child abuse or sexual assault.

How and when should a physical examination be carried out?

After a sexual assault women often feel very fearful of undergoing a physical examination. This is understandable, so it is important to make the woman feel as in control of the situation as possible and to offer her the choice of a female doctor, should she want one. She should also be able to have a friend or relative present, if she so desires. The patient should be prepared and explanations given before beginning any examination or procedure and before moving from examination of one area of the body to another.[11]

The purpose of the physical examination is twofold: to assess the patient for physical injuries; and to collect evidence for forensic evaluation and possible legal proceedings. Physical examination and evidence collecting are therefore done congruently.

BOX 17.1 Needs of sexual assault survivors

Sexual assault survivors need:
- to be believed
- to be listened to
- their doctor to have a non-judgmental attitude
- to be supported
- validation of their experiences
- safety
- privacy
- to have control—especially over whether or not to undergo an examination or pursue legal prosecution
- confidentiality
- respect.

BOX 17.2 Important items to cover when taking a history from a woman who has been assaulted

- Number of assailants
- Age and identifying information for each assailant
- Date, time and location of the alleged assault
- Circumstances of the assault
- Details of sexual contact (such as penile, digital or object penetration) and route (such as vaginal, oral or anal intercourse), as well as documentation of any ejaculation or urination by the assailant
- Whether condoms were used
- Type of physical restraints used, such as weapons, drugs or alcohol
- Whether there was any other violent contact, such as punching or hitting
- Activities of the victim after the assault, such as change of clothing, bathing, douching, drinking/eating, dental hygiene, urination or defecation, or other sexual contact
- Gynaecological history—last menstrual period, contraceptive use, pregnancy history, last consensual sexual encounter, any recent episode of gynaecologic infection and pelvic surgery
- Time of history taking and examination

With consent, the physical examination involves assessment for physical injuries and the collection of evidence for forensic evaluation and possible legal proceedings.

Valuable evidence may be gathered from clothing that a woman was wearing at the time of the assault. Clothing can be collected up to 1 month after the incident, provided the items have not been laundered. Only the victim should handle her clothes. Items of clothing should be placed in paper bags, not plastic bags, since plastic may promote bacterial growth on blood or semen stains.[12]

If she presents immediately after the attack and has not changed or showered ask the woman to undress over a sheet or pieces of butcher's paper or newspaper so that anything that falls off the clothing can be collected.

When commencing the examination, the woman's general condition should be noted (particularly if she presents immediately after the attack), giving particular attention to her state of dress or undress, her demeanour and conscious state, whether she is orientated and whether her speech is normal.

The examination should then proceed in an orderly fashion, with non-threatening areas examined first in order to build trust and confidence. The presence of foreign bodies such as soil or grass should be noted as well as any injuries. The scalp, ears, face (nose, eyes, cheeks and lips) and mouth (tongue, throat, palate and teeth) are examined. Traumatic asphyxiation from choking may result in ruptured retinal vessels on ophthalmoscopy, and petechiae on the neck and head. Common signs of oral trauma include a torn frenulum of the upper lip, broken teeth, torn lingual frenulum and contusions of the uvula, hard and soft palate.[13]

Next examine the neck, trunk (chest, breasts, ribs and abdomen), upper limbs (including cubital fossae, hands, fingers and fingernails) and lower limbs looking for signs of extragenital trauma. The most commonly injured extragenital areas are the mouth, throat, wrist, arms, breasts and thighs.[14] Document the presence, size and location of bruises, lacerations, bite marks and scratches.

Examination of the genitalia should occur last, giving time for confidence to build in the patient. Take the time to cover the rest of the woman's body while doing this examination, so as to provide her with as much dignity as possible. It is important to conduct the genital examination in a routine fashion,

starting with the pubic area and noting the state of the vulva, perineum, introitus and posterior fourchette, the hymen, buttocks and anus, before doing a vaginal examination with a speculum (lubricated with warm water only) and examining the vaginal walls and cervix. Rape may not cause any obvious genital injury and it is important to remember that absence of genital injury does not imply consent or exclude penetration,[15] and that many women who have consensual sex can have small grazes or fissures at the posterior fourchette.

If the patient consents, photograph the area(s) of trauma, incorporating a size reference such as a ruler in the area being photographed. If consent is refused, diagrams can be used to record the location of any findings during the examination (Fig 17.2) and to describe the injuries as they are seen (e.g. grazes on both knees, scabbed and crusted).

It is important to warn the woman that contusions may not become visible for at least 48 hours.[16] She may like to return to see you for further examination and documentation of those injuries at that time.

How common are injuries in cases of sexual assault?

Retrospective studies of women attending an emergency department for management after sexual assault have found that injuries are present in about half of people reporting sexual assault, with non-genital injuries more common than genital injuries.[17–20] The absence of extragenital or genital trauma, however, does not mean that a sexual assault did not occur.

Box 17.3 lists some facts relating to sexual assault.

What specimens should be collected?

There is much confusion over what exactly needs to be collected for the purposes of evidence at future legal proceedings. However, it is really quite simple if the collection of evidence is separated from screening for STIs.

The swabs used for the collection of forensic specimens are plain cotton swabs, wetted with either

---

BOX 17.3 Some facts about sexual assault

- Weapons are used in only 9% of attacks.
- Approximately 40% occur in the victim's home.
- Nearly 90% are premeditated.
- In less than 20% there are multiple assailants.
- Rape occurs primarily between the hours of 8 pm and 2 am.

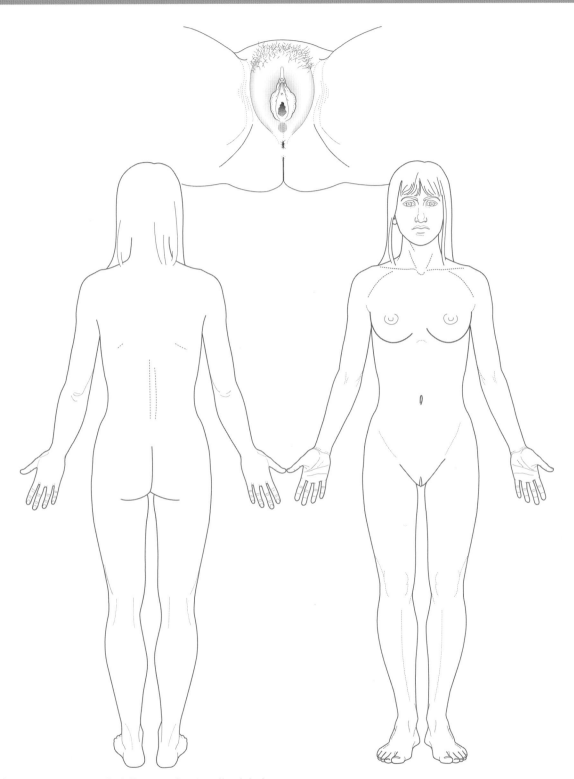

FIGURE 17.2 Anatomical diagrams for recording injuries

a little tap water or normal saline. These are rubbed on a part of the body (e.g. nipple, upper arm), a smear is made on a clean glass slide and both the smear and swab are then air-dried. The swab should not be placed in transport media.

All specimens must be appropriately labelled with the name of the patient, the date and time the specimen was collected and the site from which the specimen was taken. After packing in containers, the slide and swab are placed in a specimen bag, which should be sealed, preferably with a bradma or sticky label bearing the date and time and initialed by the doctor. Specimens should be refrigerated until collected by a police officer. When they are handed over, record the name of the officer taking the specimens and the time and date they are taken.

Swabs are generally taken from areas that have been directly affected by the rape. As part of evidence collection, the oral cavity should be swabbed. If oral penetration took place, swab the oropharynx for gonorrhoea testing[21] and the mouth for semen. Sperm have been recovered from the oral cavity up to six hours after an assault, even if the teeth were brushed or mouthwash was used.[22]

Scrapings should be collected from underneath all ten fingernails, because they may reveal skin, blood, hair, trace fibres and secretions that may help identify the assailant.[23] Pubic hair can be combed, and the hair and debris collected are placed in an envelope. Secretions pooled in the posterior fornix can be aspirated and placed in a sterile container.

What medical problems can arise from a sexual assault?

The exact risk of developing an STI after a sexual assault is difficult to quantify because:

- many women will have previously undetected disease
- many women are offered prophylactic antibiotics immediately after the sexual assault, potentially altering the incidence detected at follow-up visits.
- many women fail to return for follow-up and therefore fail to be diagnosed.[24]

The risk of transmission of STIs depends on the local prevalence of STIs (i.e. in the community to which the assailant(s) belong(s)), condom usage, the number of sexual contacts (assailants) and the nature of the sexual acts involved.[24] Risk is higher when the assault has involved penetrative sex and ejaculation. Genital and non-genital injuries may facilitate the transmission of blood-borne viruses.

The most common infections found in victims are those that are most prevalent in the general community—*Chlamydia*, *Trichomonas* and gonorrhoea.[24] There are reports of the transmission of HIV[25] and HBV[26] as a result of a sexual assault. The risk of HIV acquisition from one sexual encounter has been estimated at <1–2% (0.1–0.2% for receptive vaginal and 1–2% for penile–anal exposure).[27] Epidemiological studies indicate that high-risk assaults are those that include anal rape, trauma (including that resulting from sexual violence), bleeding, defloration or multiple assailants, and that high-risk assailants are those known to have HIV or risk factors, such as injecting drug users, men who have sex with men, or those from a high prevalence area for HIV.[28] Human papilloma virus may also be transmitted but becomes apparent only when visible genital warts emerge or on a Pap smear some months after the attack.

Risk of transmission of STIs as a result of a sexual assault depends on the local prevalence.

The other major risk to the woman is that of becoming pregnant as a result of the sexual assault. One study found an overall pregnancy rate of 5% per assault (the majority of pregnancies occurring in adolescent girls and young women usually in the context of family abuse or date rape).[29] The real risk of pregnancy, however, is dependent on the timing of the assault in relation to where the woman is in her menstrual cycle and whether there is concurrent use of long-acting contraceptives. A young woman who is vaginally assaulted between 6 days prior to ovulation and 1 day after ovulation and who is not currently using a non-coitus-dependent method of contraception (such as oral contraceptives, Depo-Provera®, implants or an IUD) may experience a pregnancy risk approaching 30%.[30]

What diagnostic tests should be carried out in relation to these risks?

When a woman presents immediately after a sexual assault, diagnostic testing is carried out in two phases. Initially, tests should be performed to ascertain if the woman is already pregnant or suffering from an STI. Follow-up testing weeks to months later will tell whether or not she has become pregnant or picked up an STI as a result of the assault. The testing schedule is given in Table 17.1.

TABLE 17.1 Screening recommendations for sexually transmissible infections (From Mein et al[10])

Infection	Test	Site (take specimen according to history)
HIV	HIV antibody	Blood
Hepatitis B	Hepatitis B surface antigen (HbsAg), core antibody (anti-HBc) and surface antibody (anti-HBs)	Blood
Syphilis	Rapid plasma reagin (RPR) + treponema pallidum haemagglutination assay (TPHA)	Blood
Chlamydia	Polymerase chain reaction	Endocervical swab, first-void urine or high vaginal swab
Gonorrhoea	Polymerase chain reaction or micros-copy, culture and sensitivity (M, C and S)	Endocervical swab, first-void urine, rectal swab* or throat swab*
Trichomonas	Microscopy, culture and sensitivity (M, C and S)	High vaginal swab

*M, C and S only, as PCR is not validated for these sites.

Can any preventive actions be offered?

Unfortunately only a small percentage of women return for follow-up after their initial contact with a doctor following a sexual assault. Because of this, and also in an effort to minimise the psychological sequelae of such attacks, prophylactic management is offered at the initial visit in an attempt to avoid pregnancy and/or the acquisition of an STI.

When should emergency contraception be offered?

Emergency contraception should be offered to all women who were not using contraception at the time of the assault. The most effective form of emergency contraception in this scenario consists of either levonorgestrel (if taken within the first 72 hours after the sexual assault) or the IUD, which can successfully prevent pregnancy up to 5 days after the assault. Further details about the regimens to use are given in the chapter on contraception. Just as for any woman using emergency contraception, follow-up is crucial, and a repeat urine pregnancy test should be carried out 2 weeks after her next bleed or approximately 6 weeks after the assault.

When should prophylaxis against STIs be offered?

GPs should offer prophylaxis for STIs if:

- there is evidence that the assailant was infected
- symptoms of infection are present on examination
- poor follow-up is anticipated
- the patient requests prophylaxis.

Because of the potential for serious consequences, the prophylaxis should be against gonorrhoea, *Chlamydia* and syphilis. Trichomoniasis should be treated only if seen on the wet mount examination.

If the patient was not previously immunised, hepatitis B virus vaccine should be given at the initial visit, then repeated at 1 and 6 months. Hepatitis B immune globulin should be reserved for use in patients who have been exposed within 14 days and who present with a high-risk exposure history, such as having an assailant who is a known intravenous drug user or having more than one assailant.

Pretest HIV counselling must be given. The theory behind treatment is to prevent infection by treating patients during a 'window of opportunity'. If the assailant cannot be apprehended and tested, as in most cases, the victim's infection status may not be known for several months. Not only may this delay foster anxiety and fear, but lifestyle changes may be necessary (e.g. need for condom use or abstaining from intercourse, postponing planned pregnancies, discontinuing breastfeeding). Therefore treatment must be made on a case-by-case basis, benefits must be weighed against lifestyle changes, and cost and potential drug toxicity must be considered. Table 17.2 (p 320) summarises the prophylactic medications that can be used.

What psychological sequelae can occur as a result of sexual assault?

The mental health effects of rape are profound. As early as 1974, a landmark study described the 'rape trauma syndrome', identifying rape as a predisposing cause of post-traumatic stress disorder (PTSD).[31] More recently sexual violence has been recognised as a 'trauma' that can precipitate an acute stress disorder as well as PTSD.

The mental health effects of rape are profound.

Acute stress reaction

This consists of:

- persistently re-experiencing the rape through thoughts, dreams and flashbacks, or distress on exposure to reminders of the assault

- symptoms of anxiety and increased arousal, such as insomnia, irritability, poor concentration, hypervigilance and exaggerated startle response
- dissociative symptoms, such as reduced emotional responsiveness, numbness, a reduction in awareness and contact with surroundings, derealisation, depersonalisation and difficulty recalling part or all of the assault.[32]

Post-traumatic stress disorder

If symptoms occur or continue beyond 1 month, the patient has post-traumatic stress disorder. PTSD is an anxiety disorder that is precipitated by a trauma. The essential feature of PTSD is that its development is anchored to a traumatic event of an extreme nature. Most survivors of trauma will develop an acute core constellation of PTSD symptoms: re-experiencing, avoidance and arousal. PTSD is diagnosed if these symptoms, together with social and occupational impairment, persist 4 weeks beyond the trauma itself. The DSM-IV-TR criteria for a diagnosis of PTSD are given in Box 17.4.

Unfortunately the prevalence of PTSD is high after rape. The immediate consequence of rape is that 95% of the victims develop PTSD symptoms within 1 to 2 weeks of the crime. At 3 months post rape, nearly half continue to meet PTSD criteria.[33]

Are there any other health effects of sexual assault?

Women who have been sexually assaulted often present further down the track with a range of symptoms and conditions such as dyspareunia, pelvic pain, irritable bowel symptoms, weight management issues, premenstrual disorder symptoms, migraine headaches or fibromyalgia.[34–37] Few women make the connection between the violence they have experienced in their lives and their current symptoms, with many feeling that the trauma has no bearing on the present complaint.[38]

Victims of sexual assault can also develop psychiatric conditions other than PTSD, such as depression, anxiety, somatisation, obsessive

---

TABLE 17.2 Suggested prophylaxis for sexually transmissible infections (treatment for high risk is shown in bold type) (From Mein et al[10])

STI	Treatment
Chlamydia	Azithromycin (1 g orally)
Hepatitis B	Hepatitis B vaccine (1 mL intramuscularly)
	For high risk add: hepatitis B immune globulin (400 IU intramuscularly*)
Gonorrhoea (only if high risk)	Ceftriaxone (250 mg intramuscularly)
	OR, where local gonococcal sensitivities permit: 20 ciprofloxacin (500 mg orally)
	OR: amoxycillin (3 g orally) and probenecid (1 g orally)
Syphilis (if high risk)	Benzathine penicillin (1.8 g intramuscularly)
HIV (if high risk)	Phone local infectious diseases or sexual health physician urgently
Other STIs	Consult local infectious diseases or sexual health physician

*Available from Commonwealth Serum Laboratories
STI = sexually transmitted infection

BOX 17.4 The DSM-IV-TR criteria for a diagnosis of post-traumatic stress disorder (From American Psychiatric Association[32])

There must be a traumatic event that meets the following (criterion A):
- The person experiences or witnesses an event involving actual or threatened death or injury, or threat to physical integrity of self or others, considered to be outside the range of normal human experience.
- The person's response involves intense fear, helplessness or horror.

There must also be symptoms from each of the following three categories:
- re-experiencing (recurrent, intrusive distressing thoughts, images, dreams, flashbacks, psychological reactivity) (criterion B)
- avoidance/numbing (active avoidance of trauma-related thoughts, feelings, activities, loss of interest, detachment from others, numbed feelings, foreshortened future) (criterion C)
- Increased arousal (sleep disturbance, irritability, concentration problems, hypervigilance, and exaggerated startle response) (criterion D).

Symptom duration: symptoms must persist for more than 1 month and cause clinically significant distress or impairment in personal, social and occupational functioning.

compulsive disorder, panic, paranoia, substance use disorders, eating disorders and borderline personality disorder.[39-44] Sexual dysfunction is also a relatively common occurrence after a sexual assault.[45]

What kind of follow-up should there be?

Because of the immediate concerns generated by a sexual assault (injuries, pregnancy, STIs and acute distress) and the long-term consequences of sexual assault, GPs should stay involved in the care of the patient and offer follow-up. Initially this should occur a couple of days after the attack and then at 1, 3, 6 and 12 months for hepatitis B/HIV follow-up. While GPs can offer supportive counselling and advice about medical issues, the patient can also be referred for cognitive behaviour therapy, which is recommended by management guidelines for post-traumatic stress disorder no matter how much time has passed since the trauma occurred.[46] If, however, the degree of psychological trauma is more extensive, professional long-term psychiatric care can be planned.[11]

Summary of key points
- The role of the GP in cases of sexual assault is to:
  - assess and treat all injuries
  - collect forensic evidence
  - identify and prevent STIs
  - assist in the prevention of pregnancy
  - minimise psychological sequelae.

- Acquiring patient consent and building up trust and confidence are paramount when undertaking forensic examinations of survivors of sexual assault.
- After a sexual assault, many women suffer from an acute stress reaction, which may persist and develop into PTSD.

INTIMATE PARTNER VIOLENCE

Why should doctors be concerned about intimate partner violence?

Intimate partner violence (IPV) is, unfortunately, an all too common event in our society, resulting in significant morbidity and sometimes mortality. Women look to their family doctor for support and assistance, seeing their GP as someone they can trust and who may be able to have some impact on their situation. Doctors therefore have a critical role to play in the identification, treatment and prevention of IPV. Through early intervention and appropriate referral we can contribute to:

- the prevention of damaging effects to victims and other family members of continuing and escalating violence
- limiting the likelihood of the repetition of violence in future generations
- reducing the health consequences and therefore the costs associated with chronic IPV.

CASE STUDY: 'You can't blame it on the alcohol this time'

Margaret had booked a 10-minute appointment. She was in her 50s and well groomed. Margaret had been married to Richard for 27 years, had two grown children and had helped her husband in the family business. She recalled that he had been physically violent towards her at the commencement of the marriage but that this had settled down after a while. Last year, the violence had recommenced and she decided to leave the marriage. That was when things became worse. She had left and gone to live with her daughter. Richard was desperate for reconciliation and had asked her to talk to him over dinner. She noted that he had drunk only half a glass of wine with his meal. When they arrived back at their daughter's house, however, he had grabbed her in a headlock and threatened her, saying he was going to kill her. He slammed her head against the car window and the dashboard and laughed as he said she couldn't blame it on the alcohol this time. She finally managed to get out of the car, and as she ran across the driveway he drove the car into her knocking her to the ground.

Margaret talked for 45 minutes. She told her GP of her efforts to get an intervention order and that this was not renewed and that he had assaulted her again 2 weeks later. She related how her husband had threatened to commit suicide and how her son (who worked with his father) was pressuring her to go back to the marriage, and she cried through the entire consultation. All this had come about 18 months after being diagnosed with breast cancer and having a lumpectomy.

Margaret was clearly not coping. She felt confused, paralysed with indecision and very threatened. Her solicitor had told her that she may need antidepressants and she had come to ascertain whether this was the case. On questioning, she disclosed tearfulness, apathy, lack of appetite and loss of weight. She was unable to sleep, felt like she was 'losing it' and that it was all her fault. Clearly the antidepressants were a viable option, but Margaret needed more help than just medication.

How common is IPV?

Intimate partner violence occurs 'behind closed doors'. For many years it was thought to be an issue between a husband and a wife, a private matter. Research conducted over the last 20 years, however, has made us understand just how common IPV really is. Community-based surveys indicate that up to 1 in 4 women have experienced IPV.[47,48] Between 5% and 20% of women attending general practice report experiencing IPV in the last year.[9,49,50] Less than one-fifth of these had discussed the issue with their doctor,[9] an indication of the vast amount of under-reporting in this area.

The prevalence of IPV in women attending other healthcare settings is similarly high. In large prospective emergency department studies, 37–54% of women seen in the emergency department had been abused by an intimate partner at some point in their lives.[51,52] In one of these studies, 11% of the women seen in an emergency department presented as a result of acute abuse.[51] In studies of pregnant women, estimates of prevalence of abuse during pregnancy range from 0.9 to 20.1% (with most studies finding 4–8%).[53]

What barriers exist to diagnosing the signs and symptoms of IPV?

Unfortunately, despite the high prevalence of IPV found in our patients, doctors consistently fail to recognise it. This means that the entity of IPV remains hidden and disguised, with little chance of being exposed and then treated.

> Despite the high prevalence of IPV among our patients, doctors consistently fail to recognise it.

Considering the chronic nature of IPV, it is important that each incident that raises a doctor's suspicion of the diagnosis is recorded for future reference. When patients do not disclose, it may be only when the doctor sees that they have several entries of presentations suggestive of IPV that they put the puzzle together and make the diagnosis. It is even more important that this happens where doctors are working in group practice or in the hospital setting, because when a diagnosis of abuse

---

CASE STUDY: 'He'll never do this to me again.'

Sandy was a 34-year-old woman with a 5-year-old son. She had separated some months ago and today had gone to pick up her son (who was on an access visit) at the agreed time from her ex-husband's house. With their son watching, her ex had thrown her to the ground, bashed her head to the ground repeatedly, punched her in the face and picked her up and thrown her against a wall. During the assault Sandy had crashed against a window that broke and cut her wrist. As she drove her car out of the driveway while getting away, she had hit her ex-husband's car. The next thing she knew the police were at her door laying charges against her for wilful damage to her ex-husband's property. They must have seen the bruises and injuries on her face and neck but they did not help her by taking a statement about the violence she had experienced nor did they put her in touch with the branch of the police who may have been able to assist her.

It is not for a GP to judge whether or not there was provocation involved, but rather to deal with the situation that you are confronted with. In Sandy's case, she had attended a local GP in an attempt to get her injuries seen to and to obtain any medical care necessary. To her surprise, having told the GP how she had sustained the injuries, she was asked to leave. The GP said he did not want to get involved in the situation.

Sandy was in need of medical assessment. When she finally undressed in front of another GP for an examination (some 24 hours after the incident had occurred), the bruising was evident. She had bruises over her cheek, jaw and breasts, scratches on her arms and legs and classic finger-grip bruising on her upper arms. Her neck was in spasm and she had a cut consistent with the window break over her forearm.

The GP's task was clear: to document these injuries carefully, as this would be the only testament to the incident that would be objective in court. Sandy was a pretty tough lady. She had lots of support from her sister and parents, had found a solicitor and was going to take out an intervention order that afternoon. The GP voiced concern for the welfare of her son, who had been witness to the assault. She explained that she had already mentioned this to the solicitor, who had advised that this would be taken into account in the access orders.

As she left Sandy said, 'Don't worry about me, Doc, I'm okay. He'll never do this to me again. I've got my family helping me now and I'll get all the legal stuff sorted out. I just feel sorry for all the other women out there. I couldn't get the police to help and the doctor turned me away. If it was hard for me, then God help them'.

is missed, treatment is likely to be inappropriate and potentially harmful.[54]

In one study of a family practice in which the prevalence of IPV was 7% for physical abuse and 23% for emotional abuse, only 1% of doctors' files documented the abuse.[55] In another study of 492 patients who completed a questionnaire after presenting at a hospital emergency department (ED), 22% admitted to being victims of IPV, but ED records identified only 5% of these victims.[56] It may be that some doctors, even if aware of the abuse experienced by their patients, still fail to document it. However, documentation is essential for the patient in case legal action ensues.

The most common reasons given by doctors for failure to uncover IPV are patient unresponsiveness, lack of physician initiative and infrequent visits by the patients.[57] Doctors perceive spouse abuse to be a complex and multifaceted problem.[58] Many feel powerless to deal with IPV and fear that in broaching the subject they are 'opening Pandora's box'.[59]

In some cases the close identification by doctors with patients of similar background may preclude the consideration of IPV as a differential diagnosis.[59] For some doctors, especially female ones, IPV may feel too close for comfort, with some practitioners having experienced IPV themselves or in their extended family. Dealing with patients' intimate partner violence issues therefore exposes their own fear of vulnerability and lack of control.[59]

Lack of training of doctors in the area of IPV,[59,60] makes it difficult to overcome a fear of offending patients by asking questions about a subject culturally defined as 'private'.[59] Some feel reluctant to accept a patient's claims of IPV without corroboration from an outside source.[59] For many, the tyranny of short consultations and a tight schedule make them feel that they will be unable to cope with the demands of disclosure.[49,58]

How can GPs conceptualise IPV in such a way that they approach it in a more constructive fashion?

It is important to acknowledge that most GPs will feel a sense of powerlessness when dealing with IPV and feel that intervention is useless and unrewarding. We tend to feel out of control when dealing with this issue, as we try to squeeze it into 10-minute consultations and still achieve positive outcomes. Enormous frustration arises from the fact that few of our patients leave the violent relationships they are in, despite our urgings for them to do so.

GPs may find it helpful to conceptualise IPV as a chronic disease, in which a GP can't cure the problem but can be supportive of the woman.

One way to overcome these feelings is to conceptualise IPV as a chronic disease. In this way we can accept the fact that the woman may be dealing with this problem for many years or even perhaps all her life. It allows us to recharacterise our role from a curative one to a supportive one. We can ask the patient to involve other professionals such as lawyers, social workers and psychologists, in a multidisciplinary way. This spreads the burden of care, as well as enabling the GP to get support or to 'debrief' with another professional who knows about the case.

Why does it happen?

Intimate partner violence is an abuse of power. It is the domination, coercion, intimidation and victimisation of one person by another by physical, sexual or emotional means within an intimate relationship.[61] While the causes are complex (Table 17.3), two factors seem to be necessary in an epidemiological sense: the unequal position of women in a particular relationship (and in society) and the normative use of violence in conflict.[62]

Societies exist in which violence is rare and violence against women virtually non-existent. Low-violence cultures share certain key characteristics,

TABLE 17.3 Causes of intimate partner violence (Adapted from Zolotor et al[100])

Level	Risk factors
The individual victim[118, 119,120]	Female gender, young age, history of IPV, history of sexual assault, history of child abuse victimisation, heavy alcohol or drug use, unemployment, depression, and racial or ethnic minority status
The relationship[121]	Income or educational disparity and male control of relationship (psychological or economical)
The community[122]	Poverty, poor social cohesion and weak sanctions, including minimal legal penalties or rare successful prosecutions
The society at large	Traditional gender norms and general acceptance of violence for conflict resolution.

which include strong sanctions against interpersonal violence, community support for victims, flexible gender roles for women and men, equality of decision making and resources in the family, a cultural ethos that condemns violence as a means of resolving conflict, and female power and autonomy outside the home.[63]

What are the health consequences of IPV?

Despite the fact that so few incidents reputedly involve medical intervention, IPV has been shown to have many important adverse effects on the physical and mental health of women, both acutely and in the long term (Box 17.5).

General health and use of medical care

Women often have to wait long periods of time before seeking medical attention. Their partner may prevent them from leaving the house for fear that someone might find out about the violence he has perpetrated.

Women also use non-trauma services more frequently for treatment of the consequences of IPV. These include psychiatric services, women's clinics and after-hours clinics. This might be because of the inability to access trauma services or because they are fearful of drawing attention to themselves and the nature of the injuries. They may not to go to their own family doctor because they are embarrassed, or fear disclosure or lack of confidentiality.

Several surveys have now looked at the types of symptoms and symptom complexes suffered by victims of IPV compared with those experienced by other women.[64–68] The symptoms more commonly found in battered women are:

- low levels of general health
- a great number of symptoms overall
- digestive problems such as diarrhoea, constipation, nausea and 'spastic colon'
- loss of appetite, eating binges and bulimia
- abdominal pain
- pelvic pain
- headaches and migraines
- fainting spells
- back pain and chronic neck pain.

Compared with non-victims, victimised women report more distress and less wellbeing, make physician visits twice as frequently and incur 2.5 times greater outpatient costs.[69]

Frequent attendance with non-specific symptoms should alert GPs to the possibility of intimate partner violence.

> **BOX 17.5 The health consequences of intimate partner violence**
>
> **General health problems**
> - Lower levels of general health
> - A greater number of symptoms overall
> - Digestive problems such as diarrhoea, constipation, nausea and 'spastic colon'
> - Loss of appetite, eating binges and bulimia
> - Abdominal pain
> - Pelvic pain
> - Headaches and migraines
> - Fainting spells
> - Back pain and chronic neck pain
>
> **Injuries**
> More commonly seen on the chest, abdomen, face, head and neck
> Multiple injuries are more common than isolated ones
>
> **Reproductive health**
> - Sexually transmitted diseases
> - Vaginal bleeding and infection
> - Decreased sexual desire
> - Genital irritation
> - Pain on intercourse
> - Chronic pelvic pain
> - Urinary tract infection
> - Pregnancy complications
>   - Increased unwanted or unplanned pregnancies and terminations
>   - Increased risk of: having poor weight gain, anaemia, infections or preterm labour; bearing a low-birth-weight infant; experiencing postnatal depression
>   - More likely to engage in behaviours harmful to health, such as smoking, drinking excessive amounts of alcohol and substance misuse
>
> **Mental health**
> - Increased number of suicide attempts
> - Poor mental health status
> - Depression and anxiety
> - Somatisation
> - Post-traumatic stress disorder
> - Drug and alcohol abuse

Suicide and homicide

At the most extreme end of the spectrum, IPV can result in death. Between 40% and 60% of murders of women are undertaken by intimate partners,[70,71] a figure that may well be higher in less-industrialised countries. Murder is most likely to occur when women attempt separation. In addition, women who have been in abusive relationships are also more likely to commit suicide or to attempt it.[72]

Injuries

Battered women are more likely to have injuries to their chest and abdomen as well as to their face, head and neck.[73] In contrast, non-abusive injuries occur more commonly to the extremities—the hands, forearms, feet and knees. The battered woman is also likely to have multiple injuries rather than isolated ones. GPs often fail to see the extent of injuries suffered by battered women because the site of the injuries is concealed by make-up or clothing.

Injuries as a result of physical abuse are more likely to be central (chest, abdomen, head and neck) and multiple.

Reproductive health

Gynaecological problems—the most consistent, longest lasting and largest physical health difference between battered and non-battered women[74]—are three times more prevalent in victims of IPV than in other women.[67] The problems suffered include sexually transmissible infections, vaginal bleeding and infection, decreased sexual desire, genital irritation, pain on intercourse, chronic pelvic pain and urinary tract infection.[67,68,75,76]

Sexual abuse frequently goes hand in hand with physical abuse in relationships characterised by IPV. In these situations there is often a recurring history of forced sex as well as verbal sexual denigration, refusal to use condoms and refusal to allow the woman to use other forms of contraception,[77] leading to a higher prevalence of sexually transmissible infections, HIV and unintended pregnancies in IPV victims.[78,79]

Pregnancy is a time when women are at high risk of IPV. When women are asked at an interview in the third trimester of pregnancy, the prevalence ranges from 7.4 to 20.1%.[53] Such violence has an enormous impact, not only on the mother but also on the developing fetus, and may translate into later child abuse or indeed fetal or infant mortality.[80] The strongest predictor of violence occurring during pregnancy is a prior history of abuse.[81] Furthermore, women abused during pregnancy are at even greater risk of violence in the postpartum period.[82]

Pregnancy is a time when women are at high risk of intimate partner violence.

The number of unwanted or unplanned pregnancies and terminations is higher among women experiencing IPV.[83,84] Those who continue with their pregnancy often obtain minimal or late antenatal care.[85,86] They are at increased risk of having poor weight gain, anaemia, infections, preterm labour, bearing a low-birth-weight infant and experiencing postnatal depression.[85] They are also more likely to engage in behaviours harmful to health, such as smoking, drinking excessive amounts of alcohol and substance misuse.[87] All of these consequences may be involved in developing the weak but significant relationship between violence experienced in pregnancy and low birth weight.[88]

Mental health

Many GPs have already made the connection (confirmed by research) that IPV results in an increased prevalence of poor mental health status,[68] depression, anxiety, somatisation[89] and post-traumatic stress disorder (PTSD).[90] Depression and PTSD, which have substantial comorbidity, are the most prevalent mental health sequelae of IPV, together with drug and alcohol abuse.[91]

The direct effect of IPV on the mental health of women can become confused with the long-term psychological impact of childhood forms of abuse,[92] which many women also suffer. One study examining the contributions of both childhood and adulthood victimisation found that past childhood abuse and current adulthood abuse were equivalently associated with more physical symptoms, higher scores for depression, anxiety, somatisation, low self-esteem, and higher rates of attempted suicide and substance abuse. Women who had experienced childhood abuse and who were also experiencing current adulthood abuse had the highest levels of these poor health outcomes.[93]

How does IPV present in general practice?

Intimate partner violence presents in general practice in the form of the symptoms and symptom complexes described above. Few women will present to their GP and spontaneously disclose the existence of IPV in their relationship. Patients are reluctant to disclose violence unless they are specifically asked about it.[9] This may be because of fear, denial and disbelief, emotional bonds to their partner, commitment to marriage, hope for change, staying for the sake of the children, 'normalisation' of violence, social isolation, depression, stress, and feeling that they will not be believed or that services will not be able to help.[94,95]

Few present to police or IPV services in the first instance.[96] They are more likely to seek help from family or friends, general practitioners, personal and relationship counsellors, child specialists, psychiatrists, teachers, hospital staff, solicitors, family support services, self-help groups, church representatives or charity organisations.[95] Rather than seeking help for their symptoms, many women seek assistance with what they perceive as the reason behind the abuse (e.g. marital conflict, their partner's mental health, a drug and alcohol or gambling problem) or want information about how to deal with the violence.[95]

GPs should think about intimate partner violence in women who:

- are under 40 years of age
- have a past history of child abuse or have a child who is currently being abused
- have gone through recent separation or divorce
- are socially isolated
- have an accompanying partner who is overattentive
- present frequently
- delay in seeking treatment or are non-compliant.[97]

Another reason for GPs to suspect a history of IPV is if they find themselves wanting to write out a prescription for psychotropic medication, as women who have experienced severe violence in the past year are 2.8 times more likely to have used a psychotropic medication during that time.[98]

General practice as an opportunity

General practice provides a safe, confidential and powerful opportunity to confront IPV. Unlike when using IPV services, women do not have to identify themselves to others as 'battered' when they go to see their GP. Visiting a doctor is also a socially acceptable way of seeking help, and less likely to draw the attention of the perpetrator. GPs are also in an ideal position to offer help to the woman. In most cases, the woman and her family are probably well known to the GP, who should also be familiar with the local services that can assist the woman, should she wish it.

General practice provides a safe, confidential and powerful opportunity to confront intimate partner violence.

Should I be screening for IPV among my patients?

Because the prevalence of IPV is relatively high and the consequences so significant, many organisations—including the American Medical Association, American Academy of Family Physicians, and American College of Obstetricians and Gynecologists—have advocated routine screening for IPV in primary-care settings. In contrast, the US Preventive Services Task Force (USPSTF) gave screening for IPV

> a recommendation of level I (insufficient evidence), citing methodologic problems with many studies and lack of proved efficacy of interventions to assist patients (successful intervention for IPV in adults was defined as shelter use or leaving the abusive relationship).[99]

Many are critical of the UPSTF approach, however, saying that, although evidence does not exist to prove definitively that knowing about IPV reduces harm, common sense and prior experience suggest that knowing about such a difficult, potentially dangerous situation would be helpful towards understanding and assisting patients with health problems and may even prevent needless deaths.[100]

In line with this approach, more recent guidelines[101] recommend that family practitioners routinely ask all pregnant adult and adolescent women about partner violence, but otherwise ask only patients with symptoms of partner violence and those with symptoms of abusive behaviour (case finding). This is because of the high prevalence in pregnant women and adolescents, the opportunities for early intervention provided by regular antenatal checkups, the particular risks to pregnant women and potential adverse pregnancy outcomes.

In practice, screening may produce several benefits:

- The fact that she is being asked about IPV suggests to the woman that the GP will be sympathetic if she discloses.
- Often patients do not make a connection between the abuse they are suffering and the health problems they present with. Detecting IPV makes the connection clearer for the doctor who can then explain the aetiology of the symptoms to the patient.
- Screening and detection lessens the chance of inappropriate management being instituted.
- It allows for the protection of children who are at risk of abuse.

Screening for intimate partner violence makes the woman aware that the GP is interested in hearing about intimate partner violence. It also alerts her to the fact that there may be a connection between her health problems and the violence she is experiencing and allows for the protection of children who are at risk of abuse.

Interestingly women are very supportive of screening, with 77% in favour of routine screening about IPV by their own GP.[103] Qualitative studies are clear about women's preferences in relation to IPV screening, as indicated in Box 17.6.

What screening questions should a GP ask?

While different questionnaires, whether delivered at interview or in written form, have been tested by researchers, women respond best when asked direct questions and when screening occurs in a private, confidential and face-to-face encounter.[105]

Screening can take place when a GP meets a patient for the first time, or the opportunity can be taken with the occurrence of a new life event, such as when the doctor becomes aware of the fact that the patient has entered into a new relationship or has become pregnant. GPs should also screen if they are suspicious that intimate partner violence is occurring.

It is often helpful to frame the questions in a way that normalises the fact that you are asking about IPV. Here are some examples.

- I ask all my patients about violence in their relationships; does your partner ever hit you, hurt you or threaten you?
- I want to make sure that each of my patients is safe in her/his relationships. Does anyone you know ever hit you, hurt you or threaten you?

Screening for IPV—smoking as an analogy[102]

When primary-care physicians routinely ask about smoking as part of patient history taking, they do not do so in the belief that asking the question will stop their patients from smoking. Instead, knowledge of smoking status may guide the physician to undertake more frequent monitoring of cardiovascular and pulmonary health status, including measurement of blood pressure, evaluation of exercise tolerance and so on. Similarly, asking about IPV and obtaining a positive response identifies an opportunity for prevention of health-related sequelae.

BOX 17.6 Expectations of healthcare providers by women exposed to intimate partner violence (From Feder et al[104])

Women want healthcare professionals to:
- be non-judgmental and compassionate and keep confidentiality
- understand the complex, long-term nature of IPV and to understand its social and psychological ramifications
- to avoid medicalising the issue and to raise it in a confident, unrushed manner
- confirm that the violence was unacceptable and undeserved and that abuse was not their fault
- bolster their confidence and allow them to progress at their own pace
- avoid putting them under pressure to disclose, leave the relationship or press charges
- allow them to share in decision making

- Feeling that a person close to you does not respect you or treat you well can be so difficult. How do your partner/family members treat you?

Other examples of direct questions include:

- Does your partner ever hit you, hurt you or threaten you in any way?
- Has your partner ever forced you to have sex when you didn't want to?
- Are you ever frightened of your partner?
- Has anyone ever hit you, hurt you or threatened you in the past?

Less direct but sometimes helpful are the following:

- What happens when you and your partner disagree? How do you settle disagreements?
- How do you feel your partner/family members treat you?
- Tell me more about your home environment.
- Do you feel safe at home?

Patients who are being abused may still choose not to disclose, despite being asked. GPs should not feel disheartened by this, nor should they feel that it is a negative outcome if they suspect that the woman is being battered. The fact that the woman has been asked will register with her and she may disclose at a subsequent visit. She may also discuss the fact that she was asked about IPV by her GP with friends or family, thereby helping to bring this issue more into the open.

She has just disclosed that her partner beats her. What then?

Follow-up after disclosure involves assessment of the patient, intervention and documentation (Box 17.7).

A GP's role in dealing with patients who are experiencing intimate partner violence involves detection and provision of support, education, safety planning and referral.

After disclosure the doctor should assess the immediate risk of homicide or injury (including the perpetrator's use of and access to weapons), degree of readiness for change and safety of children (after explaining limits of confidentiality). The patient should also be examined if there has been an acute violent event.

Intervention involves four major components:

- showing support
- providing education
- safety planning
- referral.

How can a GP show support?

One study asking women what was the most important feature of their encounter with healthcare providers found that it was validation of their

---

BOX 17.7 Guideline recommendations for the management of intimate partner violence in general practice (From Victorian Government Department of Justice[101])

Initial response
- Acknowledge and validate disclosure.
- Express the unacceptability of any abusive behaviour but not of the patient. Encourage a patient who has disclosed their abuse of a partner to take responsibility for their behaviour and change.
- Ensure and emphasise confidentiality within limits of harm to herself or others. Monitor personal and professional attitudes to patient and patient's partner for management bias.
- Offer education and support.

Safety
- If previously seeing the couple, consider referring one partner to a colleague.
- Assess the patient's safety and the risk of harm to themselves and others.
- Assess whether anyone else is using abusive behaviour against an abused woman.
- Ask about any weapons.
- Discuss a basic safety plan with abused patients.

Children and parenting
- Discuss any parenting concerns in the partner-abuse context.
- Assess the risk to and adult perception of the impact on the children.
- Consider the risk to the children's lives and children's perception of the impact on their lives.
- Consider the children's access to significant supportive others.
- Offer referral of the children to therapeutic support services.

- Report children at risk according to mandatory laws.
- Consider the patient's level of fear about the children's removal.
- Assess patient's level of social support.
- Offer options for referrals (including referral of certain types of men who abuse to accredited behaviour change programs when available).
- Do not offer couple counselling in the practice.
- Provide ongoing monitoring of the woman, her partner and their children for safety and progress.

Documentation
- Document comprehensively and carefully.
- Ensure that posters and leaflets in the clinic waiting area offer support and referral for patients.
- Seek own and staff family violence training for management of all family members experiencing partner violence.
- Ensure that the patient's file is confidential and cannot be accessed by other family members.
- Use a clinic protocol for monitoring danger to the patient and other family members by any clinician seeing patient.
- Ensure that quality assurance and accreditation includes the needs and confidentiality of these patients.
- Ensure that staff safety protocol includes the risk from and needs of these patients.
- Ensure interagency collaboration for the benefit of the patient, her partner and their children.

experience. Validation provided 'relief' and 'comfort', 'planted a seed' and 'started the wheels turning' towards changing the way they perceived their situations and moving them towards safety.[106]

Immediately after disclosure the GP should praise the patient. This might sound strange, but it takes a lot of courage for women (or men) to divulge this kind of information to a stranger, even to a doctor. It may feel natural to take her hand in yours, look her in the eye and tell her what great courage she is showing in talking openly about the violence she has experienced. She should be told that she is very strong if she has dealt with all of this alone to date and that this strength will sustain her.

What education can a GP provide?

Next reassure the woman about how common these problems are. Explain that IPV always occurs 'behind closed doors', that no one acknowledges its existence but that doctors, and especially GPs, see it all too commonly in women from all social, economic and ethnic backgrounds. One useful way to express this is to tell the woman how many other women you have seen that week suffering in similar circumstances. If the woman has children, it is important to make her aware of how IPV can affect children.

> Explain to women that intimate partner violence is a very common problem.

Many myths exist among women and in society in general about the nature of IPV; it is important to try to demystify the area by explaining to women how violence is a tool used to obtain power in relationships, not an irrational act that is uncontrollable. When consulting, it may be helpful to use an anecdote to convey this message. It involves burly policemen. Tell the woman, 'You may think that he is out of control when he is being violent towards you, but what do you think he would do if in the middle of the violence five burly policemen walked into the room?' Usually the woman responds, 'He would probably stop'. Then say, 'Exactly … so it is under his control, isn't it?'

The issue of responsibility is the hardest message to get across to patients involved in IPV situations, whether you are talking to the victim or the perpetrator. It is important to make a woman understand that her partner needs to take responsibility for his/her violence before it will stop. Aggressive and violent behaviour will not stop in a week and may not stop in a month. It may take several months or years before change occurs, if it ever does. The cessation of behaviours associated with the violence, such as gambling or drinking, may assist, but this is no guarantee that the violence will end.

How can a GP help with safety planning?

The third issue that needs to be dealt with during the consultation is the woman's safety and that of any children who may be involved. A woman is generally very aware of the degree of danger she is in and you need to get an accurate assessment of this. If she feels acutely threatened, it is best to call a refuge or women's shelter and get the woman to safety immediately. This can be arranged by ringing the refuge directly during the consultation. If there is less danger, then perhaps staying with family or friends may be sufficient. Another alternative is to seek legal advice about the availability of intervention orders that can be obtained through a court. A woman should be made aware that the time of departure from a violent relationship is the time when she and her children are in the greatest danger of harm from her partner and she needs to be prepared for this, preferably by always being in the company of another adult or someone who can offer some protection.

> The time of departure from a violent relationship is the time when a woman and her children are in the greatest danger of harm from her partner.

While it may be useful to provide written information to the patient, GPs should always ask the patient if it is safe for her to take the information home. If found by the perpetrator, the written material may provoke further violence.

Why is documentation important?

One of the most important duties a GP can undertake in IPV cases is to document accurately the circumstances of the woman and any injuries she has sustained. Not only will this provide the woman with one of few available sources of evidence, should the matter become a legal one, but it will also inform all providers who are in contact with the patient and the medical record of this crucial health problem. This is especially important for those GPs working in a group practice or large clinic, when the patient may out of necessity see one of the other health practitioners working in the practice.

What is the relationship between IPV and child abuse?

The likelihood of co-existent child abuse in families where there is IPV is high,[107,108] and children can be affected both physically (being subject to physical and sexual violence) and mentally (from verbal abuse or neglect, being witness to the violence or its after-effects or by feeling guilty or in some way responsible for the fact that they cannot stop the violence). Primary-care providers are, in some ways, uniquely poised to consider the dynamics of family violence in an entire family unit. In some cases, the best interests of the child and parent victims may not be served in the same way.[100]

If child abuse is clearly present and the non-offending parent has been unable to improve her own or her chidlren's safety, GPs are obliged to report the matter to child protection services.[109]

What if the perpetrator is also my patient?

This scenario arises commonly in general practice when a family has been seeing one GP on a regular basis. Having both the victim and perpetrator as patients does not present a conflict of interest, however. Both patients have a right to autonomy, confidentiality, honesty and quality care. Patients should be dealt with independently. Physicians should not discuss the possibility of domestic abuse with the male partner without the prior consent of the abused female partner. Joint counselling is generally inadvisable. If the physician feels unable to deal effectively with either patient because of the dual relationship, referral to another qualified physician is preferred.[110] Confidentiality becomes critical if the woman has disclosed and is fearful of her partner finding out (with the caveat that if children are being abused their rights to protection are paramount).

GPs should not discuss the possibility of domestic abuse with the male partner without the prior consent of the abused female partner.

In some cases the woman will ask the GP to engage her male partner in discussion about his violent behaviour. This can be done in a number of ways.[111] Patients can be asked directly if they have trouble with anger or whether they have done anything when angry that they later regretted. This type of question can be incorporated into questions about general lifestyle issues such as smoking and drug/alcohol use.[112] Opportunities such as when male patients make non-specific comments about their female partners can also be used. Placing written information about local perpetrator-treatment programs in the waiting rooms or as posters behind toilet doors may also spur patients to discuss their behaviours.

GPs can feel extraordinarily reluctant to raise IPV issues with known perpetrators, but ignoring it is essentially acting in collusion with the perpetrator and is not a neutral action.[111] Few perpetrators will identify IPV as their problem. In most cases, they will deny it or try to minimise it, and their behaviour is notoriously difficult to change.[113]

Often men are motivated to change their violent behaviour when they realise it may be affecting their children. Counselling perpetrators of IPV should therefore include explanations as to how persistent fear and threats of violence adversely affect the physical, emotional, behavioural, cognitive and social aspects of child development.[114]

What about perpetrator-treatment programs?

Often perpetrators will only engage in these programs because they have been directed by a court to do so, or because their partner is threatening to leave the relationship or has already left.

Most treatment programs focus on encouraging perpetrators to take responsibility for their actions. The most useful models for treatment programs are those using cognitive behaviour therapy and a 'pro-feminist' educational program[113] where:

- the safety and autonomy of victims is a priority
- there is education of perpetrator and victims, and the sociocultural context of the violence is discussed
- the need for participants to take responsibility for their own behaviour is emphasised
- the program is clearly linked with the criminal justice system, so that perpetrators know the consequences of using violence and victims are aware of their right to be protected.

Unfortunately, attrition rates are high, with up to 40% dropping out.[115] In those completing programs, violence does stop for a period, although in some cases the nature of the violence changes from physical to verbal or psychological abuse.[111] One more encouraging study found that two-thirds of men completing a program remained free from subsequent violence at 18 months, but in this study less than half the men who started the program finished it.[116]

Summary of key points

- Up to 20% of women attending general practitioners have experienced intimate partner violence in the last year.
- Many of the barriers to diagnosing and dealing with intimate partner violence lies with the doctor and not the patient.
- Women who are victims of intimate partner violence suffer from worse general health, use medical care more, have more gynaecological problems and worse mental health than women who are not victims.
- General practice consultations provide safe, confidential and powerful opportunities to tackle the issue of intimate partner violence.
- GPs should screen their patients for intimate partner violence and offer support, education, safety planning and referral if necessary.
- GPs should be aware of the effects of intimate partner violence on children and the likelihood of co-existing child maltreatment.

TIPS FOR PRACTITIONERS

- Useful advice for women who have experienced a sexual assault:
  - Try not to bottle up your feelings.
  - Talk to family and friends whom you can trust about what happened, how you feel and how they can help you. If you are unable to do this, there are local and national helplines, agencies and organisations to contact that offer emotional support, medical assistance and information about the criminal justice process.
  - Take care of yourself. Give yourself time to absorb the shock of this experience. Try to get adequate rest and sleep, eat regularly and take moderate exercise.
  - Avoid using alcohol or drugs to 'switch off' your mind. While these may give temporary relief, in the long term they can have adverse effects.
  - Do not blame yourself. The blame for sexual violence must rest with those who perpetrate such acts, not with you.
- When recording a history, the GP should use terms such as 'alleged sexual assault' or 'sexual assault by history', not 'she was raped' as rape is not a medical term but rather a legal term and so should not enter the lexicon of a medical report.
- The absence of extragenital or genital trauma does not mean that a sexual assault did not occur.

- The swabs used for the collection of forensic specimens are plain cotton swabs wetted with either a little tap water or normal saline. These are rubbed on a part of the body (e.g. nipple, upper arm), a smear is made on a clean glass slide, and both the smear and swab are then air-dried. The swab should not be placed in transport media.
- GPs should conceptualise intimate partner violence as chronic disease and therefore one where a cure is rarely achievable, where long-term follow-up is needed and where the patient is best assisted by a multidisciplinary team.
- When screening for intimate partner violence, try to contextualise and normalise your questions.
- Useful tips to use in consultations with perpetrators[117]:
  - Be direct.
  - Ask how disagreements or situations of conflict are resolved.
  - Focus on the abusive conduct rather than the explanations or rationalisations.
  - Make the connection between the perpetrator's behaviour and the victim's injuries (e.g. 'When you hit her on Saturday night you broke her nose. That is criminal assault').
  - Help the perpetrator to see that intimate partner violence is a healthcare issue and that it negatively affects him as well as his partner and children.
  - Ask what effect he thinks his violence has on his wife and children and how it might have changed his relationship with them.
  - Ask if he wants his children to learn about violence in relationships from him.
  - Discuss options for treatment and referral.

REFERENCES

1. Gise LH, Paddison P. Rape, sexual abuse, and its victims. Psychiatr Clin North Am 1988; 11:629–648.
2. Groth AN, Burgess AW. Sexual dysfunction during rape. N Engl J Med 1977; 297:764–766.
3. DeLaHunta E, Baram D. Sexual assault. Clin Obstet Gynecol 1997; 40:648–660.
4. Brickman J, Briere J. Incidence of rape and sexual assault in an urban Canadian population. Int J Women's Stud 1984; 7:195–206.
5. Beebe DK. Emergency management of the adult female rape victim. Am Fam Physician 1991; 43:2041–2046.
6. Kilpatrick DG, Best CL, Veronen LJ, et al. Mental health correlates of criminal victimization. A random community survey. J Consult Clin Psychol 1985; 53:866–873.
7. DiVasto PV, Kaufman A, Rosner L, et al. The prevalence of sexually stressful events among females in the general population. Arch Sex Behav 1984; 13:59–67.

8. Walch AG, Broadhead WE. Prevalence of lifetime sexual victimization among female patients. J Fam Pract 1992; 35:511–516.

9. Mazza D, Dennerstein L, Ryan V. Physical, sexual and emotional violence against women: a general practice-based prevalence study. Med J Aust 1996; 164:14–17.

10. Mein JK, Palmer CM, Shand MC, et al. Management of acute adult sexual assault. Med J Aust 2003; 178(5):226–230.

11. Martin CA, Warfield MC, Braen GR. Physician's management of the psychological aspects of rape. JAMA 1983; 249: 501–503.

12. Petter L, Whitehill D. Management of female sexual assault. Am Fam Physician 1998; 59:920–926.

13. Dwyer B. Rape: psychological, medical and forensic aspects of emergency management. Emergency Medicine Reports 1995; 16:105–116.

14. Kobernick ME, Seifert S, Sanders AB. Emergency department management of the sexual assault victim. J Emerg Med 1985; 2:205–214.

15. White C, McLean I. Adolescent complainants of sexual assault; injury patterns in virgin and non-virgin groups. J Clin Forensic Med 2006; 13(4):172–180.

16. Rogers D. Physical aspects of alleged sexual assaults. Med Sci Law 1996; 36:117–122.

17. Sugar NF, Fine DN, Eckert LO. Physical injury after sexual assault: findings of a large case series. Am J Obstet Gynecol 2004; 190(1):71–76.

18. Riggs N, Houry D, Long G, et al. Analysis of 1076 cases of sexual assault. Ann Emerg Med 2000; 35:353–362.

19. Cartwright PS. Factors that correlate with injury sustained by survivors of sexual assault. Obstet Gynecol 1987; 70:44–46.

20. Bowyer L, Dalton ME. Female victims of rape and their genital injuries. Br J Obstet Gynaecol 1997; 104:617–620.

21. Hampton HL. Care of the woman who has been raped. N Engl J Med 1995; 332:234–237.

22. Enos WF, Beyer JC. Management of the rape victim. Am Fam Physician 1978; 18:97–102.

23. Rambow B, Adkinson C, Frost T, et al. Female sexual assault: medical and legal implication. Ann Emerg Med 1992; 21: 727–731.

24. Lamba H, Murphy SM. Sexual assault and sexually transmitted infections: an updated review. Int J STD AIDS 2000; 11:487–491.

25. Murphy S, Kitchen V, Harris JR, et al. Rape and subsequent seroconversion to HIV. Br Med J 1989; 299:718.

26. Crowe C, Forster GE, Dinsmore WW, et al. A case of acute hepatitis B occurring four months after multiple rape. Int J STD AIDS 1996; 7:133–134.

27. Gostin LO, Lazzarini Z, Alexander D, et al. HIV testing, counselling, and prophylaxis after sexual assault. JAMA 1994; 271:1436–1444.

28. Fisher M, Benn P, Evans B, et al. UK Guideline for the use of post-exposure prophylaxis for HIV following sexual exposure. Int J STD AIDS 2006; 17(2):81–92.

29. Holmes MM, Resnick HS, Kilpatrick DG, et al. Rape-related pregnancy: estimates from a national sample of women. Am J Obstet Gynecol 1996; 175:320–324.

30. Wilcox AJ, Weinberg CR, Baird DD. Timing of sexual intercourse in relation to ovulation: effects on the probability of conception, survival of the pregnancy, and sex of the baby. N Engl J Med 1995; 333:1517–1521.

31. Burgess AW, Homstrom LL. Rape trauma syndrome. Am J Psychiatry 1974; 131:981–986.

32. American Psychiatric Association. Diagnostic and statistical manual of mental disorders. 4th edn, text revision. Washington, DC: American Psychiatric Press; 2000.

33. Foa EB, Riggs DS. Posttraumatic stress disorder following assault: theoretical considerations and empirical findings. Curr Dir Psychol Sci 1995; 4:61–65.

34. Boisset-Pioro MH, Esdaile JM, Fitzcharles M-A. Sexual and physical abuse in women with fibromyalgia syndrome. Arthritis Rheum 1995; 38:235–241.

35. Felitti VJ. Long-term medical consequences of incest, rape and molestation. South Med J 1991; 84:328–331.

36. Rapkin AJ, Kames LD, Darke LL, et al. History of physical and sexual abuse in women with chronic pelvic pain. Obstet Gynecol 1990; 76:92.

37. Koss MP, Heslet L. Somatic consequences of violence against women. Arch Fam Med 1992; 1:53–59.

38. Brady KT. Posttraumatic stress disorder and comorbidity: recognizing the many faces of PTSD. J Clin Psychiatry 1997; 58 (Suppl 9):12–15.

39. Atkeson BM, Calhoun KS, Resick PA, et al. Victims of rape: recent empirical findings. Am J Orthopsychiatry 1979; 49:658–669.

40. Becker JV, Skinner LJ, Abel GG, et al. Depressive symptoms associated with sexual assault. J Sex Marital Ther 1984; 10:185–192.

41. Kilpatrick DG, Veronen LJ, Resick PA. Psychological sequelae to rape: assessment and treatment strategies. In: Doleys DM, Meredith RL, Ciminero AR, eds. Behavioral medicine: assessment and treatment strategies. New York; Plenum Press; 1982.

42. Wonderlich SA, Crosby RD, Mitchell JE, et al. Eating disturbance and sexual trauma in childhood and adulthood. Int J Eat Disord 2001; 30:401–412.

43. Creamer M, Burgess P, McFarlane AC. Post-traumatic stress disorder: findings from the Australian National Survey of Mental Health and Well-being. Psychol Med 2001; 31: 1237–1247.

44. Sansone RA, Sansone LA, Wiederman M. The prevalence of trauma and its relationship to borderline personality symptoms and self-destructive behaviours in a primary care setting. Arch Fam Med 1995; 4:439–442.

45. Van Berlo W, Ensink B. Problems with sexuality after sexual assault. Annu Rev Sex Res 2000; 11:235–257.

46. National Collaborative Centre for Mental Health. Post-traumatic stress disorder. The management of PTSD in adults and children in primary and secondary care. National Clinical Practice Guideline 26. London: 2005. Online. Available: http://www.nice.org.uk/nicemedia/live/10966/29772/29772.pdf [accessed 25.06.09].

47. Kelleher P, Kelleher C, O'Connor M. Making the links: towards an integrated strategy for the elimination of violence against women in intimate relationships with men. Dublin: Women's Aid, 1995.

48. Johnson H, Sacco VF. Researching violence against women: Statistics Canada's national survey. Can J Criminol 1995; 37:281–304.

49. Hamberger LK, Saunders D, Hovery M. Prevalence of domestic violence in community practice and rate of physician inquiry. Fam Med 1992; 24:283–287.

50. Marais A, Villiers PD, Moller A, et al. Domestic violence in patients visiting general practitioners: prevalence, phenomenology, and association with psychopathology. S Afr Med J 1999; 89:635–640.

51. Abbott J, Johnson R, Koziol-McLain J, et al. Domestic violence against women: incidence and prevalence in an emergency department population. JAMA 1995; 273: 1763–1767.

52. Dearwater S, Coben J, Campbell J, et al. Prevalence of intimate partner abuse in women treated at community hospital emergency departments. JAMA 1998; 280:433–438.

53. Gazmararian JA, Lazorick S, Spitz A, et al. Prevalence of violence against pregnant women: a review of the literature. JAMA 1996; 275:1915–1920.

54. Council on Scientific Affairs, American Medical Association. Violence against women: relevance for medical practitioners. JAMA 1992; 267:3184–3189.

55. Martins R, Holzapfel S, Baker P. Wife abuse: are we detecting it? J Womens Health 1992; 1:77–80.
56. Goldberg WG, Tomlanovich MC. Domestic violence victims in the emergency department. New findings. JAMA 1984; 251:3259–3264.
57. Ferris LE, Tudiver F. Family physicians' approach to wife abuse: a study of Ontario, Canada, practices. Fam Med 1992; 24:276–282.
58. Brown JB, Sas G. Focus groups in family practice research: an example study of family physicians' approach to wife abuse. Fam Pract Res J 1994; 14:19–28.
59. Sugg NK, Inui T. Primary care physicians' response to domestic violence. Opening Pandora's box. JAMA 1992; 267:3157–3160.
60. Kurz D, Stark E. Not so benign neglect: the medical response to battering. In: Yllo K, Bograd M (eds). Feminist perspectives on wife abuse. Newbury Park, California: Sage Publications; 1988:249–266.
61. Australian Medical Association. Position statement on domestic violence. Canberra: Australian Medical Association; 1998.
62. Jewkes R. Intimate partner violence: causes and prevention. Lancet 2002; 359:1423–1429.
63. Heise LL. Gender-based abuse: the global epidemic. In: Dan AJ (ed). Reframing women's health: multidisciplinary research and practice. Thousand Oaks, CA: Sage Publications; 1994:233–250.
64. Leserman J, Li D, Drossman DA, et al. Selected symptoms associated with sexual and physical abuse among female patients with gastrointestinal disorders: the impact on subsequent health care visits. Psychol Med 1998; 28: 417–425.
65. Plichta SB. Violence and abuse: implications for women's health. In: Falik MK, Collins KS (eds). Women's health, the Commonwealth Fund survey. Baltimore, MD: The Johns Hopkins University Press; 1996.
66. Campbell J, Jones AS, Dienemann J, et al. Intimate partner violence and physical health consequences. Arch Intern Med 2002; 162:1157–1163.
67. McCauley J, Kern DE, Kolodner K, et al. The 'battering syndrome': prevalence and clinical characteristics of domestic violence in primary care internal medicine practices. Ann Intern Med 1995; 123:737–746.
68. Coker AL, Smith PH, Bethea L, et al. Physical health consequences of physical and psychological intimate partner violence. Arch Fam Med 2000; 9:451–457.
69. Koss MP, Koss PG, Woodruff WJ. Deleterious effects of criminal victimization on women's health and medical utilization. Arch Intern Med 1991; 151:342–347.
70. Crawford M, Gartner R, Dawson M. Intimate femicide in Ontario, 1991–1994. Toronto: Women We Honour Action Committee; 1997.
71. Brock K, Stenzel A. When men murder women: an analysis of 1997 homicide data—females murdered by males in single victim/single offender incidents. Washington, DC: Violence Policy Center; 1999.
72. Bergman B, Brismar B. Suicide attempts by battered wives. Acta Psychiatr Scand 1991; 83:380–384.
73. Grisso JA, Schwarz DF, Hirschinger N, et al. Violent injuries among women in an urban area. N Engl J Med 1999; 341:1899–1905.
74. Campbell JC. Health consequences of intimate partner violence. Lancet 2002; 35:1331–1336.
75. Letourneau EJ, Holmes M, Chasendunn-Roark J. Gynecologic health consequences to victims of interpersonal violence. Women's Health Issues 1999; 9:115–120.
76. Schei B, Bakketeig LS. Gynaecological impact of sexual and physical abuse by spouse: a study of a random sample of Norwegian women. Br J Obstet Gynaecol 1989; 96: 1379–1383.
77. Campbell JC, Soeken K. Forced sex and intimate partner violence: effects on women's health. Violence Against Women 1999; 5:1017–1035.
78. Wingood G, DiClemente R. The effects of an abusive primary partner on the condom use and sexual negotiation practices of African-American women. Am J Public Health 1997; 87:1016–1018.
79. Wingood GM, DiClemente RJ, Raj A. Adverse consequences of intimate partner abuse among women in non-urban domestic violence shelters. Am J Prev Med 2000; 19:270–275.
80. Jejeebhoy SJ. Associations between wife-beating and fetal and infant death: impressions from a survey in rural India. Stud Fam Plann 1998; 29:300–308.
81. Resnick HS, Acierno R, Kilpatrick DG. Health impact of interpersonal violence. 2: medical and mental health outcomes. Behav Med 1997; 23:65–78.
82. Gielen AC, O'Campo P, Faden R, et al. Interpersonal conflict and physical violence during the childbearing year. Soc Sci Med 1994; 39:781–787.
83. Evins G, Chescheir N. Prevalence of domestic violence among women seeking abortion services. Women's Health Issues 1996; 6:204–210.
84. Glander SS, Moore ML, Michielutte R, et al. The prevalence of domestic violence among women seeking abortion. Obstet Gynecol 1998; 91:1002–1006.
85. Parker B, McFarlane J, Soeken K. Abuse during pregnancy: effects on maternal complications and birth weight in adult and teenage women. Obstet Gynecol 1994; 84:323–328.
86. Norton LB, Peipert JF, Zierler PH, et al. Battering in pregnancy: an assessment of two screening methods. Obstet Gynecol 1995; 85:321–325.
87. Amaro H, Fried L, Cabral H, et al. Violence during pregnancy and substance use. Am J Public Health 1990; 80:575–579.
88. Murphy CC, Schei B, Myhr TL, et al. Abuse: a risk factor for low birth weight? A systematic review and meta-analysis. CMAJ 2001; 164:1567–1572.
89. Jaffe P, Wolfe D, Wilson S, et al. Emotional and physical health problems of battered women. Can J Psychiatry 1986; 31:625–629.
90. Golding JM. Intimate partner violence as a risk factor for mental disorders: a meta-analysis. J Fam Violence 1999; 14:99–132.
91. Ratner PA. The incidence of wife abuse and mental health status in abused wives in Edmonton, Alberta. Can J Public Health 1993; 84:246–249.
92. Widom C. Post-traumatic stress disorder in abused and neglected children grown up. Am J Psychiatry 1999; 156:1223–1229.
93. McCauley J, Kern D, Kolodner K, et al. Clinical characteristics of women with a history of childhood abuse. JAMA 1997; 277:1362–1368.
94. Head C, Taft A. Improving general practitioner management of women experiencing domestic violence: a study of the beliefs and experiences of women victim/survivors and of GPs. Canberra: Department of Health, Housing and Community Services; 1995.
95. Keys Young. Against the odds: how women survive domestic violence. Office of the Status of Women: Canberra; 1998.
96. Roberts G. Domestic violence victims in the emergency department. Brisbane: University of Queensland; 1995.
97. Eisenstat S, Bancroft L. Domestic violence. N Engl J Med 1999; 341:886–892.
98. Mazza D. An analysis of the relationship between psychotropic drug use and a current or past history of physical and or sexual abuse. MD thesis, University of Melbourne, 1996.

99. US Preventive Services Task Force. Screening for family and intimate partner violence: recommendation statement. Ann Fam Med 2004; 2(2):156–160.

100. Zolotor AJ, Denham AC, Weil A. Intimate partner violence. Prim Care 2009; 36(1):167–179, x.

101. Victorian Government Department of Justice. Management of the whole family when intimate partner violence is present: guidelines for primary care physicians. 2006. Online. Available: http://www.racgp.org.au/guidelines/intimatepartner abuse [accessed 05.06.09].

102. Janssen P, Dascal-Weichhendler H, McGregor M. Assessment for intimate partner violence: where do we stand? J Am Board Fam Med 2006; 19(4):413–415.

103. Bradley F, Smith M, Long J, et al. Reported frequency of domestic violence: cross sectional survey of women attending general practice. Br Med J 2002; 324:271.

104. Feder GS, Hutson M, Ramsay J, et al. Women exposed to intimate partner violence: expectations and experiences when they encounter health care professionals: a meta-analysis of qualitative studies. Arch Intern Med 2006; 166(1):22–37.

105. Kimberg L. Addressing intimate partner violence in primary care practice. Medscape Women's Health eJournal 2001; 6(1). Online. Available: http://www.medscape.com/viewarti cle/408937 [accessed 23.02.09].

106. Gerbert B, Abercrombie P, Caspers N, et al. How health care providers help battered women: the survivor's perspective. Women Health 1999; 29:115–135.

107. Bair-Merritt MH, Blackstone M, Feudtner C. Physical health outcomes of childhood exposure to intimate partner violence: a systematic review. Pediatrics 2006; 117(2):e278–e290.

108. Lee LC, Kotch JB, Cox CE. Child maltreatment in families experiencing domestic violence. Violence Vict 2004; 19(5):573–591.

109. Hegarty K, Taft A, Feder G. Violence between intimate partners: working with the whole family. BMJ 2008; 337:a839.

110. Ferris L, Norton P, Dunn E, et al. Guidelines for managing domestic abuse when male and female partners are patients of the same physician. JAMA 1997; 278:851–857.

111. Romans SE, Poore MR, Martin JL. The perpetrators of domestic violence. Med J Aust 2000; 173:484–488.

112. Platt FW. Domestic violence: the perpetrators are our patients too. Arch Intern Med 1996; 156:2626.

113. Robertson N. Stopping family violence programmes; enhancing the safety of battered women or producing better educated batterers? NZ J Psychol 1999; 28:68–78.

114. Perry BD, Azad I. Post-traumatic stress disorders in children and adolescents. Curr Opin Pediatr 1999; 11:310–316.

115. Shepard M. Predicting batterer recidivism five years after community intervention. J Fam Violence 1992; 7:167–178.

116. Edleson JL, Syers M. The effects of group treatment for men who batter: an 18–month follow-up study. Res Soc Work Pract 1991; 1:227–243.

117. Gardyne H. The general practitioner and partner abuse. Auckland: Public Health Promotion, Auckland Healthcare; 1995.

118. Tjaden P, Thoennes N. Full report of the prevalance, incidence, and consequences of violence against women: findings from the national violence against women survey. Washington DC: US Department of Justice; 2000.

119. McCloskey LA, Lichter E, Ganz ML, et al. Intimate partner violence and patient screening across medical specialties. Acad Emerg Med 2005; 12(8):712–722.

120. Lehrer JA, Buka S, Gortmaker S, et al. Depressive symptomatology as a predictor of exposure to intimate partner violence among US female adolescents and young adults. Arch Pediatr Adolesc Med 2006; 160(3):270–276.

121. Bowen E, Heron J, Waylen A, et al. Domestic violence risk during and after pregnancy: findings from a British longitudinal study. BJOG 2005; 112(8):1083–1089.

122. Zolotor AJ, Runyan DK. Social capital, family violence, and neglect. Pediatrics 2006; 117(6):e1124–e1131.

Index

Page numbers followed by 'f' denote figures, by 't' denote tables and by 'b' denote boxes.